Nutrition Concepts and Medical Nutrition Therapy

by Susan Davis Allen, MS, RD

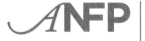 Association of
Nutrition & Foodservice
Professionals

Association of Nutrition & Foodservice Professionals
406 Surrey Woods Dr.
St. Charles, IL 60174
800.323.1908
www.ANFPonline.org

ISBN 0-9753476-8-3

Printed in the United States of America

Acknowledgements

Julie Abernathy, DTR, CDM, CFPP
China Grove, NC

Joan Bahr, MS, RD, CDE
Platteville, WI

Marian Benz, MS, RD, CDE, CD
Wauwatosa, WI

Michael Braun, MS, RD, CD
Madison, WI

Janet Burtch, CDM, CFPP
Toledo, OH

Jolene Campbell, MEd, RD, LDN
Baltimore, MD

Sharon Doughten, MS, RD, LD
Cleveland, OH

Juanita Gunnell, MS, RD, LDN
Dallas, NC

Linda Handy, MS, RD
San Marcos, CA

Carol Hill, RD, LD, CSG
Ankeny, IA

Cindra Holland, RD, LD
Perrysburg, OH

Laura Horn, MEd, RD, LD
Cincinnati, OH

Kay Jarrett, RD, LDN
Jacsonville, NC

Floristene Johnson, MS, RD, LD
Desoto, TX

Judy Kaplan, MS, RD, LD
Cleveland, OH

Tama S. Krause, MS, RD, LMNT
Norfolk, NE

M. Theresa Leo, RD, MAS, LDN
Morgantown, PA

Fran Lukacik, RD, MS, CDM, CFPP
Lafayatte Hill, PA

J.J. Marcano, RD, LDN, CSG
Ambler, PA

Linda Eck Mills, MBA, RD, LDN, FADA
Bernville, PA

Monica Perry, RD, LD
Boise, ID

Marla Prytz, MS, RD, CD
Rice Lake, WI

Ruby Puckett, MA, FCSI
Gainesville, FL

Beth Ringlein, BA, AOS
Milan, OH

Tim Roberts, PhD, RD, LD
Auburn University, AL

Brenda Rubash, RD, LD
Laporte, MN

Becky Rude, MS, RD, CDM, CFPP
Grand Forks, ND

Joanne Seid, RD, MS
Valhalla, NY

Sharon Smith, RD, LD
St. Paul, MN

Loretta Spangler, RD, LMNT
Ewing, NE

Jane Valentine, MS, RD, LD
Champaign, IL

Linda Waite, MS, RD, LD, CDM, CFPP
Quincy, IL

Meshele Wyneken, RD
Fort Wayne, IN

Mary Louise Zernicke, MS, RD, MPH, CSG
Berkeley, CA

This textbook is dedicated to Mrs. Bernice Judd, Lancaster, Wisconsin, who at 100 years old, still demonstrates that eating well assures well-being in later years.

We would like to express our appreciation to many individuals who have contributed to the development of this textbook, including Sue Grossbauer, RD, Karen Eich Drummond, EdD, RD, FADA and Linda S. Eck, MBA, RD, FADA.

In addition, we would like to recognize the contribution of the review team who generously invested their professional expertise and valuable time to offer many recommendations for achieving the educational objectives of this textbook.

Furthermore, the ongoing efforts of the developers of the Nutrition and Foodservice Professional Training Curriculum, Susan Davis Allen, MS, RD, Marion Benz, MS, RD, CDE, CD, Becky Rude, MS, RD, CDM, CFPP, Katherine Church, RD and the Certifying Board for Dietary Managers have done much to focus the development of this textbook.

We also wish to express gratitude to Mercy Ehrler for the graphic design and production and Sue Moen for editing this textbook.

Finally, thank you to Pam Himrod, MS, RD, CDM, CFPP, ANFP Director of Professional Development and the ANFP staff for their support, direction and ongoing commitment to enhancing the profession, and their dedication to the members of Association of Nutrition & Foodservice Professionals.

A Personal Invitation

We at Association of Nutrition & Foodservice Professionals (ANFP) would like to extend a personal invitation to every student enrolled in the Nutrition & Foodservice Professional Training Program to join ANFP. We recognize the value of your career choice, and would like to offer you the many benefits of ANFP membership. As a student, you are welcome to join today and establish your professional footing through your participation in this professional association.

Association of Nutrition & Foodservice Professionals is a national not-for-profit association established in 1960 that today has 15,000 professionals dedicated to the mission: "promoting career development, setting standards for foodservice best practices, and enhancing and strengthening the overall profession of foodservice management."

ANFP's core values are:

- Professionalism
- Integrity
- Advocacy
- Best Practices

ANFP members work in hospitals, long-term care, schools, correctional facilities, and other non-commercial settings. The association provides foodservice reference, publications and resources, employment services for members, continuing education and professional development, and certification programs. ANFP monitors industry trends and legislative issues, and publishes one of the industry's most respected magazines, *Nutrition & Foodservice Edge*.

The ANFP national and regional meetings also offer a unique opportunity to enjoy timely educational sessions and network with colleagues. ANFP also provides industry leadership in the area of food protection and offers online resources about food safety and sanitation.

For more information about ANFP, please contact Association of Nutrition & Foodservice Professionals by telephone at 800.323.1908 or 630.587.6336; or visit the ANFP website at www.ANFPonline.org to join online.

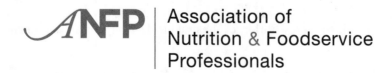

Table of Contents

CHAPTER 1

Food Preferences and Customs

Overview and Objectives

To provide nutritional care, Certified Dietary Managers need to understand what motivates people to eat, and how clients choose their foods. Certified Dietary Managers also need to recognize cultural, religious, and regional influences on food choices.

After completing this chapter, you should be able to:

✓ Investigate factors that affect food intake

✓ Classify reasons why people eat

✓ Identify food customs of various racial, ethnic, or religious groups

✓ Compare nutritional intake of various racial, cultural, and religious groups

✓ Modify a menu for an ethnic, racial, or religious preference

Food and its components are essential for life. In this book, you will read a great deal about nutrition science. As you will examine in later chapters, food provides many **nutrients**. Without these nutrients, we could not survive. However, food means more than survival to people. We do not eat based on science alone. A professor once explained that if we ate food based on science alone, we could all eat the same diet such as our pets do. Can you imagine eating the same diet every day and in the same form such as dry dog food? Most of us have complex reasons for choosing the foods we do.

To be successful in helping your clients attain good health, you have to do more than provide healthy food. You will have to investigate the factors that affect the food intake of your clients. Let's take a closer look at some of the factors that influence what foods we choose, and how we feel about dietary choices. These factors include: cultural heritage, regional trends, religious practices, social and emotional meanings, availability of food, personal taste, aesthetic influences, attitudes and values, lifestyle, and personal health.

Cultural Heritage

First, consider food as part of our culture. To understand this aspect of food, try asking yourself some questions. What does turkey and dressing with cranberry sauce mean to you? Many people will answer: Thanksgiving. This food has become part of a cultural tradition. Now, think about a wedding

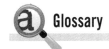 **Glossary**

Nutrients
Components in food that are essential to good health

celebration. What food will always be served? Most people will answer: a wedding cake. Or, in China, the answer may be: roasted pig. Now, try another question. What food has become a symbol of American heritage and pride? Many people will answer: apple pie. From these examples, you can see that we regard food choices as cultural symbols. The meaning of these foods is much deeper than a sum of protein, carbohydrate, fat, vitamins, and minerals—the sheer nutritional values.

Many food choices arise from what we learn through our own cultural experiences. Holidays, festivals, and important events each have associated foods. In addition, daily food choices vary by culture. Traditional German cuisine, for example, is likely to include sausage, schnitzel, spaetzel, beer, and other specialties. Japanese cuisine includes sushi, tempura, and rice. Swedish cuisine may include pancakes, even at meals other than breakfast. Mexican cuisine includes staples such as tortillas, rice, and refried beans. Creole cuisine, popular in New Orleans, represents a synthesis of French cooking with locally available foods, and the influences of Caribbean and Spanish cultures.

Cultural contributions to cuisine include the choices of ingredients, the style of preparation, the equipment used to cook food, the seasonings, and styles for displaying and serving. Dining itself is also cultural. Washing hands at the table with a warm, moist cloth is a common practice in some cultures. Choices for dining room décor, table settings, eating utensils, ambiance, music, lighting, accepted dress, and even the timing of meals all reflect cultural patterns.

As a land of immigrants, the U.S. enjoys multi-faceted cultural diversity. Our food choices are as rich and complex as our population itself. See Figure 1.1 for cultural food influences. Here are more examples of cultural and ethnic food influences.

Hispanics/Latinos. The United States Census Bureau defines Hispanics as those who indicate their origin to be Mexican, Puerto Rican, Cuban, Central or South American (e.g., Dominican, Nicaraguan, Colombian) or other Hispanic origin. The largest of these is the Mexican-American population, which represents at least two-thirds of all Hispanics/Latinos. According to a national survey conducted by the U.S. Department of Agriculture, "Hispanics tend to eat more rice, but less pasta and ready-to-eat cereals than their non-Hispanic white counterparts. Hispanics are also likely to consume vegetables, especially tomatoes, although they have a slightly higher consumption of fruits. Compared to non-Hispanic whites, Hispanics are more than twice as likely to drink whole milk, but much less likely to drink low-fat or skim milk. Hispanics are also more likely to eat beef, but less likely to eat processed meats such as hot dogs, sausage, and luncheon meats." Legumes and corn in combination are a good source of protein and cheese is a frequent ingredient in foods.

East Indian Americans. Staples of the Indian diet include rice, beans, lentils, and bread. Rice is usually served steamed and mixed with flavorings. Indian breads include chapatis, round flatbread made of whole wheat flour; and naan, a bread that uses yeast. India's religious beliefs have also influenced the diet

Figure 1.1   Cultural Influences on Food Intake in the United States

Group	Grains	Vegetables	Fruits	Meat	Dairy
Hispanic/Latino	Tortillas (may be made with lard), rice	Cactus, cassava, chayote, jicama, peppers, pinto beans, tomatoes (salsa)	Avocado, bananas, guava, mango, papaya, plantain, citrus fruits	Chorizo (sausage and other processed meat), goat meat, tongue, pork	Goat cheese, goat milk, whole milk
Asian (China, Japan, Korea, Southeast Asia)	Rice noodles	Garlic, ginger, mung beans, sprouts, bamboo shoots, bok choy, cabbage, carrots	Mango, banana, citrus fruit, coconut, pineapple	Small amounts of meat especially fish; eggs, tofu	Soy milk
Middle Eastern	Couscous, tahini, pita bread, filo dough	Tomatoes, olives, lentils, hummus, grape leaves, eggplant	Dates, figs, citrus fruits	Small amounts of lamb, fish, chicken	Yogurt, feta cheese
East Indian	Rice, whole wheat flat bread (naan)	Red lentils, pigeon peas, legumes, curries	Coconut, watermelon, mango	Many East Indian people are vegetarian; some mutton chicken, fish	Milk, butter, yogurt

Please note that this is not meant to be an exact list of foods. All of these cultures have diets that vary from one region/country to another.

of Indians (e.g. Hindus believe that cows are sacred so they do not eat beef). Chicken or lamb, in moderation, is augmented with vegetables, dried beans, lentils and split peas. Curry powder, a mixture of spices, is often used to flavor Indian foods. The heart of Indian cooking is the combination of spices that gives each dish its unique flavor. Indian cuisine has become increasingly popular during the first decade of the 21st Century with over 1200 Indian food products now available in the U.S.

Chinese Americans. Vegetables, rice and noodles, fruits, and foods made from soybeans (such as tofu and soy milk) are very important foods in the Chinese-American diet. Plain rice is served at all meals. Sometimes fried rice is served. Pork, poultry, and fish are popular and used in small amounts to flavor the rice. Foods are often seasoned with soy sauce, which is high in sodium. (Low-sodium versions can be purchased). Corn oil, sesame oil, and peanut oil are used. Tea is the main beverage and it is always enjoyed black—without sugar, cream, or milk. Cow's milk and dairy products are not used often. Fruits are important and few sweets are eaten.

Japanese Americans. Some people are surprised to learn that Japanese food is quite different in appearance and taste from Chinese food. While Chinese food is often stir-fried, Japanese food is often simmered, boiled, steamed, or broiled. Also, Japanese foods are not as highly seasoned as Chinese dishes. Sushi, a rice wrapped in seaweed has become a popular food choice in the U.S. in the past decade. Rice is the staple of many Japanese-American diets, along with a variety of noodles. As in Chinese cooking, soybean products, such as soy sauce, are important. Seafood is generally more popular than meat and

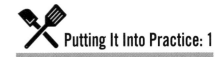

Putting It Into Practice: 1

As a new Certified Dietary Manager, you want to recognize the cultural differences of your customers. What is the first step to implementing a cultural change movement in your facility?

(Check your answer at the end of this chapter)

poultry. Vegetables, such as watercress and carrots, are an important part of most meals. Tea is the most popular beverage, especially green tea, an excellent source of antioxidants.

Middle Eastern Americans. Foods of choice in a traditional Middle Eastern diet include yogurt, cheeses (such as feta and goat cheese), lamb, poultry, chick peas, lentils, lemons, eggplant, pine nuts, olives, and olive oil. A Greek specialty is baklava, a baked dessert made with nuts, honey, and filo dough. Common cooking styles are grilling, frying, and stewing.

Cultural Change Movement

How many times do we as Americans get together socially without food? A culture change movement is spreading across the U.S. that involves many of these cultural contributions. This culture change movement is transforming nursing home care from an institutional setting to a home setting. With the increase in the 'senior' population, nursing care facilities will have to focus on the opportunities to make choices and allow customers to express preferences. As we have seen in this chapter, these choices are fundamental to our basic quality of life.

Regional Trends

Part of the cultural heritage unique to the U.S. is the development of regional culinary trends. Often, these trends reflect a mix of native cultures, foods that are grown and harvested in the area, and ethnic traditions contributed by settlers and immigrants over time. For example, New England is known for maple syrup, Boston beans, brown bread, and cranberry muffins. Maine is recognized for lobster. Blueberries are important in New Jersey and in the Midwest, where many are grown. In Pennsylvania and parts of Ohio, the Pennsylvania Dutch heritage gives rise to scrapple (a loaf made from meat scraps, broth, and flour), homemade noodles, and shoofly (molasses) pie.

Vidalia onions are a hallmark of Georgia's cuisine and are the official state vegetable. Peanuts and peaches are also key crops in Georgia. Florida is known for key limes and key lime pie, coquina soup, and other specialties. Kuchen is the official state dessert in South Dakota. Most people associate Idaho with potatoes, and New Orleans with Creole cuisine, such as jambalaya, "dirty" rice, and gumbo. Barbecued meats and pickled okra have special significance in Texas. In the Southwest (Arizona, New Mexico, Oklahoma, Texas), Mexican-style foods such as burritos and tacos are popular. Garlic is so important in California that the town of Gilroy celebrates an annual garlic festival. In fact, food celebrations, such as strawberry harvest festivals, maple syrup festivals, and many others are key events in all parts of the country.

Religious Practices

Religious beliefs, along with religious customs and rituals, can exert strong influence on eating habits. Fasting is one practice that many religions observe. The length of time one fasts varies with his/her religion and can range from one day to a month. Some Muslims observe Ramadan, which lasts for one month and fasting occurs from sun up to sun down. Think about how this practice

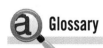

Glossary

Kosher
Fit, proper or in agreement with religious law. Kosher meat means the animal has been slaughtered in a special way. Usually Kosher foods have been blessed by a rabbi.

Comfort Food
Any food that imparts a unique sense of emotional well-being such as chicken soup

might affect Muslim clients in a long-term care facility. The following information explains several religious beliefs and food laws.

Jewish Dietary Laws. The Jewish dietary laws are called kashrut or keeping **kosher**. Some Jews follow all the Jewish dietary laws all the time; others follow the laws not at all or to varying degrees, perhaps only on special holidays. The word kosher means fit, proper, or in agreement with religious law. Basic concepts of Jewish dietary law include the following:

✓ Pig and pork products are not kosher so they are not eaten. Also, birds of prey are not kosher (this includes wild chickens and turkey). Domestic chicken, turkey, goose, pheasant, and duck are fine.

✓ According to Jewish dietary laws, only fish with both fins and scales are considered kosher. All finfish are acceptable, but shellfish, crustaceans, and fish-like mammals are not allowed. This includes shrimp, lobster, oysters, clams, scallops, crab, catfish, shark, and frog. Fish do not have to be koshered like meats and poultry.

✓ Meat and meat products may not be cooked or served with any dairy products. For example, chicken a la king and creamed chipped beef are forbidden unless made with nondairy products. Pots and pans in which meat is cooked and dishes on which it is served may not be used for dairy products. Separate sets of utensils and dishes are necessary. Dairy products may be eaten from one to six hours after meat is eaten (the amount of time depends upon an individual's traditions).

✓ All fruits, vegetables, and starches are considered kosher as well as *pareve* (meaning neutral) so they can be served with meat or dairy meals. A food-service operation offering kosher food must be sure that all aspects of the operation are in accordance with kosher dietary laws.

Social and Emotional Meanings

Eating has many social and emotional meanings to us. In the heritage of every human culture, a meal is enjoyed with family and friends and is often an event unto itself. Even the food preparation can be a social event complete with rituals and traditions. With today's fast-paced lifestyles, however, more people eat while doing something else—such as while working, driving, or walking. Companionship, though, makes a meal more satisfying. We can see how important this is by thinking about food and social events. Food is always part of a celebration. Food is part of courtship and dating. People go to restaurants to have fun together. When a visitor comes to your home or place of work, the custom is to offer food or drink. Food is fundamental to hospitality.

Emotionally, foods can represent comfort. Many adults associate particular foods with happy childhood memories, or talk about the favorites that "mom (or dad or another family member) used to make." Food that is very familiar and part of long-standing habits can also be comforting and is called a **comfort food**. Which foods provide comfort vary from one person to the next, but some foods have built a reputation for comfort. For some people, mashed potatoes and fried chicken are comfort foods. Other comfort foods may include things like chocolate cake, or grilled cheese sandwiches and cream of tomato soup.

Figure 1.2   Religious Dietary Practices

Religion	Dietary Practice or Laws	Underlying Principle
Buddhism	Avoid animal products, sometimes even fish; many Buddhists are vegetarians; fasting practiced by monks.	Like many other religions, plant foods or foods of the earth are considered most wholesome.
Eastern Orthodox Christianity	Restrictions on meat and fish during fasting which for the strict Orthodox Christian can be over half of each year.	Fasting, especially on holy days, is part of their faith.
Hinduism	Beef is not eaten. Other meat and fish are restricted or avoided including pork, poultry and shellfish. Many are strict vegetarians or vegans. They also practice fasting.	The cow is considered a sacred animal so eating beef is forbidden. Dairy products are allowed.
Islam	Pork or birds of prey are excluded. Alcohol, coffee, tea, and other stimulants are avoided. Eating for health is important. Fasting is considered to have a cleansing effect.	Following prescribed dietary laws is an important part of their faith.
Judaism	Pork and shellfish are excluded. Meat and dairy are not allowed to be served at the same meal. Leavened bread such as yeast bread is also restricted. Fasting promotes spiritual growth.	Following prescribed dietary laws is an important part of their faith.
Mormonism	Strict Mormons avoid alcohol and caffeinated beverages including coffee, tea and chocolate. Fasting is practiced and plant-based foods are highly encouraged.	Addictive behaviors are believed to cause poor physical and emotional health. Fasting promotes spiritual growth.
Rastafarianism	Foods may only be slightly cooked so meats and canned foods are excluded. Most seafood is restricted.	Foods that are permitted are Biblical based or I-tal which means slightly cooked.
Roman Catholicism	Red meat is restricted on certain days such as Fridays during Lent. Fasting is practiced by some.	Fasting and food restrictions are observed according to the church calendar.
Seventh-Day Adventist	Pork and most meat and fish is excluded; eating a plant-based diet is prescribed. Low-fat dairy products and eggs are allowed	Eating and drinking is done to 'honor God' and preserve one's health.

Source: Adapted from www.faqs.org/nutrition/pre-sma/religion-and-dietary-practices.html.

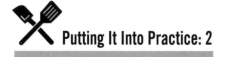

Putting It Into Practice: 2

One of your customers observes Orthodox Jewish customs. How would you adjust your menus to accommodate this customer?

(Check your answer at the end of this chapter)

Whatever a person associates with good feelings and family routines can become a comfort food.

When someone is not feeling well, the value of comfort foods increases. Often, a food that is well tolerated has emotional meaning, too. Chicken soup, for example, not only has some medicinal value for someone suffering from a cold, it may also feel emotionally soothing. Sometimes, food as comfort plays a strong role in an individual's nutrition. Food has such powerful emotional overtones that it can take on its own meaning. Some people eat when they feel lonely, nervous, or stressed.

Social and emotional meanings of food can exert strong influence on the foods each of us choose to eat. Meanings such as these play an important role in dietary care. Because food is not just "chow," we all need a comfortable social environment, companionship, and a certain amount of familiar fare to feel satisfied from a meal. In fact, research shows that in a long-term care environment, residents eat better when they are with others and in a relaxed environment.

Availability of Food

Another factor that influences food choices is simply what is available. This relates to cash on hand and what food a person can afford to buy. It relates to the ability to go shopping. Someone who cannot go to a grocery store on a regular basis is more likely to rely on canned and dried foods that store well in a cupboard. Someone who has access to a garden during the growing season may eat a great deal of fresh vegetables.

Availability also relates to local crops. Certain foods are more available in some areas than others. In coastal areas, fresh seafood may be key to the cuisine because it is caught close by. Pineapple is used extensively in Hawaii, because it is fresh and readily available. This distinction is blurring somewhat with the globalization of the U.S. food supply. Today, American consumers can enjoy food from anywhere in the world. However, price factors affect choices, and some imported foods may not be as fresh or as economical as local specialties.

Another aspect of availability comes into play when an individual is eating away from home, or when home is an institution. If someone else is providing meals, the menu dictates what foods are available. Preferred foods may not be options. An individual will then choose something else. Over time, this can vastly alter a person's dietary habits and nutritional state. In particular, if preferred foods are not available, some individuals simply will not eat adequately.

Personal Taste

Personal taste is really a combination of biology and preferences we develop. The biological sense of taste arises from contact of food with the tongue and soft palate, where taste buds sense four types of tastes—bitter, sweet, sour and salty.

From the tongue and soft palate, taste sensations transfer to the brain, where we process them. One misconception is that certain parts of the tongue sense certain tastes—such as the tip of the tongue for sweetness, or the sides of the tongue for saltiness. Actually, this is not true. Experts say that tastes buds can sense all flavors on all areas of the tongue. How the brain interprets these signals and puts them together may vary from one person to another. Taste has its basis in taste genes, which were recently identified.

Along with what the taste buds sense, other factors contribute to our sense of taste. Smell is very important. The aroma of good food enhances taste tremendously. Conversely, someone suffering from a cold virus and stuffy nose may notice that food doesn't have much "flavor." This is because sense of smell is reduced. An unpleasant smell can ruin a meal. Another component of taste is called mouthfeel. This describes how food feels in the mouth as we eat it. Mouthfeel can be crunchy or smooth, creamy or lumpy. This has a strong impact on what we describe as the taste of food.

In general, we all tend to select foods that taste good to us. Preferences vary considerably. Many develop from habit, as well as from individual variations in how we sense the flavors of foods. While cultural influences and food habits are part of the picture, biology is another part.

Aesthetic Influences

Sometimes, for holiday fun, people change the color of food. Think of St. Patrick's Day and green food. Green milkshakes are commonly available at this time. Many people enjoy green shakes because they taste like mint. We think of "green" and "mint" as belonging together. But what happens when we color mashed potatoes or cheese sauce green? These foods may not be appealing. Why? Because they just don't look right. Some people may even associate green in these foods with mold. Clearly, we have expectations about how food should look. Most of the time, we don't even think about these expectations.

The visual impact of food and the way it is presented is quite powerful. For example, maybe you really enjoy beef stew. The colorful assortment of shapes and flavors can be very attractive—brown chunks of meat, creamy-white potatoes, orange carrot slices, and light-green celery bits. Now, what happens if you blenderize the stew and put it in a cup? Will you enjoy the food in the same way? It may now look like a medium brown-colored sludge. The flavors, though, haven't changed. Most of us will say this doesn't sound appealing.

Again, this example demonstrates our need for visual appeal when we eat. As it turns out, this example represents a key challenge in providing dietary care. Sometimes, clients are unable to chew or swallow well, and need to receive blenderized food. A Certified Dietary Manager may be called upon to overcome this aesthetic disadvantage when serving pureed food.

In addition, some people will respond strongly to whether foods are mixed together or presented separately. This can be personal choice, but can also have cultural influences. For example, a person raised in traditional Appalachian culture may never have seen a casserole. A person influenced by traditional Japanese culinary practices will expect to see each food separate from others, and may feel uncomfortable with mixed dishes.

Color of food is just one factor in the aesthetic impression food conveys. Presentation is also significant. How food looks on a plate—or in a bowl—influences how we believe it will taste. How is meat sliced? How are fruit pieces cut? Does the food have appealing shapes? What sauces and garnishes appear? What kind of dishware, trays, and table settings provide the backdrop for the meal? The finest chefs give tremendous attention to these details. Much like the first impressions we form of people we meet, the visual first impressions of meals affect how much we enjoy them.

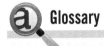

Glossary

Functional Foods
Foods that convey health benefits beyond the nutrients

Phytochemicals
Phyto means plant so these are chemicals in plants thought to provide special health benefits

Vegan Diet
A diet containing no animal foods

Lacto-Vegetarian
A diet excluding all animal foods except dairy

Ovo-lacto Vegetarian
A diet excluding animal foods except dairy and eggs

Attitudes and Values

What do you think of when you hear these words: Broccoli? Tomatoes? Fresh blueberries? These are among the foods believed to impart special health benefits as part of a new understanding of **functional foods**. These foods are also said to contain **phytochemicals**. An example is tomatoes, which contain lycopene, a naturally-occurring chemical. Lycopene is touted as a preventative for cancer and heart disease. Today, many people choose foods such as tomatoes, soybean products, garlic, blueberries, or many others specifically to achieve health benefits. See *Nutrition in the News* at the end of this chapter for more details about how a desire for health affects eating patterns.

Some individuals choose foods with the idea of losing weight, or gaining weight and building muscle. Some are motivated by physical performance. Sometimes, a desire to avoid diseases in the future affects food choices. For example, one person may avoid eggs and butter and eat fish to reduce a risk of heart disease.

In addition, we tend to assign value judgments to food. Some reflect a sense of status. It's easy to picture this idea when we think of caviar or high-priced champagne. These are perceived as "high-status" foods because of their price tags. Some people may perceive a meal made from dried beans as "low-status" because it is inexpensive. Value assignments and attitudes also affect the range of foods a person will try. Ask yourself: How do you feel about eating crawdads, or escargot (snails), or frogs' legs, or turtle soup, or rabbit meat, or dog meat, or venison? Some people may consider some of these delicacies, while others may reject them, often based on attitudes towards foods or what they represent. Political convictions may play a role in food choices, too. For example, some consumers may boycott particular products based on company practices.

The choice to follow a **vegetarian diet** can also stem from attitudes and values. Some vegetarians avoid fish and seafood. Some avoid all animal products, including milk, cheese, and eggs. A diet with no animal products is called a **vegan diet**. People may identify themselves as a certain type of vegetarian such as a vegan, **lacto-vegetarian**, or **ovo-lacto vegetarian**. If a client identifies themselves as a vegetarian, further questions are needed to determine what food product they include or exclude. Some people choose to avoid animal foods out of values and convictions regarding animal rights and humane treatment, while others choose vegetarian diets for health or religious reasons.

Value judgments also come into play as consumers evaluate special food categories, like genetically engineered foods and organic foods. To make genetically engineered foods, scientists take a selected gene from one plant (or animal) and place it into the genetic structure of another to change its characteristics. In food crops, a gene may be changed to improve resistance to pests and improve crop yields, or to improve shelf life after harvest, or to produce yeast that makes bread rise better, or to enhance nutritional components of a food. Most genetically engineered foods do not require special marketing approval from the Federal Department of Agriculture (FDA) or any other government agency to reach the market.

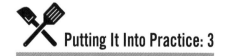

Putting It Into Practice: 3

Your menu for the noon meal follows. How would you adjust the meal to accommodate a lacto-vegetarian?

- Cream of tomato soup
- Grilled tuna sandwiches with whole grain bread
- Pickle slices
- Fresh watermelon cubes
- Oatmeal cookie

(Check your answer at the end of this chapter)

The burgeoning organic foods trend is another current food issue that affects many consumers' food choices. **Organic foods** are grown without genetic engineering, without use of inorganic (chemically synthesized) growth hormones, antibiotics, pesticides, herbicides, or fertilizers. Part of the idea of growing food organically is conservation of soil, water, and other natural resources. Some consumers embrace this concept out of concern for environmental protection. Organic farmers may use organic fertilizers and natural pest control (insect traps, predator insects to eliminate harmful insects, etc.). They may practice crop rotation. Organic foods, according to their legal definition enacted with the National Organic Standards Program in 2002, contain at least 95% organic ingredients. Foods that meet this requirement can bear a USDA Organic Seal (See Figure 1.3).

Yet another food term that elicits value judgments from many consumers is natural foods. **Natural foods**, as defined by the U.S. Food Safety and Inspection Service, contain no artificial ingredients or added color and are only minimally processed. For some, the natural foods trend has become part of consumer backlash to today's advanced field of food technology. In a related vein, some consumers choose foods based on distance of transport—wanting locally grown foods. Or, they choose based on packaging—preferring minimal packaging to protect the environment.

Note that knowledge and education can be critical factors shaping dietary choices, too. While the U.S. population devotes a great deal of attention to nutrition and food issues, reported facts can seem confusing. Nutrition advice can even seem contradictory. Knowledge may be incomplete, and not everyone is a nutrition scientist. Thus, some attitudes and values can evolve out of ignorance or uncertainty.

As part of the natural foods movement, there is emphasis today on sustainability. In 1989, the World Commission on Environment and Development

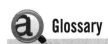

Glossary

Organic Foods
Grown without genetic engineering, without use of inorganic hormones, antibiotics, pesticides, herbicides, or fertilizers

Natural Foods
Contain no artificial ingredients or added color and are only minimally processed

Therapeutic Diets
Dietary changes dictated by health conditions

Figure 1.3	USDA Organic Food Symbol

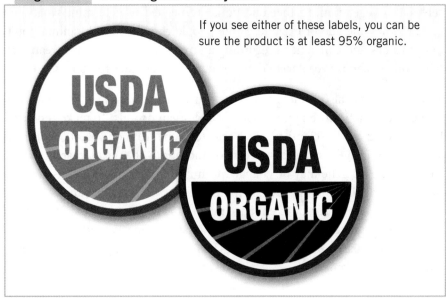

If you see either of these labels, you can be sure the product is at least 95% organic.

(Brundtland Commission) proposed the following definition of sustainability: "to meet the needs of the present without compromising the ability of future generations to meet their own needs." That means foodservice uses methods, materials, and systems that won't harm the environment or deplete natural resources.

Sustainability includes a focus on purchasing foods locally. The farther food travels from the farm to the table, the more opportunity for foodborne illness and nutrient loss from the food. Farmer's markets are commonplace today, as are Community Share Associations (CSAs), where customers purchase a share in a community garden or a farmer's garden in exchange for delivery of local produce every week. A 2009 article by Huang and Gregoire, reported 10 percent of hospital foodservice directors are routinely offering locally grown foods. There are some issues to fully implementing sustainability such as:

✓ Lack of year-round availability

✓ Working with multiple vendors

✓ Licensure or approval status of local vendors

✓ Consistency in products

✓ Delivery times

In spite of these concerns, the emphasis on sustainability will bring about additional change in health care facilities.

Lifestyle

A critical factor driving food choices today is lifestyle. According to the National Restaurant Association (NRA), eating out is big business—estimated at over $491 billion for the year 2007. This includes fast food dining and eating on-the-run. In fact, a report from the NRA in 2000 indicates that 41 percent of all cellular phone users use their phones to make restaurant takeout or delivery orders. This is a powerful reflection of the lifestyle issues that have molded dietary habits in America.

Personal Health

Aside from health beliefs, many personal diets are affected by health status. As an example, one person may be diagnosed with diabetes and face prescribed dietary changes. Another may be diagnosed with high blood cholesterol levels and be advised to follow a low-fat diet. In this book, you will become familiar with many dietary changes dictated by health conditions. As a group, these are called **therapeutic diets**. Some individuals follow therapeutic diets more meticulously than others. In general, though, dietary advice offered by a physician, Registered Dietitian, or other health professional is likely to influence food choices.

At the same time, a person who is not feeling well may suffer a loss of appetite. A person taking one of many common medications may experience changes in how foods taste. One person may avoid what used to be favorite foods, or even develop a new list of food preferences based on medical changes. Yet another medication may increase a person's sense of hunger or thirst, bringing on a

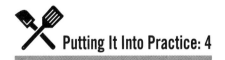

Putting It Into Practice: 4

Your facility is interested in beginning a sustainability effort. What are the first steps to take?

(Check your answer at the end of this chapter)

round of unplanned dietary changes. One person may have experienced loss of teeth or other dental conditions that affect ability to chew. Chronic pain can significantly reduce appetite. A person with a neurological disorder may find an ordinary diet difficult to swallow. Physical disability, psychological illness or depression, and many medical factors affect food intake. Many women experiencing premenstrual syndrome (PMS) may face food cravings late in the menstrual cycle. Most likely, there is a biological basis for these cravings. Similar findings relate to food cravings during pregnancy. These are all examples of ways in which personal health status may result in dietary changes.

Finally, a dietary practice that sometimes occurs among low-income groups is called pica. Pica is the practice of eating items that are not actually food—such as laundry starch, clay, or paste. Some researchers believe that pica occurs most often among women or children who lack iron in their bodies. Ironically, though, eating these items does not improve nutritional state.

Nutrition Versus Diet

In all, it's clear there is a big difference between nutrition and diet. **Nutrition** is the science of how components in food nourish the body. These components include carbohydrates, fats, proteins, vitamins, and minerals. A **diet** is the foods and beverages a person consumes. The original Greek meaning of diet was "manner of living." Any person's diet reflects individual choices stemming from cultural heritage, regional trends, religious practices, social and emotional meanings, availability of food, personal taste, aesthetic influences, attitudes and beliefs, lifestyle, and personal health. In addition, dietary choices tend to become habit for most people. Dietary choices include not only what a person chooses to eat, but also what foods a person chooses to avoid.

Nutrition alone can, in theory, be provided by chemical formulations. However, we do not generally choose to obtain nutrition in this way, due to the powerful meaning of food to us as humans. Instead, we enjoy a rich, personal experience related to food. Thus, to provide nutritional care, a Certified Dietary Manager must consider both nutrition and diet to develop plans that will help clients maintain or improve health. An effective dietary plan weaves comfortably into personal dietary choices. It respects heritage and preferences. It supports habits that have become meaningful for each of us as individuals. A critical factor driving food choices today is lifestyle.

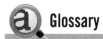 **Glossary**

Nutrition
The science of how components in food nourish the body

Diet
The foods and beverages a person consumes

2010 Food and Health Survey

Consumer Attitudes Toward Food Safety, Nutrition, and Health

The International Food Information Council Foundation's 2010 Food & Health Survey takes an extensive look at what Americans are doing regarding their eating and health habits, and food safety practices. When it comes to calories consumed versus calories burned, most Americans (58 percent) do not make an effort to balance the two; a large majority of people (77 percent) are not meeting the U.S. Department of Health and Human Services' Physical Activity Guidelines.

Executive Summary and Key Trends

The 2010 *Food & Health Survey: Consumer Attitudes Toward Food Safety, Nutrition & Health*, commissioned by the International Food Information Council Foundation, is the fifth annual national quantitative study designed to gain insights from consumers on important food safety, nutrition, and health-related topics. The research provides the opportunity to gain insight on how consumers view their own diets, their efforts to improve them, how they balance diet and exercise, and their actions when it comes to food safety practices.

There is now more of a need than ever to understand consumers' perceptions of nutrition and food safety issues. The *2010 Dietary Guidelines for Americans* will target, for the first time, an overweight and obese American population and advocate a "total diet" approach. There also are ongoing initiatives to address childhood obesity from the White House to Main Street, including First Lady Michelle Obama's *Let's Move* initiative. Landmark healthcare legislation was signed into law requiring calorie counts at restaurant chains. And, there is pending food safety legislation before the U.S. Congress.

While the *Food and Health Survey* highlights that many different messages about the importance of a healthful lifestyle are being heard, the *Survey* also shows disconnects in consumers' awareness of the relationship between diet, physical activity, and calories. Although weight loss and physical activity are top of mind with Americans, the *Survey* provides valuable insights into consumer beliefs and behaviors with regards to food safety, safe food handling, and consumer food shopping preferences, among other topics.

This *Survey* offers the important voice and insights of the consumer for the health professionals, government officials, educators, and other interested individuals who seek to improve the lives of Americans.

The following are key findings from 2010 with comparisons to results from the 2006 through the 2009 editions of the *Food & Health Survey*.

Overall Health Status: Americans' perceptions of their health status remains steady from previous years with 38 percent indicating their health is "excellent" or "very good." Although there was no significant change from year to year, Americans' degree of satisfaction with their health status remains relatively high with 57 percent indicating "extremely satisfied" or "somewhat satisfied."

Weight: Americans' concern with their weight status remains unchanged since last year, and continues to be a strong factor influencing the decision to make dietary changes and remain physically active. Most Americans (70 percent) say they are concerned about their weight status, and the vast majority (77 percent) is trying to lose or maintain their weight. When asked what actions they

(Continued...)

are taking, most Americans say they are changing the *amount* of food they eat (69 percent); changing the *type* of foods they eat (63 percent); and engaging in *physical activity* (60 percent). Further, 65 percent of Americans report weight loss as a top driver for improving the healthfulness of their diet; 16 percent report improving their diet to maintain weight. Americans are more singularly focused on making dietary changes for losing weight, rather than a variety of other motivators, as has been true in the past. In addition, losing or maintaining their weight is the top motivator (35 percent) for Americans who are physically active.

Diet and Physical Activity: Two-thirds of Americans (64 percent) report making changes to improve the healthfulness of their diet. The primary driver for making these changes is "to lose weight" (65 percent). Other drivers for making dietary changes have significantly decreased since previous years, including "to improve overall well-being "(59 percent vs. 64 percent in 2009) and "to improve physical health" (56 percent vs. 64 percent in 2008). The specific types of dietary changes they most often report are changing the *type* of food they eat (76 percent), changing the *amount* of food they eat (70 percent), and changing *how often* they eat (44 percent). Americans' reports of their physical activity levels show that, on average, 63 percent are physically active, and 68 percent of those who are physically active report being "moderately" or "vigorously" active three to five days a week. However, among those who are active, slightly more than half (56 percent) do not include any strength training sessions. Further, a large majority of Americans (77 percent) are not meeting the U.S. Department of Health and Human Services' *Physical Activity Guidelines*.

Calorie and Energy Balance: Few Americans (12 percent) can accurately estimate the number of calories they should consume in a day for a person their age, height, weight, and physical activity. Of those who say they are trying to lose or maintain weight, only 19 percent say they are keeping track of calories. Additionally, almost half of Americans do not know how many calories they burn in a day (43 percent) or offer inaccurate estimates (35 percent say 1000 calories or less). When it comes to calories consumed versus calories burned, most Americans (58 percent) do not make an effort to balance the two.

Dietary Fats: Americans are confused about the differences among dietary fats. While Americans who have "heard" of these various types of dietary fats are reducing their consumption of saturated and trans fats (64 percent are trying to consume less *trans* fats and saturated fats), less than half (43 percent) state they consume more Omega-3 fatty acids, and only a quarter (26 percent) state that they are consuming more Omega-6 fatty acids. Americans also seem to be less focused on dietary fat when looking at the Nutrition Facts Panel. When looking at the Nutrition Facts Panel listing of dietary fats, Americans are less frequently focusing on: total fat (62 percent vs. 69 percent in 2009); saturated fat (52 percent vs. 58 percent in 2008); *trans* fat (52 percent vs. 59 percent in 2008); and calories from fat (51 percent vs. 57 percent in 2007).

Carbohydrates and Sugars: Americans who have "heard" of the various types of carbohydrates and sugars are trying to consume more fiber (72 percent) and whole grains (73 percent) in their diets, but remain confused about the benefits of consuming more complex carbohydrates. Americans generally agree with the statement that "moderate amounts of sugar can be part of an overall healthful diet," however, this sentiment declined to 58 percent from 66 percent in 2009.

Protein: New to this year's *Survey* were questions about protein. Close to half of Americans say they are trying to consume more protein. Moreover, Americans are twice as likely to say protein is found in animal sources (56 percent) vs. plant sources (28 percent). The majority of Americans (68 percent) believe protein helps build muscle.

Sodium: Another new topic to this year's *Survey* was sodium. More than half of Americans (53 percent) are concerned with the amount of sodium in their diet. Six in ten Americans regularly purchase reduced/lower sodium foods. Among those that do purchase reduced/

(Continued...)

2010 Food and Health Survey (Continued)

lower sodium foods, the most cited items include canned soup (58 percent), snacks (48 percent), and canned vegetables (41 percent).

Low-Calorie Sweeteners: Nearly four in ten Americans (38 percent) agree that low-calorie/artificial sweeteners can play a role in weight loss or weight management, and one-third of Americans (34 percent) also agree that low-calorie/artificial sweeteners can reduce the calorie content of foods. Consistent with these data, one-third of Americans (32 percent) say they consume low-calorie/artificial sweeteners to help with calorie management.

Caffeine: Nearly three-quarters of Americans (72 percent) report consuming caffeine in moderation this year, significantly more than in 2009 (66 percent). There are also significantly fewer Americans (10 percent vs. 16 percent in 2009) who say they have either eliminated caffeine from their diet or say they consume more than the average person (18 percent in 2010 vs. 22 percent in 2008). Those who say they consume caffeine in moderation are more likely to perceive their health as "very good" or "excellent."

Food Additives: The majority of Americans (61 percent) agree with at least two out of five statements provided regarding food additive facts or benefits. Those with the highest percent agreement include: "Food additives extend the freshness of food/act as a preservative" (57 percent), "Food additives can add color to food products" (54 percent), and "Food additives can help keep or improve the flavor of food products" (47 percent).

Food Safety: For the past three years, consumer confidence in the safety of the U.S. food supply has remained steady with nearly half of Americans (47 percent) rating themselves as confident in the safety of the U.S. food supply. Those not confident fell significantly (down to 18 percent from 24 percent in 2009) and those who are neither confident nor unconfident increased to 35 percent from 26 percent in 2009.

As in previous years, we see consistency in consumers' beliefs that food safety is primarily the responsibility of government (74 percent) and industry (70 percent). Overall, approximately one-third of Americans (31 percent) see food safety as a shared responsibility

among five or more stakeholder groups including farmers/producers, retailers and themselves.

Safe Food Handling: While still high, there continues to be a decline in basic consumer food safety practices such as washing hands with soap and water (89 percent vs. 92 percent in 2008). These same declines are also relevant in microwave food safety practices, where 69 percent vs. 79 percent in 2008 of Americans follow all the cooking instructions. Although a significant number of Americans (84 percent) use their microwave to prepare packaged products such as soup, popcorn, and frozen meals where microwave cooking instructions are clearly indicated, an even larger number of Americans (92 percent) cite the main reason for using the microwave is to reheat leftovers, foods, and/or beverages.

Consumer Information Sources and Purchasing Influences: In addition to information gathered on the Nutrition Facts Panel and the food label, consumers were asked about their awareness and use of the U.S. Department of Agriculture's *MyPyramid* food guidance system. While 85 percent of Americans say they are aware of *MyPyramid*, only 29 percent of individuals report having used *MyPyramid* in some way.

Consistent with previous years, taste remains the biggest influence on purchasing decisions (86 percent), followed by price, healthfulness (58 percent) and convenience (56 percent). The importance of price continues to have a large impact on consumers' food and beverage purchasing decisions (73 percent in 2010 vs. 64 percent in 2006).

Food Labeling: Similar to previous years, Americans say they are actively using the Nutrition Facts Panel (68 percent), the expiration date (66 percent), and, increasingly, the brand name (50 percent vs. 40

(Continued...)

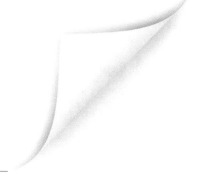

2010 Food and Health Survey *(Continued)*

percent in 2008) and allergen labeling (11 percent vs. 6 percent in 2008). Among consumers who use the Nutrition Facts Panel, they rank calories as the top piece of information they use (74 percent), followed by sodium content (63 percent vs. 56 percent in 2009). Fewer Americans, however, are looking at total fat content (62 percent vs. 69 percent in 2009) and sugars (62 percent vs. 68 percent in 2008).

Food Purchasing Influences: The vast majority of Americans (88 percent) conduct the bulk of their food shopping at a supermarket/grocery store. Roughly three-quarters of Americans are satisfied with the healthfulness of products offered at their supermarket/grocery store (73 percent) and warehouse membership club (80 percent).

The full Survey findings and Web casts are available on the International Food Information Council Foundation's website: www.foodinsight.org.

About the International Food Information Council Foundation

Our Mission: The International Food Information Council Foundation is dedicated to the mission of effectively communicating science-based information on health, food safety and nutrition for the public good.

Additional information on the Foundation is available on the "About" section of our Web site: www.foodinsight.org.

END OF CHAPTER

Putting It Into Practice Questions & Answers

1. As a new Certified Dietary Manager, you want to recognize the cultural differences of your customers. What is the first step to implementing a cultural change movement in your facility?

   A. *Talk to residents! What do they like/want? What would they do regarding food choices and meal times if they didn't live in your facility?*

2. One of your customers observes Orthodox Jewish customs. How would you adjust your menus to accommodate this client?

   A. *Offer alternatives when pork or shellfish are served; separate meat from dairy products including cooking and serving dishes; avoid serving dairy and meat products in the same meal.*

3. Your menu for the noon meal follows. How would you adjust the meal to accommodate a lacto-vegetarian? Cream of tomato soup, grilled tuna sandwiches with whole grain bread, pickle slices, fresh watermelon cubes, oatmeal cookie.

   A. *Substitute grilled cheese sandwich for the grilled tuna.*

4. Your facility is interested in beginning a sustainability effort. What are the first steps to take?

   A. *Contact other healthcare facilities in the area to see what they are doing.*

   Visit a farmer's market or a 'locally grown food store' to determine availability.

   Focus on one area of sustainability at a time such as implementing locally grown foods.

Identify Nutrition Concepts

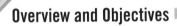

CHAPTER 2

Overview and Objectives

A Certified Dietary Manager needs to select and recommend foods according to established nutrition principles. In addition, a Certified Dietary Manager needs to be able to apply guides and tools to assess nutritional adequacy. After completing this chapter, you should be able to:

- ✓ Discuss the importance of good nutrition
- ✓ Select types of carbohydrate
- ✓ Select types of lipids
- ✓ Explore health effects of protein
- ✓ Distinguish between vitamins and minerals
- ✓ Identify the role of water as a nutrient
- ✓ Define phytochemicals and functional foods
- ✓ Select the best food sources of specific vitamins and minerals
- ✓ Calculate daily fluid requirement
- ✓ Differentiate between different food guides
- ✓ Analyze own intake for the leader nutrients

This chapter helps you look at the total diet. The total diet is about consuming food. The Dietary Guidelines Advisory Committee (DGAC) defines "total diet" as "the combination of foods and beverages that provide energy and nutrients and constitute an individual's complete dietary intake, on average, over time. This encompasses various foods and food groups, their recommended amounts and frequency, and the resulting eating pattern." With so many foods from which to choose, what is the best combination of nutrients while consuming food?

Sound nutrition advice combined with food consumption advice is available from both government and private agencies. We will look at several in this chapter.

- ✓ Dietary Guidelines
- ✓ MyPyramid
- ✓ USDA Food Plans
- ✓ Healthy People Campaign
- ✓ Dietary Reference Intakes (DRIs)

Health Concerns

Early nutrition scientists focused on identifying essential nutrients. A few decades ago, nutrition advice centered on encouraging intake of certain foods to prevent deficiencies and enhance growth. Today, however, nutrition scientists devote a great deal of research to an opposite problem: nutritional excess and imbalance. The Surgeon General's Report on Nutrition and Health in 1988 became a kind of turning point for nutritional planning. The report concluded that over-consumption of certain nutrients—not deficiency—should be our chief nutritional concern. Generally, the over-consumed nutrients are macronutrients. Some studies of over-consumption focus on fats and types of fats, as well as overall caloric intake.

The American government tracks what we eat, the nutritional content, and the related health concerns. Two such surveys were combined in 2002 to become What We Eat in America (WWEIA), NHANES. These two agencies conducted national food surveys: USDA's Continuing Survey of Food Intakes by Individuals (CSFII) and HHS' NHANES (National Health and Nutrition Examination Survey). The most recent data release was 2005-2006 and Figure 2.1 shows the top food sources of calories.

Figure 2.1   Top Food Sources of Calories Per Day for Adults

Pizza — 98
Yeast Breads — 114
Chicken/CKN Dishes — 121
Soda/Energy Drinks — 129
Grain Based Desserts — 139
Other — 1598

Based on 2,199 Calories per Day. According to the NHANES, 2005-2006.

Specifically, the survey found that Americans eat too many calories and too much solid fats, added sugars, refined grains, and sodium. Americans also eat too little dietary fiber, vitamin D, calcium, potassium, and unsaturated fatty acids (specifically omega-3s), and other important nutrients that are mostly found in vegetables, fruits, whole grains, low-fat milk and milk products, and seafood.

Obesity is a major public health challenge, not only in the United States, but world-wide. According to the Surgeon General's Report in 2010, "obesity contributes to an estimated 112,000 preventable deaths in the U.S. annually." Figure 2.2 shows the obesity trends over the past 30 years and illustrates that the trend is a concern not just for adults but also young children and teens. Because of the dramatic increase in childhood obesity, the White House convened a Task Force on Childhood Obesity (including 12 federal agencies) in 2010 in order to make recommendations to address childhood obesity.

Figure 2.2   Obesity Trends Over the Past 30 Years

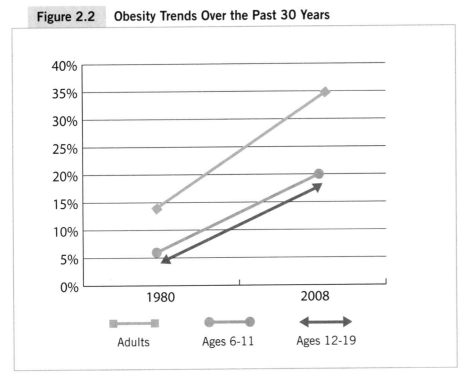

Source: CDC, Surgeon General

Being overweight is measured through **body mass index** (**BMI**). BMI is used to express weight adjusted for height. BMI is calculated as weight in kilograms divided by height in meters squared. There are many charts available where one can just enter height in inches and weight in pounds to pinpoint BMI. **Overweight** is defined as being at a BMI of 25-29.9. **Obesity** is defined as being at a BMI of 30 or greater.

According to the Dietary Guidelines Advisory Committee report on Energy Balance and Weight Management, 2010, the conditions listed in Figure 2.3 are health risks associated with overweight and obesity and with a sedentary life style. Note the health risks that are the same.

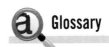 **Glossary**

Body Mass Index (BMI)
A method of determining degree of overweight that takes into consideration both weight and height

Overweight
Having a body mass index of 25 to 29.9

Obesity
Having a body mass index (BMI) of 30 or greater

Figure 2.3   Health Risks Associated with Overweight, Obesity, and Sedentary Life Style

Overweight and Obesity Health Risks	Sedentary Life Style Health Risks
• Type 2 Diabetes (T2D)	• Type 2 Diabetes (T2D)
• Hypertension	• Hypertension
• Cardiovascular Disease (CVD)	• Coronary Artery Disease
• Stroke	• Stroke
• Certain Kinds of Cancer	• Certain Kinds of Cancer
• Osteoarthritis	• Osteoporosis
• Gall Bladder Disease	• Depression
• Sleep Apnea	• Decreased Health-Related Quality of Life
• Dyslipidemia	• Overweight and Obesity
	• Decreased Overall Fitness

Note that some of the health risks are the same in both categories.

Obesity is influenced by many factors. For each individual, body weight is the result of a combination of genetic, metabolic, behavioral, environmental, cultural, and socioeconomic influences. However, based on a growing amount of evidence provided by the Dietary Guidelines Advisory Committee, there are two factors that have a significant impact on the obesity epidemic:

✓ The food environment

✓ Amount of physical activity

The food environment is associated with a lower intake of fruits and vegetables and an increased body weight. Food environment includes the distance from a supermarket that offers a large variety of fruits and vegetables and the density

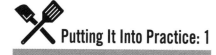

Putting It Into Practice: 1

If a client had a BMI of 25.5, how would they be classified?

(Check your answer at the end of this chapter)

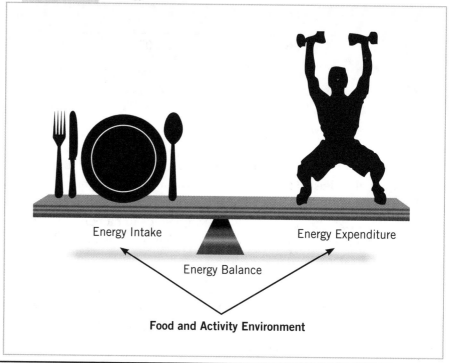

Figure 2.4   Energy Balance

Energy Intake   Energy Expenditure

Energy Balance

Food and Activity Environment

of fast food restaurants in the area where you live. "The strongest documented relationship between fast food and obesity is when one or more fast-food meals are consumed per week." There is also a direct relationship between portion size and body weight. An important addition in the discussion on food environment is the amount of screen time (amount of time spent watching TV, the computer, or video games) for both adults and children. "The strongest association with overweight and obesity is with television screen time."

There is solid evidence to indicate that we consume too many calories in comparison to the current level of physical activity. While food alone does not cause, cure, or control obesity, weight control is a nutritional issue. When we consume more than we use, we gain weight. Exercise is very important in managing weight and preventing disease. Exercising regularly helps a person:

✓ Achieve a healthy balance of energy consumed and energy used (see Figure 2.4)

✓ Prevent heart disease by strengthening the heart and cardiovascular system

✓ Reduce the risk of developing breast cancer, colon cancer, and other forms of cancer through weight control

It is obvious from the information above that we need both dietary goals and physical activity goals to maintain energy balance. Figure 2.5 provides physical activity goals and facts on inactivity.

Dietary Guidelines

How can we manage our food environment with so many foods from which to choose? How can we evaluate our diet, plan adequate menus or advise others about how to choose health-promoting foods? The Center for Nutrition Policy and Promotion, an organization of the U.S. Department of Agriculture, was established in 1994 to improve the nutrition and well-being of Americans. The Center focuses its efforts on two primary objectives:

1. Advance and promote dietary guidance for all Americans, and

2. Conduct applied research and analyses in nutrition and consumer economics

---

Figure 2.5   Physical Activity Goals and Facts on Inactivity

Physical Activity and Inactivity

* It is recommended that Americans accumulate at least 30 minutes (adults) or 60 minutes) (children) of moderate physical activity most days of the week. More may be needed to prevent weight gain, to lose weight, or to maintain weight loss.

* Less than $1/3$ of adults engage in the recommended amounts of physical activity.

* Many people live sedentary lives; in fact, 40 percent of adults in the United States do not participate in any leisure time physical activity.

* 43 percent of adolescents watch more than 2 hours of television each day.

* Physical activity is extremely helpful in maintaining weight loss, especially when combined with healthy eating.

Source: US Surgeon General, American Cancer Society

The Center produces six core products to support its objectives; those starred below will be addressed in this chapter.

✓ Dietary Guidelines for Americans*

✓ **MyPyramid** Food Guidance System*

✓ Healthy Eating Index

✓ U.S. Food Plans*

✓ Nutrient Content of the U.S. Food Supply

✓ Expenditures on Children by Families

Dietary Guidelines for Americans

The **Dietary Guidelines** for Americans 2010 supports a total diet approach to achieving dietary goals. They are issued jointly by the U.S. Department of Agriculture (USDA) and the U.S. Department of Health and Human Services (DHHS). According to the USDA, "The Guidelines provide authoritative advice for people two years and older about how good dietary habits can promote health and reduce risk for major chronic diseases. They serve as the basis for federal food and nutrition education programs."

The Guidelines are intended to "summarize and synthesize knowledge regarding individual nutrients and food recommendations into a pattern of eating that can be adopted by the public," says the USDA. They are updated every five years based on new scientific information.

Dietary Guidelines 2010 list recommendations under nine groups. Each group contains a series of key recommendations, including some for specific population groups. See Figure 2.6.

With the 2010 Dietary Guidelines, Americans are being urged to "achieve their recommended nutrient intakes by consuming foods within a total diet that meets but does not exceed energy needs." This begins with Americans being aware of what and how much they consume every day while self monitoring their physical activity levels. It is important to remember that beverages count in our calorie intake. This is especially true today with the dramatic increase in sport and juice drinks. Portion control plays a very important part in managing our total diet. Excessive portions are common today in restaurants.

The 2010 Dietary Guidelines focus specifically on reducing calories from <u>so</u>lid <u>f</u>ats and <u>a</u>dded <u>s</u>ugars, called **SoFAS**. SoFAS represent about 35 percent of our daily calorie intake and are responsible for our increased saturated fat and cholesterol intakes. See Figure 2.7 for examples of SoFAs that represent major food sources in today's diets.

It is important to remember that these are guidelines and that putting the guidelines into practice is the responsibility of each person. Three of the core products produced by the USDA's Center for Nutrition Policy and Promotion provide Americans with specific eating patterns that incorporate current research.

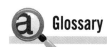

Glossary

Dietary Guidelines
Guidelines issued jointly by the U.S. Department of Agriculture (USDA) and the U.S. Department of Health and Human Services (DHHS) to provide advice, promote health, and reduce risk for major chronic diseases

SoFAS
A new term in the 2010 Dietary Guidelines that refers to <u>so</u>lid <u>f</u>ats and <u>a</u>dded <u>s</u>ugars

MyPyramid
Also developed by the USDA and DHHS provides a personalized plan about how to eat and apply the Dietary Guidelines

Figure 2.6   Dietary Guidelines for Americans 2010

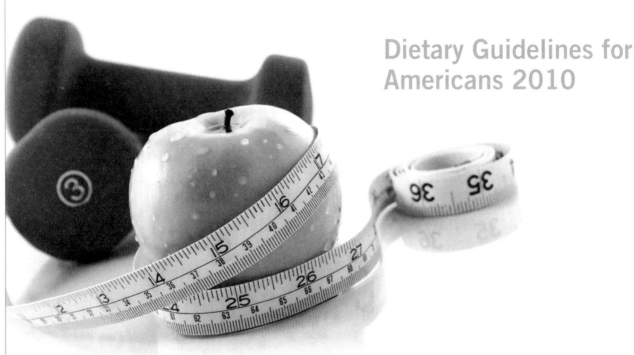

Dietary Guidelines for Americans 2010

Executive Summary

Eating and physical activity patterns that are focused on consuming fewer calories, making informed food choices, and being physically active can help people attain and maintain a healthy weight, reduce their risk of chronic disease, and promote overall health.

The *Dietary Guidelines for Americans, 2010* exemplifies these strategies through recommendations that accommodate the food preferences, cultural traditions, and customs of the many and diverse groups who live in the United States.

By law (Public Law 101-445, Title III, 7 U.S.C. 5301 et seq.), *Dietary Guidelines for Americans* is reviewed, updated if necessary, and published every 5 years. The U.S. Department of Agriculture (USDA) and the U.S. Department of Health and Human Services (HHS) jointly create each edition. *Dietary Guidelines for Americans, 2010* is based on the Report of the *Dietary Guidelines Advisory Committee* on the *Dietary Guidelines for Americans, 2010* and consideration of Federal agency and public comments.

Dietary Guidelines recommendations traditionally have been intended for healthy Americans ages 2 years and older. However, *Dietary Guidelines for Americans, 2010* is being released at a time of rising concern about the health of the American population. Poor diet and physical inactivity are the most important factors contributing to an epidemic of overweight and obesity affecting men, women, and children in all segments of our society. Even in the absence of overweight,

poor diet and physical inactivity are associated with major causes of morbidity and mortality in the United States. Therefore, the *Dietary Guidelines for Americans, 2010* is intended for Americans ages 2 years and older, including those at increased risk of chronic disease.

Dietary Guidelines for Americans, 2010 also recognizes that in recent years nearly 15 percent of American households have been unable to acquire adequate food to meet their needs.[1] This dietary guidance can help them maximize the nutritional content of their meals. Many other Americans consume less than optimal intake of certain nutrients even though they have adequate resources for a healthy diet. This dietary guidance and nutrition information can help them choose a healthy, nutritionally adequate diet.

The intent of the Dietary Guidelines is to summarize and synthesize knowledge about individual nutrients and food components into an interrelated set of recommendations for healthy eating that can be adopted by the public. Taken together, the Dietary Guidelines recommendations encompass two overarching concepts:

(Continued...)

Figure 2.6   Dietary Guidelines for Americans 2010 *(Continued)*

- **Maintain calorie balance over time to achieve and sustain a healthy weight.** People who are most successful at achieving and maintaining a healthy weight do so through continued attention to consuming only enough calories from foods and beverages to meet their needs and by being physically active. To curb the obesity epidemic and improve their health, many Americans must decrease the calories they consume and increase the calories they expend through physical activity.

- **Focus on consuming nutrient-dense foods and beverages.** Americans currently consume too much sodium and too many calories from solid fats, added sugars, and refined grains.[2] These replace nutrient-dense foods and beverages and make it difficult for people to achieve recommended nutrient intake while controlling calorie and sodium intake. A healthy eating pattern limits intake of sodium, solid fats, added sugars, and refined grains and emphasizes nutrient-dense foods and beverages—vegetables, fruits, whole grains, fat-free or low-fat milk and milk products,[3] seafood, lean meats and poultry, eggs, beans and peas, and nuts and seeds.

A basic premise of the Dietary Guidelines is that nutrient needs should be met primarily through consuming foods. In certain cases, fortified foods and dietary supplements may be useful in providing one or more nutrients that otherwise might be consumed in less than recommended amounts. Two eating patterns that embody the Dietary Guidelines are the USDA Food Patterns and their vegetarian adaptations and the DASH (Dietary Approaches to Stop Hypertension) Eating Plan.

A healthy eating pattern needs not only to promote health and help to decrease the risk of chronic diseases, but it also should prevent foodborne illness. Four basic food safety principles (Clean, Separate, Cook, and Chill) work together to reduce the risk of foodborne illnesses. In addition, some foods (such as milks, cheeses, and juices that have not been pasteurized, and undercooked animal foods) pose high risk for foodborne illness and should be avoided.

The information in the *Dietary Guidelines for Americans* is used in developing educational materials and aiding policymakers in designing and carrying out nutrition-related programs, including Federal food, nutrition education, and information programs. In addition, the *Dietary Guidelines for Americans* has the potential to offer authoritative statements as provided for in the Food and Drug Administration Modernization Act (FDAMA).

The following are the *Dietary Guidelines for Americans, 2010* Key Recommendations, listed by the chapter in which they are discussed in detail. These Key Recommendations are the most important in terms of their implications for improving public health.[4] To get the full benefit, individuals should carry out the Dietary Guidelines recommendations in their entirety as part of an overall healthy eating pattern.

(Continued...)

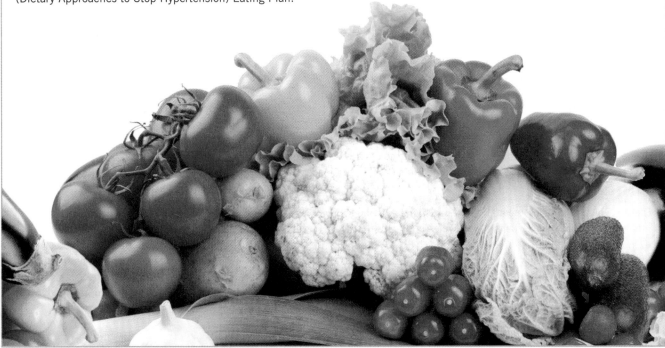

Figure 2.6   Dietary Guidelines for Americans 2010 *(Continued)*

Key Recommendations

Balancing Calories to Manage Weight

- Prevent and/or reduce overweight and obesity through improved eating and physical activity behaviors.

- Control total calorie intake to manage body weight. For people who are overweight or obese, this will mean consuming fewer calories from foods and beverages.

- Increase physical activity and reduce time spent in sedentary behaviors.

- Maintain appropriate calorie balance during each stage of life—childhood, adolescence, adulthood, pregnancy and breastfeeding, and older age.

Food and Food Components to Reduce

- Reduce daily sodium intake to less than 2,300 milligrams (mg) and further reduce intake to 1,500 mg among persons who are 51 and older and those of any age who are African American or have hypertension, diabetes, or chronic kidney disease. The 1,500 mg recommendation applies to about half of the U.S. population, including children, and the majority of adults.

- Consume less than 10 percent of calories from saturated fatty acids by replacing them with monounsaturated and polyunsaturated fatty acids.

- Consume less than 300 mg per day of dietary cholesterol.

- Keep trans fatty acid consumption as low as possible by limiting foods that contain synthetic sources of trans fats, such as partially hydrogenated oils, and by limiting other solid fats.

- Reduce the intake of calories from solid fats and added sugars.

- Limit the consumption of foods that contain refined grains, especially refined grain foods that contain solid fats, added sugars, and sodium.

- If alcohol is consumed, it should be consumed in moderation—up to one drink per day for women and two drinks per day for men—and only by adults of legal drinking age.[5]

Foods and Nutrients to Increase

Individuals should meet the following recommendations as part of a healthy eating pattern while staying within their calorie needs.

- Increase vegetable and fruit intake.

- Eat a variety of vegetables, especially dark-green and red and orange vegetables and beans and peas.

- Consume at least half of all grains as whole grains. Increase whole-grain intake by replacing refined grains with whole grains.

- Increase intake of fat-free or low-fat milk and milk products, such as milk, yogurt, cheese, or fortified soy beverages.[6]

- Choose a variety of protein foods, which include seafood, lean meat and poultry, eggs, beans and peas, soy products, and unsalted nuts and seeds.

- Increase the amount and variety of seafood consumed by choosing seafood in place of some meat and poultry.

(Continued)

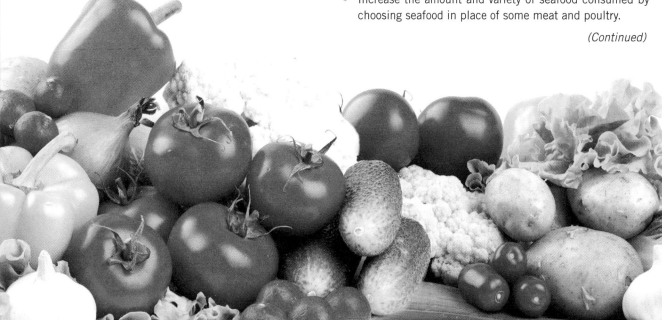

| **Figure 2.6** | **Dietary Guidelines for Americans 2010** *(Continued)* |

- Replace protein foods that are higher in solid fats with choices that are lower in solid fats and calories and/or are sources of oils.
- Use oils to replace solid fats where possible.
- Choose foods that provide more potassium, dietary fiber, calcium, and vitamin D, which are nutrients of concern in American diets. These foods include vegetables, fruits, whole grains, and milk and milk products.

Recommendations for Specific Population Groups

Women capable of becoming pregnant[7]

- Choose foods that supply heme iron, which is more readily absorbed by the body, additional iron sources, and enhancers of iron absorption such as vitamin C-rich foods.
- Consume 400 micrograms (mcg) per day of synthetic folic acid (from fortified foods and/or supplements) in addition to food forms of folate from a varied diet.[8]

Women who are pregnant or breastfeeding[7]

- Consume 8 to 12 ounces of seafood per week from a variety of seafood types.
- Due to their high methyl mercury content, limit white (albacore) tuna to 6 ounces per week and do not eat the following four types of fish: tilefish, shark, swordfish, and king mackerel.
- If pregnant, take an iron supplement, as recommended by an obstetrician or other health care provider.

Individuals ages 50 years and older

- Consume foods fortified with vitamin B12, such as fortified cereals, or dietary supplements.

Building Healthy Eating Patterns

- Select an eating pattern that meets nutrient needs over time at an appropriate calorie level.
- Account for all foods and beverages consumed and assess how they fit within a total healthy eating pattern.
- Follow food safety recommendations when preparing and eating foods to reduce the risk of foodborne illnesses.

Footnotes

1. Nord M, Coleman-Jensen A, Andrews M, Carlson S. Household food security in the United States, 2009. Washington (DC): U.S. Department of Agriculture, Economic Research Service. 2010 Nov. Economic Research Report No. ERR-108. Available from http://www.ers.usda.gov/publications/err108.

2. Added sugars: Caloric sweeteners that are added to foods during processing, preparation, or consumed separately. Solid fats: Fats with a high content of saturated and/or trans fatty acids, which are usually solid at room temperature. Refined grains: Grains and grain products missing the bran, germ, and/or endosperm; any grain product that is not a whole grain.

3. Milk and milk products also can be referred to as dairy products.

4. Information on the type and strength of evidence supporting the Dietary Guidelines recommendations can be found at http://www.nutritionevidencelibrary.gov.

5. See Chapter 3, Foods and Food Components to Reduce, for additional recommendations on alcohol consumption and specific population groups. There are many circumstances when people should not drink alcohol.

6. Fortified soy beverages have been marketed as "soymilk," a product name consumers could see in supermarkets and consumer materials. However, FDA's regulations do not contain provisions for the use of the term soymilk. Therefore, in this document, the term "fortified soy beverage" includes products that may be marketed as soymilk.

7. Includes adolescent girls.

8. "Folic acid" is the synthetic form of the nutrient; whereas, "folate" is the form found naturally in foods.

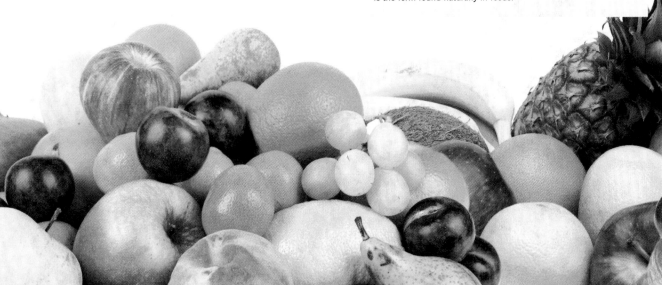

Source: Diet Instructions. Becky Dorner & Associates, Inc. Used with permission.

Figure 2.7 Examples of Solid Fats and Added Sugars in Current American Diets

Solid Fats	Added Sugars

Solid Fats

- Grain-based desserts, including cakes, cookies, pies, doughnuts, and granola bars
- Regular cheese
- Sausage, franks, bacon, and ribs
- Pizza
- Fried white potatoes, including french fries and has-browns
- Dairy-based desserts such as ice cream

SoFAS

Added Sugars

- Soda
- Grain-based desserts
- Fruit drinks
- Dairy-based desserts
- Candy

Eating Plans

An eating plan or eating pattern is designed to integrate dietary recommendations and current research into a healthy way to eat for most individuals. These eating patterns are not weight loss diets, but rather illustrative examples of how to eat in accordance with the Dietary Guidelines. Three eating plans based on the Dietary Guidelines are:

✓ MyPyramid /Choose MyPlate

✓ DASH diet (covered in Chapter 5)

✓ USDA Food Patterns

MyPyramid

The myPyramid plan, developed by the USDA and the Department of Health and Human Services, provides practical guidance about how to eat. It offers a pattern for making dietary choices, based on sound nutrition. It is not designed as a therapeutic diet to address specific health conditions. However, for the general healthy public over the age of two, it represents solid "basic nutrition" advice that can help individuals choose foods that will contribute to health, balance calorie intake with physical activity, and consume nutrient-dense foods.

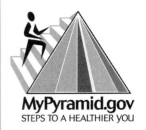

MyPyramid.gov
STEPS TO A HEALTHIER YOU

The myPyramid plan is presented as "a personalized plan" because it is scalable across a range of target calorie levels. How many calories does a person need? This depends on age, sex, and level of physical activity.

The myPyramid Website at www.myPyramid.gov has an interactive page that takes into account your age, sex, height, weight, and how much physical activity you usually do. This will help you design your own personal eating plan or pattern.

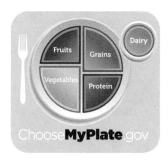

ChooseMyPlate.gov

Serving Sizes from MyPyramid

Grains = 1 oz.*

Veggies = 1 cup, 2 cup leafy greens

Fruits = 1 cup, ½ cup dried

Milk = 1 cup, 1½ oz. cheese

Meat = 1 oz., 1 egg, 1 Tbsp. peanut butter, ¼ cup dry beans

Oils = 1 tsp.

* In the 2011 Choose MyPlate campaign, half of your grains should be whole grains.

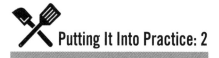

Putting It Into Practice: 2

In the menu below, what would the sources of SoFAS be?

- Tomato soup
- Grilled cheese sandwiches on white bread
- Pickle slices
- Birthday cake

(Check your answer at the end of this chapter)

Ten Tips—Choose MyPlate

The Choose MyPlate plan illustrates ten recommendation/categories as follows:

1. **Balance Calories**—Find out how many calories YOU need for a day as a first step in managing your weight. Go to www.ChooseMyPlate.gov to find your calorie level. Being physically active also helps you balance calories.

2. **Enjoy Your Food, But Eat Less**—Take the time to fully enjoy your food as you eat it. Eating too fast or when your attention is elsewhere may lead to eating too many calories. Pay attention to hunger and fullness cues before, during, and after meals. Use them to recognize when to eat and when you've had enough.

3. **Avoid Oversized Meals**—Use a smaller plate, bowl, and glass. Portion out foods before you eat. When eating out, choose a smaller size option, share a dish, or take home part of your meal.

4. **Foods to Eat More Often**—Eat more vegetables, fruits, whole grains, and fat-free or 1% milk and dairy products. These foods have the nutrients you need for health—including potassium, calcium, vitamin D and fiber. Make them the basis for meals and snacks.

5. **Make Half Your Plate Fruits and Vegetables**—Choose red, orange, and dark-green vegetables like tomatoes, sweet potatoes and broccoli, along with other vegetables for your meals. Add fruit to meals as part of main or side dishes or as dessert.

6. **Switch to Fat-Free or Low-Fat (1%) Milk**—They have the same amount of calcium and other essential nutrients as whole milk, but fewer calories and less saturated fat.

7. **Make Half Your Grains Whole Grains**—To eat more whole grains, substitute a whole-grain product for a refined product—such as eating whole wheat bread instead of white bread or brown rice instead of white rice.

8. **Foods to eat Less Often**—Cut back on foods high in solid fats, added sugars, and salt. They include cakes, cookies, ice cream, candies, sweetened drinks, pizza, and fatty meats like ribs, sausages, bacon and hot dogs. Use these foods as occasional treats, not everyday foods.

9. **Compare Sodium in Foods**—Use the Nutrition Facts label to choose lower sodium versions of foods like soup, bread and frozen meals. Select canned foods labeled "low sodium," "reduced sodium," or "no salt added."

10. **Drink Water Instead of Sugary Drinks**—Cut calories by drinking water or unsweetened beverages. Soda, energy drinks, and sports drinks are a major source of added sugar and calories in American diets.

Now take a look at Figure 2.8, which shows how many servings from each food group are recommended at several different calorie levels. The Choose MyPlate website at www.choosemyplate.gov lists intake patterns for additional calorie levels.

Figure 2.8   Sample myPyramid Servings at Three Calorie Levels

Calorie Level	Fruits	Vegetables	Grains	Meat & Beans	Milk	Oils	Discretionary Calories
1600	1.5 cups	2 cups	5 oz-eq	5 oz-eq	3 cups	5 tsp.	132
2200	2 cups	3 cups	7 oz-eq	6 oz-eq	3 cups	6 tsp.	290
2800	2.5 cups	3.5 cups	10 oz-eq	7 oz-eq	3 cups	8 tsp.	426

Source: USDA and DHHS

Servings and Portions

What is a serving? A serving is a measurement used for keeping track of amounts of food designated in an eating plan. This is different from a portion. A portion is the total amount of food served or consumed at any point in time. A portion can be larger (or smaller) than a serving. For example, consider the Choose MyPlate guide for a person targeting 2,200 calories per day. The suggested intake from the Grains group is 7 servings. To meet that total, a person may choose many different combinations and amounts of grains foods, such as:

✓ 1 cup of ready-to-eat whole-grain cereal at breakfast (1 serving), plus

✓ 2 slices of rye bread at lunch in a sandwich (2 servings), plus

✓ Several crackers (1 serving) for a snack, plus

✓ 1½ cups of rice or pasta at dinner (3 servings)

This would provide a total of seven servings from this group for a day.

For mixed foods, you can estimate food groups of the main ingredients. For example, a generous serving of pizza would count in the Grains group (crust), the Milk group (cheese), and the Vegetable group (tomato). A serving of beef stew would count in the Meats and Beans group and the Vegetable group. Figure 2.9 provides examples of counting mixed dishes in the Choose MyPlate plan.

A food pyramid approach provides a simple tool that is readily understood. Most people can select their own food choices from within each food group and make personal dietary choices that contribute to good health. The pyramid image is easy to conceptualize and makes a good educational tool as well. Note that myPyramid, like other food guides, is not absolute. As you will learn in later chapters, an individual's nutritional needs vary throughout the stages of life. In addition, medical conditions can affect what constitute "ideal" dietary choices for any individual. In later chapters, you will learn more about how diets may need to be modified for certain disease states.

USDA Food Pattern

The USDA Food Pattern (see Figure 2.10) is the recommended daily intake amounts from each food group or subgroup at all calorie levels. Recommended intakes from vegetable subgroups are per week. This food pattern can be used to plan menus for school foodservice, correctional facilities, and healthcare facilities. Additional food patterns are available online at: www.fns.usda.gov/cnd/menu/menu_planning.doc

Healthy People Campaign

The U.S. Department of Health and Human Services (DHHS) sets science-based, 10-year national objectives for promoting health and preventing disease. Healthy People 2020 is the current edition. There are 38 categories of objectives that range from A (Access to Health Services) to V (Vision). Figure 2.11 shows the objectives for the *Nutrition and Weight Status* category. The purpose of these objectives is to provide direction for diverse groups of people

Figure 2.9   Examples of Counting Mixed Dishes

Food and Sample Portion	Amount From Food Group in This Portion					
	Grains Group	Vegetable Group	Fruit Group	Milk Group	Meat & Beans Group	Estimated Total Calories
Cheese Pizza—Thin Crust (1 slice from medium pizza)	1 oz.-eq.	1/8 cup	0	½ cup	0	215
Macaroni and Cheese (1 cup made from package mix)	2 oz.-eq.	0	0	½ cup	0	260
Tuna Noodle Casserole (1 cup)	1½ oz.-eq.	0	0	½ cup	2 oz.-eq.	260
Chicken Pot Pie (8 oz. pie)	2½ oz.-eq.	¼ cup	0	0	1½ oz.-eq.	500
Beef Taco (2 tacos)	2½ oz.-eq.	¼ cup	0	¼ cup	2 oz.-eq.	370
Egg Roll (1)	½ oz.-eq.	1/8 cup	0	0	½ oz.-eq.	150
Chicken Fried Rice (1 cup)	1½ oz.-eq.	¼ cup	0	0	1 oz.-eq.	270
Stuffed Peppers with Rice and Meat (½ pepper)	½ oz.-eq.	½ cup	0	0	1 oz.-eq.	190
Clam Chowder-New England (1 cup)	½ oz.-eq.	1/8 cup	0	½ cup	2 oz.-eq.	165
Cream of Tomato Soup (1 cup)	½ oz.-eq.	½ cup	0	½ cup	0	160
Large Cheeseburger	2 oz.-eq.	0	0	1/3 cup	3 oz.-eq.	500
Peanut Butter & Jelly Sandwich (1)	2 oz.-eq.	0	0	0	2 oz.-eq.	375
Tuna Salad Sandwich (1)	2 oz.-eq.	¼ cup	0	0	2 oz.-eq.	290
Chef Salad (3 cups—no dressing)	0	1½ cups	0	0	3 oz.-eq.	230
Pasta Salad with Vegetables (1 cup)	1½ oz.-eq.	½ cup	0	0	0	140
Apple Pie (1 slice)	2 oz.-eq.	0	¼ cup	0	0	280

Source: USDA and DHHS

to combine their efforts and work as a team. Whatever phase of healthcare or foodservice you are in, achieving these objectives should be part of your efforts.

Dietary Modifications

Today's nutrition advice indicates a need to make some adjustments to the usual American diet. Here are more tips for making changes for each of the macronutrients.

Carbohydrate

The Dietary Guidelines for Americans recommend using sugars only in moderation. Foods containing large amounts of refined sugars should be eaten in moderation by most healthy people and sparingly by people with low calorie needs. For very active people with high calorie needs, sugars can be an additional source of calories. The following tips can help reduce sugar in the diet:

✓ Instead of regular soft drinks or powdered drink mixes, choose diet soft drinks, 100 percent fruit juices, bottled waters such as seltzer, or iced tea made without added sugar or with nonnutritive sweeteners.

✓ Instead of sweet desserts such as cake, emphasize fruits in desserts. Fresh fruit can be baked (as in baked apples), poached (as in poached pears), broiled, or made into compote. Choose canned fruits that are packed in fruit juice (not syrup).

✓ Make your own cakes, cookies, pies, and other baked goods and reduce the sugar by one-quarter to one-third. It usually does not affect the quality of the product. Use recipes that contain fruits to sweeten, and sweet spices such as cinnamon, nutmeg, and cloves.

✓ Try a cookie that uses less sugar, such as graham crackers, vanilla wafers, ginger snaps, or fig bars.

✓ Choose 100 percent pure fruit juices. They do not contain added sugars. Products labeled as fruit drinks, fruit beverages, or flavored drinks usually contain only small amounts of fruit juice and much refined sugar.

✓ Choose unsweetened breakfast cereals. Choose cereals with less than four grams of sugar per serving, unless the sugar comes from a dried fruit such as raisins. Top cereals with fresh fruit.

✓ Jams, jellies, and pancake syrup contain considerable amounts of refined sugar. For less refined sugar and calories, select jams and jellies made without (or with less) sugar, and pancake syrup labeled "reduced calorie." Other toppings for toast or pancakes are chopped fresh fruit, applesauce, part-skim ricotta cheese, and fruit.

Choose MyPlate: Mixed Dishes

Some mixed foods also contain a lot of fat, oil, or sugar, which adds calories. The values listed in Figure 2.9 are estimates based on how these foods are often prepared. The estimated total calories in each dish are also shown. The amounts in an item you eat may be more or less than these examples.

✓ Instead of sweetened breakfast pastries such as Danish, try a bagel, English muffin, roll, or fruited muffin and make them whole grain.

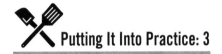

Putting It Into Practice: 3

How would you change the following menu to reduce the total daily sugar intake?

Breakfast
- Sugar-coated flakes
- Low-fat milk
- Whole-wheat toast
- Orange juice drink

Lunch
- Roast beef
- Mashed potatoes
- Steamed green beans
- Apple pie squares

Dinner
- Turkey sandwich
- Canned peaches
- Low-fat milk
- Oatmeal cookie

(Check your answer at the end of this chapter)

Figure 2.10 **USDA Food Patterns**

Recommended daily intake amount[1] from each food group or subgroup at all calorie levels. Recommended intakes from vegetable subgroups are per week.

Energy Level of Pattern[2]	1000	1200	1400	1600	1800	2000	2200	2400	2600	2800	3000	3200
Fruits	1 c	1 c	1½ c	1½	1½	2 c	2 c	2 c	2½ c	2½ c	2½ c	2½ c
Vegetables	1 c	1½ c	1½ c	2 c	2½ c	2½ c	3 c	3½ c	3½ c	3½ c	4 c	4 c
Dark green vegetables	½ c/wk	1 c/wk	1 c/wk	1½ c/wk	1½ c/wk	1½ c/wk	2 c/wk	2 c/wk	2½ c/wk	2½ c/wk	2½ c/wk	2½ c/wk
Red/Orange vegetables	2½ c/wk	3 c/wk	3 c/wk	4 c/wk	5½ c/wk	5½ c/wk	6 c/wk	6 c/wk	7 c/wk	7 c/wk	7½ c/wk	7½ c/wk
Cooked dry beans & peas	½ c/wk	½ c/wk	½ c/wk	1 c/wk	1½ c/wk	1½ c/wk	2 c/wk	2 c/wk	2½ c/wk	2½ c/wk	3 c/wk	3 c/wk
Other vegetables	1½ c/wk	2½ c/wk	2½ c/wk	3½ c/wk	4 c/wk	4 c/wk	5 c/wk	5 c/wk	5½ c/wk	5½ c/wk	7 c/wk	7 c/wk
Grains	3 oz eq	4 oz eq	5 oz eq	5 oz eq	6 oz eq	6 oz eq	7 oz eq	8 oz eq	9 oz eq	10 oz eq	10 oz eq	10 oz eq
Whole grains	1½ oz eq	2 oz eq	2½ oz eq	3 oz eq	3 oz eq	3 oz eq	3½ oz eq	4 oz eq	4½ oz eq	5 oz eq	5 oz eq	5 oz eq
Other grains	1½ oz eq	2 oz eq	2½ oz eq	2½ oz eq	3 oz eq	3 oz eq	3½ oz eq	4 oz eq	4½ oz eq	5 oz eq	5 oz eq	5 oz eq
Meat and beans	2 oz eq	3 oz eq	4 oz eq	5 oz eq	5 oz eq	5½ oz eq	6 oz eq	6½ oz eq	6½ oz eq	7 oz eq	7 oz eq	7 oz eq
Milk	2 c	2 c	2 c	3 c	3 c	3 c	3 c	3 c	3 c	3 c	3 c	3 c
Oils	15 g	17 g	17 g	22 g	24 g	27 g	29 g	31 g	34 g	36 g	44 g	51 g
Maximum SoFAS[3] limit, Calories (% total calories)	137 (14%)	137 (11%)	137 (10%)	121 (8%)	161 (0%)	258 (13%)	266 (12%)	330 (14%)	362 (14%)	395 (14%)	459 (15%)	596 (19%)

1 Food group amounts shown in cup (c) or ounce equivalents (oz. eq). Oils are shown in grams (g). Quantity equivalents for each food group are:

- Grains, 1 ounce equivalent is: ½ cup cooked rice, pasta, or cooked cereal; 1 ounce dry pasta or rice; 1 slice bread; 1 small muffin (1 oz.); 1 oz. ready-to-eat cereal.

- Fruits and vegetables, 1 cup equivalent is: 1 cup raw or cooked fruit or vegetable; 1 cup fruit or vegetable juice, 2 cups leafy salad greens.

- Meat and beans, 1 ounce equivalent is: 1 ounce lean meat, poultry, fish; 1 egg, ¼ cup cooked dry beans; 1 Tbsp. peanut butter; ½ ounce nuts/seeds.

- Milk, 1 cup equivalent is: 1 cup milk or yogurt, 1½ ounces natural cheese such as Cheddar cheese or 2 ounces of processed cheese.

2 Food intake patterns at 1000, 1200, and 1400 calories meet the nutritional needs of children ages 2 to 8 years. Patterns from 1600 to 3200 calories meet the nutritional needs of children 9 years of age and older and adults. If a child ages 2 to 8 years needs more calories and, therefore, is following a pattern at 1600 calories or more, the recommended amount from the milk group can be 2 cups per day. Children ages 9 years and older and adults should not use the 1000, 1200, or 1400 calorie patterns.

3 SoFAS are calories from solid fats and added sugars.

Figure 2.11   Healthy People 2020 Nutrition and Weight Status Objectives

- Increase the proportion of adults who are at a healthy weight.
- Reduce the proportion of adults who are obese.
- Reduce iron deficiency among young children and females of childbearing age.
- Reduce iron deficiency among pregnant females.
- Reduce the proportion of children and adolescents who are overweight or obese.
- Increase the contribution of fruits to the diets of the population aged 2 years and older.
- Increase the variety and contribution of vegetables to the diets of the population aged 2 years and older.
- Increase the contribution of whole grains to the diets of the population aged 2 years and older.
- Reduce consumption of saturated fat in the population aged 2 years and older.
- Reduce consumption of sodium in the population aged 2 years and older
- Increase consumption of calcium in the population aged 2 years and older.
- (Developmental) Increase the proportion of worksites that offer nutrition or weight management classes or counseling.
- Increase the proportion of physician office visits that include counseling or education related to nutrition or weight.
- Eliminate very low food security among children in U.S. households.
- (Developmental) Prevent inappropriate weight gain in youth and adults.
- Increase the proportion of primary care physicians who regularly measure the body mass index of their patients.
- Reduce consumption of calories from solid fats and added sugars in the population aged 2 years and older.
- Increase the number of States that have State-level policies that incentivize food retail outlets to provide foods that are encouraged by the Dietary Guidelines.
- Increase the number of States with nutrition standards for foods and beverages provided to preschool-aged children in childcare.
- Increase the percentage of schools that offer nutritious foods and beverages outside of school meals.

✓ Use less refined sugars in coffee, tea, cereals, etc., or use sugar substitutes.

✓ Try fresh or dried fruit for a sweet snack instead of candy.

General recommendations for fiber intake are from 20 to 35 grams daily. The Daily Value used for Nutrition Facts Labeling is 25 grams. For children, use the "age + 5" rule, which recommends that children consume an amount of fiber equal to their age plus an additional 5 grams of fiber. Unfortunately, the average American takes in less than 20 grams of fiber a day. Figure 2.12 lists good sources of fiber. When increasing fiber intake, do so slowly to avoid problems with cramps, diarrhea, and excessive gas. Also, it's important to chew foods well and drink at least 8 to 10 glasses of water each day, because fiber takes water out of the body. Make at least half of your grains whole grains.

Fat

The Dietary Guidelines for Americans recommend a diet moderate in total fat and low in saturated fat and cholesterol. Guidelines generally suggest that no more than 30 percent of daily calories should come from fat. Figure 2.13 gives some examples of fat levels corresponding to various calorie levels. Additional recommendations for Americans without cardiovascular disease include:

✓ No more than 10 percent of total calories should be in the form of saturated fat with an eventual goal of <7 percent.

✓ Avoid trans-fatty acids from processed food sources.

✓ Cholesterol intake should be less than 300 milligrams daily.

✓ Increase total amount of fish consumption to two times per week, especially those fish high in omega-3 fatty acids.

This advice does not apply to infants and toddlers below the age of two years. After age two, children should gradually adopt a diet that, by about five years of age, contains no more than 30 percent of calories from fat. As they begin to consume fewer calories from fat, children should replace these calories by eating more grain products, fruits, vegetables, low-fat milk products or other calcium-rich foods, beans, lean meat, poultry, fish, or other protein-rich foods.

Meat, poultry, fish, and shellfish contain saturated fat and/or cholesterol. Luckily, some choices are quite low in saturated fat. In general, poultry is low in saturated fat, especially when the skin is removed. When buying fresh ground turkey or chicken, find a product that says "light meat" or "breast" on the label. Poultry products that include the skin and/or dark meat and are much higher in fat. Goose and duck are also high in fat. Most fish is lower in saturated fat and cholesterol than meat and poultry. Fatty fish (such as salmon and tuna) are rich in omega-3 fatty acids, which may protect against heart disease and certain forms of cancer. Shellfish varies in cholesterol content.

Figure 2.14 lists lean cuts of meat. High-fat processed meats, such as many luncheon meats and sausages, provide a hefty 60 to 80 percent of their calories from fat, much of which is saturated. Other examples of these processed meats are bacon, bologna, salami, hot dogs, and sausage. In some cases, these processed meats are made from turkey or chicken and are lower in fat. Look for low-fat processed meats. Organ meats, like liver, sweetbreads, and kidneys are relatively low in fat. However, these meats are high in cholesterol.

When cooking meats, poultry, and fish, use cooking methods that use little or no fat, such as roasting, broiling, grilling, boiling, stir frying or poaching. Do not fry. When making pan gravy, refrigerate the drippings first so the fat will solidify and can be removed. One may also extend meat with pasta or vegetables for hearty dishes. For less saturated fat and cholesterol and more variety, dried beans or legumes are an excellent meat alternative.

Figure 2.12 Good Sources of Fiber and Fiber Grams per Standard Serving Size

Breakfast Cereals (1 cup)	Vegetables (½ cup)	Fruits
Bran-type Cereals 10	Broccoli. .3	Apple . . . .<1
Raisin Bran-type Cereals 8	Brussels Sprouts. 3	Banana .3
Whole Wheat Breakfast Cereals 4	Cabbage 2	Blackberries (1 cup) 8
Whole Oat Breakfast Cereals 2	Carrots. .3	Cherries (10 each) 2
	Cauliflower. 2	Dates (10 each) 6
	Peas 4	Figs (10 each) 2
Breads and Pastas (1 ounce)	Potatoes with Skin (1 each). 5	Grapefruit 2
Whole Wheat Bread 2	Spinach, raw . . . .<1	Kiwi Fruit. 3
Bran Muffin 5	Sweet Potatoes (1 each) 3	Orange. .3
Whole Wheat Pasta. 1-6		Pear 4
		Prunes (1 cup) 16
Dried Beans and Peas (½ cup)		Raspberries (1 cup) 8
All Cooked Beans and Peas 7		Strawberries (1 cup) 3

Figure 2.13 Recommended Fat and Saturated Fat Intake

Total Daily Calories	Saturated Fat @ 10%	Saturated Fat @ 7%	Total Fat @ 30%
1200	13 grams	9 grams	40 grams
1500	17 grams	12 grams	50 grams
1800	20 grams	14 grams	60 grams
2000	22 grams	15.5 grams	67 grams
2200	24 grams	17 grams	73 grams
2400	27 grams	19 grams	80 grams
2600	29 grams	20 grams	86 grams
2800	31 grams	22 grams	93 grams
3000	33 grams	23 grams	100 grams

Although many people believe that meats have the highest cholesterol and saturated fat content, dairy products can also be high in saturated fat and cholesterol. As dairy products are often added to foods like casseroles, cakes, or pies, it's easy to eat a significant amount of them without knowing it. Both 1% percent and skim milk provide much less saturated fat and cholesterol and fewer calories than whole milk, as shown in Figure 2.15.

Often, when people cut back on meat, they replace it with cheese, thinking they are cutting back on their saturated fat and cholesterol. They couldn't be more wrong. Because most cheeses are prepared from whole milk or cream, they are also high in saturated fat and cholesterol. Cheeses are particularly high in saturated fat (Figure 2.15). Fortunately, manufacturers offer low-fat versions of cheese favorites like cheddar, Swiss, and mozzarella. They use skim milk and vegetable oils to replace some of the cream and other fat. The result is reduced fat or fat free cheese. (Please see Chapter 10 for terms used on food labels and their exact definitions.)

Americans love ice cream. Ice cream is made from whole milk and cream and therefore contains a considerable amount of saturated fat and cholesterol. Some frozen desserts such as ices, popsicles, and sorbet are generally made without fat. Ice milk contains less fat and saturated fat than regular ice cream, as does frozen low-fat yogurt. With the wide variety of frozen desserts, it's a good idea to read nutrition labels.

Egg yolks are high in cholesterol. The average large egg yolk contains 213 milligrams of cholesterol, about two-thirds of the suggested daily intake. For less cholesterol and fat, use egg substitutes with less than 60 calories per one-quarter cup serving, or egg whites, which contain no cholesterol. Two egg whites can be substituted for one egg in most recipes.

Most breads and bread products contain only small amounts of fat, with less than two grams per slice or serving—that is, if we don't spread margarine or mayonnaise on them. Some breads typically have significant fat added in their

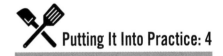

Putting It Into Practice: 4

Your daily calorie intake is 1800 calories. To help meet the new recommendations of 7% of the calories from saturated fat, what changes would you make to the following meal?

- 4 ounce roast beef with gravy
- ½ cup mashed potatoes
- ½ cup steamed broccoli with cheese sauce
- 1 cup 2% milk
- ½ cup ice cream with chocolate sauce

(Check your answer at the end of this chapter)

Figure 2.14 Lean Cuts of Meat

Beef	Veal	Pork	Lamb
• Eye of the Round • Top Round	• Shoulder • Ground Veal • Cutlets • Sirloin	• Tenderloin • Sirloin • Top Loin	• Leg-shank

preparation. Examples include biscuits, croissants, cornbread, and muffins. Also note that most granolas are high in fat. Commercial cakes, pies, cookies, donuts, and pastry are often high in fat, saturated fat, and calories. In addition, some are quite high in cholesterol. Tasty alternatives include angel food cake, sponge cake, fig bars, ginger snaps, and baked goods made with little or no fat. Recipe substitution ideas appear in Figure 2.16. Many desserts can also be made with less fat. Simply reduce the fat called for by one-fourth to one-third the original amount.

Protein

Proteins are especially important because they provide both energy (4 calories per gram) and essential amino acids. Unlike fats, the amount required per day is based on grams of protein per kilogram of body weight. The Recommended Dietary Allowance (RDA) for protein is 0.8 g protein/kg body weight/day for ages 19 and above. Average protein intake for most Americans is considered adequate but as Americans decrease their calorie intake to fight obesity, the percentage of calories from protein may need to increase, especially from a high quality protein source. See Figure 2.17 on how the percentage of calories from protein changes for a 150-pound person based on the total daily calorie intake.

Figure 2.15 Comparison of Milk, Poultry, Meat and Cheese

Food	Total Fat	Saturated Fat	Cholesterol	Calories
Milk				
Skim Milk	0.4 grams	0.3 grams	4 milligrams	86
1% Milk	2.6 grams	1.6 grams	10 milligrams	102
2% Milk	4.7 grams	2.9 grams	18 milligrams	121
Whole Milk	8.2 grams	5.1 grams	33 milligrams	150
Chicken **Roasted Chicken, no skin, light meat, 3 ounces**	—	1 gram	64 milligrams	4 grams
Meat **Beef, top round, broiled, 3 ounces**	—	3 grams	73 milligrams	8 grams
Cheese **Natural Cheddar, 1 ounce**	—	6 grams	30 milligrams	9 grams

Source: National Institutes of Health

Figure 2.16 Lower Fat Baking Substitutions

Instead of this...	Use this...
1 cup shortening	2/3 cup vegetable oil
1 whole egg	2 egg whites
1 cup sour cream	1 cup reduced-fat sour cream
1 cup whole milk	1 cup skim milk
1 tablespoon cream cheese	1 tablespoon light cream cheese
1 cup cream	1 cup low-fat yogurt
1 ounce baking chocolate	3 tablespoons cocoa and 1 tablespoon vegetable oil
Some of the butter or oil in a baked product	Fruit-based butter and oil replacements

High quality protein sources are animal proteins. In the past few years, many consumers have adopted high-protein diets for weight-loss purposes. This has resulted in some Americans consuming diets high in protein, especially animal sources. According to the Report of the DGAC on the Dietary Guidelines for Americans 2010, "long term studies of weight loss or maintenance of weight loss find no differences among diets lower or higher in protein." Eating too much protein has no benefits. In fact, eating excess protein from animal products may add excessive fat and calories.

Lower quality protein sources are plant based. If you are choosing a vegetarian diet, it is important to consume complementary protein sources such as beans and rice. Review the complementary protein sources in Chapter 3. Consuming lower-quality proteins is of greater concern when protein needs are high such as pregnancy, lactation, childhood, and during illness or injury. The Report of the DGAC on the Dietary Guidelines for Americans, 2010, found moderate evidence linking a plant-protein diet to lower blood pressure.

The best way to manage protein intake is to follow the Dietary Guidelines and Choose MyPlate. Also, note that many of the recommendations for reducing dietary fat and saturated fat are based on following recommended portion sizes.

Dietary Reference Intakes (DRIs)

Since 1941, the Food and Nutrition Board of the National Academy of Sciences has been preparing recommendations on nutrient intakes for Americans. Contemporary studies address topics ranging from the prevention of classical nutritional deficiency diseases to the reduction of risk of chronic diseases such as osteoporosis, cancer, and cardiovascular disease. In partnership with Health Canada, the Food and Nutrition Board has responded to these developments by making fundamental changes in its approach to setting nutrient reference values. This partnership issued the first of its new standards in 1997, replacing Recommended Dietary Allowances (RDAs). Dietary Reference Intakes is the inclusive name given to the new approach.

Figure 2.17 Changes in Protein Needs by Calorie Level

Calorie Level	% of Calories
1200	18
1500	14.4
1800	12
2000	10.8
2500	8.5
Protein needs for 150 lb. person @ 0.8gm/kg = 54 grams	
That amount stays the same regardless of the calorie level.	

Dietary Reference Intakes (DRIs) is a generic term used to refer to four types of reference values: Estimated Average Requirement, **Recommended Dietary Allowance**, **Adequate Intake**, and **Tolerable Upper Intake Level**. Dietary reference intakes are designed for various age and gender groups, because nutrient needs vary from childhood through adulthood, and some needs vary between males and females.

Estimated Average Requirement (EAR)

The EAR is the intake value that is estimated to meet the requirement defined by a specified indicator of adequacy in 50 percent of a specific group (age and gender group). A requirement is how much is needed in the diet to prevent symptoms of deficiency. A deficiency is the illness that occurs over time when a nutrient is not present in adequate amounts. For example, not eating enough vitamin C causes the deficiency disease scurvy. Not having enough vitamin D causes the deficiency disease rickets. Scurvy and rickets are examples of nutrient deficiency illnesses. At the EAR level of intake, 50 percent of the specified group would not have its needs met. In other words, if everyone consumed exactly the EAR levels of nutrients, some people would actually develop nutrient deficiencies. Thus, the EAR is designed only for setting a benchmark for baseline nutrient requirements. An EAR is not intended for use in evaluating an individual's dietary intake.

Recommended Dietary Allowance (RDA)

A Recommended Dietary Allowance (RDA) is the amount of a nutrient that is adequate to meet the known nutrient needs of practically all healthy persons. Contrary to popular belief, an RDA is not a minimum daily requirement. It is a dietary recommendation. To develop RDAs, scientists first reviewed research studies that indicated what minimum levels of nutrients might be required to prevent nutrient deficiencies. Then, they padded the requirements to account for additional factors that might affect requirements. They also padded the numbers to account for the difference between the amount of a nutrient consumed and the amount the body can actually use. These scientists used statistics to calculate individual variations in nutrient needs, and projected figures that would address the needs of most healthy people. Thus, an RDA is truly a recommendation about how much of a nutrient to consume through food. If everyone consumed exactly the RDA levels of nutrients, very, very few people in that group would develop nutrient deficiencies. Also, RDAs are for healthy individuals. RDAs do not always apply to someone who is suffering from a chronic illness or who has special medical conditions. Unlike the EAR, an RDA is a goal for groups of individuals.

Adequate Intake (AI)

For some nutrients, we simply don't know enough to set a meaningful RDA. We lack the scientific research that backs up the calculation of requirements. When this is the case, we use an Adequate Intake value. For example, we do not have a great deal of information about the physiological requirements for choline. Instead of setting an RDA, experts have designated an AI for choline. An AI represents a scientific judgment. We cannot be certain that an AI covers the nutrient needs of groups or individuals, but the AI value seems to be a reasonable point of reference based on what we know. When the only standard we have for a nutrient is an AI, it is fine to apply the AI to both groups and individuals.

Tolerable Upper Intake Level (UL)

The UL is the maximum level of daily nutrient intake that is unlikely to pose risks of adverse health effects. ULs have been developed for some nutrients as safety guidelines. For example, these points of reference are helpful in determining whether the doses of nutrients contained in nutritional supplements represent safe intakes.

As you might guess, setting dietary reference intakes is a complex task. Scientists are working to develop figures we can refer to when assessing individuals' diets and planning menus. Due to the enormity of this undertaking, the Dietary Reference Intake project has been divided into seven nutrient groups, which are updated intermittently.

How can I use the Dietary Reference Intakes?

The RDAs were developed to assess the diets of groups of people rather than individuals. Use the DRIs to plan and evaluate the diets of your facility. Because our bodies store nutrients for later use, we don't need to eat the RDAs every day. The USDA has a website that lists the current DRI tables (http://fnic.nal.usda.gov/interactiveDRI/). Log on to use their interactive tool to calculate daily nutrient recommendations for yourself or your client for dietary planning based on the Dietary Reference Intakes (DRIs). See Appendix B for the DRI, RDA, and AI.

Daily Fluid Requirement

Water is an essential nutrient. In the past, there was no dietary guideline or Dietary Reference Intake for water. Some people have even referred to it as the "forgotten nutrient." Since nearly all of our bodily systems depend on water and proper hydration, let's look at the recommendation for water and how to calculate daily fluid requirement. How much we need depends upon our health, our physical activity, and even where we live. We lose about 10 cups of water each day through breathing, sweating, and urine and bowel movements. Most physicians recommend drinking 8-10, 8-ounce glasses of water each day. We get about 20 percent of our fluid from food (refer to Figure 3.20 in Chapter 3).

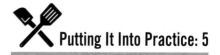

Putting It Into Practice: 5

Your client is a strict vegetarian (vegan). How would you adjust the menu below to make sure they are receiving a complete protein source?

- Chicken tacos with lettuce and tomato
- Pickle chips
- Apple slices
- Oatmeal cookie

(Check your answer at the end of this chapter)

Sources of water from food plus the eight to ten glasses of water would help us replace what we lose each day. In our efforts to fight the obesity epidemic, replacing other fluids such as soda, sport drinks, and juice with water will help reduce calories. Currently, we consume over 130 calories each day from soda, sport drinks, and juice. One pound of fat is equivalent to 3500 calories. By substituting water for soda, sport drinks, and juice, we could lose over one pound each month with no other changes. For additional information on calculating fluid requirements, see Chapter 10.

Food or Supplements?

A common nutritional question concerns multivitamin preparations or supplements. Should you rely on a balanced diet or pills to ensure good nutrition? While nutrition science is quite advanced, we are only beginning to understand the many components of foods that are active in the human body. The emerging concept of functional foods makes this quite evident (see *Nutrition in the News* at the end of this chapter). Beyond vitamins, minerals, protein, lipids, and carbohydrates, foods provide other natural chemicals. Some appear to offer health benefits. Already, some functional ingredients in foods have been incorporated into nutritional supplements. But this is not a complete answer for sound nutrition. The bottom line is that real food is preferable to chemical formulations. In real food, provided through a balanced diet and based on established dietary guidance, we can obtain necessary nutrients, as well as compounds we may not understand very well as yet. Real food also gives people pleasure, offers fiber (not present in all supplemental products) and water. It provides a sense of satiety or fullness when we eat it.

Multivitamins or nutritional supplements can be important for an individual who wishes to ensure adequate nutrition, or who needs to correct a deficiency. Iron supplements, for example, may be important to supplement dietary intake of iron. Iron-deficiency anemia is common in the U.S., and it is not easy for everyone to consume adequate iron through food. Calcium is another nutrient that may be worth supplementing—especially for adult women. The AI level is not easy for every woman to achieve, and calcium plays a role in preventing osteoporosis. These are just examples of situations in which supplementation may be useful. However, it's prudent to consider supplements as what they are—*supplements*—not *replacements* for healthy eating habits. It is also important to review DRIs for nutrients, and pay particular attention to the UL levels for nutrients. Excessive supplementation of some nutrients can cause health problems.

The Dietary Guidelines emphasize real foods over nutrition supplements, saying, "A basic premise of the Dietary Guidelines is that nutrient needs should be met primarily through consuming foods. Foods provide an array of nutrients and other compounds that may have beneficial effects on health. In certain cases, fortified foods and dietary supplements may be useful sources of one or more nutrients that otherwise might be consumed in less than recommended amounts. However, dietary supplements, while recommended in some cases, cannot replace a healthful diet." Figure 2.18 provides guidelines for maximizing nutrient loss during cooking.

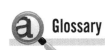

Glossary

Dietary Reference Intakes
Generic terms that encompass four types of reference values: Estimated Average Requirement, Recommended Dietary Allowance, Adequate Intake, and Tolerable Upper Intake Level

Recommended Dietary Allowance (RDA)
The amount of a nutrient adequate to meet the known nutrient needs of practically all healthy persons

Adequate Intake (AI)
A scientific judgment on the amount of some nutrients for which a specific RDA is not known

Tolerable Upper Intake Level (UL)
The maximum level of a daily nutrient that is considered safe

In all, a diet is complex. So much information about nutrition bombards us that it can be challenging to make dietary choices. Reliance on Choose My-Plate and the Dietary Guidelines for Americans is an excellent way to assure a healthy diet. For menu planning and in-depth assessment, the DRIs offer science-based standards of reference.

Figure 2.18 Tips for Protecting Nutrients

- Minimize storage time. Do not store foods longer than necessary.

- Keep foods wrapped or covered in storage.

- Do not soak foods in water unless absolutely necessary. If you need to soak a food, use as little water as possible. If practical, add the water to your product (e.g. a soup).

- Cut and cook vegetables in large pieces to minimize contact between surface area and air.

- To cook vegetables, steam rather than boil. This helps them retain nutrients.

- Cook vegetables as soon as possible after cutting.

- Use raw vegetables (rather than cooked) as practical.

- Avoid adding baking soda to vegetables during cooking. Some people use this practice to retain color. However, it destroys thiamin and vitamin C.

- Avoid overcooking food, as heat can destroy vitamins (especially vitamin C). Cook just until tender.

- Do not rinse rice before cooking.

- Do not brown undercooked rice before adding water. This destroys thiamin.

- After cooking rice, pasta, or other grain-based foods, do not rinse; just drain.

- Store food away from light or in dark containers. This is important for milk, since riboflavin and B vitamin in milk is destroyed by light.

- In foodservice operations, cook food as close to service times as possible. Cook in small batches as appropriate. For example, steamed vegetables may be prepared in small batches throughout an extended meal service time.

- Minimize holding time as much as possible. Keep foods covered during holding.

Source: USDA

Functional Foods Fact Sheet: Antioxidants

October 15, 2009

Background

Plant foods, such as fruits, vegetables, and whole grains contain many components that are beneficial to human health. Research supports that some of these foods, as part of an overall healthful diet, have the potential to delay the onset of many age-related diseases. These observations have led to continuing research aimed at identifying specific bioactive components in foods, such as antioxidants, which may be responsible for improving and maintaining health.

Antioxidants are present in foods as vitamins, minerals, carotenoids, and polyphenols, among others. Many antioxidants are often identified in food by their distinctive colors—the deep red of cherries and tomatoes; the orange of carrots; the yellow of corn, mangos, and saffron; and the blue-purple of blueberries, blackberries, and grapes. The most well-known components of food with antioxidant activities are vitamins A, C, and E; carotene; the mineral selenium; and more recently, the compound lycopene.

Health Effects

The research continues to grow regarding the knowledge of antioxidants as healthful components of food. Oxidation, or the loss of an electron, can sometimes produce reactive substances known as free radicals that can cause oxidative stress or damage to the cells. Antioxidants, by their very nature, are capable of stabilizing free radicals before they can react and cause harm, in much the same way that a buffer stabilizes an acid to maintain a normal pH. Because oxidation is a naturally occurring process within the body, a balance with antioxidants must exist to maintain health.

Research

While the body has its defenses against oxidative stress, these defenses are thought to become less effective with aging as oxidative stress becomes greater. Research suggests there is involvement of the resulting free radicals in a number of degenerative diseases associated with aging, such as cancer, cardiovascular disease, cognitive impairment, Alzheimer's disease, immune dysfunction, cataracts, and macular degeneration. Certain conditions, such as chronic diseases and aging, can tip the balance in favor of free radical formation, which can contribute to ill effects on health.

Consumption of antioxidants is thought to provide protection against oxidative damage and contribute positive health benefits. For example, the carotenoids lutein and zeaxanthin engage in antioxidant activities that have been shown to increase macular pigment density in the eye. Whether this will prevent or reverse the progression of macular degeneration remains to be determined. An increasing body of evidence suggests beneficial effects of the antioxidants present in grapes, cocoa, blueberries, and teas on cardiovascular health, Alzheimer's disease, and even reduction of the risk of some cancers.

Until recently, it appeared that antioxidants were almost a panacea for continued good health. It is only as more research has probed the mechanisms of antioxidant action that a far more complex story continues to be unraveled. Although recent research has attempted to establish a causal link between indicators of oxidative stress and chronic disease, none has yet been validated. A new area of research, led by the study of the human genome, suggests that the interplay of human genetics and diet may play a role in the development of chronic diseases. This science, while still in its infancy, seeks to provide an understanding of how common dietary nutrients such as antioxidants can affect health through gene-nutrient interactions.

(Continued...)

Functional Foods Fact Sheet: Antioxidants *(Continued)*

Examples of Functional Components*		
Class/Components	**Source***	**Potential Benefit**
CAROTENOIDS		
Beta-carotene	Carrots, Various Fruits	Neutralizes free radicals which may damage cells; Bolsters cellular antioxidant defenses
Lutein, Zeaxanthin	Kale, Collards, Spinach, Corn, Eggs, Citrus	May contribute to maintenance of healthy vision
Lycopene	Tomatoes and Processed Tomato Products	May contribute to maintenance of prostate health
FLAVONOIDS		
Anthocyanidins	Berries, Cherries, Red Grapes	Bolster cellular antioxidant defenses; May contribute to maintenance of brain function
Flavanols—Catechins, Epicatechins, Procyanidins	Tea, Cocoa, Chocolate, Apples, Grapes	May contribute to maintenance of heart health
Flavanones	Citrus Foods	Neutralize free radicals which may damage cells; Bolster cellular antioxidant defenses
Flavonols	Onions, Apples, Tea, Broccoli	Neutralize free radicals which may damage cells; Bolster cellular antioxidant defenses
Proanthocyanidins	Cranberries, Cocoa, Apples, Strawberries, Grapes, Wine, Peanuts, Cinnamon	May contribute to maintenance of urinary tract health and heart health
ISOTHIOCYANATES		
Sulforaphane	Cauliflower, Broccoli, Brussels Sprouts, Cabbage, Kale, Horseradish	May enhance detoxification of undesirable compounds and bolster cellular antioxidant defenses
PHENOLS		
Caffeic Acid, Ferulic Acid	Apples, Pears, Citrus Fruits, Some Vegetables	May bolster cellular antioxidant defenses; May contribute to maintenance of healthy vision and heart health
SULFIDES/THIOLS		
Diallyl Sulfide, Allyl Methyl Trisulfide	Garlic, Onions, Leeks, Scallions	May enhance detoxification of undesirable compounds; May contribute to maintenance of heart health and healthy immune function
Dithiolthiones	Cruciferous Vegetables—Broccoli, Cabbage, Bok Choy, Collards	Contribute to maintenance of healthy immune function

(Continued...)

Functional Foods Fact Sheet: Antioxidants *(Continued)*

Examples of Functional Components *(continued)**		
Class/Components	**Source***	**Potential Benefit**
WHOLE GRAINS		
Whole Grains	Cereal Grains	May reduce risk of coronary heart disease and cancer; May contribute to reduced risk of diabetes

Chart adapted from International Food Information Council Foundation: Media Guide on Food Safety and Nutrition: 2004-2006.
* Not a representation of all sources

There still remains a lack of direct experimental evidence from randomized trials that antioxidants are beneficial to health, which has led to different recommendations for different populations. For example, the use of supplemental-carotene has been identified as a contributing factor to increased risk of lung cancer in smokers.However, because the risk has not been indicated in non-smokers, these studies suggest that a precaution regarding the use of supplemental-carotene is not warranted for non-smokers. If supplementation is desired, the use of a daily multivitamin-mineral supplement containing antioxidants has been recommended for the general public as the best advice at this time.

A recent review of current literature suggests that fruits and vegetables in combination have synergistic effects on antioxidant activities leading to greater reduction in risk of chronic disease, specifically for cancer and heart disease. For some time, health organizations have recognized the beneficial roles fruits and vegetables play in the reduced risk of disease and developed communication programs to encourage consumers to eat more antioxidant-rich fruits and vegetables. The American Heart Association recommends healthy adults "Eat a variety of fruits and vegetables. Choose 5 or more servings per day." The American Cancer Society recommends to "Eat 5 or more servings of fruits and vegetables each day." The World Cancer Research Fund and the American Institute for Cancer Research 1997 Report Food, Nutrition and the Prevention of Cancer: A Global Perspective states, "Evidence of dietary protection against cancer is strongest and most consistent for diets high in vegetables and fruits." The potential for antioxidant-rich fruits and vegetables to help improve the health of Americans led the National Cancer Institute (NCI) to start the, "5-A-Day for Better Health" campaign to promote consumption of these foods.

Given the high degree of scientific consensus about consumption of a diet that is high in fruits and vegetables—particularly those which contain dietary fiber and vitamins A and C; the Food and Drug Administration (FDA) released a health claim for fruits and vegetables in relation to cancer. Food packages that meet FDA criteria may now carry the claim "Diets low in fat and high in fruits and vegetables may reduce the risk of some cancers." In addition the FDA, in cooperation with NCI, released a dietary guidance message for consumers, "Diets rich in fruits and vegetables may reduce the risk of some types of cancer and other chronic diseases." Most recently the Dietary Guidelines for Americans stated, "Increased intakes of fruits, vegetables, whole grains and fat-free or low-fat milk and milk products are likely to have important health benefits for most Americans."

Antioxidant research continues to grow and emerge as new beneficial components of food are discovered. Reinforced by current research, the message remains that antioxidants obtained from food sources, including fruits, vegetables and whole grains, are potentially active in disease risk reduction and can be beneficial to human health.

(Continued...)

The Bottom Line

Most research indicates that there are overall health benefits from antioxidant-rich foods consumed in the diet. The results of clinical trials with antioxidant supplements have yet to provide conclusive indication of health benefits. Current recommendations by the U.S. government and health organizations are to consume a varied diet with at least five servings of fruits and vegetables per day and 6-11 servings of grains per day, with at least three of those being whole grains.

Examples of Antioxidant Vitamins and Minerals			
Vitamins	**Dietary Reference Intake***	**Antioxidant Activity**	**Sources**
Vitamin A	300-900 µg/d	Protects cells from free radicals	Liver, Dairy Products, Fish
Vitamin C	15-90 mg/d	Protects cells from free radicals	Bell Peppers, Citrus Fruits
Vitamin E	6-15 mg/d	Protects cells from free radicals; Helps with immune function and DNA repair	Oils, Fortified Cereals, Sunflower Seeds, Mixed nuts
Selenium	20-55 µg/d	Hepls prevent cellular damage from free radicals	Brazil Nuts, Meats, Tuna, Plant Foods

Chart adapted from Food and Nutrition Board Institute of Medicine DRI reports and National Institute of Health Office of Dietary Supplements

* DRIs provided are a range for Americans ages 2-70

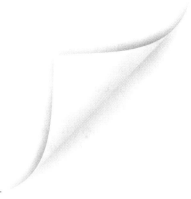

END OF CHAPTER

 Putting It Into Practice Questions & Answers

1. If a client had a BMI of 25.5, how would they be classified?

   A. *The client would be classified as overweight, which is a BMI between 25 and 29.*

2. In the menu below, what would the sources of SoFAS be?

   - Tomato soup
   - Grilled sandwiches on white bread
   - Pickle slices
   - Birthday cake
   - Cheese

   A. *SoFAS are Saturated Fats and Added Sugars. The sources of SoFAS in this menu could be the saturated fat in tomato soup if cream or whole milk is used. It would be saturated fat in the cheese in the sandwich, which could be decreased if a low-fat cheese is used. The added sugars would be the pickle slices, if they are sweet pickles, and the birthday cake. The birthday cake may also be a source of saturated fats depending upon the fat used in the cake mix. Cakes made with oils will have less saturated fats.*

3. How would you change the following menu to reduce the total daily sugar intake?

Breakfast	Lunch	Dinner
Sugar-coated flakes	Roast beef	Turkey sandwich
Low-fat milk	Mashed potatoes	Canned peaches
Whole-wheat toast	Steamed green beans	Low-fat milk
Orange juice drink	Apple pie squares	Oatmeal cookie

   A. *Substitute a whole grain cereal for the sugar-coated flakes and 100 percent orange juice in place of the orange drink. Substitute a baked apple for the apple pie squares for lunch. For dinner, use peaches canned in their own juice instead of a heavy syrup.*

4. Your daily calorie intake is 1800 calories. To help meet the new recommendations of 7 percent of the calories from saturated fat, what changes would you make to the following meal?

   - 4 oz. roast beef with gravy
   - ½ cup mashed potatoes
   - ½ cup steamed broccoli with cheese sauce
   - 1 cup 2% milk
   - ½ cup ice cream with chocolate sauce

   A. *Substitute roast turkey with non-fat gravy for the roast beef. Delete the cheese sauce on the broccoli and use a sprinkle of shredded cheese instead as a garnish. Replace the ice cream with ice milk.*

5. Your client is a strict vegetarian (vegan). How would you adjust the menu below to make sure they are receiving a complete protein source?

   - Chicken tacos with lettuce and tomato
   - Pickle chips
   - Apple slices
   - Oatmeal cookie

   A. *Use corn tortillas for the taco shells and replace the chicken with refried beans. Corn and beans are complementary protein sources that together provide the essential amino acids. Replace the cookie with a granola bar made without eggs or milk.*

CHAPTER 3

Use Basic Nutrition Principles

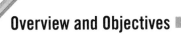

Overview and Objectives

In order to plan and implement menus, a Certified Dietary Manager needs to master nutrition concepts. An understanding of basic nutrients is also essential for planning modified diets. Certified Dietary Managers apply information from the six nutrient categories.

After completing this chapter, you should be able to:

✓ Identify six groups of nutrients

✓ Define calorie

✓ List the energy content of nutrients

✓ Differentiate between simple and complex carbohydrates

✓ Explain nutrient density of foods

✓ Calculate energy content of a simple food

We eat foods for many different reasons. Most of us have strong feelings about food based on a combination of reasons. Most of us also care about our body.... how we feel and look. If you are one of those people, then you already have a relationship with nutrition. Nutrition is all about how food nourishes our body. It is the nutrients in the food we eat that, when properly combined, provide optimum health.

Nutrition is also about energy, which affects both how we look and feel. We need energy every day to work and play. That energy comes either directly or indirectly from the sun in the form of nutrients in food. Plants convert the sun's rays into stored energy and when we eat plant foods, our bodies release that energy. Animals that eat plant foods get their energy the same way, so both plant and animal foods provide us with energy.

Nutrients or food components supply our bodies with energy, promote the growth and maintenance of tissues, and regulate body processes. There are about 50 known nutrients that are categorized into six groups:

✓ Carbohydrates

✓ Lipids (includes fats and oils)

✓ Proteins

✓ Vitamins

✓ Minerals

✓ Water

The functions of each group of nutrients are shown in Figure 3.1.

Most foods are a mixture of carbohydrates, proteins, and lipids, and contain smaller quantities of other nutrients, such as vitamins, minerals, and water. It's been said many times: "You are what you eat." Indeed, the nutrients you eat are in your body. Water accounts for about 50-70 percent of body weight. Lipids (fats) account for about 4-27 percent of body weight, and protein accounts for about 14-23 percent of body weight. Carbohydrates comprise only 0.5 percent. (Even though carbohydrates are important nutrients, most do not remain as carbohydrates in the body.) The remainder of body weight includes minerals, such as calcium in bones, and traces of vitamins.

Most, but not all, nutrients are considered essential nutrients. **Essential nutrients** either cannot be made in the body or cannot be made in the quantities needed by the body; therefore, we must obtain them through food. Thus, "essential" in this term means it is essential that we consume these nutrients; they are essential components of our diets. Carbohydrates, vitamins, minerals, water, and some parts of lipids and proteins are considered essential. Note that we do not usually eat nutrients by themselves. Nutrients are components of foods.

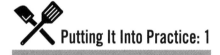

Putting It Into Practice: 1

As you review the food label for yogurt below, how many of the six nutrient categories can you locate?

(Check your answer at the end of this chapter)

Food Label for Greek Yogurt

Amount Per Serving	% of Daily Value
Total Fat 0 g	0%
Saturated Fat 0 g	0%
Trans Fat 0 g	0%
Cholesterol 0 mg	0%
Sodium 65 mg	3%
Total Carbohydrate 20 g	7%
Dietary Fiber < 1 g	4%
Sugars 19 g	
Protein 14 g	22%
Vitamin A 2%	Vitamin C 2%
Calcium 20%	Iron 0%

Figure 3.1   Functions of Each Group of Nutrients

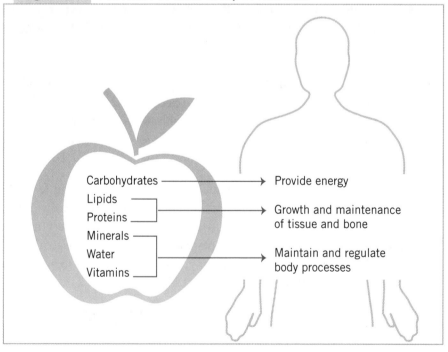

SECTION A | Energy Nutrients

Some nutrients provide energy. These are called **energy-yielding nutrients**—carbohydrates, lipids (fats), and protein. A **calorie** is a unit of measurement of heat or energy. Although we use the term calorie in our speech, and will use it in this book, calorie is actually a shortened form of the term "kilocalorie", which means 1,000 calories. Of the nutrients, only carbohydrates, lipids, and protein provide energy as follow:

✓ Carbohydrates: 4 calories per gram

✓ Lipids (Fat and Oils): 9 calories per gram

✓ Protein: 4 calories per gram

A **gram** is a unit of weight; there are 28 grams in one ounce. Vitamins, minerals, and water do not have any calories. Alcohol, although not a nutrient, provides seven calories per gram.

As you can see in Figure 3.1, energy-yielding nutrients also serve as building blocks for body tissue and bone. This is particularly true of proteins and lipids (fats). Because these nutrients give our bodies energy and they are used for building body tissue and bone, we need large amounts of these nutrients. The other three categories of nutrients—vitamins, minerals, and water—do not provide calories. Now, let's take a close look at the six nutrient categories, starting with those that provide calories—carbohydrates, lipids, and protein.

Carbohydrates

Carbo means carbon, and *hydrate* means water. Carbohydrates (CHO) contain carbon and the two chemical elements that make up water: hydrogen and oxygen. The main function of carbohydrates is to provide energy to the body. In fact, the central nervous system, including the brain and nerve cells, relies almost exclusively on a form of carbohydrate called glucose for energy.

Carbohydrates fall into two categories: **simple carbohydrates** (commonly called sugars), and complex carbohydrates (commonly called starch and fiber). All digestible forms of CHO are converted to glucose in the body. The number of molecules of glucose linked together determines the type of carbohydrates. If a food is a simple sugar, you will know it because it literally melts in your mouth. It also has fewer glucose molecules linked together. Think of foods that you know of that are high in sugar (i.e. frostings, marshmallows, hard candy). Notice that these are also the not-so-nutritious foods. Complex carbohydrate foods include nutritious foods such as whole grain breads and cereals, fruits and vegetables, dried beans and peas. They are complex because there are many sugar molecules linked together. To better understand carbohydrates, let's take a closer look at simple and complex carbohydrates.

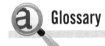

Glossary

Essential Nutrient
The six categories of nutrients that we must obtain through food. Not enough of these nutrients can be made in the body

Energy-Yielding Nutrients
Those nutrients that provide energy or calories to the body (carbohydrates, lipids, protein)

Calorie
A measurement of heat or energy. Foods that provide energy provide calories

Gram
A unit of weight. There are 28 grams in one ounce

Glucose
A single sugar used for energy; sometimes called blood sugar or dextrose

Simple Carbohydrates
Those that are usually found in foods as a sugar and contain one or two molecules of sugar

Monosaccharide
Simple carbohydrate containing one sugar molecule

Disaccharide
Simple carbohydrate containing two sugar molecules

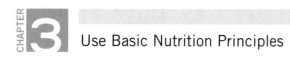
Figure 3.2	Six Sugar Molecules Important in Nutrition	
Sugar Molecule	**Characteristics**	**Known As**
Glucose	Mono (one) saccharide	Blood sugar in the body; commonly found in nature and used for energy
Fructose	Mono (one) saccharide	Fruit sugar or the sugar in honey
Galactose	Mono (one) saccharide	Combines with lactose as milk
Sucrose	Di (two) saccharide comprised of glucose and fructose	Table sugar
Lactose	Di (two) saccharide comprised of glucose and galactose	Milk sugar
Maltose	Di (two) saccharide comprised of two molecules of glucose	Malt sugar

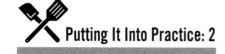

Putting It Into Practice: 2

Knowing that there are 28 grams to an ounce can help us determine how many calories we are adding during cooking. For example, if you are adding one ounce of butter, and you know that butter is a fat, how many calories are you adding?

(Check your answer at the end of this chapter)

Simple Carbohydrates (Sugars)

Simple carbohydrates are so named because their chemical structure is fairly simple. In fact, the simple carbohydrates are building blocks for the complex carbohydrates. There are six forms of simple carbohydrates or sugars that are nutritionally important (see Figure 3.2).

When you eat a food containing a single glucose molecule or **monosaccharide**, it is absorbed immediately into the blood stream. In the body, glucose is called blood sugar because it circulates in the blood at a relatively constant level. **Glucose** is the most used sugar in the body. It is the preferred energy source for brain functions, the nervous system, and for performing physical activity.

When you eat **disaccharides**, your body must break them down or digest them first. Enzymes split the two sugar molecules apart so they can be more easily absorbed into the blood stream. Because of the need for every cell to use glucose, carbohydrate is an essential nutrient. There is no substitute for carbohydrate in the body.

Sugar in Food

As we have discovered, carbohydrate is the essential fuel for our bodies. It is also important because of the sweet taste it imparts to foods. The sugars listed in Figure 3.2 also have differing levels of sweetness. Fructose, also called fruit sugar, is found in ripe fruits and honey and is a very sweet sugar. Fructose is more than twice as sweet as glucose. Some chemicals that provide a sweet taste are not sugars at all. Instead, they are artificial sweeteners.

There are two types of sugar in the food we eat. There are naturally occurring sugars in fruits and dairy products and there are added sugars. Sweeteners come in different forms, from powdered and crystalline to syrup (see Figure 3.3). Some are not sugars at all. Sucralose and aspartame, for example, are artificial sweeteners not sugars. However, they can substitute for sugars in food by providing a sweet taste. For more information on artificial sweeteners, see *Nutrition in the News* (Facts About Low-Calorie Sweeteners) at the end of this chapter.

Besides sweetening foods, sugars prevent spoilage in jams and jellies and perform several functions in baking, such as browning the crust and retaining moisture in baked goods. Sugar also acts as a food for yeast in breads. When yeast "eats" sugar, carbon dioxide (a gas) is produced. Carbon dioxide makes bread rise and gives it an airy texture.

In addition to occurring naturally in some foods, sugar is often added to foods to sweeten them. Added sugars are often table sugar, high fructose corn syrup, or corn syrup. Although a natural sugar, honey is primarily fructose and glucose, the same two components as table sugar. Honey and table sugar both contribute only energy and no other nutrients in significant amounts. Because honey is more concentrated, it has twice as many calories as the same amount of table sugar. Fruits are an excellent source of natural sugar. Canned fruits are packed in four different ways: in water, fruit juice, light syrup, and heavy syrup. Both light syrup and heavy syrup have sugar added, with heavy syrup containing more added sugar. Dried fruits are much more concentrated sources of sugar than fresh fruits because they contain much less water. Lactose, or milk sugar, is present in large amounts in milk, ice cream, ice milk, sherbet, cottage cheese, cheese spreads and other soft cheeses, eggnog, and cream. Hard cheeses contain only traces of lactose.

As you review Figure 3.3, note that sucrose and corn sweeteners are the most frequently used sugars. Added sugars are used to sweeten soft drinks, breakfast cereals, candy, baked goods such as cakes and pies, syrups, jams and jellies. One-quarter of the sugar consumed in the U.S. is in soft drinks. While table sugar consumption has dropped over the past 15 years, consumption of high fructose corn syrup has increased almost 250 percent, according to figures from the U.S. Department of Agriculture. Figure 3.4 lists the sugar content of some foods.

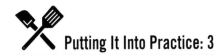

Putting It Into Practice: 3

What would you tell a diabetic client who proudly states that she doesn't eat sugar because she only purchases foods that are "sucrose-free?"

(Check your answer at the end of this chapter)

Figure 3.3   Common Forms of Added Sugars

Form of Sugar	Description
Table Sugar (granulated sugar, sucrose)	Obtained in crystalline form from cane and beets. Is about 99.9% pure and is sold in granulated or powdered form.
Corn Sweeteners	Corn syrup and other sugars made from corn.
Corn Syrup	Made from cornstarch; mostly glucose; only 75% as sweet as sucrose; less expensive than sucrose; used extensively in baked goods; also used in canned goods.
High Fructose Corn Syrup	Corn syrup treated with an enzyme that converts glucose to fructose, which results in a sweeter product. Used in soft drinks, baked goods, jelly, syrups, fruits, and desserts.
Brown Sugar	Sugar crystals contained in a molasses syrup with natural flavor and color; 91 to 96% sucrose.
Molasses	Thick syrup left over after making sugar from sugar cane. Brown in color with a high sugar concentration.
Tubinado Sugar	Sometimes viewed incorrectly as raw sugar. Produced by separating raw sugar crystals and washing them with steam to remove impurities.

Figure 3.4   **Sugar Content of Foods**

Food/Portion	Teaspoons of Sugar
Dairy	
Skim Milk, 1 cup	3
Swiss Cheese, 1 ounce	Less than 1
Vanilla Ice Cream, ½ cup	4
Meat, Poultry, and Fish	
Meat, Poultry, or Fish, 3 ounces	0
Eggs	
Egg, 1	0
Grains	
White Bread, 1 slice	Less than 1
English Muffin, 1	Less than 1
White Rice, Cooked, ½ cup	Less than 1
Circular-shaped oat cereal, 1 cup	Less than 1
Honey-flavored circular-shaped oat cereal, 1 cup	3
Square-shaped oatmeal cereal, 1 cup	2
Fruits	
Apple, 1 medium	4.5
Banana, 1 medium	7
Orange, 1 medium	3
Raisins, ½ ounce	2.5
Vegetables	
Broccoli, ½ cup raw chopped	Less than 1 gram
Mixed Vegetables, 1/3 cup chopped	Less than 1 gram
Beverages	
Cola soft drink, 12 fluid ounces	10
Cakes, Cookies, Candies, and Pudding	
Brownie, 1 average	6
Chocolate Graham Crackers, 8	2
Chocolate Chip Cookies, 3	3
Lemon Drops, 4 pieces	2.5
Candy coated chocolate pieces, 70 pieces	7
Vanilla Pudding, ½ cup	6
Sweeteners	
White Sugar, 1 Tablespoon	4
Honey, 1 Tablespoon	4
High Fructose Corn Syrup, 1 Tablespoon	4

Source: USDA

Sugarless gums and many sugar-free products use sweeteners such as sorbitol or mannitol. These substances are called sugar alcohols. Sorbitol is 60 percent as sweet as sucrose, with about the same number of calories per gram. Sorbitol is used in such products as sugarless hard and soft candies, chewing gums, jams, and jellies. Xylitol, another sugar alcohol, is about as sweet as table sugar and is absorbed very slowly. A third sugar alcohol, mannitol, is poorly digested, so it does not contribute a full four calories per gram. It occurs naturally in pineapple, olives, sweet potatoes and carrots, and is added to sugarless gums. Both mannitol and sorbitol, when taken in large amounts, can cause diarrhea. Products whose reasonably foreseeable consumption may result in a daily ingestion of 50 grams of sorbitol or 20 grams mannitol must bear the labeling statement, "Excess consumption may have a laxative effect."

Sugar on the Food Label

Sugar content is now reported on the nutrition label of food. Both the naturally occurring sugars in food, such as the fruit sugar or milk sugar, as well as added sugars, such as table sugar, are reported on the food label. These are lumped together so it is difficult to determine the amount of added sugars. Read the food label carefully and look for the sugars listed in Figure 3.3. Limit foods that are high in added sugars.

Complex Carbohydrates: Starches

Whereas simple sugars are chemically made up of one or two units of monosaccharides, **starch** is more complex. Chemically, starches and fiber—both forms of complex carbohydrates—consist of many glucose molecules strung together. This is why we refer to them as complex. Another term for complex carbohydrates is polysaccharides. *Poly* means many, so a polysaccharide is made up of many glucose units. A single starch molecule (or chain) may contain 300 to 1,000 or more glucose molecules. The giant molecules are packed side by side in a plant root or seed, providing energy for the plant. All starches are plant materials.

Figure 3.5   A Grain of Rice

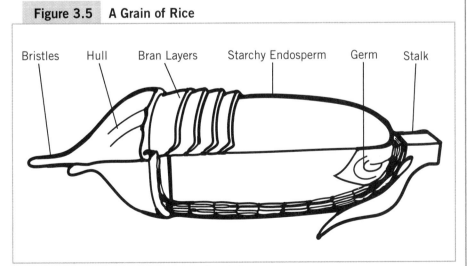

Bristles   Hull   Bran Layers   Starchy Endosperm   Germ   Stalk

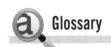 **Glossary**

Starch
A polysaccharide made up of many molecules of sugar; plant materials that are digestible

Figure 3.6   Sources of Starch

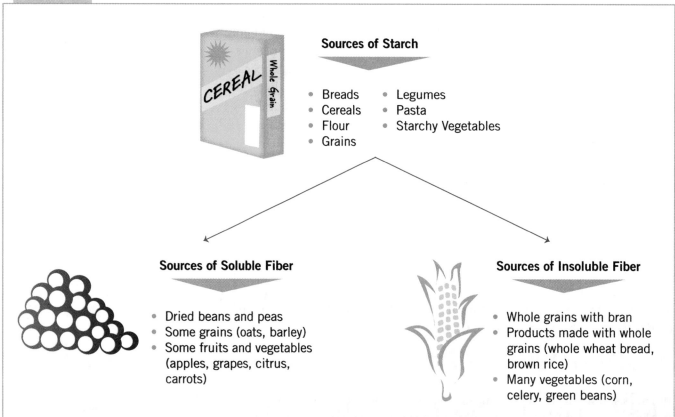

Sources of Starch

- Breads
- Cereals
- Flour
- Grains
- Legumes
- Pasta
- Starchy Vegetables

Sources of Soluble Fiber

- Dried beans and peas
- Some grains (oats, barley)
- Some fruits and vegetables (apples, grapes, citrus, carrots)

Sources of Insoluble Fiber

- Whole grains with bran
- Products made with whole grains (whole wheat bread, brown rice)
- Many vegetables (corn, celery, green beans)

Cereal grains, which are the fruits or seeds of cultivated grasses, are rich sources of starch. Examples include wheat, corn, rice, rye, barley, and oats. Wheat and other grains consist of three parts: the starchy endosperm, the vitamin-rich germ, and the bran—the protective outer coat that contains fiber. Figure 3.5 is a diagram of a grain of rice. Cereal grains are used to make breads, breakfast cereals, and pastas. Starches are also found in potatoes, vegetables, and dried beans and peas. Figure 3.6 identifies common sources of starch in the diet.

Starches are a key component of a healthful diet. As you might guess from the chemical structure, a starch molecule is a terrific way for the body to store sugar for future use. In fact, this is one way the body uses starch. Some starch breaks down immediately after a meal and is used as sugar (glucose) to fuel body functions. But blood sugar (glucose) sometimes goes the other way. Extra sugar in the body may be built back into starch and stored for energy in the future. The body's form of stored starch is called **glycogen**. Glycogen is stored in muscles and in the liver. Glycogen is not really a food component; it is a special form of carbohydrate the body makes.

Complex Carbohydrates: Dietary Fiber

The term **dietary fiber** describes a variety of carbohydrate compounds from plants that are not digestible. Like starch, most fibers are chains of glucose units bonded together, but what's different is that the chains can't be broken down or digested. In other words, most fiber passes through the stomach and intestines unchanged and is excreted in the feces. Unlike sugars or starches, fiber does not give rise to sugar in the body. Fiber was called roughage a few generations ago. Fiber is found only in plant foods where it supports the plant's stems, leaves, and seeds.

There are two major types of fiber—insoluble and soluble. **Soluble fiber** simply means fiber that dissolves in water, forming a gel. **Insoluble fiber** is the tough, fibrous part of plants that is not digestible.

Soluble fibers include gums, mucilages, pectin, and some hemicelluloses. These are components of foods such as apples, oats, and dried beans (see Figure 3.6). In the body, they slow down the movement of food through the lower digestive tract. They slow down the release of glucose from other foods into the body, which may be beneficial to someone with diabetes who needs to control blood sugar. They also help control blood cholesterol levels.

Insoluble fibers include cellulose, lignin, and some hemicelluloses. These fibers occur in bran (wheat bran, corn bran, whole grain breads) and vegetables. Insoluble fibers form the structures of plants, such as skins, and the bran of the wheat kernel. You have seen insoluble fiber in the skin of whole kernel corn and the strings of celery. Insoluble fibers speed up the movement of food through the lower digestive tract and can help prevent constipation. Like soluble fibers, they also slow down the release of glucose from other foods into the body. People need both types of dietary fiber for proper nutrition and digestion.

The amount of fiber in a plant varies from one kind of plant to another and may vary within a species or variety, depending on growing conditions and maturity of the plant at the time of harvest. Like starch, fiber is found abundantly in plants, especially in the outer layers of cereal grains and the fibrous parts of legumes (dried beans and peas), fruits, vegetables, nuts, and seeds. Fiber is not found in animal products such as meat, poultry, fish, dairy products, and eggs. Most plant foods contain both soluble and insoluble fibers.

Whenever the fiber-rich bran and the vitamin-rich germ are left on the endosperm of a grain, the grain is called whole grain. Examples of whole grains include whole wheat, whole rye, bulgur (whole wheat grains that have been steamed and dried), oatmeal, whole cornmeal, whole hulled barley, popcorn, and brown rice. The milling of whole wheat to produce white flour removes the bran and germ and leaves behind mostly starch.

By law, white flour and other refined grain products must be **enriched**, meaning that certain nutrients (thiamin, riboflavin, niacin, and iron) are added in amounts approximately equivalent to those originally present in the whole grain but lost through milling. Enrichment does not replace the fiber removed by milling, it only replaces some of the nutrients lost. Whole wheat flour retains most of the original nutrients and has more fiber, vitamin B6, magnesium, and zinc than enriched white flour.

As a general rule, unrefined foods contain more fiber than refined foods because fiber is usually removed in processing. For example, raw apples contain much fiber in the skin, but the skin is removed to make applesauce or canned sliced

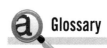

Glossary

Glycogen
A stored form of starch used for quick energy by the body

Dietary Fiber
A polysaccharide made up of many molecules of sugar; plant materials that are NOT digestible by the body

Soluble Fiber
Fiber that forms a gel when combined with water (i.e. fruits, oats, dried beans)

Insoluble Fiber
Outer covering (bran) of plants or fibrous inner parts that are NOT soluble in water (i.e. bran, celery, corn)

Enriched
Adding the B-Vitamins and iron back into refined flour and grain products

apples. Whole foods contain a greater variety of fibers, as well as many other nutrients. Purified fibers in large amounts can be harmful, and certain purified fibers may not have the same effect in the body as the actual fiber in food.

Since insoluble fiber holds water and speeds the movement of wastes through the intestines, stools produced by a high fiber diet tend to be bulkier and softer and pass more quickly and more easily through the intestines. A diet high in insoluble fiber helps prevent and treat hemorrhoids and diverticulosis, a disease of the large intestine in which the intestinal walls become weakened and bulge out into pockets. Insoluble fibers may also reduce the risk of colon cancer.

Studies indicate that soluble fibers play a role in reducing the level of cholesterol in the blood. Eating soluble fiber may help lower blood cholesterol when part of an overall health plan that includes eating less fat and cholesterol. Soluble fiber helps people with diabetes maintain control of their blood sugar levels. Lastly, fiber-rich foods usually require more chewing and provide an increased sense of fullness or satiety, so they are excellent choices for anyone trying to lose weight.

Lipids

Lipids is the scientific name for a diverse family of compounds that are characterized by their insolubility in water and include fats, oils, and cholesterol. Except for cholesterol, these compounds are important for providing energy and for helping the body absorb fat-soluble vitamins (discussed later in this chapter). Fats and oils are the most plentiful lipids in nature. It is customary to call a lipid a fat if it is a solid at room temperature and an oil if it is a liquid at the same temperature. Lipids from animal sources, such as butter, are usually solid, whereas oils are liquid and generally of plant origin (such as corn oil). A few exceptions to this rule of thumb include coconut oil and palm kernel oil. These are fats from plant sources that may be solid at room temperature. We commonly speak of "animal fats" and "vegetable oils." For the purposes of this book, we will use the word "fat" to refer to both fats and oils.

In recent years there has been much discussion about how much fat and cholesterol we eat, what kind of fat we eat, and the relationship between dietary fats and cholesterol and cardiovascular (heart and artery) disease. A high level of blood cholesterol has been identified as one of the major risk factors for having a heart attack or a stroke. This is important because diet, particularly fat intake, influences blood cholesterol levels.

Functions of Lipids

Fat serves a variety of functions. Some fat is needed in the diet to provide the essential fatty acids. Fat in food also contains the fat-soluble vitamins (A, D, E, and K). Fat also provides a concentrated source of energy (9 calories per gram). About 15-20 percent of the weight of healthy normal-weight men is fat, and about 18-25 percent for women. At least half of fat deposits are located just beneath the skin, where they help to cushion body organs (acting like shock absorbers) and provide insulation (to help maintain a constant body temperature). Lipids are also an important component of cells, including the cell

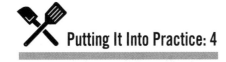

Putting It Into Practice: 4

A client complains he is always hungry 30 minutes after he eats. What foods would you suggest he add to his diet that would increase satiety and delay the onset of hunger?

(Check your answer at the end of this chapter)

membrane (the outer layer of the cell). Because fats slow digestion and the emptying of the stomach, they delay the onset of hunger. In addition to creating a feeling of fullness, fats increase the palatability of foods by enhancing their aroma, taste, flavor, juiciness, and tenderness.

Triglycerides

The bulk of the body's fat tissue is in the form of **triglycerides**, and most of the fats in foods are also in the form of triglycerides. Figure 3.7 shows what a triglyceride looks like. It is composed of three fatty acids attached to glycerol. Each fatty acid is made up of carbon atoms joined like links on a chain. The carbon chains vary in length, with most fatty acids containing 4 to 20 carbon atoms. Each carbon has hydrogen attached, much like charms on a charm bracelet.

Figure 3.7 A Triglyceride Molecule

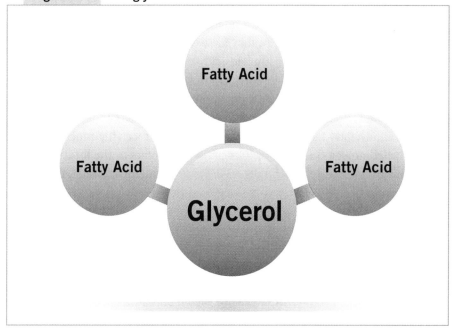

Types of Fatty Acids

Fatty acids may be one of three different types:

✓ Saturated

✓ Monounsaturated

✓ Polyunsaturated

These terms relate to chemistry. "Saturated" describes the chemical structure. When each carbon atom in the chain holds as many hydrogen atoms as it can (two), it is called a saturated fatty acid. A **saturated fatty acid** is therefore filled, or saturated, with hydrogens. When a double bond forms between two neighboring carbons, two hydrogens are missing, so the carbons are not saturated. This type of fatty acid is called an **unsaturated fatty acid**. A fatty acid that contains one double bond in the chain is a **monounsaturated fatty acid** (mono means one). A fatty acid containing more than one double bond is a **polyunsaturated fatty acid (PUFA)**. *Poly* means many, so this term means that

 Glossary

Lipids
A category that is both fats, such as butter and shortening; and oils, such as olive oil or canola oil

Triglycerides
A common form of fats and foods comprised of three fatty acids and glycerol

Saturated Fatty Acid
A fatty acid that is filled with hydrogen, making it solid or semi-solid at room temperature and is found in foods like butter, cream, coconut oil

Unsaturated Fatty Acid
A fatty acid that contains one or more double bonds

Monounsaturated Fatty Acid
A fatty acid that contains one double bond and is found in foods like olive oil, almonds, most hydrogenated margarines

Polyunsaturated Fatty Acid (PUFA)
A fatty acid that contains more than one double bond and is found in foods like corn oil, soybean oil, soft margarines

Trans-Fatty Acid
A fatty acid where the hydrogen atoms have been chemically rearranged, found in hydrogen atoms that have been chemically rearranged; and are found in hydrogenated oils, margarines, and shortening

Hydrogenated
A process of adding hydrogen to oils in order to make them more solid

the fatty acid is unsaturated in many places. Another fatty acid, **trans-fatty acid**, has its hydrogen atoms in an unusual location. Trans-fatty acids are made during the process in which vegetable oils are partially **hydrogenated** to make them more solid. Hydrogenated oils are used in margarines and shortening. See Appendix F for a list of fatty acids in fats and oils.

Hydrogenated oils are used in margarines and shortening to extend the shelf life of the fat. The health risk of trans-fat has been widely publicized in the past decade. The consumption of trans-fat increases your "bad" LDL cholesterol, and at the same time, decreases your "good" HDL cholesterol. A law that went into effect in 2008 requires that trans-fat be listed on the Nutrition Facts panel of all foods. Some states have banned all trans-fat use in food products. Trans-fatty acids are found in vegetable shortenings and some margarines. Trans-fatty acids are also found in foods that contain shortening or margarines, such as crackers, cookies, and foods fried in partially hydrogenated fats.

Two of the fatty acids in food are considered to be **essential fatty acids (EFA).** Because the body can't make EFA, they are essential in our diets. The names of the two essential fatty acids are linoleic acid and linolenic acid. Linoleic acid is polyunsaturated and is found in corn, cottonseed, soybean, and safflower oil. It is also found in nuts, seeds, and whole grain products. Linolenic acid is also polyunsaturated and appears in some vegetable oils such as canola, walnut, soybean oils, and in fatty fish. Another type of fatty acid receiving much attention today is called omega-3 fatty acid. "Omega-3" just refers to the location of the first double bond in the chain. Omega-3 is a type of polyunsaturated fatty acid.

Triglycerides in Foods

The fat in our diets is both visible and invisible. When we think about fats, most of us think about only the visible fats—butter, margarine, and cooking oils. But much of the fat in the diet comes from less visible sources—the fatty streaks in meat, the fat under the skin of poultry, the fat in milk and cheese, the fat in many baked goods, fried foods, nuts, and the fat contained in many processed foods such as candy, chips, crackers, canned soups, and convenience frozen dinners. Unprocessed cereal grains, fruits and vegetables (except avocados and olives), flour, pasta, breads, and most cereals have little or no fat.

All fats in foods are made up of mixtures of fatty acids. If a food contains mostly saturated fatty acids, it is considered a key source of saturated fat. If it contains mostly polyunsaturated fatty acids, it is a key source of polyunsaturated fat. Monounsaturated fats contain mostly monounsaturated fatty acids. Regardless of the type of fat used—saturated, monounsaturated or polyunsaturated—it is still nine calories per gram.

Animal fats are generally more saturated than liquid vegetable oils. Saturated fat raises blood cholesterol more than anything else in the diet. Animal products are a major source of saturated fat in the typical American diet. The fat in whole dairy products (like butter, cheese, whole milk, ice cream and cream) contains high amounts of saturated fat. Saturated fat is also concentrated in the fat that surrounds meat and in the white streaks of fat in the muscle of meat (marbling). Well-trimmed cuts from certain sections of the animal, such as the

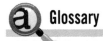
Glossary

Essential Fatty Acid (EFA)
Fatty acids that cannot be made by the body

Figure 3.8   Make the Right Choice With Healthy Dietary Fats

Right Type of Fat	Increase Your Intake of These Foods
Polyunsaturated Fats	Most low-fat or soft margarines, soybean oil, corn oil, sunflower oil, safflower oil, walnuts, sunflower seeds
Monounsaturated Fats	Peanuts and peanut oil, olive oil, canola oil, almonds, avocado, some seeds
Omega 3-Fatty Acids	Cold water finfish, flaxseed products, flaxseed oil, walnuts
Wrong Type of Fat	**Decrease Your Intake of These Foods**
Saturated Fats	Animal products, high-fat cheese and other dairy products, lard, butter, coconut and palm oil
Trans Fats	Foods fried in trans fat oils, foods made with partially hydrogenated oils, shortening, some margarines
Dietary Cholesterol	Eggs, animal products, shellfish

round, are lower in saturated fat than well-marbled, untrimmed meat. Poultry, when the skin is removed, and most fish are lower in saturated fat.

A few vegetable fats—coconut oil, cocoa butter, and palm oil—are high in saturated fat. These may be used for commercial deep-fat frying and in foods such as cookies and crackers, whipped toppings, coffee creamers, cake mixes, and even frozen dinners. Chocolate products, such as chocolate candy bars and baking chips, contain cocoa butter and sometimes also palm kernel oil or palm oil.

Recommendations for Daily Fat Intake

There are specific recommendations for how much of these fats we should consume. Total fat intake should be no more than 30 percent of your total calories. Of that 30 percent, less than 10 percent should come from saturated fat. The American Heart Association recommends less than one gram per day of trans-fat and less than 300 milligrams per day of dietary cholesterol. See Figure 3.8 for ways to choose healthy fats.

Cholesterol

Cholesterol is a type of sterol the body needs and is made by the liver, so it is technically not an essential nutrient. The body uses cholesterol to build cell membranes and brain and nerve tissues. Cholesterol also helps the body produce steroid hormones needed for body regulation, bile acids needed for digestion, and a form of vitamin D.

Cholesterol is found only in foods of animal origin: egg yolks, meat, poultry, fish, milk, and milk products. Egg yolk and organ meats (liver, kidney, sweetbread, brain) are major sources of cholesterol. One egg yolk contains about 10 times as much cholesterol as one ounce of meat. Cholesterol is found in both the lean and fat sections of red meat, and the meat and skin of poultry. In milk products, cholesterol is mostly in the fat, so lower fat products contain less cholesterol. Egg whites and foods that come from plants have no cholesterol. Figure 3.9 shows the cholesterol content of selected foods.

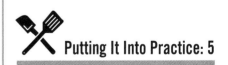

Putting It Into Practice: 5

What's wrong with this picture?
A grocery store recently hung a sign in front of their sunflower oil section. The sign said 95% fat and cholesterol free.

(Check your answer at the end of this chapter)

Figure 3.9   Cholesterol in Foods

Food/Portion	Cholesterol (milligrams)
Liver, braised, 3 ounces	333
Egg, whole, 1	213
Beef, short ribs, braised, 3 ounces	80
Beef, ground, lean, broiled medium, 3 ounces	74
Beef, top round, broiled, 3 ounces	73
Chicken, roasted, without skin, light meat, 3½ ounces	75
Haddock, baked, 3 ounces	63
Mackerel, baked, 3 ounces	64
Swordfish, baked, 3 ounces	43
Shrimp, moist heat, 3 ounces	167
Milk, whole, 8 ounces	33
Milk, 2% fat, 8 ounces	18
Milk, 1% fat, 8 ounces	10
Skim Milk, 8 ounces	4
Cheddar Cheese, 1 ounce	30
American Processed Cheese, 1 ounce	27
Cottage Cheese, low fat, ½ cup	5

Source: National Institutes of Health

Protein

Carbohydrate and fat can both be independent food sources, such as sugar or butter, or they can be combined into food sources such as cookies. Protein is rarely found by itself; it is usually found in combination with fat. The word protein comes from a Greek word that means "of prime importance." Protein has been considered to be "of prime importance" for centuries because of the essential functions in our bodies. Most people eat too much protein, resulting in a diet also higher in fat.

To most Americans, the term "protein" means meat, poultry, or fish. While these foods are all excellent sources of protein, there are other less well-known sources such as dried beans and peas, whole grains, and vegetables. Protein-rich meats, poultry, and fish rank high in the diets of Americans. In other parts of the world, plant-based protein sources are the foundation of the diet.

Like carbohydrates and fats, proteins contain carbon, hydrogen, and oxygen. But unlike these other nutrients, proteins contain the chemical element nitrogen. **Amino acids** are the nitrogen-containing building blocks of proteins. Proteins are strands of amino acids (Figure 3.10). This allows for an endless number of combinations and sequences in the amino acid chains and, therefore, a great variety of proteins in plants and animals.

Each protein has a unique sequence of amino acids or protein building blocks and a unique way of bending and coiling that is necessary for the protein to function normally. Different tissues in the body, such as hair and skin, each have their own characteristic proteins. Some amino acids, called **essential**

Glossary

Amino Acids
Building blocks of proteins

Enzymes
Catalysts that speed up chemical reactions and are made from protein

Essential Amino Acids
Cannot be made in the body

Nonessential Amino Acid
Is able to be made in the body

Hormones
Chemical messengers such as the thyroid hormone

Antibodies
Blood proteins required for an immune response to foreign bodies

Figure 3.10   Amino Acids-Building Blocks of Proteins

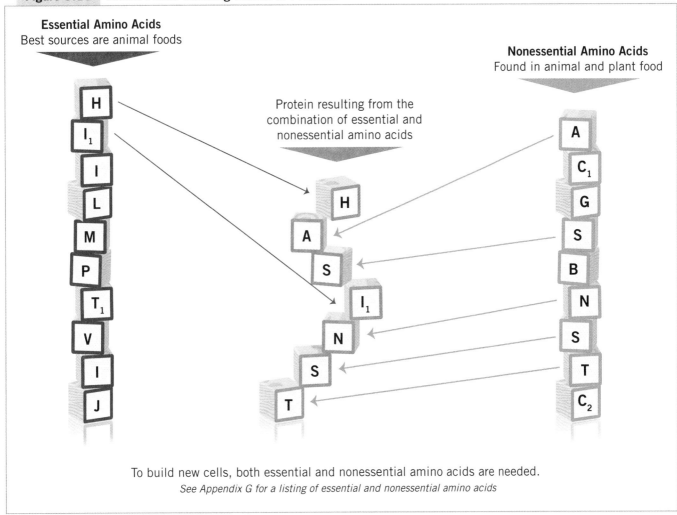

Essential Amino Acids
Best sources are animal foods

Nonessential Amino Acids
Found in animal and plant food

Protein resulting from the combination of essential and nonessential amino acids

To build new cells, both essential and nonessential amino acids are needed.
See Appendix G for a listing of essential and nonessential amino acids

amino acids, must be provided by food because the body can't make them. Other amino acids are considered **nonessential amino acids** because they can be made by the human body. If we don't consume essential amino acids regularly, our body isn't able to synthesize proteins. In Figure 3.10, you can see that if the H amino acid wasn't available, the body couldn't make the protein.

Functions of Protein

Building. Amino acids are required by the body for building new cells. For instance, proteins are found in the skin, bone, cartilage, and muscles. The greatest amounts of proteins are needed when the body is building new cells rapidly, such as during infancy, pregnancy, or when a mother is nursing a child. Building cells is also important after burns, surgery, healing, or for new hair or nails.

Amino acids are combined to build **enzymes**, some of the most important proteins formed in cells. Enzymes act as a catalyst that helps make the chemical reactions in our bodies. **Hormones**, chemical messengers which regulate metabolism, are built from amino acids.

Proteins build **antibodies** that fight infection. Antibodies travel in the blood, where it is their job to attack any foreign bodies that do not belong, such as a virus, bacteria, or a toxin. Antibodies actually combine with these foreign bodies, producing an immune response that helps ward off harmful infections.

Maintaining. Besides building cells, protein also maintains tissues by replacing worn-out cells. Our bodies are sloughing cells daily that need to be replaced whether they are red blood cells, cells lining our intestinal tract, or skin cells.

Proteins also assist in maintaining water and electrolyte balance. There must be a constant amount of fluid maintained both inside and outside of our cells. Proteins are important in the maintenance of fluid levels. **Edema** is a condition that occurs if this fluid maintenance system fails.

Proteins assist in maintaining an acid-base balance within our bodies. Blood proteins keep the blood neutral, meaning it is neither too acidic nor too basic. Normal processes of the body produce acids and bases that can cause major problems in the blood and in the body, such as coma and death. The blood proteins buffer these acids and bases to keep the blood pH neutral.

Providing Energy. Because the functions just described are so important to healthy bodies, protein isn't considered a major source of energy. However, protein does provide four calories per gram so if the diet does not supply enough calories from carbohydrates or fats, proteins are used for energy at the expense of tissue building and maintenance functions. Some amino acids can be converted to glucose, the sole fuel of the brain.

Unlike fat, the body has little protein reserves so we need to consume protein daily. However, if more protein, and subsequently more calories, are eaten than are needed by the body, the extra proteins are used for energy or are converted to body fat and stored in fat cells. The daily recommended amount of protein is 0.8 grams per kilogram of body weight per day. That converts to about 40-60 grams of protein per day; the average daily protein intake is 100 grams.

During digestion, proteins are broken down into amino acids that are then absorbed into the blood. Amino acids travel through the blood into the body's cells. There is an amino acid pool in the body that provides the cells with a supply of amino acids for making protein. The amino acid pool refers to the overall amount of amino acids distributed in the blood, the organs (such as the liver), and the body's cells. Amino acids from foods, as well as amino acids from body proteins that have been dismantled, stock these pools. In this manner, the body recycles its own proteins. If there is a shortage of a nonessential amino acid during production of a protein, the cell will make it and add it to the protein strand. If there is a shortage of an essential amino acid, the protein can't be completed.

Protein deficiency in the U.S. is usually due to illness, injury, or economic factors. Protein deficiency may cause wasting of muscles, weight loss, delayed wound healing, lowered immunity due to fewer antibodies being made, and edema. Edema is the abnormal pooling of fluid in the tissues, causing swelling

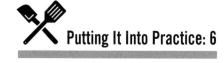

Putting It Into Practice: 6

If a client weighs 120 pounds, what is her daily protein requirement?

(Check your answer at the end of this chapter)

Figure 3.11 Complete and Complementary Proteins

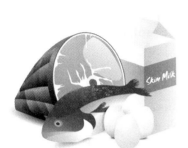 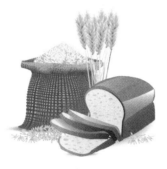 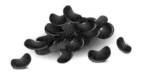 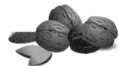

Complete Proteins
Animal sources contain all essential amino acids

Complementary Proteins
Not complete—Combine foods from two or more of these categories throughout the day to provide essential amino acids.

Meat, Dairy Products, Eggs

Grains
Whole grain bread, barley, corn, cornmeal, oats, rice, pasta

Legumes
Dried beans and peas, peanuts, soy products

Seeds/Nuts
Nut butters, nuts, sunflower seeds, sesame seeds

of the part of the body where the pooling occurs. Edema is often seen in malnutrition because protein helps to maintain fluid balance. In protein deficiency, fluids collects outside the cells. With appropriate nutritional intervention, extra protein can be given where there is a loss of body protein due to burns, surgery, stress, infections, skin breakdown, and similar situations. Protein deficiency commonly occurs in developing countries where children do not have enough to eat. It is rarely seen without a deficiency of calories and other nutrients as well. **Protein-calorie malnutrition** is the name for a group of diseases characterized by both protein and energy deficiency. Protein-calorie malnutrition is also called Protein Energy Malnutrition (PEM). Protein-deficiency disease is called kwashiorkor, and energy-deficiency disease is called marasmus. Kwashiorkor is characterized by retarded growth and development, a protruding abdomen due to edema, peeling skin, a loss of normal hair color, irritability, and sadness. Marasmus is characterized by gross underweight, no fat stores, and wasting away of muscles. There is no edema, as seen in kwashiorkor, and individuals are apathetic. Whereas marasmus is usually associated with severe food shortage, prolonged semi-starvation, or early weaning, kwashiorkor is associated with poor protein intake.

Sources and Quality of Protein

Protein occurs in almost all foods of animal and plant origin. Animal sources of protein in the American diet include meat, poultry, seafood, eggs, milk, and cheese. Plant sources include legumes, cereal grains, and products made with them, such as bread and ready-to-eat cereals, vegetables, nuts, and seeds. The legumes (beans, peas, and lentils) contain larger amounts and better quality proteins than other plant sources. Fruits contain very little protein. Animal sources of protein almost always have fat, especially saturated fat, while plant sources contain very little fat.

 Glossary

Edema
Abnormal pooling of fluid in the tissues causing swelling

Complete Protein
Foods that contain all of the essential amino acids

Incomplete Protein
Foods that lack either the amount or type of amino acid needed for growth and maintenance of tissues

Complementary Proteins
Two or more incomplete protein foods that, when eaten within the same day, provide essential amino acids

Protein-Calorie Nutrition
A name for a group of diseases characterized by both protein and calorie deficiency

The quality of a particular protein depends on its content of essential amino acids. Food proteins providing all of the essential amino acids in the proportions needed by the body are called **complete or high-quality proteins**. Meat, poultry, fish, milk and milk products, and eggs are all sources of complete proteins. Animal proteins are much better absorbed than plant proteins; over 90 percent of the amino acids are absorbed into the body. Complete protein has a high biological value (BV). BV measures how effectively the body can use a particular protein source. Plant proteins are usually low in one or more of the essential amino acids and are called **incomplete proteins**. The amino acid that is in short supply is called the limiting amino acid. Plant proteins are not absorbed as well as animal proteins. About 80 percent of the protein in legumes is absorbed, while 60 to 90 percent of the protein in cereal grains and other plant foods is absorbed. Although plant proteins are incomplete proteins, they are the major source of protein for many people around the world. To **complement proteins** means to eat either some animal protein (such as milk or eggs) with vegetable protein, or to combine two plant sources, such as grains and legumes, so that the essential amino acids deficient in one are present in the other. See Figure 3.11 for examples of complete and complementary proteins.

SECTION B Vitamins

Vitamins

Vitamins are essential in small quantities for growth and good health. Vitamins are similar to each other because they are made of the same elements—carbon, hydrogen, oxygen, and sometimes nitrogen or cobalt. They are different in that their elements are arranged differently, and each vitamin performs one or more specific functions in the body. In the early 1900s, scientists thought they had found the compounds needed to prevent two diseases caused by vitamin deficiencies: scurvy and pellagra. These compounds originally were believed to belong to a class of chemical compounds called amines. Their name comes from the Latin *vita*, or life, plus *amine*—vitamine. Later, the "e" was dropped when it was found that not all of the substances were amines. At first, no one knew what they were chemically, and they were identified by letters. Later, what was thought to be one vitamin turned out to be many, and numbers were added; the vitamin B complex is the best example (for example, vitamin B1 and vitamin B6). When they were found unnecessary for human needs, some vitamins were removed from the list, which accounts for some of the gaps in the numbers. For example, vitamin B8, adenylic acid, was later found not to be a vitamin. Others, originally designated differently from each other, were found to be one and the same. For example, vitamins H, M, S, W, and X were all shown to be biotin. Let's start with some basic facts about vitamins.

✓ Very small amounts of vitamins are needed by the human body, and very small amounts are present in foods. Some vitamins are measured in I.U.s (international units), a measure of biological activity; others are measured

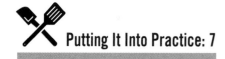

Putting It Into Practice: 7

Based on new research, what two vitamins and their food sources would be important for the mental health of the elderly?

(Check your answer at the end of this chapter)

in weight in micrograms (μg) or milligrams (mg). Some vitamins, such as vitamin D, can be measured in both I.U.s and micrograms. To illustrate how small these amounts are, remember that one ounce is 28.3 grams. A milligram is 1/1000 of a gram, and a microgram is 1/1000 of a milligram.

✓ Although vitamins are needed in small quantities, the roles they play in the body are enormously important.

✓ Vitamins must be obtained through foods because they are either not made in the body or not made in sufficient quantities.

✓ There is no perfect food that contains all the vitamins in just the right amounts. The best way to assure an adequate intake of vitamins is to eat a varied and balanced diet.

✓ Vitamins do not have any calories, so they do not directly provide energy to the body. However, they are involved in how the body uses energy and performs many of its necessary functions.

✓ Some substances considered to be vitamins in foods are not actually vitamins, but rather are precursors. In the body, the precursor is chemically changed to the active form of the vitamin, under proper conditions.

Vitamins are classified according to how soluble they are in either fat or water. Figure 3.12 lists the fat-soluble and water-soluble vitamins. The fat-soluble vitamins generally occur in foods containing fat and can be stored in the body, in fat tissue. The water-soluble vitamins are not stored appreciably in the body.

Now let's take a closer look at 13 vitamins.

Vitamin A

Vitamin A is involved in many different functions. It plays a role in the formation and maintenance of healthy skin and hair, as well as in proper bone growth and tooth development in children. Vitamin A is also needed for the immune system to work properly (for fighting infections) and for maintenance of the protective linings of the lungs, intestines, urinary tract, and other organs. Vitamin A is essential for normal reproduction and, when eaten generously in

Figure 3.12 Vitamins—Quick Glance

Category	Vitamin Name	
Fat Soluble	Vitamin A	
	Vitamin D	
	Vitamin E	
	Vitamin K	
Water Soluble	Vitamin C	Folate
	B Vitamins	Vitamin B12
	Thiamin	Pantothenic Acid
	Riboflavin	Biotin
	Niacin	Vitamin B6

the form of fruits and vegetables, may protect against certain forms of cancer. Vitamin A is well-known for its part in helping us see properly. Vitamin A is necessary for the health of the eye's cornea, the clear membrane that covers the eye. Without enough vitamin A, the cornea becomes cloudy and dry. Vitamin A is also necessary for night vision, the ability for eyes to adjust after seeing a flash of bright light at night. In night blindness, it takes longer than normal to adjust to dim lights. This is an early sign of vitamin A deficiency. If the deficiency continues, it can eventually lead to blindness.

The form of vitamin A found in fruits and vegetables is actually a precursor of vitamin A called beta carotene. In the body, beta carotene is converted to vitamin A. Beta carotene often gives foods an orange color. It occurs in dark green vegetables, such as spinach, and deep orange fruits and vegetables, such as apricots, carrots, and sweet potatoes (see Figure 3.13).

Figure 3.13 Vitamin A in Foods

Food/Portion	Retinol Equivalents
Liver, Beef, 3 oz.	9,011
Sweet Potato, baked, 1 small	2,488
Carrots, raw, 1	2,025
Spinach, cooked, ½ cup	875
Squash, butternut, ½ cup	857
Cantaloupe, ¼ melon	516
Milk, 2%, 1 cup	140
Apricots, dried, 4 large halves	127
Broccoli, cooked, ½ cup	110
Egg Yolk, 1	97
Cheese, Cheddar, 1 oz.	86
Margarine, fortified, 1 tsp.	47
Peach, 1 medium	47
Orange, 1 medium	27

Source: USDA

Other sources of vitamin A include animal products such as liver (a very rich source), egg yolk, butter, milk, fortified margarine, cream, cheese, and fortified cereals. Low-fat and skim milks are often fortified with vitamin A because the vitamin is removed from the milk when the fat is removed. **Fortified** foods have one or more nutrients added. Most ready-to-eat and instant-prepared cereals are also fortified with vitamin A. Retinol, the active form of vitamin A found in animal foods, is used in fortification.

Nutrient needs for vitamin A are expressed in retinol equivalents (REs). Retinol equivalents measure the amount of retinol the body will actually obtain from eating foods with various forms of vitamin A, e.g. retinol or beta carotene.

Because the body stores vitamin A, it is not absolutely necessary to eat a good source every day. Vitamin A deficiency is not often seen in the U.S. Unfortunately,

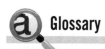
Glossary

Fortified
Foods that have one or more nutrients added

Antioxidant
'Anti' means against and 'oxidant' means oxygen so antioxidant prevents oxygen from destroying important substances

it is of concern in third-world countries where a lack of vitamin A causes poor growth, infection, blindness, and death. Although there may not be agreement on exactly how much vitamin A can be considered a toxic dose, excessive use of vitamin A may cause dry, scaly skin, bone pain, soreness, stunted growth, liver damage, nausea, and diarrhea. Megadoses (more than 10 times the estimated nutrient need) are particularly dangerous for pregnant women and children.

Vitamin D

Vitamin D differs from the other fat-soluble vitamins in that it can be made in the body and it acts more like a hormone than like a vitamin. Acting like a hormone or chemical messenger, vitamin D maintains blood calcium and phosphorus levels so that there is enough calcium and phosphorus present for building bones and teeth. Vitamin D also helps the body absorb calcium and phosphorus from the digestive tract. Only small amounts of vitamin D are found in most foods. For this reason, milk is usually fortified with vitamin D. Other significant food sources of vitamin D include liver, egg yolks, and fish liver oils. Fortunately, many people make enough vitamin D to meet ongoing needs. When ultraviolet rays shine on the skin, a cholesterol-like compound is converted into a vitamin D precursor and absorbed into the blood. The precursor is then transformed into vitamin D. A light-skinned person needs only 10 to 15 minutes of sun each day to make enough vitamin D; a dark-skinned person needs several hours. Vitamin D deficiency, which is rare in the U.S., causes rickets in children and infants. In rickets, bones are soft and pliable because they lack enough calcium and phosphorus to become strong. When this happens, several problems develop: bowlegs, knock knees, chest deformities, and curving of the spine. Deficiency may also occur in adults who have little exposure to the sun and low intakes of vitamin D, calcium, and phosphorus. It is referred to as osteomalacia and is seen in the Middle East and the Orient. It is characterized by soft bones that break easily and bend easily as well, causing deformities of the spine, for example.

New research over the past decade suggests vitamin D may provide protection from osteoporosis, hypertension (high blood pressure), cancer, dementia, and several autoimmune diseases. Although further research is needed, three new studies released in 2010, show both vitamins D and E might protect against dementia and Parkinson's Disease. The Adequate Intake (AI) levels of vitamin D have been established by the U.S. Institute of Medicine of the National Academy of Sciences. Recommendations are: 5 micrograms (200 IU or International Units) daily for all individuals (male, female, pregnant/lactating women) under the age of 50. For all individuals age 50-70 years, 10 micrograms daily (400 IU) is recommended. For those who are over 70 years, 15 micrograms daily (600 IU) is suggested.

Vitamin D, when taken in excess, is the most toxic (poisonous) of all the vitamins. Toxicity symptoms include nausea, vomiting, diarrhea, fatigue, and thirst. It can lead to calcium deposits in the heart and kidneys that can cause severe health problems. Young children and infants are especially susceptible to the toxic effects of too much vitamin D; megadoses can cause growth failure.

Vitamin E

Vitamin E has an important function in the body as an antioxidant. **Antioxidants** combine with oxygen so oxygen is not available to oxidize, or destroy, important substances. Vitamin E prevents destruction of cells. Today, scientists suggest that antioxidants can slow down the normal aging process and provide important protection against cancer. Both vitamin E and vitamin C are considered antioxidant vitamins. Vitamin E is important for the health of the cell (especially the red blood cells), the proper functioning of the immune system, and the metabolism of vitamin A.

Vitamin E is widely distributed in plant foods. Rich sources include vegetable oils, margarine and shortening made from vegetable oils, and wheat germ. In oils, vitamin E acts like an antioxidant and thereby prevents the oil from going rancid or bad. Other good sources include whole grain cereals, green leafy vegetables, nuts, and seeds. Animal foods are poor sources, except for liver and egg yolk. Vitamin E deficiency is rare, as is toxicity due to large doses of vitamin E.

Vitamin K

Vitamin K has an essential role in the production of proteins involved in blood clotting. When the skin is broken, blood clotting is vital to prevent excessive blood loss. Vitamin K is also involved in calcium metabolism. Vitamin K appears in certain foods and is also made in the body. There are billions of bacteria which normally live in the intestines, and some of them produce vitamin K. It is thought that the amount of vitamin K produced by the bacteria is significant and may meet about half of the body's need. Food sources of vitamin K provide the balance. Excellent sources of vitamin K include green leafy vegetables such as kale, spinach, cabbage, and liver. Other sources include milk and eggs. A deficiency of vitamin K is rare in adults. An infant is normally given this vitamin after birth to prevent bleeding because the intestines do not yet have the bacteria to produce vitamin K.

Water-Soluble Vitamins

The water-soluble vitamins include vitamin C and the B-complex vitamins. The B vitamins work in every cell of the body where they function as coenzymes. A coenzyme works with an enzyme to make it active. An enzyme boosts chemical reactions in the body to support all kinds of body functions. The body stores only limited amounts of water-soluble vitamins; excesses are excreted in the urine. Nevertheless, many water-soluble vitamins taken in excess (e.g. through massive supplementation) can cause toxic side effects.

Vitamin C

Vitamin C (also called ascorbic acid) is important in forming collagen, a protein that gives strength and support to bones, teeth, muscle, cartilage, blood vessels, and skin tissue. It has been said that vitamin C acts like cement, holding together our cells and tissues. Vitamin C also helps absorb iron into the body and strengthens resistance to infection. Like vitamin E, vitamin C is an important antioxidant, preventing the oxidation of vitamin A and polyunsaturated fatty acids in the intestine. Its antioxidant properties have made vitamin

C widely used in foods as an additive to preserve freshness. It may appear on the food label as sodium ascorbate, calcium ascorbate, or simply ascorbic acid.

Foods rich in vitamin C include citrus fruits (oranges, grapefruits, limes, and lemons) and tomatoes. Good sources include white potatoes, sweet potatoes, tomatoes, broccoli, and other green and yellow vegetables, as well as cantaloupe and strawberries (Figure 3.14). There is little or no vitamin C in meats or dairy foods. Some juices are fortified with vitamin C, as are most ready-to-eat cereals. Certain situations raise the body's need for vitamin C. These include pregnancy and nursing, growth, fevers, infections, burns, fractures, surgery, cancer, heavy alcohol intake, and cigarette smoking. Megadoses of vitamin C often cause nausea, abdominal cramps, and diarrhea. Megadoses of vitamin C can also interfere with clotting medications (such as warfarin and dicoumarol) and cause incorrect urine test results for diabetes. A deficiency of vitamin

Figure 3.14 Vitamin C in Foods

Food/Portion	Vitamin C (milligrams)
Fruits	
Orange, 1	80
Kiwi, 1 medium	75
Cranberry Juice Cocktail, ¾ cup	67
Orange Juice, from concentrate, ½ cup	48
Papaya, ½ cup cubes	43
Strawberries, ½ cup	42
Grapefruit, ½	41
Grapefruit Juice, canned, ½ cup	36
Cantaloupe, ½ cup cubes	34
Tangerine, 1	26
Mango, ½ cup, slices	23
Honeydew Melon, ½ cup cubes	21
Banana, 1	10
Apple, 1	8
Nectarine, 1	7
Vegetables	
Broccoli, chopped, cooked, ½ cup	49
Brussels Sprouts, cooked, ½ cup	48
Cauliflower, cooked, ½ cup	34
Sweet Potato, baked, 1	28
Kale, cooked, chopped, ½ cup	27
White Potato, baked, 1	26
Tomato, 1 fresh	22
Tomato Juice, ½ cup	22
Cereals	
Corn Flakes, 1 cup	15

Source: USDA

Putting It Into Practice: 8

You notice that it is the cook's practice to cook the vegetables and put them into the steam table a minimum of two hours prior to plating on the trayline. What would you recommend to the cook to increase the vitamin content of the cooked vegetable?

(Check your answer at the end of this chapter)

C causes a disease called scurvy. Symptoms of scurvy include bleeding gums, weakness, growth failure, delayed wound healing, easy bruising, and iron-deficiency anemia. Many of these symptoms are due to the faulty formation of collagen. Vitamin C deficiency is of some concern in the U.S. and is sometimes seen in elderly individuals, or among individuals who have inadequate diets. Of all the vitamins, vitamin C is the most fragile and the most easily destroyed during preparation, cooking, or storage.

Thiamin, Riboflavin, and Niacin

Thiamin, riboflavin, and niacin all play key roles as coenzymes in energy metabolism. Coenzymes are chemical compounds that help enzymes work. As mentioned earlier, enzymes are specialized proteins that speed up specific chemical reactions in the body. These vitamins are essential to release energy from glucose, fatty acids, and amino acids. Thiamin also plays a vital role in the normal functioning of the nervous system and appetite. Riboflavin is important for healthy skin and normal functioning of the eyes. Niacin is needed for the maintenance of healthy skin and the normal functioning of the nervous system and digestive tract. Because thiamin, riboflavin, and niacin all help release energy from food, the need for these vitamins increase as calorie intake rises.

Thiamin is widely distributed in foods, but mostly in moderate amounts. Pork is an excellent source of thiamin. Other sources include liver, dry beans and peas, peanuts, peanut butter, seeds, and whole grain and enriched breads and cereals.

Milk is a major source of riboflavin; yogurt and cheese are also good sources. Other sources include organ meats like liver (very high in riboflavin), whole grain and enriched breads and cereals, and some meats.

The main sources of niacin are meat, poultry, and fish. Organ meats are quite high in niacin. All foods containing complete protein, such as those just mentioned and also milk and eggs, are good sources of the precursor of niacin, tryptophan. Tryptophan is an amino acid present in some of these foods that is converted to niacin (with the help of riboflavin and vitamin B6). Whole-grain and enriched breads and cereals supply niacin.

A thiamin deficiency causes a disease called beriberi, which is characterized by poor appetite, depression, confusion, weakness, wasting, heart problems, and deterioration of the nervous system. Thiamin deficiency is not common in developed countries, except in alcoholics, who get most of their calories from alcohol rather than from food. Most deficiencies of B vitamins include more than just one vitamin, so it is not surprising to find riboflavin lacking, along with thiamin. Because the symptoms of a thiamin deficiency are more severe, the signs of a riboflavin deficiency (cracks at the corner of the mouth, skin rash, poor healing, burning and itching eyes) may never be seen. Niacin deficiency still occurs in poor urban areas, possibly because there is poor intake of complete protein sources that contribute much of the niacin in the diet. The effects of pellagra, the niacin-deficiency disease, are easy to remember as the "4 Ds"—diarrhea, dermatitis (skin inflammation), dementia, and ultimately death. Niacin deficiency first appears as fatigue, poor appetite, indigestion, and a skin rash. Later, nervous system symptoms appear, including confusion and disorientation.

Toxicity is not a problem with these vitamins, except for niacin. Nicotinic acid, a form of niacin, has been prescribed by physicians to lower elevated blood cholesterol levels. Unfortunately, it has some undesirable side effects. Starting at doses of 100 milligrams, typical symptoms include flushing, rashes, tingling, itching, hives, nausea, diarrhea, and abdominal discomfort. Flushing of the face, neck, and chest lasts for about 20 minutes after taking a large dose. More serious side effects of large doses include liver malfunction, high blood sugar levels, and abnormal heart rhythm.

Whole grains, enriched breads, and cereals supply the majority of the starch in many diets today. It is important to understand that grains are an excellent source of vitamins, but processing results in both vitamin and mineral losses. Processing removes the germ and the bran from the grain taking with it many vitamins and minerals that are not replaced through enrichment or fortification (see Figure 3.15).

Figure 3.15 Processing Effects on Grain

Vitamins & Minerals Lost During Processing	Vitamins & Minerals Replaced With Enrichment
Thiamin	Thiamin
Riboflavin	Riboflavin
Niacin	Niacin
Vitamin B6	Iron
Folate	
Pantothenic Acid	
Vitamin E	
Fiber	
Iron	
Magnesium	
Copper	
Calcium	
Zinc	
Manganese	
Potassium	

Vitamin B6

Vitamin B6 plays an important role as part of a coenzyme involved in carbohydrate, fat, and protein metabolism. It is particularly important in protein metabolism. Vitamin B6 is also used to make red blood cells, which transport oxygen around the body. It helps convert tryptophan, an amino acid, to niacin. The need for vitamin B6 is directly related to protein intake. As the intake of protein increases, the need for vitamin B6 increases.

Good sources of vitamin B6 include organ meats, meat, poultry, and fish. Vitamin B6 also appears in plant foods; however, it is not as well absorbed from these sources. Good plant sources include whole grains, potatoes, some fruits (such as bananas and cantaloupe), and some green leafy vegetables (such as broccoli and spinach). Fortified ready-to-eat cereals are also good sources of vitamin B6. Deficiency of vitamin B6 causes muscle twitching, rashes, greasy skin, and a type of anemia called microcytic anemia, a small cell anemia. Excessive use of vitamin B6 (more than two grams daily for two months or more) can cause irreversible nerve damage and symptoms such as numbness in hands and feet and difficulty walking.

Folate

Folate is also called folic acid, its synthetic form used in fortified foods and supplements. Folate is part of a coenzyme used to make new cells, including red blood cells, white bloods cells, and digestive tract cells. A deficiency of folate can cause megaloblastic anemia, a condition in which the red blood cells are oversized and function poorly. Other symptoms may include digestive tract problems, such as diarrhea and mental depression. During pregnancy, the need for folate increases because of its vital role in producing new cells. Folate is needed both before and during pregnancy to help reduce the risk of certain serious and common birth defects called neural tube defects, which affect the brain and spinal cord. The tricky part is that neural tube defects can occur in an embryo before a woman realizes she's pregnant. Luckily, folate occurs naturally in a variety of foods, including liver; dark-green leafy vegetables such as collards, turnip greens, and Romaine lettuce; broccoli and asparagus; citrus fruits and juices; whole grain products; wheat germ; and dried beans and peas, such as pinto, navy, and lima beans, and chick-peas and black-eyed peas. By law, many grain products are fortified with folate. This gives women another way to get sufficient folate.

Vitamin B12

Vitamin B12, also called cobalamin and cyanocobalamin, is present in all body cells. Along with folate, vitamin B12 is involved in making new cells in the body and in the growth of healthy red blood cells. It also helps in the normal functioning of the nervous system by maintaining the protective cover around nerve fibers. Vitamin B12 is different from other vitamins in that it is found only in animal foods such as meat, poultry, fish, shellfish, eggs, milk, and milk products. Plant foods do not contain any vitamin B12. Vegetarians who do not eat any animal products will need to include fortified soy milk in their diet, or take supplements.

Vitamin B12 is also different from other vitamins in that it requires a compound called intrinsic factor (produced in the stomach) to be absorbed. A deficiency of vitamin B12 in the body is usually not due to poor intake, but rather due to a problem with absorption. When there is a problem with absorption of vitamin B12, pernicious anemia develops. Pernicious anemia results in macrocytic anemia, as seen when there is a folate deficiency. Therefore, folate supplementation may mask the symptoms of pernicious anemia. Pernicious anemia is also characterized by deterioration in the functioning of the nervous system that, if untreated, could cause significant and sometimes irreversible damage. Therapy includes vitamin B12 injections.

Pantothenic Acid and Biotin

Both pantothenic acid and biotin are involved in energy metabolism. Pantothenic acid is part of a coenzyme used in energy metabolism. Biotin is part of a coenzyme used in energy metabolism, fat synthesis, amino acid metabolism, and glycogen synthesis. Both pantothenic acid and biotin are widespread in foods, and deficiency is rare. There is no known toxicity of either pantothenic acid or biotin.

Vitamins in Food Preparation

Food preparation and storage techniques affect the vitamin content of food. Using too much water, too high a temperature, or too long a time to cook vegetables significantly reduces the content of vitamins B and C. Because vitamin A is fat soluble, adding butter or margarine to vegetables during cooking and then pouring off the cooking water also reduces the vitamin A content of the cooked vegetable. Some chefs use baking soda to enhance the color of vegetables. This process significantly reduces the vitamin content of vegetables. Use batch cooking (cooking small amounts of vegetables immediately prior to service) to minimize vitamin loss for vegetables. Vitamin loss can be diminished during storage by keeping dairy products at a constant, cold temperature and out of the light. Thawing and refreezing causes nutrient loss as well as loss of quality. Figure 3.16 summarizes the functions and food sources of vitamins.

SECTION C | Minerals

If you were to weigh all the minerals in the body, they would only amount to four or five pounds. We need only small amounts of minerals in the diet, but they perform enormously important jobs—such as building bones and teeth, regulating heartbeat, and transporting oxygen from the lungs to tissues.

Some minerals are needed in relatively large amounts in the diet—over 100 milligrams daily. (A paper clip weighs about 1 gram. A milligram is 1/1000 of a gram.) These minerals are called **major minerals** and include calcium, chloride, magnesium, phosphorus, potassium, sodium, and sulfur. Other minerals, called **trace minerals** or trace elements, are needed in smaller amounts—less than 100 milligrams daily. Iron, fluoride, and zinc are examples of trace minerals. Figure 3.17 lists major and trace minerals.

Minerals have some distinctive properties not shared by other nutrients. For example, whereas over 90 percent of the carbohydrate, fat, and protein in the diet is absorbed into the body, the percentage of minerals absorbed varies tremendously. As examples, only 5-10 percent of dietary iron is normally absorbed; about 30 percent of calcium is absorbed; yet almost all of dietary sodium is absorbed. Unlike some vitamins, minerals are not easily destroyed in storage or preparation. Like vitamins, minerals can be toxic when consumed in excessive amounts.

 Glossary

Major Minerals
Calcium, chloride, magnesium, phosphorous, potassium, sodium and sulfur

Trace Minerals
Minerals needed in less than 100 ml daily

Figure 3.16 Vitamins: Functions and Food Sources

Vitamin	Functions	Food Source
Vitamin A	Forming skin, hair, teeth, protective linings; immune function	Orange/yellow vegetables and fruits, dark green vegetables, dairy products
Vitamin D	Aids absorption of calcium and phosphorous; bone health; used in hormones	Fortified milk, liver, egg yolks, fish liver oil
Vitamin E	Antioxidant; protects red and white blood cells	Vegetable oils, margarine, shortening, seeds, nuts, wheat germ, whole grain and fortified breads and cereals, soybeans
Vitamin K	Blood clotting; makes protein used in making bones	Dark green leafy vegetables, cabbage, intestinal bacteria
Vitamin C	Antioxidant; formation of collagen; wound healing; iron absorption; functioning of immune system	Citrus fruits, bell peppers, kiwifruit, broccoli, strawberries, tomatoes, potatoes, juices and cereals fortified with vitamin C
Thiamin	Coenzyme in energy metabolism; functioning of nervous system; normal growth	Pork, sunflower seeds, wheat germ, peanuts, dry beans, whole grain and enriched/fortified breads and cereals
Riboflavin	Coenzyme in energy metabolism; healthy skin; normal vision	Milk and milk products, whole grain and enriched/fortified breads and cereals, some meats, eggs
Niacin	Coenzyme in energy metabolism; healthy skin; normal functioning of nervous system	Meat, poultry, fish, whole grain and enriched/fortified breads and cereals, eggs
Vitamin B6	Coenzyme in carbohydrate, fat, and protein metabolism; synthesis of blood cells	Meat, poultry, fish, fortified cereals, some leafy green vegetables, potatoes, bananas, watermelon
Folate	Formation of new cells	Green leafy vegetables, legumes, orange juice, enriched/fortified breads and cereals
Vitamin B12	Activation of folate; normal functioning of the nervous system	Meat, poultry, seafood, eggs, dairy products, fortified breads and cereals
Pantothenic Acid	Energy metabolism	Widespread
Biotin	Energy metabolism; carbohydrate, fat, and protein metabolism	Widespread

Figure 3.17 Minerals—Quick Glance

Category	Mineral			
Major Minerals *(Body contains five teaspoons or 25 grams)*	Calcium Magnesium	Potassium Sulphur	Chloride Phosphorus	Sodium
Trace Minerals *(Body contains less than ½ teaspoon or 3 grams)*	Iron Copper	Iodine Zinc	Manganese Fluoride	Selenium

Calcium and Phosphorus

Calcium and phosphorus are used for building bones and teeth and are the most abundant minerals in the body. They give rigidity to the structures. Bone is being constantly rebuilt, with new bone being formed, and old bone being taken apart, every day. Teeth are also rebuilt, but at a much slower rate.

Calcium also circulates in the blood and appears in other body tissues, where it helps blood clot, muscles contract (including the heart muscle), and nerves transmit impulses. Calcium helps maintain normal blood pressure and immune defenses.

Phosphorus is involved in the release of energy from fats, proteins, and carbohydrates during metabolism, and in the formation of genetic material and many enzymes. Phosphorus also helps in the absorption and transport of fats and assists in keeping blood chemistry neutral. Phosphorus has the ability to buffer or neutralize both acids and bases.

The major sources of calcium are milk and milk products. Not all milk products are as rich in calcium as milk (Figure 3.18). As a matter of fact, butter, cream, and cream cheese contain very little calcium. Other good sources of calcium include canned salmon and sardines (containing bones), oysters, calcium-fortified foods such as orange juice, and greens such as broccoli, collards, kale, mustard greens, and turnip greens. Other greens such as spinach, beet greens, Swiss chard, sorrel, and parsley are rich in calcium but also contain a binder (called oxalic acid) that prevents calcium from being absorbed. Dried beans and peas and certain shellfish contain moderate amounts of calcium but are usually not eaten in sufficient quantities to make a significant contribution. Meats and grains are poor sources.

Even though only about 30 percent of the calcium we eat is absorbed, the body absorbs more calcium (up to 60 percent) when it is needed—such as during growth and pregnancy, and also when there is inadequate calcium in the diet. Vitamin D aids in calcium absorption.

Phosphorus is widely distributed in foods and is not likely to be lacking in the diet. Milk and milk products are excellent sources. Good sources are meat, poultry, fish, eggs, legumes, and whole grain foods. Fruits and vegetables are generally low in this mineral. Compounds that include phosphorus are used in processed foods, especially soft drinks.

When there isn't enough calcium in the diet, calcium is removed from the bones, a problem that over time will weaken the bone structure and lead to a disease called osteoporosis or adult bone loss. Sometimes individuals who are aware of the problems of osteoporosis take calcium supplements. Many calcium supplements provide mixtures of calcium with other compounds, such as calcium carbonate, a good source of calcium. There are also powdered forms of calcium-rich sources, such as bone meal and dolomite (a rock mineral). These are dangerous, as they may contain lead and other elements in amounts that would constitute a risk. Calcium supplements should not be taken without guidance from a physician or Registered Dietitian.

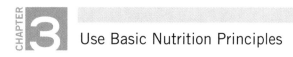
Figure 3.18 Calcium in Selected Foods

Food	Calcium Content (mg)	Food	Calcium Content (mg)
Milk		**Yogurt**	
Milk, skim, 8 oz.	302	Yogurt, low-fat, 1 cup	415
Milk, 2%, 8 oz.	297	Yogurt, low-fat with fruit, 1 cup	345
Milk, whole, 8 oz.	291	Yogurt, frozen, 1 cup.	200
Cheese		**Miscellaneous**	
Cottage cheese, creamed, 1 cup	147	Ice Cream, 1 cup	176
Swiss, 1 oz.	272	Cheeze Pizza, ¼ of 14" pie	332
Parmesan, 1 oz.	390	Macaroni and Cheese, ½ cup.	181
Cheddar, 1 oz.	204	Orange Juice, calcium-fortified, 8 oz.	300
Mozzarella, 1 oz.	183	Tofu, 3½ oz.	128
American, 1 oz.	174	Dried Navy Beans, cooked, 1 cup	95
Fish		**Vegetables**	
Sardines with Bones, 3 oz.	372	Turnip Greens, frozen and cooked, 1 cup	249
Oysters, 1 cup	226	Kale, frozen and cooked, 1 cup	179
Shrimp, 3 oz.	98	Mustard Greens, 1 cup	104
		Broccoli, frozen and cooked, 1 cup.	94

Source: USDA

Sodium

Sodium is a critical mineral that helps the body maintain water balance and acid-base balance. It also plays an important role in helping contract muscles and transmit nerve impulses. Meat, poultry, fish, eggs, and milk are high in natural sodium when compared to fruits and vegetables, but are still quite low compared to processed foods.

Deficiency of sodium is not a problem in the U.S. The estimated minimum requirement is 500 mg per day. The sodium intake of Americans is easily six times this amount—varying from three to eight grams daily. According to the 2010 Dietary Guidelines, Americans are consuming too much sodium. This may be due to consuming too many processed foods. To reduce dietary sodium, limit processed foods, salt added during cooking, and at the table.

Potassium

Potassium is an **electrolyte** found mainly inside the body's cells. In the cell, potassium is needed for making protein. Along with sodium, it helps maintain water balance and acid-base balance. Potassium is also needed to release energy from carbohydrates, fats, and proteins. In the blood, potassium assists in muscle contraction, helps maintain a normal heartbeat, and helps send nerve impulses.

Potassium is distributed widely in foods, both plant and animal. Unprocessed, whole foods are the best sources of potassium, such as fruits and vegetables (winter squash, potatoes, oranges, and grapefruits), milk, grains, meat, poultry, fish, and legumes.

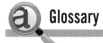 **Glossary**

Electrolyte
Compounds that contain both potassium and chloride. They can separate when in contact with water and are required for fluid balance in the body

Diuretics
A chemical that causes the body to increase urine output

A potassium deficiency is very uncommon in healthy people, but may result from dehydration or from using a certain class of blood pressure medications called **diuretics**. Diuretics cause increased urine output and some cause an increased excretion of potassium as well. Symptoms of a deficiency include weakness, nausea, and abnormal heart rhythms that can be very dangerous, even fatal.

Excessive potassium is equally dangerous and megadoses of it can cause numbness, abnormal heart rhythms, and cardiac failure, in which the heart stops beating. It is not recommended to take potassium supplements without the advice of a physician. Some salt substitutes contain potassium instead of sodium. Some healthcare facilities require a doctor's order to give salt substitutes to a client. A good alternative to using salt substitutes is a packet of herbs and spices that help flavor foods without sodium or potassium.

Chloride

Chloride is another important electrolyte in the body. It helps maintain water balance and acid-base balance. Chloride is also part of hydrochloric acid, found in quite high concentration in the juices of the stomach. Hydrochloric acid aids in protein digestion. The most important source of chloride in the diet is sodium chloride or salt. If sodium intake is adequate, there will be ample chloride as well.

Magnesium

Magnesium is found in all body tissues, with about 60-70 percent being in the bones, and the remainder in the muscles and other soft tissues. It is an essential part of many enzyme systems responsible for energy conversions in the body. Magnesium is used in building bones and teeth and works with calcium, potassium, and sodium to contract muscles and transmit nerve impulses. Magnesium also has a role in making protein.

Magnesium is a part of the green pigment called chlorophyll that is found in plants. Good sources include green leafy vegetables, nuts (especially almonds and cashews), seeds, whole grain cereals, and legumes such as soybeans. Seafood is also a good source. Deficiency symptoms are rare.

Sulfur

Sulfur is found in three of the amino acids. The protein in hair, skin, and nails is particularly rich in sulfur. Sulfur is also a part of two vitamins, thiamin and biotin. High protein foods supply plentiful amounts of sulfur and a deficiency is not known to occur.

SECTION D Trace Minerals and Water

Most of the trace minerals do not occur in the body in their free form, but are bound to organic compounds on which they depend for transport, storage, and function. Our understanding of many trace minerals is just starting to emerge. All the trace minerals are toxic in excess.

Fluoride

Fluoride is the term used for the form of fluorine as it appears in drinking water and in the body. The terms fluoride and fluorine are used interchangeably. Fluoride contributes to solid tooth formation and results in a decrease of dental caries (cavities), especially in children. There is also evidence that fluoride helps retain calcium in the bones of older people.

The major source of fluoride is drinking water. Some supplies of drinking water are naturally fluoridated, and many supplies of water have fluoride added, usually at a concentration of one part fluoride to one million parts water. In nearly all areas where **fluoridation** of water has been introduced, the incidence of dental caries in children has been reduced by 50 percent or more. In areas where there is too much natural fluoride in the water, teeth become discolored, but there are no undesirable health effects.

Iodine

Iodine is required in extremely small amounts for the normal functioning of the thyroid gland. The thyroid gland is located in the neck and is responsible for producing important hormones that maintain a normal level of metabolism in the body. These hormones are essential for normal growth and development.

With a deficiency of dietary iodine, thyroid enlargement (called goiter) occurs. Iodine-deficiency goiter was common in certain inland areas of the U.S. where the soil contains little iodine. (Foods grown along the seacoast are goods sources of iodine as well as saltwater fish and shellfish.) Iodized salt was introduced in 1924 to combat iodine deficiencies. Iodine also finds its way accidentally into milk, because cows receive drugs containing iodine and feed containing iodine—and into baked goods through iodine-containing compounds used in processing.

Iron

Iron is an important part of compounds necessary for transporting oxygen to the cells and making use of the oxygen when it arrives. It is widely distributed in the body, where much of it is in the blood as the *heme* portion of hemoglobin. Hemoglobin is the oxygen carrier found in red blood cells. Iron is also part of the protein myoglobin in muscles, which makes oxygen available for muscle contraction. Iron works with many enzymes in energy metabolism.

Liver is an excellent source of iron. Other sources are meats, egg yolks, seafood, green leafy vegetables, legumes, dried fruits, and whole grain and enriched breads and cereals.

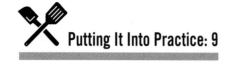

Putting It Into Practice: 9

For clients who have an iron deficiency, what are two dietary practices that would improve iron absorption?

(Check your answer at the end of this chapter)

The ability of the body to absorb and utilize iron from different foods varies from 3 percent for some vegetables to up to 30 percent from red meat. The form of iron in animal foods such as meat, poultry, and fish is absorbed and utilized more readily than iron in plant foods. The presence of these animal products in a meal increases the availability of iron from other foods, as well. The presence of vitamin C in a meal also increases iron absorption. Some foods actually decrease iron consumption: coffee, tea, calcium supplements, wheat bran, and other forms of fiber. The body adjusts its own iron absorption according to need. The body absorbs iron more efficiently when iron stores are low and during growth spurts or pregnancy.

The most common indication of poor iron status is **iron-deficiency anemia**, a condition in which the size and number of red blood cells are reduced. This condition may result from inadequate intake of iron or from blood loss. Symptoms of iron-deficiency anemia include fatigue, pallor, irritability, and lethargy. Iron-deficiency anemia is a real concern in the U.S., more so for women than men. Iron requirements are higher for women of childbearing age than for men, because women have to replace menstrual blood losses.

Selenium

It was not known that selenium was an essential mineral until 1979. Selenium is part of an enzyme that acts like an antioxidant and prevents oxidative damage to tissues, much like vitamin E. Excellent sources include seafood, meat, and liver. Because selenium is sometimes found in the soil, whole grains may be a good source of selenium as well. Deficiency in the U.S. is rare, and selenium can be toxic in large amounts.

Zinc

Zinc is involved in enzymes that promote at least 50 metabolically important reactions in the body. Zinc assists in wound healing, bone formation, development of sexual organs, and general growth and maintenance of all tissues. Zinc is also important for taste perception and appetite.

Protein-containing foods are all good sources of zinc, particularly meat, shellfish, eggs, and milk. Whole grains and some legumes are good sources as well, but zinc is much more readily available in animal foods. In general, iron and zinc are both found in the same foods.

Children, pregnant and premenopausal women, and the elderly are most at risk for being deficient in zinc. Children who are deficient in zinc typically have poor growth and little appetite. Other symptoms of zinc deficiency include diarrhea, impaired immune response, slowed metabolism, loss of taste and smell, confusion, and poor wound healing. Too much zinc interferes with copper metabolism and can cause other serious problems.

Other Trace Minerals

Chromium participates in carbohydrate and fat metabolism. Chromium actually works with insulin to get glucose into the body's cells. A chromium deficiency results in a condition much like diabetes, in which the glucose level in

Glossary

Fluoridation
The addition of fluoride to municipal water systems

Iron-Deficiency Anemia
A condition resulting from insufficient dietary iron intake or blood loss

the blood is abnormally high. Good sources of chromium are liver, meat, the dark meat of poultry, whole grains, and brewer's yeast.

Cobalt is a part of vitamin B12 and is therefore needed to form red blood cells. We take in the cobalt we need by eating vitamin B12-rich foods. (Remember that vitamin B12 is found only in animal foods.)

Copper is necessary along with iron for the formation of hemoglobin. As a part of many enzymes, it also helps make the protein collagen, assists in wound healing, and keeps nerves healthy. Copper occurs in most unprocessed foods. Organ meats, meats, shellfish, whole grain cereals, nuts, and legumes are rich sources. Copper deficiency is generally not a problem (except in cases of malnutrition), and excessive copper intake can be toxic.

Manganese is needed for blood formation and bone structure, and as part of many enzymes involved in energy metabolism. Manganese is found in many foods, especially whole grains, legumes, nuts and seeds, and green leafy vegetables. A deficiency is unknown.

Molybdenum is a cofactor in a number of enzyme systems and is possibly involved in the metabolism of fats. Deficiency does not seem to be a problem.

As time goes on, more trace minerals will probably be recognized as essential to human health. There are currently several trace minerals that are essential to animals and are likely to be essential to humans as well. They include arsenic, nickel, silicon, and boron. Figure 3.19 summarizes this section on minerals.

What about Vitamin and Mineral Supplementation?

Many people in the U.S. arbitrarily take a vitamin/mineral supplement daily. But, a multivitamin is a poor substitute if you don't eat a healthy, balanced diet like the one proposed in the U.S. Food Pyramid. The National Institute of Health Office of Medical Applications of Research and the Office of Dietary Supplements convened a panel in 2006 to assess the evidence on the safety and effectiveness of vitamin/mineral supplements. The panel recommended the following:

✓ "A calcium and vitamin D supplement for postmenopausal women to protect bone health

✓ Anti-oxidants and zinc for non-smoking adults with intermediate-stage, age-related macular degeneration

✓ Folate for women of childbearing age to prevent neural tube defects."

The best insurance is to eat a healthy, balanced diet because food has other benefits besides just the vitamins and minerals. Phytochemicals are one example. If you are ill or have a chronic condition, see your physician about taking supplements. If you choose to take supplements, follow these three simple rules:

✓ Take a low-potency supplement (e.g. not more than 100 percent of the Dietary Reference Intake (DRI)

✓ Take a multi-vitamin/mineral supplement, not single supplements

✓ Take a multi-vitamin/mineral supplement that only contains chemicals for which there is an DRI

Water

Nothing survives without water, and virtually nothing takes place in the body without water playing a vital role. While variations may be great, the average adult's body weight is generally 50 to 60 percent water—enough, if it were bottled, to fill 40 to 50 quarts. For example, in a 150-pound man, water accounts for about 90 pounds, fat about 30 pounds, with proteins, carbohydrates, vitamins and minerals making up the balance. Men generally have more water

Figure 3.19 Minerals: Functions and Food Sources

Mineral	Functions	Food Sources
MAJOR MINERALS		
Calcium	Mineralization of bones and teeth; blood clotting; muscle contraction; transmission of nerve impulses	Milk and milk products, calcium-set to calcium-fortified foods, broccoli, collards, kale, mustard greens, turnip greens, legumes, whole wheat bread
Phosphorus	Mineralization of bones and teeth; energy metabolism; formation of DNA and many enzymes; buffer	Milk and milk products, meat, poultry, eggs, legumes
Magnesium	Energy metabolism; formation of bones and maintenance of teeth; muscle contraction, nerve transmission; immune system	Green leafy vegetables, potatoes, nuts, legumes, whole grain cereals
Sodium	Water balance; acid-base balance; buffer; muscle contraction; transmission of nerve impulses	Salt, processed foods, MSG
Potassium	Water balance; acid-base balance; buffer; muscle contraction; transmission of nerve impulses	Many fruits and vegetables (potatoes, oranges, grapefruit), milk and yogurt, legumes, meats
Chloride	Water balance; acid-base balance; part of hydrochloric acid in stomach	Salt
Sulfur	Part of some amino acids; part of thiamin	Protein foods
TRACE MINERALS		
Copper	Iron metabolism; formation of hemoglobin; collagen formation; energy release	Seafood, whole grain breads and cereal, legumes, nuts, seeds
Fluoride	Strengthening of developing teeth	Water (naturally or artificially fluoridated), tea, seafood
Iodine	Normal functioning of thyroid gland; normal metabolic rate; normal growth and development	Iodized salt, saltwater fish
Iron	Part of hemoglobin and myoglobin; part of some enzymes; energy metabolism; needed to make amino acids	Red meats, shellfish, legumes, whole grain and enriched breads and cereals, green leafy vegetables
Selenium	Activation of antioxidant	Seafood, meat, liver, eggs, whole grains and vegetables (if soil is rich in selenium)
Zinc	Cofactor of many enzymes; wound healing; DNA and protein synthesis; bone formation; development of sexual organs; general growth and maintenance; taste perception and appetite	Protein foods; legumes, dairy products, whole grain products, fortified cereals
Chromium	Works with insulin	Liver, meats, whole grains, nuts

than women. Some parts of the body have more water than others. Human blood is about 92 percent water; muscle and the brain are about 75 percent; and bone is about 22 percent.

The body uses water for virtually all its functions—digestion, absorption, circulation, excretion, transporting nutrients, building tissue, and maintaining temperature. Almost all of the body's cells depend on water to perform their functions. Water carries nutrients to the cells and carries away waste materials to the kidneys. Water is needed in each step of the process of converting food into energy and tissue. Digestive secretions are mostly water, acting as a solvent for nutrients. Water in the digestive secretions softens, dilutes, and liquifies the food to facilitate digestion. It also helps move food along the gastrointestinal tract.

Water serves as an important part of lubricants, helping to cushion the joints and internal organs, keeping body tissues such as the eyes, lungs and air passages moist, and surrounding and protecting the fetus during pregnancy.

The body gets rid of the water it doesn't need through the kidneys and skin and, to a lesser degree, from the lungs and gastrointestinal tract. The largest amount is excreted as urine by the kidneys. About a pint to more than two quarts a day are excreted as urine. The amount of urine reflects, to some extent, the amount of fluid intake of the individual, although no matter how little water one consumes, the kidneys will always excrete a certain amount each day to eliminate waste products generated by the body's metabolic actions. In addition to the urine, air released from the lungs contains some water. Evaporation that occurs from the skin (when sweating or not sweating) contains water as well. See Figure 3.20 for food sources of water. See Figure 3.21 for factors that upset water balance.

Figure 3.20 Food Sources of Water

Percent	Food Sources
100	Coffee, tea, (brewed)
95-99	Clear broth; boiled vegetables such as celery, cabbage, cauliflower, broccoli; cucumber slices; iceberg lettuce; pumpkin; beer
90-94	Cider, cola drinks, lemonade, canned juice, skim milk, most broth-based soups, green peppers
80-89	Whole milk, wines, spaghetti canned in tomato sauce, boiled potatoes, canned grapefruit, fresh orange juice, strawberries, low-fat yogurt, eggplant, mango, cooked spinach, peas, stewed apples
70-79	Milkshake, yogurt, mashed potato, baked beans, sweet potato, cooked oatmeal, rice, poached fish, peaches, banana, boiled egg, cottage cheese
50-69	Pizza, fried and scrambled egg, tuna in oil, stewed prunes, most beef and poultry, cheese spread, cream
30-49	Pork, lunch meat, cheddar cheese, processed cheese, hazelnuts
10-29	Most other nuts, salad dressings, honey syrup
<10	Peanut butter, candy and sugar, oils, potato chip

Glossary

Nutrient Density
The amount of nutrients a food contains relative to its calorie (energy) content

Empty Calories
Calories that provide little or no nutrient density

Figure 3.21   Factors that Upset Water Balance

Surgery

Physical Activity

Illness with Prolonged Vomiting, Diarrhea or Fever

Amount of Alcohol Consumed

Diuretic Consumption

Pregnancy/Breast Feeding

Hot Weather or Hot Environments

Increased Intake of Fiber, Salt, Protein, or Sugar

SECTION E   Nutrient Density

Foods vary in how rich they are in nutrients. Foods that are nutrient-rich relative to their calorie (energy) content are said to be of high **nutrient density**. For example, one cup of broccoli has 25 calories and proportionally high levels of vitamins and minerals. It has a high nutrient density. In contrast, one cup of cola has 100 calories and no vitamins. You can think of calories as a "price" paid for vitamins, minerals, and other essential nutrients. If you pay a high price for a small amount of nutrients when you eat a particular food, that food is not nutrient dense. Sometimes people use the term **empty calories** to describe a food that has low nutrient density. See the sample in Figure 3.22. In the "price" analogy, if you pay a low price (caloric intake) and receive many nutrients, the food you are consuming is nutrient-dense. Sound dietary habits rely on nutrient-dense foods for many of the daily food choices.

Figure 3.22   Example of Empty Calories

Homemade Cupcake with Icing

INFORMATION PER SERVING: Serving Size = 1 Cupcake

Calories 170	Vitamin A................................ *
Fat.............................5 grams	Vitamin C................................ *
Sodium..............110 milligrams	Calcium .... *
Carbohydrates ....30 grams	Iron .... *
Protein ....2 grams	

* Less than 2% of recommended intakes

You are paying a high calorie price for very little of the essential nutrients, except those we already eat too much of.

Facts About Low-Calorie Sweeteners

Low-calorie sweeteners (sometimes referred to as non-nutritive sweeteners, artificial sweeteners, or sugar substitutes) are ingredients added to foods and beverages to provide sweetness without adding a significant amount of calories. In fact, they can also play an important role in a weight management program that includes both good nutrition choices and physical activity.

Low-calorie sweeteners have a long history of safe use in a variety of foods and beverages, ranging from soft drinks to puddings and candies to table-top sweeteners. They are some of the most studied and reviewed food ingredients in the world today and have passed rigorous safety assessments. In the U.S., the most common and popular low-calorie sweeteners permitted for use in foods and beverages today are:

- acesulfame potassium (ace-K)
- aspartame
- neotame
- saccharin
- stevia sweeteners
- sucralose

When added to foods and beverages, these low-calorie sweeteners provide a taste that is similar to that of table sugar (sucrose), and are generally several hundred to several thousand times sweeter than sugar. They are often referred to as "intense" sweeteners. Because of their intense sweetening power, these sweeteners can be used in very small amounts and thus add only a negligible amount of calories to foods and beverages. As a result, they can substantially reduce or completely eliminate the calories in certain products such as diet beverages, light yogurt and sugar-free pudding. In addition, many low-calorie sweeteners do not contribute to cavities or tooth decay. The following are some helpful facts about the safety, benefits, and uses of low-calorie sweeteners.

FACT: Low-calorie sweeteners are reviewed for safety by the federal government before being approved for use in foods and beverages.

Low-calorie sweeteners are thoroughly tested and carefully regulated by U.S. and international regulatory authorities, as well as scientific organizations, to ensure the safety of foods, beverages and other products that contain them. Also, food and beverage manufacturers are required to list low-calorie sweeteners in the ingredients list on the product label.

The Acceptable Daily Intake (ADI) must be determined by the U.S. Food and Drug Administration (FDA) prior to approval for any food ingredient, including low-calorie sweeteners, for use in foods and beverages in the U.S. The ADI is the amount of an ingredient (expressed in milligrams per kilogram of body weight) that a person can safely consume every day over a lifetime without risk. The ADI is set at one one-hundredth of the amount that has been found not to produce any adverse health effects in key animal studies. Therefore, it would be very difficult for a person to consume enough of any low-calorie sweetener to reach the ADI. In fact, current intake of each low-calorie sweetener is well below the ADI.

FACT: All approved low-calorie sweeteners can be safely consumed by the general population, including people with diabetes, pregnant women, and children.

One exception is people who have a rare hereditary condition called phenylketonuria (PKU), which means they cannot metabolize phenylalanine, a component of aspartame. All products containing aspartame must carry a statement warning people with PKU of the presence of aspartame on the label.

For people with diabetes who must control their blood-sugar levels through careful monitoring of their sugar

(Continued...)

Facts About Low-Calorie Sweeteners *(Continued)*

and carbohydrate intake, low-calorie sweeteners can offer a sweet alternative that does not affect blood glucose levels.

In addition, pregnant women and children can safely consume foods and beverages sweetened with low-calorie sweeteners. Current low-calorie sweetener consumption in children is well below the Acceptable Daily Intake (ADI) for all approved low-calorie sweeteners. However, pregnant women and young children are not encouraged to restrict their calorie intake, so they should talk with their healthcare provider and/or Registered Dietitian about ensuring that dietary plans including low-calorie sweeteners still meet the desired calorie and nutrient goals.

FACT: Low-calorie sweeteners do not cause or increase the risk of cancer.

Studies have repeatedly shown that low-calorie sweeteners do not cause or increase the risk of developing cancer. The following discusses cancer research conducted on each approved low-calorie sweetener.

Ace-K. Acesulfame potassium (ace-K) has been thoroughly tested in several longterm animal studies which used amounts of ace-K that were far higher than any person could potentially consume, and no evidence of cancer or tumors was found.

Aspartame. The vast majority of the research conducted over the last three decades has concluded that aspartame does not cause cancer. The National Cancer Institute (NCI) recently concluded that aspartame is not associated with increased risk of cancer, even among individuals with high aspartame intakes. In September 2007, a panel of experts published a safety report on aspartame which found "no credible evidence that aspartame is carcinogenic" (Magnuson, 2007). While two recent studies by a group of Italian researchers reported a link between aspartame and cancer in rats, the FDA found "significant shortcomings" in the design and interpretation of both studies. FDA subsequently stated that it does not plan to change its position on the safety of aspartame, and the European Food Safety Authority (EFSA) published an official opinion of the same tone in April 2009.

Neotame. Prior to its approval as a general-purpose sweetener in 2002, more than 100 scientific studies were conducted on neotame, including cancer studies. Human studies were also conducted and "no significant effects of neotame were observed."

Saccharin. While saccharin's safety has been the subject of ongoing controversy, the sweetener has been established as safe for many years. Studies conducted several decades ago found a link between saccharin consumption and bladder cancer in rats, which raised concerns. This caused FDA to propose a ban on saccharin in 1977 and require a warning label on products containing saccharin. However, since then, researchers have concluded that the finding on bladder cancer in the rats do not apply to humans. (NCI, 2006). Other human studies on saccharin have found no consistent evidence to link saccharin with bladder cancer in humans. As of 2001, products containing saccharin no longer have to carry a warning label.

Stevia sweeteners. Several studies conducted on stevia sweeteners since the 1980s have shown that they are not associated with cancer. Recent research confirmed the conclusions of earlier research that steviol glycosides, the primary components of stevia sweeteners, do not pose a cancer risk. Additionally, in June 2008, the Joint Expert Committee on Food Additives (JECFA) completed a multi-year review of all the available scientific data on high purity steviol glycosides, and concluded that they are safe for use as general purpose sweeteners.

Sucralose. Extensive research on sucralose and health has been conducted over the last two decades. Comprehensive toxicology studies designed to meet the highest scientific standards have clearly demonstrated that sucralose is not cancerous.

(Continued...)

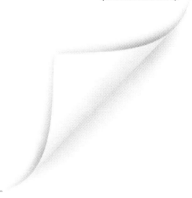

Facts About Low-Calorie Sweeteners *(Continued)*

FACT: Low-calorie sweeteners do not cause or increase the risk of other health conditions.

Low-calorie sweeteners are often inaccurately linked to adverse health effects, such as seizures, infertility, stomach ailments, and possible effects on kidney and liver function. However, the existing body of research does not support such effects. Health authorities around the world have verified that low-calorie sweeteners are safe. The following information on each low-calorie sweetener demonstrates that they do not cause or increase the risk of these or other health conditions.

Ace-K. There is a large body of scientific evidence that supports the safety of ace-K for use in foods and beverages. Throughout more than 15 years of extensive use, there have been no documented health problems in humans from consuming ace-K. The FDA has concluded that the safety of ace-K is consistent with research findings from other countries. EFSA's re-examination of the sweetener in 2000 reaffirmed its safety.

Aspartame. Both the French Food Safety Agency and EFSA re-evaluated and re-confirmed the safety of aspartame in 2002. In addition, the review by Magnuson, et al (2007) examined over 500 scientific studies, articles, and reports published over the last 25 years looking at mechanisms of aspartame absorption and metabolism, worldwide consumption levels, and toxicology data. Based on their review, the panel concluded that aspartame does not cause cancer, seizures, or other adverse effects on behavior, cognitive function, or neural function. In addition, EFSA again convened a Panel in 2009 to review all available evidence on aspartame safety and concluded that aspartame does not cause cancer or genotoxic effects, and there is no reason to revise the previously established ADI for aspartame.

Neotame. Of over 100 scientific studies conducted on neotame, no link has been found between neotame consumption and adverse health conditions, including toxicity, developmental and reproductive problems, or cancer.

Saccharin. Saccharin has been evaluated by credible health and science organizations and confirmed to be safe. The American Dietetic Association (ADA), American Cancer Society (ACS), and American Medical Association (AMA) all agree that saccharin is safe and acceptable for use.

Stevia sweeteners. The safety of stevia sweeteners for human consumption has been established through rigorous peer-reviewed research, including metabolism and pharmacokinetic studies, general and multi-generational safety studies, intake studies and human studies. This research is consistent with JECFA's review of steviol glycosides, completed in 2008, which concluded that steviol glycosides are safe for human consumption.

Sucralose. More than 100 scientific studies have been conducted over a 20-year period on sucralose, looking at a variety of health conditions, such as toxicity, cancer, reproductive health, kidney health, brain and blood disorders, children's health, and nutrition. These studies have demonstrated that sucralose does not cause adverse health effects and is safe for use as a sweetening ingredient. The research on sucralose's safety has also been reviewed by scientific and regulatory bodies including JECFA and EFSA, both of which concluded it is safe for human consumption.

FACT: Low-calorie sweeteners can help with weight management and do not cause weight gain.

As Americans face increasing obesity rates, low-calorie sweeteners can offer help with weight management. Research indicates that people who incorporate foods and beverages sweetened with low-calorie sweeteners into their diet in place of calorie-containing sweeteners actually consume fewer calories than those who do not. Additionally, since they are not deprived of sweets, individuals consuming low-calorie sweeteners may feel more satisfied with their eating plans, helping them to lose weight and keep it off.

(Continued...)

Facts About Low-Calorie Sweeteners *(Continued)*

In one recent study, researchers at Purdue University found that consumption of saccharin led to increased appetite and weight gain in rats. However, due to a known affinity for saccharin of rats, small sample size, and other flaws in the study design, many experts agree that the results cannot be applied to humans. While a few studies have suggested that low-calorie sweeteners may cause cravings and/or lead to weight gain, these studies have not changed the overall scientific consensus that low-calorie sweeteners can aid in weight management.

Clinical studies conducted in humans over the past 20 years have shown that low-calorie sweeteners can help with weight loss and/or maintenance. A 2006 review of aspartame's role in weight management demonstrated a weight loss of 0.2 kg/week (or 0.4 lb/week) when aspartame-sweetened products were substituted for those sweetened with sugar. Similar findings were seen in a 1997 study published in the American Journal of Clinical Nutrition. Experts agree that successful weight management requires more than just calorie reduction—moderation, along with eating a balanced diet and regular exercise, is key to reaching an optimal weight.

More on the Six Low-Calorie Sweeteners

Each low-calorie sweeter has a slightly different set of characteristics:

Acesulfame-Potassium (Ace-K)—Ace-K is a combination of an organic acid and potassium, and is 200 times sweeter than sugar. It is a popular sweetener used in low-calorie sweetener blends to create an optimal flavor profile in foods and beverages.

Ace-K was approved by the U.S. Food and Drug Administration (FDA) in 1988 for use in numerous food products and as a tabletop sweetener. In 1998, the FDA extended its approval to beverages, and finally as a general purpose sweetener in 2003. Ace-K is approved for use in nearly 90 countries.

Ace-K is not broken down by the body and is eliminated unchanged by the kidneys. It has no effect on serum glucose, cholesterol or triglycerides, and people with diabetes may safely include products containing ace-K in their diet.

Aspartame—Discovered in 1965, aspartame is used in foods and beverages in more than 100 countries worldwide. FDA approved aspartame for use in foods in 1981, followed by beverages in 1983. In 1996, it received approval as a general purpose sweetener.

Aspartame is a molecule consisting of two amino acids—phenylalanine and aspartic acid. People who have a rare hereditary condition called phenylketonuria (PKU) cannot metabolize phenylalanine; therefore, all products containing aspartame must carry a statement warning people with PKU of the presence of aspartame on the label.

Aspartame provides four calories per gram. However, it is used in very small amounts, contributing negligible calories to the diet. Aspartame is approximately 180 times sweeter than sugar. It is not heat-stable and is not suggested for use in cooking or baking.

Neotame—Neotame is also a derivative of aspartic acid and phenylalanine. It is approximately 7,000 to 8,000 times sweeter than sugar, although some report a sweetening power of up to 13,000 times that of sugar. It is partially absorbed, but rapidly metabolized and excreted from the body.

Neotame was approved by FDA in July 2002 as a general purpose sweetener. Neotame has also received favorable evaluation by JECFA and is approved for use in other countries, including most parts of Eastern Europe, Australia, Russia, Mexico and several South American countries.

Because of the extraordinary sweetening power of a small amount of neotame, the level of exposure to phenylalanine as it is released into the bloodstream is considered clinically insignificant. Therefore, products sweetened with neotame are not required to carry a statement on the label alerting persons with PKU to the presence of phenylalanine.

(Continued...)

Facts About Low-Calorie Sweeteners *(Continued)*

Low-Calorie Sweeteners At-A-Glance			
Sweetener	Date Approved	Sweeter Than Sugar	Brand Name(s)
Ace-K	1988	200x	Sunett®, Sweet One®
Aspartame	1981	180x	NutraSweet®, Equal®, others
Neotame	2002	7,000x	n/a
Saccharin	Years prior to 1958	300x	Sweet 'N Low®, Sweet Twin®, Sugar Twin®, others
Stevia Sweeteners	2008	200x	Truvia™, PureVia™, Sun Crystals®
Sucralose	1998	600x	Splenda®

Sources: Comprehensive Reviews in Food Science and Food Safety, IFT, 2006 Food and Chemical Toxicology, 2008

Saccharin—Originally discovered in 1878, saccharin is considered the oldest of the low-calorie sweeteners approved for food and beverage use. Today, saccharin is still used safely and widely and often in combination with other sweeteners. Saccharin is 300 times sweeter than sugar, although some reports have indicated it can be up to 700 times sweeter than sugar. It is not broken down by the body and is eliminated without providing any calories. Saccharin is heat stable, therefore making it suitable for cooking and baking.

Stevia sweeteners—The stevia plant is native to South America, and today, it can be found growing in many countries including China, Brazil, Argentina, Paraguay, India and South Korea. Hundreds of foods and beverages consumed around the world are sweetened with stevia sweeteners.

Stevia sweeteners are highly purified steviol glycosides, which make up the sweetest part of the stevia plant. In December 2008, the FDA stated it had no questions regarding the conclusion of an expert panel that steviol glycosides are generally recognized as safe (GRAS) for use as general purpose sweeteners. Prior to this, stevia (in its unpurified form) was only permitted for use as a dietary supplement in the U.S. Stevia sweeteners are natural, contain zero calories, and are 200-300 times sweeter than sugar.

Stevia sweeteners are approved for food and beverage use in several countries and can be found in the U.S. in many food and beverage products, including some juice and tea beverages, as well as some tabletop sweeteners.

Sucralose—In 1998, FDA approved sucralose for use in 15 food and beverage categories—the broadest initial approval ever given to a food additive. In 1999, FDA extended the approval to all categories of foods and beverages as a general-purpose sweetener.

Six hundred times sweeter than sugar, the intense sweetness of sucralose is made from a process that begins with regular table sugar (sucrose); however, it is not sugar. It is produced through a process whereby three hydrogen-oxygen groups on the sugar molecule are replaced with three chlorine atoms. Sucralose is not recognized by the body as a carbohydrate. It is poorly absorbed and is excreted unchanged from the body. As a result, sucralose provides no calories. Because sucralose is very stable, it can be used almost anywhere sugar is used, including in cooking and baking.

Facts About Low-Calorie Sweeteners *(Continued)*

REFERENCES

Blackburn GL, Kanders BS et al. The effect of aspartame as part of a multidisciplinary weight-control program on short- and long-term control of body weight [abstract]. Am J Clin Nutr. 1997;65:409-418.

Carakostas M.C., Curry L.L., Boileau A.C., Brusick D.J. Overview: The history, technical function and safety of rebaudioside A, a naturally occurring steviol glycoside, for use in food and beverages. *Food and Chemical Toxicology*. 2008;46:S1-S10.

de la Hunty A, Gibson S, Ashwell M. A review of the effectiveness of a spartame in helping with weight control. *Nutrition Bulletin*. 2006;31:115-128.

European Commission, Health and Consumer Protection Directorate (2002). *Opinion of the Scientific Committee on Food: Update on the Safety of Aspartame*. http://www.food. gov.uk/multimedia/pdfs/ aspartameopinion.pdf

European Food Safety Authority. Question number EFSA-Q-2005-122. *The EFSA Journal*, (2006), v 356, p 1-44. http://www.efsa.europa.eu/cs/ BlobServer/Scientific_ Opinion/afc_op_ej356_aspartame_en1.pdf? ssbinary=true

French Food Safety Agency (2002). *Assessment Report*. http://www.aspartame.org/pdf/AFSSA-Eng.pdf

International Food Information Council Foundation. A Look at Low Calorie Sweeteners. *Food Insight*. (September/October 2005). http://www.ific.org/ foodinsight/2005/so/lcsfi505.cfm

International Food Information Council Foundation. *Gestational Diabetes and Low-Calorie Sweeteners: Answers to Common Questions* (November 2004). http://www.ific.org/ publications/brochures/gestdiabetes.cfm

International Food Information Council Foundation. *IFIC Review, Low-Calorie Sweeteners and Health* (October 2000). http://www.ific.org/publications/reviews/sweetenerir.cfm

International Food Information Council Foundation. *The Lowdown on Low-Calorie Sweeteners* Continuing Professional Education (CPE) module (January 2008). http://www.ific.org/ adacpe/lcscpe.cfm

International Food Information Council Foundation. *Sugar Alcohols Fact Sheet* (September 2004). http://www.ific.org/ publications/factsheets/sugaralcoholfs.cfm

International Food Information Council Foundation. US Food and Drug Administration. *Food Ingredients and Colors*. (November 2004). http://www.ific.org/publications/brochures/ foodingredandcolorsbroch.cfm

Journal of the American Dietetic Association (2004). Position of the American Dietetic Association: Use of Nutritive and Nonnutritive Sweeteners. p 255- 275. http://www.eatright. org/cps/rde/xchg/ada/hs.xsl/advocacy_adap0598_ENU_ HTML.htm

Kroger, M., Meister, K., Kava. (2006). Low calorie sweeteners and other sugar substitutes: A review of the safety issues. *Comprehensive Reviews in Food Science and Food Safety*. Vol. 5, p 35-47. http://members.ift.org/NR/rdonlyres/DA941122- 00F5-49AA-8BC3-27E32F80B746/0/crfsfsv5n2p3547.pdf

Magnuson BA, Burdock GA et al. Aspartame: A Safety Evaluation Based on Current Use Levels, Regulations, and Toxicological and Epidemiological Studies. *Critical Reviews in Toxicology*. 2007;37:629-727. National Cancer Institute (NCI). "Artificial Sweeteners and Cancer: Questions and Answers." National Cancer Institute Fact Sheet. Revised 10/2006. http://www.cancer.gov/cancertopics/factsheet/Risk/ artificialsweeteners (accessed 7/11/07).

Soffritti, M., Belpoggi, F., Esposti, D.D., Lambertini, L. Aspartame induces lymphomas and leukemias in rats. *Eur. J. Oncol*. 2005;vol. 10, n. 2.

Soffritti M, Belpoggi F et al. Life-Span Exposure to Low Doses of Aspartame Beginning during Prenatal Life Increases Cancer Effects in Rats. *Environ Health Perspect*. 2007;115: 1293–1297.

Swithers SE, Davidson TL. A Role for Sweet Taste: Calorie Predictive Relations in Energy Regulation. *Behavioral Neuroscience*. 2007;122:161-173.

Putting It Into Practice Questions & Answers

1. As you review the food label for yogurt to the right, how many of the six nutrient categories can you locate?

   A. *There are four of the six nutrient categories in the yogurt itself although there are five nutrient categories listed on the label: total fat, of which there is 0% in the yogurt; the saturated fat, trans fat and cholesterol are all part of the total fat. There are three minerals listed: sodium, calcium, iron. There are two types of carbohydrate, dietary fiber and sugar. Protein is listed, as well as two vitamins—Vitamin A and vitamin C.*

Food Label for Greek Yogurt

Amount Per Serving	% of Daily Value
Total Fat 0 g	0%
Saturated Fat 0 g	0%
Trans Fat 0 g	0%
Cholesterol 0 mg	0%
Sodium 65 mg	3%
Total Carbohydrate 20 g	7%
Dietary Fiber < 1 g	4%
Sugars 19 g	
Protein 14 g	22%

Vitamin A 2%	Vitamin C 2%
Calcium 20%	Iron 0%

2. Knowing that there are 28 grams to an ounce can help us determine how many calories we are adding during cooking. For example, if you are adding one ounce of butter, and you know that butter is a fat, how many calories are you adding?

   A. *1 oz. = 28 grams | Fat has 9 calories per gram | 9 x 28 = 252 calories*

3. What would you tell a diabetic client who proudly states that she doesn't eat sugar because she only purchases foods that are "sucrose-free?"

   A. *Explain to the client that sucrose is only one kind of sugar. Show her the listing of the different types of sugar besides sucrose that might be in prepared products. If she is able to read small print, have her find all of the kinds of sugar on a label of a prepared product.*

4. A client complains that he is always hungry 30 minutes after he eats. What foods would you suggest he add to his diet that would delay the onset of hunger?

   A. *Foods that are high in protein and fat provide more satiety than carbohydrate foods. In other words, they stay in the stomach longer because they take longer to digest. Add more fat in the form of gravies, salad dressing, or butter/margarine if he is not on a calorie restricted diet. If he is, add lean protein such as white meat chicken or turkey. If he drinks milk, include milk or high protein Greek yogurt with his dinner meal.*

5. What's wrong with this picture? A grocery store recently hung a sign in front of their sunflower oil section. The sign said "95% fat and cholesterol free." What should the sign say?

   A. *Sunflower oil is actually 100% fat so a sign that says it is 95% fat free is incorrect. Since sunflowers are plants, the oil would be cholesterol free. What the sign should have said is: 95% Saturated fat and cholesterol free. See Appendix F in the back of the text for a listing of the amount of saturated fat, monounsaturated fat, and polyunsaturated fat in various fat sources.*

Putting It Into Practice Questions & Answers *(Continued)*

6. If a client weighs 120 pounds, what is her daily protein requirement?

   A. *1. Determine the number of kilograms this person weighs. 120 ÷ 2.2 = 54.5 kilograms*

   2. Multiply the kilograms by the amount of protein needed per kilogram (0.8)
   54.5 × 0.8 = 43.6 or 44 grams of protein per day

7. Based on new research, what two vitamins and their food sources would be important for the mental health of the elderly?

   A. *Vitamin D and Vitamin E may prevent dementia and improve resistance to Parkinsons and Alzheimers.*

8. You notice that it is the cook's practice to cook the vegetables and put them into the steam table a minimum of two hours prior to plating on the trayline. What would you recommend to the cook to increase the vitamin content of the cooked vegetable?

   A. *Cook the vegetables just prior to service or use a batch cooking technique where only small amounts of vegetables are cooked right before service if the trayline time is lengthy. If butter or margarine is added, add the butter or margarine to the tray so the client can add it.*

9. For clients who have an iron deficiency, what are two dietary practices that would improve iron absorption?

   A. *1. Serve the food containing iron with a food containing citrus such as pork sausage with orange juice.*
   2. Serve hot tea or iced tea either one hour before or one hour after the meal. Citrus foods improve iron absorption if consumed at the same meal; tea decreases iron absorption.

CHAPTER 4

Describe the Process of Digestion

Overview and Objectives

An understanding of how digestion occurs helps a Certified Dietary Manager plan and modify menus for individuals who have unique needs.

After completing this chapter, you should be able to:

✓ Follow the path of digestion

✓ Relate digestion to nutrition

✓ Describe the organs involved in digestion

✓ Differentiate between digestion of protein, fat, and types of carbohydrate

✓ Discuss absorption and its relationship to other body systems

✓ Explain the concepts of absorption and availability of nutrients

✓ Analyze own intake for the leader nutrients

Systems of the Human Body

Digestion occurs through the digestive system. The body is made up of systems. The word system describes groups of organs working together to perform functions. Systems are made up of organs. Organs are made up of body tissues. In turn, tissues are made up of cells. Cells are the basic unit of life and the building blocks of the human body. Each cell has a cell membrane that surrounds and protects the cell. Most cells also have a nucleus, which directs the work going on in the cell. The body contains many types of cells, such as nerve cells, bone cells, muscle cells, and fat cells. Each type of cell has a unique structure related to what it does in the body.

Tissues are groups of similar cells that work together to perform a certain function. For example, epithelial tissue lines many body surfaces, and one of its functions is to protect the body. Organs are made of several kinds of tissue. Examples of body organs include the liver, stomach, intestines, gallbladder, kidney, brain, and heart. Even skin is considered an organ. Organs work together as part of body systems. Systems include:

✓ The digestive system, which digests food

✓ The circulatory system, which circulates blood and lymph (a body fluid)

✓ The musculoskeletal system, essential for body movement

✓ The nervous and endocrine (hormone) systems, which control body functions

✓ The respiratory system, responsible for breathing

✓ The immune system, which protects against illness and infection

✓ The reproductive system, responsible for new life

✓ The urinary system, which excretes waste (urine)

How the Digestive System Works

Have you ever wondered how food you eat becomes the nutrients you need? What controls what happens to the food? You do control <u>what</u> you eat but your brain and hormones let you know when you are hungry. Your brain and hormones also guide your digestive system after you've eaten. The digestive system is made up of organs and a long, looped tube from the mouth to the anus (over 30 feet long when stretched out—Figure 4.1). The digestive system feeds the rest of the body, which is why it is so important that you choose wisely. When we eat food, it goes through three different processes: digestion, absorption, and metabolism. **Digestion** is the process of breaking food into smaller components, in some cases, converting those components into nutrients, and eliminating solid wastes. That long, looped tube is known as the **gastrointestinal tract (GI tract)**. It starts in the mouth, which is connected to the throat or pharynx, esophagus, stomach, small intestine, large intestine, rectum, and anus, where solid waste leaves the body. These organs are hollow so that digested food can pass through them. The mouth, stomach, and small intestine contain a lining (called **mucosa**) that produces juices to help digest food. There is also a layer of smooth muscle in the GI tract that helps food move along and further break down food.

Other organs involved in digestion are the liver, pancreas, and gallbladder. The liver produces bile that emulsifies fat and the pancreas also produces digestive juices. These digestive juices are sent from the liver and the pancreas to the intestine through small tubes called ducts. The gallbladder is the holding tank and stores the liver's digestive juices until they are needed in the intestine. Figure 4.2 lists the organs involved in digestion.

Body cells cannot use a steak, or an apple, or a slice of bread for food. Instead, they need food in its smaller chemical units, as nutrients. Thus, to convert food into nutrients, the body needs to break it down into smaller components. This is part of what digestion is about. Essentially, the body takes food apart so that it can use the pieces to re-build exactly what it needs for life.

During the process of digestion, food is broken down two ways: mechanically and chemically. **Mechanical breakdown** is the physical breaking of food into smaller pieces. In the digestive system, this is the job of the mouth, the esophagus, and the stomach. The first part is obvious. When we chew food, we break it into smaller bites. Teeth, tongue, and jaws all help with this process. The next forms of mechanical breakdown are invisible to us. As food moves through the esophagus towards the stomach, strong muscular action breaks it down a little bit more. When food is in the stomach, it is churned into even smaller pieces.

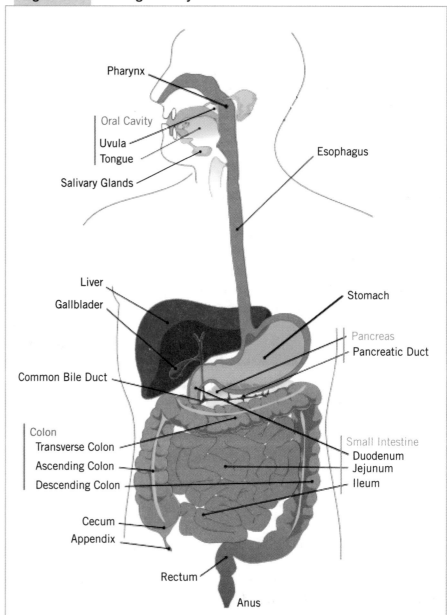

Figure 4.1 The Digestive System

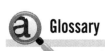 **Glossary**

Digestion
The process of breaking down food into nutrients

Gastrointestinal Tract (GI Tract)
The tubular organs from the mouth to the anus plus the liver, pancreas, and gallbladder

Mucosa
The lining of the mouth, stomach and small intestine that contain tiny glands to produce digestive enzymes

Mechanical Breakdown
Physical breaking down of food into smaller pieces using teeth, tongue, jaws, and the smooth muscles in the esophagus and stomach

Chemical Breakdown
Breakdown of food from digestive juices or enzymes

Chemical breakdown of food occurs with the help of digestive enzymes. Enzymes are substances that speed up chemical reactions and help in the breakdown of complex nutrients. Enzymes break complex proteins into simpler amino acids. They break starch into sugar, and reduce complicated sugars to simple sugars such as glucose. Enzymes also break large fat molecules down to fatty acids and glycerol. Figure 4.3 lists some of the digestive enzymes.

The digestive system starts with the mouth or oral cavity. The tongue, which extends across the floor of the mouth, moves food around the mouth during chewing and rolls it into a ball to be swallowed. There are 32 permanent teeth in the mouth that grind and break down the food. Chewing is important because it breaks the food up into smaller pieces so that enzymes can get in and do their job. Saliva, a fluid secreted into the mouth from the salivary glands, not only

Figure 4.2   Organs in the Digestive System

Organ	What Happens Here
Mouth	Chewing and mixing of food with salivary fluids
Esophagus	Delivers swallowed food to the stomach
Stomach	Food is churned and mixed with hydrochloric acid and pepsin for further breakdown. The food mixture that leaves the stomach is called chyme. Alcohol and certain drugs are absorbed from the stomach.
Duodenum (first part of the small intestines)	Mixes food with secretions from the liver and pancreas to neutralize stomach acid and further digest food. Much absorption of food occurs here.
Jejunum (second part of the small intestines)	Continues chemical digestion. Much absorption of food occurs here.
Ileum (third part of the small intestines)	Re-absorbs bile salts used to digest fats earlier in the small intestines.
Colon	Absorbs water and vitamins. Collects indigestible residue (waste) to form feces.
Rectum	Controls release of waste (feces).
Liver	Produces bile, a chemical that emulsifies fat, i.e. it breaks fat down into smaller globules so that digestive enzymes can go to work.
Gallbladder	Stores bile and secretes it into the duodenum during digestion
Pancreas	Produces many digestive enzymes

produces amylase to begin breakdown of starches, it also lubricates the food so that it may readily pass down the throat and esophagus. The mucous-like substance in saliva coats food and helps to form a mass of chewed food called a bolus. Food in the form of a bolus can safely be swallowed.

How does swallowing work? There are two steps. In the first step, the tongue pushes the bolus back towards the pharynx, or the back of the oral cavity (see Figure 4.4). Then, an involuntary muscular contraction pushes the bolus into the esophagus. Involuntary means that this occurs automatically, as a reflex. We do not consciously control this step. During this second step, the body automatically closes the respiratory passages so that we will not breathe in food. Anatomically speaking, a muscular flap called the epiglottis covers the trachea, the passageway to the lungs. From time to time, this process doesn't work. You can probably think of times when a little bit of food or drink has accidentally entered your respiratory system. This is called aspiration. In a healthy person, the result is coughing to clear it out.

Food enters the esophagus, a muscular tube about 10 inches long that connects the throat to the stomach. Food is propelled down the esophagus by rhythmic contractions of circular muscles in the wall of the esophagus. These

Figure 4.3   Examples of Digestive Enzymes

Enzyme	Where It Is	What It Does
Salivary Amylase	Mouth (made by salivary glands)	Breaks down starch and complex sugars
Pepsin	Stomach	Breaks down protein
Lipase	Secreted by the pancreas into the small intestine	Breaks down fat
Protease	Secreted by the pancreas into the small intestine	Breaks down protein

contractions are called peristalsis. Peristalsis also helps break up food into smaller and smaller particles. You might want to think of it as squeezing a marble (the bolus) through a rubber tube. Food passes down the esophagus through the lower esophageal sphincter (LES), a muscle that relaxes and contracts to move food from the esophagus into the stomach. The LES works like a gatekeeper into the stomach. Normally, it allows only a one-way movement. When a person experiences heartburn, the LES has mistakenly allowed stomach acid contents to shoot back up into the esophagus. This backflow of stomach contents is also called reflux. (Note that heartburn actually has nothing to do with the heart. It acquires its name because the discomfort sufferers feel is close to the position of the heart.)

The stomach has three digestive tasks. The first is a muscular sac that holds about one liter of food. Within the folds of the mucous membranes are digestive glands that make the enzyme pepsin, as well as hydrochloric acid. Hydrochloric acid makes stomach contents very acid (pH about 2.0, more acid than vinegar), which activates the pepsin for protein digestion. Hydrochloric acid also destroys harmful bacteria, and increases the ability of calcium and iron to be absorbed. People sometimes wonder why the stomach does not digest itself. The stomach has several forms of protection from these strong chemicals. It has a mucous lining that can neutralize hydrochloric acid, and it keeps the enzyme pepsin ready in a safer state called pepsinogen. Only after food arrives does it release acid and make pepsin active.

The second digestive task of the stomach is to churn food so that it can be passed into the first part of the small intestine. When the food is ready, it reaches a liquid consistency known as chyme. The stomach functions like a holding tank and takes approximately two to six hours to empty. A high amount of fat in a meal slows stomach emptying. Little absorption of nutrients takes place here. However, this is the site where alcohol and aspirin are absorbed.

The third digestive task of the stomach is to empty the chyme slowly into to the small intestine. Several factors determine how quickly the stomach empties, including the kind of food and the degree of muscle action. Carbohydrates are the easiest to digest and therefore spend the least amount of time in the stomach. Carbohydrate digestion begins in the mouth so it is already partly digested when it arrives in the stomach. Protein digestion begins in the stomach so protein stays in the stomach longer. Fat takes the longest to digest and stays in

Figure 4.4   Anatomy Involved in Swallowing

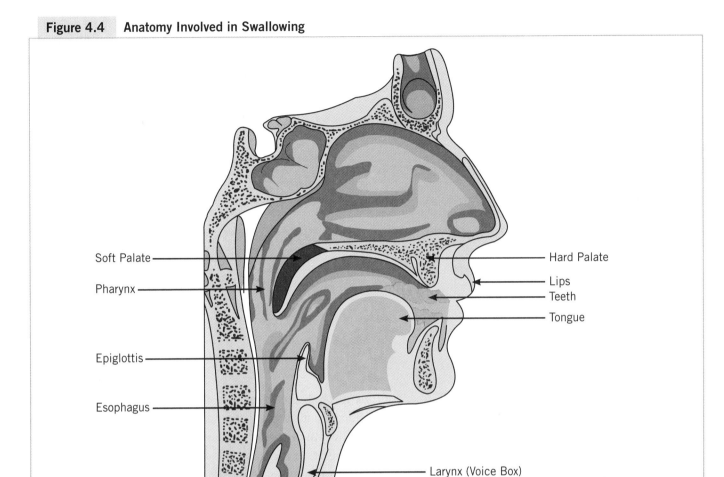

the stomach the longest. See Figure 4.5 for an estimate of the amount of time food stays in the stomach.

A specialized muscle called the pyloric sphincter allows chyme to travel from the stomach into the small intestine. The small intestine is about 20 feet long and has three parts: the duodenum, the jejunum, and the ileum. It is called the small intestine because the diameter is smaller than that of the large intestine. Like the mouth and the stomach, the small intestine adds digestive juices to food. These juices include enzymes and other chemicals produced by the pancreas. One of the chemicals is sodium bicarbonate, which simply neutralizes the acid chyme arriving from the stomach. Next is an array of digestive enzymes that convert protein to amino acids and small groups of amino acids. The duodenum, about one foot long, receives the digested food from the stomach. A small organ above the intestines, the pancreas, releases enzymes into the duodenum to help digest carbohydrate, protein, and fat.

Before enzymes can work on fat, however, the fat must be broken down into smaller parts. This is the job of bile, a compound produced by the liver and stored in the gallbladder. The gallbladder releases bile into the small intestine. Bile works like detergent, to emulsify fat. What does this mean? Imagine that your hands are greasy from rubbing oil on a turkey, or changing oil in your car.

You cannot rinse the fat off your hands with water. You use soap or detergent to split fat globules into smaller parts so you can wash them away. Bile works quite similarly. Its action produces smaller pieces of fat, so that enzymes can get at them and digest the fat. See Figure 4.6 to review digestion.

Figure 4.5   Amount of Time Food Stays in the Stomach

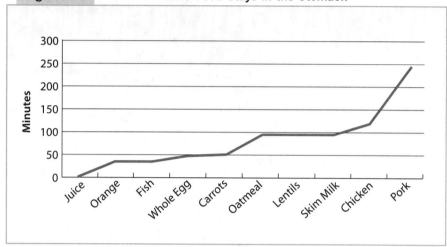

Sugar passes quickly through the stomach into the small intestine where it is broken down into glucose and fructose. Starch digestion begins in the mouth with an enzyme in saliva, then passes quickly through the stomach into the small intestine where digestion is completed. Protein foods such as meat and eggs are large molecules so the stomach must break these molecules into smaller molecules. When they are small enough, they are passed into the small intestine and broken down further into amino acids. Fat digestion begins in the stomach.

Vitamins are also absorbed through the small intestine. Fat-soluble vitamins are dissolved with the fat and stored in the liver and fatty tissues of the body. Water-soluble vitamins are not easily stored and are passed into the urine.

In the wall of the duodenum—and throughout the entire small intestine—are tiny, fingerlike projections called villi. The muscular walls mix the chyme with the digestive juices and bring the nutrients into contact with the villi for absorption. Most nutrients pass through the villi of the duodenum and jejunum into either the blood or lymph vessels, where they are transported to the liver and to the cells of the body. The duodenum connects with the second section, the jejunum, which connects to the ileum.

The large intestine or colon, which is four to five feet long, extends from the end of the ileum to the rectum. Water and some minerals are absorbed here. In addition, healthful bacteria in the colon actually manufacture vitamin K, as well as some biotin and folic acid. The body absorbs and uses these nutrients. One of the functions of the large intestine is to receive and store the waste products of digestion; in other words, it handles the material that has not entered the blood or lymph vessels. The waste accumulated here includes indigestible fiber from foods. Bacteria that are naturally present in the colon ferment some of

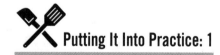

Putting It Into Practice: 1

You have a client with low blood sugar (remember, glucose is the sugar in blood). What foods would increase the blood sugar more quickly?

(Check your answer at the end of this chapter)

the fiber, producing gases. Indigestible fiber also attracts and holds water. This makes stools softer and helps prevent constipation. The large intestine stores waste material until it is released as solid feces, through the anus, the lower opening of the gastrointestinal tract.

Before the body can use any of the nutrients present in food, the nutrients must pass through the walls of the gastrointestinal tract through a process called **absorption**. Nutrients pass through the cells of the intestinal tract into the circulatory system. Two parts of the circulatory system are involved: blood and lymph. The blood and lymph are two body fluids that circulate throughout the body, delivering needed products to the cells for use. Sugars and amino acids travel into the blood, while fatty acids enter the body through the lymphatic system. Remember that fat and water do not mix. The blood is largely water-based. This is why fat cannot enter the bloodstream. Lymphatic fluid, on the other hand, can hold and carry fat. If nutrients are not absorbed into the blood or lymph at some point along the gastrointestinal tract, they are excreted in the feces.

As the blood and lymph circulate nutrients through the body, cells begin to use the nutrients in a process called metabolism. **Metabolism** refers to all the chemical processes in a cell by which nutrients are used to support life. Metabolism involves building substances (called anabolism) or breaking down substances (called catabolism). Nutrients such as glucose are split into smaller units in a catabolic reaction that releases energy to maintain body temperature or to perform work within the cell. Anabolism is the opposite of catabolism. It is the process of building substances, such as proteins, from their amino acid components.

Availability of Nutrients

An important aspect of nutrition is the bioavailability of nutrients. The term bioavailability describes how well a nutrient is absorbed and used by the body. When the process of digestion and absorption is complete, the amount of a nutrient a body actually has may differ from the amount consumed. For example, the body typically absorbs only about 10 percent of dietary iron. If the iron is from a meat source (a form called *heme iron*), absorption may rise to about 25 percent. Interestingly, studies demonstrate that individuals who have iron deficiency absorb iron more efficiently.

In addition, presence of other nutrients in the intestinal tract can have positive or negative effects on absorption. Vitamin C, for instance, seems to promote iron absorption. A person taking an iron supplement along with a glass of orange juice may enjoy better absorption and a higher bioavailability of the nutrient. Conversely, high amounts of magnesium in the gastrointestinal tract may interfere with absorption of iron and calcium. A natural compound in dark green leafy vegetables, called oxalate, can also slow down iron absorption. To absorb fat-soluble vitamins, the body generally needs some fat in the intestinal tract, too. In a food-based diet, this is easy to accomplish, because fat-soluble vitamins are found in conjunction with dietary fat.

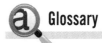

Glossary

Absorption
The process by which nutrients pass through the cells of the intestinal tract into the circulatory system

Metabolism
The chemical processes in a cell by which nutrients are used to support life

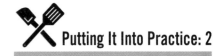

Putting It Into Practice: 2

Why is it important for us to have a bowel movement every day or two?

(Check your answer at the end of this chapter)

Figure 4.6   Digestion and Absorption Summary

Food	Digestion Locations	Outcome
Sugar	Small Intestine	Glucose
Starch	Mouth and Small Intestine	Glucose, Fructose, Galactose
Fiber	No Digestion Action	Binds some molecules; most excreted in feces
Protein	Stomach and Small Intestine	Peptides ----> Amino Acids
Fats	Milk fat begins in mouth; small amount in stomach; most is in the small intestine	Fatty Acids and Glycerol

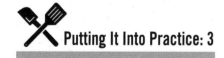

Putting It Into Practice: 3

How would you change the following meal for a person who has iron-deficiency anemia and is lactose intolerant?

- Pork Stir Fry
- Tossed salad with Blue Cheese dressing
- Butterscotch pudding parfait

(Check your answer at the end of this chapter)

Even after absorption, various factors affect how well the body can use nutrients. For example, alcohol counteracts the effects of vitamin B6 in metabolism. Many drugs, too, can affect the metabolism of nutrients. Some increase bioavailability; some decrease it.

Some people have trouble absorbing nutrients such as lactose. About three-fourths of the world population loses their ability to absorb lactose as they age. In a normal small intestine, lactose is broken down into glucose and galactose by an enzyme made in the small intestine called lactase. A person who is lactose intolerant doesn't make enough lactase or makes none at all. This may cause the person to experience pain, diarrhea, or excessive gas.

Gastrointestinal illness can affect bioavailability of nutrients, as well. If the intestines are inflamed and intestinal villi are damaged, as in Crohn's disease, adequate nutrient absorption may not take place. In another example, a poorly functioning pancreas may fail to make enough of the critical enzymes needed for digestion of protein and fat, leading to poor bioavailability of protein and fat in the body. In cases of illness, an average diet that is adequate in protein, fat, carbohydrate, vitamins, and minerals may nevertheless not be adequate to maintain good nutritional status. This is due to reduced absorption and reduced bioavailability of nutrients. For healthy people, the Recommended Dietary Allowance (RDA) levels of nutrients address ordinary factors that influence nutrient bioavailability. It's important for a Certified Dietary Manager to know, however, that established nutrient standards may not always fit the bill under various medical conditions. Thus, individual screening and assessment are important to help a Certified Dietary Manager address the unique needs of each client. Likewise, communication with medical staff and a Registered Dietitian can help assure that meals leaving the kitchen are nutritionally adequate for the population being served.

END OF CHAPTER

 Putting It Into Practice Questions & Answers

1. You have a client with low blood sugar (remember, glucose is the sugar in the blood). What foods would increase the blood sugar more quickly?

   A. *Choose foods that are digested quickly, i.e. foods high in sugar such as orange juice or hard candy.*

2. Why is it important for us to have a bowel movement every day or two?

   A. *As you have read, the digestive system is extremely important. Moving food waste all the way through the digestive system keeps the digestive system running smoothly. If food waste backs up in the rectum, the system begins to slow down. This can cause headaches, illness, or loss of appetite.*

3. How would you change this meal for a person who has iron-deficiency anemia and is lactose intolerant?
   - Pork Stir Fry
   - Tossed Salad with Blue Cheese Dressing
   - Butterscotch Pudding Parfait

   A. *Add mandarin oranges to the Pork Stir Fry. Citrus (high in vitamin C) helps to absorb iron from the pork. Replace the Blue Cheese dressing with a dressing that does not contain lactose, such as a vinaigrette. Prepare the butterscotch pudding parfait with a lactose free milk or substitute a different dessert.*

CHAPTER 5

Determine Basic Concepts of Medical Nutrition Therapy

Overview and Objectives

Medical nutrition therapy is important for the prevention and/or treatment of many diseases. A Certified Dietary Manager is often responsible for implementing therapeutic diets. Therefore, an understanding of health conditions and related diet planning is a cornerstone of the profession.

After completing this chapter, you should be able to:

✓ Review symptoms of nutritional deficiency and excess

✓ Identify basic medical nutrition terminology

✓ Define the basic concepts of medical nutritional therapy

✓ Relate basic concepts to nutritional deficiency and excess

✓ Relate basic concepts of medical nutritional therapy to diseases involving different organ systems

✓ Compare basic concepts to current diet manual or other accepted resource

✓ Explain utilization of medical nutritional therapy in long-term care and acute care settings

Diet and Health

A quote by an unknown author states, "Health is the slowest rate at which you can die." Can what you eat really affect your risk of disease? *The Report of the Dietary Guidelines Advisory Committee (DGAC) on the Dietary Guidelines for Americans, 2010,* reveals what many of us already suspect: there is a strong correlation between diet and health. Specifically, a poor diet is related to chronic diseases such as obesity, cardiovascular disease (atherosclerosis, stroke), Type 2 Diabetes, hypertension, hyperlipidemia, some cancers, and osteoporosis. These diseases are classified as problems of nutrient excess. Too much fat contributes to obesity and heart disease, while also increasing the risk of developing cancer. Too much sugar is related to Type 2 Diabetes. In the first part of the twentieth century, nutrition-related problems involved inadequate amounts of nutrients resulting in a deficiency. While those still exist today, we see these **chronic diseases** in epidemic proportions (see Figure 5.1).

As Certified Dietary Managers, you and other health professionals can provide help in dietary planning as well as serving as good individual examples. Dietary planning takes into account the actual needs of an individual or group, adjusting nutrient levels and fine tuning the balance of nutrients to promote

Figure 5.1   Leading Causes of Death—U.S., 2007

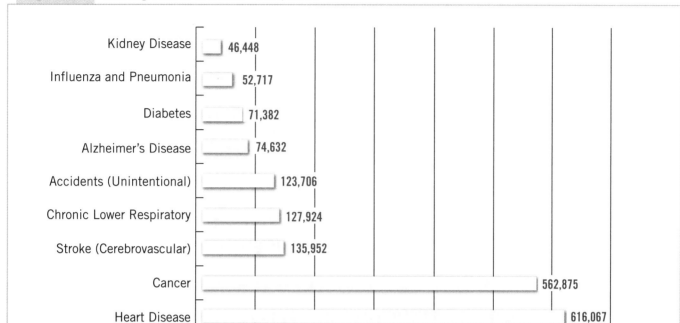

Kidney Disease — 46,448
Influenza and Pneumonia — 52,717
Diabetes — 71,382
Alzheimer's Disease — 74,632
Accidents (Unintentional) — 123,706
Chronic Lower Respiratory — 127,924
Stroke (Cerebrovascular) — 135,952
Cancer — 562,875
Heart Disease — 616,067

100,000 200,000 300,000 400,000 500,000 600,000 700,000

Thousands

Source: Centers for Disease Control and Prevention (CDC)

wellness. What exactly needs to be done can vary based on an individual's medical condition and how body systems are functioning. At times, a diet helps to compensate for unhealthy shifts in the body's metabolism and functioning. We will explore these ideas in detail throughout this chapter. This chapter is divided into four sections that addresses the following:

✓ Section A—diets for cardiac and pulmonary conditions

✓ Section B—diets for diabetes and weight management

✓ Section C—diets for gastrointestinal conditions or modified consistency

✓ Section D—renal diets and additional therapeutic needs, including cancer, renal failure, and functional disorders

Medical Nutrition Therapy (MNT)

Sometimes dietary changes are dictated by health conditions. As a group, these changes are called therapeutic or modified diets. Medical nutrition therapy is a broader term. **Medical nutrition therapy (MNT)** is the nutritional assessment and treatment of a condition, illness, or injury that places an individual at risk. It involves two components: assessment of the client's nutritional status, and treatment or intervention. Medical nutrition therapy generally focuses on individuals at risk for nutritional problems. Part of the healthcare process is to identify individuals at risk. This process is known as nutrition screening.

Treatment may include therapeutic diets, counseling, and/or the use of nutrition support. This dietary treatment goes hand-in-hand with other therapies,

 Glossary

Chronic Diseases
Degenerative diseases of body organs due in part to diet

Medical Nutrition Therapy (MNT)
Nutritional assessment and treatment for patients with an illness, disease related condition, or injury, in order to benefit the patient's own health

such as medication, surgery, physical therapy, radiation, and many others. Thus, foodservice professionals work with others on the healthcare team to address the medical therapeutic needs of patients.

A therapeutic diet is a regular diet that has been adjusted to meet a client's special nutrient needs. Diets may be adjusted to control specific nutrients. Examples include calorie-controlled diets for weight loss, fat and cholesterol-controlled diets for treatment of cardiovascular disease, and sodium-controlled diets used in hypertension or renal (kidney) disease. Even water or fluid may need to be limited—or increased—based on medical conditions. Protein needs to be limited during renal failure. Furthermore, some therapeutic diets accommodate difficulties in chewing or swallowing—such as pureed diets or dysphagia diets. Others are used in treatment of problems in the digestive system. These include clear liquid diets, very low-fat diets, and gluten-free diets. As you can already see, medical nutrition therapy is critical in the treatment of many diseases.

SECTION A Cardiac & Pulmonary Conditions

Medical Nutrition Therapy of Cardiovascular Disease

Cardiovascular disease (CVD) is a general term that refers to diseases of the heart and blood vessels. It is the number one cause of death in the U.S. About one in five Americans die of heart disease, and one in four Americans has one or more of these forms of cardiovascular disease:

✓ Coronary artery disease

✓ Stroke

✓ High blood pressure

✓ Chronic Obstructive Pulmonary Disease (COPD)

Coronary Artery Disease (CAD)

Most heart disease is the result of **atherosclerosis**, a process in which deposits of cholesterol, fat, calcium, and other substances accumulate on the inside of arteries. Atherosclerosis is also called hardening of the arteries. This process gradually reduces the amount of blood that can flow through an artery and also makes the artery less elastic and stretchy. Sometimes the buildup, also called plaque, can even close off an artery and stop blood flow completely (see Figure 5.2—Atherosclerosis).

Coronary artery disease (CAD) occurs when the coronary arteries, which supply blood to the heart, are clogged with atherosclerotic deposits. A heart attack occurs when the arteries that feed the heart muscle are blocked. In medical language, a heart attack is called a **myocardial infarction (MI)**. If part of the heart muscle is denied oxygen, it dies. A piece of the heart is damaged and no longer contracts, so the heart works less efficiently. A heart attack may develop slowly or suddenly. Major symptoms and warning signs are:

✓ Chest discomfort that lasts several minutes or longer. This may feel like pressure, squeezing, fullness or pain.

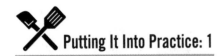

Putting It Into Practice: 1

Can you guess (a) how many, and, (b) which of the leading causes of death are directly related to diet?

(Check your answer at the end of this chapter)

✓ Discomfort in other areas of the upper body, such as one or both arms, the back, neck, jaw, or stomach.

✓ Shortness of breath

✓ Breaking out in a cold sweat

✓ Nausea or light-headedness

Many of the risk factors for coronary heart disease have nutrition connections. Let's look more closely at one of these factors—high blood cholesterol, or hyperlipidemia. Cholesterol travels through the bloodstream in little clusters of proteins and lipids called lipoproteins. Usually, we distinguish blood cholesterol measurements into two types: Low-Density Lipoproteins (LDL) and High-Density Lipoproteins (HDL).

Low-Density Lipoproteins (LDL), or "bad cholesterol," carries most of the cholesterol in the blood. Cholesterol and fat from LDLs are the main source of dangerous buildup and blockage in the arteries. Thus, the higher the LDL cholesterol level, the greater the risk of heart disease. As a memory aid, you can also think of LDL as "L= lousy" cholesterol.

Figure 5.2   Atherosclerosis

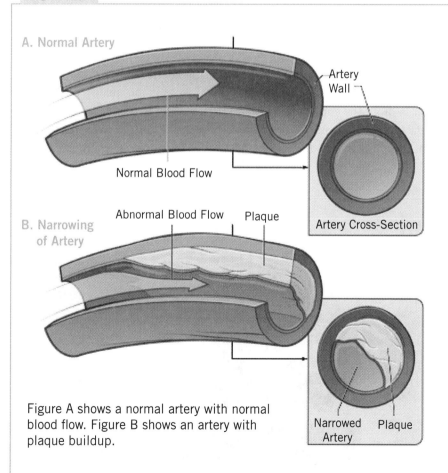

A. Normal Artery

Artery Wall

Normal Blood Flow

Artery Cross-Section

B. Narrowing of Artery

Abnormal Blood Flow   Plaque

Narrowed Artery   Plaque

Figure A shows a normal artery with normal blood flow. Figure B shows an artery with plaque buildup.

National Heart, Lung, Blood Institute: www.nhlbi.nih.gov, August 6, 2010.

 Glossary

Atherosclerosis
When plaque builds up in the arteries

Myocardial Infarction (MI)
Heart attack

Low-Density Lipoproteins (LDL)
The lipoprotein that carries most of the cholesterol in the blood—"lousy" cholesterol

High-Density Lipoproteins (HDL)
The lipoprotein that carries cholesterol away from body organs to the liver—"healthy" cholesterol

CVD
Cardiovascular disease

High-Density Lipoproteins (HDL), or "good cholesterol," carries cholesterol away from body organs and takes it to the liver for destruction. Think of HDL as cholesterol that is on its way out of the body. A high level of HDL is a favorable health indicator. As a memory aid, you can think of HDL as "H=healthy" cholesterol.

Triglyceride is the most common type of fat in the body and in food. Triglycerides are made up of three fatty acid units and one unit of glycerol. Triglyceride levels can increase from excess carbohydrates in the diet or excess alcohol. A high triglyceride level combined with low HDL cholesterol or high LDL cholesterol increases the onset of atherosclerosis.

For HDL, high numbers are better. A level less than 40 mg/dl is low and is considered a major risk factor because it increases the risk of developing heart disease. HDL levels of 60 mg/dl or more help to lower the risk. Triglyceride levels are borderline high at 150-199 mg/dl or high at over 200 mg/dl.

More than 90 million Americans have blood cholesterol levels that present risks for heart disease. Reaching and/or maintaining a normal weight, exercising, and limiting fat and cholesterol in the diet can all help adjust LDL and HDL levels to a healthier profile. Drugs are also used for this purpose. Keep in mind that the preventive goal is to reduce LDL and raise HDL. The National Cholesterol Education Program provides guidelines for cholesterol levels, shown in Figure 5.3.

Relationship between Saturated Fats and Cardiovascular Disease. To control risk factors for heart disease, the critical issue is the quality of fat in the American diet. The consumption of fats such as saturated fatty acids (SFA) and trans-fatty acids increases the risk of cardiovascular disease. Unsaturated fats, such as monounsaturated and polyunsaturated fatty acids, promote health. In

Figure 5.3 **Cholesterol Guidelines**

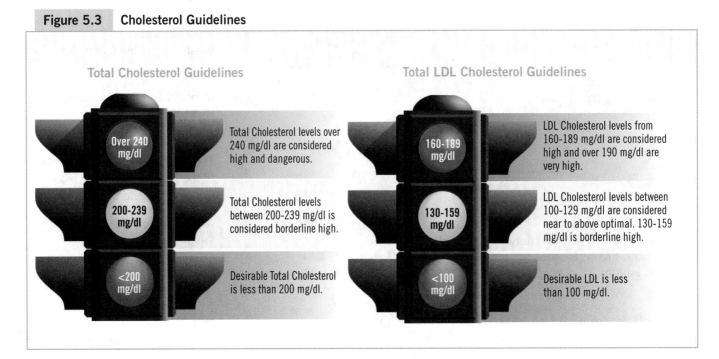

Total Cholesterol Guidelines

- Over 240 mg/dl: Total Cholesterol levels over 240 mg/dl are considered high and dangerous.
- 200-239 mg/dl: Total Cholesterol levels between 200-239 mg/dl is considered borderline high.
- <200 mg/dl: Desirable Total Cholesterol is less than 200 mg/dl.

Total LDL Cholesterol Guidelines

- 160-189 mg/dl: LDL Cholesterol levels from 160-189 mg/dl are considered high and over 190 mg/dl are very high.
- 130-159 mg/dl: LDL Cholesterol levels between 100-129 mg/dl are considered near to above optimal. 130-159 mg/dl is borderline high.
- <100 mg/dl: Desirable LDL is less than 100 mg/dl.

Figure 5.4 Comparison of Saturated Fat in Common Food Choices

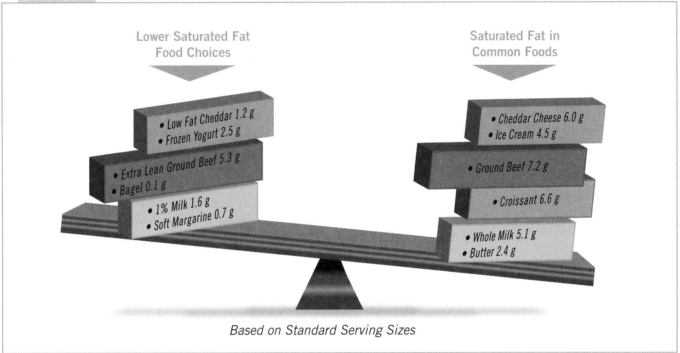

Lower Saturated Fat
Food Choices

Saturated Fat in
Common Foods

- Low Fat Cheddar 1.2 g
- Frozen Yogurt 2.5 g
- Extra Lean Ground Beef 5.3 g
- Bagel 0.1 g
- 1% Milk 1.6 g
- Soft Margarine 0.7 g

- Cheddar Cheese 6.0 g
- Ice Cream 4.5 g
- Ground Beef 7.2 g
- Croissant 6.6 g
- Whole Milk 5.1 g
- Butter 2.4 g

Based on Standard Serving Sizes

the past, recommendations have been made to limit the total amount of fat in the diet. Today, there is more evidence to indicate that decreasing saturated fat and trans-fatty acids are more effective at decreasing CVD than limiting total fat intake. It is important to note that we do not react to decreases in dietary fat in a uniform way. The effects of dietary fat are dependent on many factors such as physical activity, life style habits, and genetics.

To lower LDL cholesterol through diet, it is important to choose foods low in saturated fat and trans-fatty acids. Saturated fat is found in greater amounts in foods from animals. Decreasing animal foods or using lower fat choices will help reduce saturated fat in the diet. *The Report of the DGAC on the Dietary Guidelines for Americans, 2010* did find that a five percent decrease in consumption of SFAs, replaced by mono-or polyunsaturated fats, resulted in a reduction of CVD risk. Saturated fat should be limited to 7 percent of the diet. Figure 5.4 compares saturated fat in some common food choices.

Whenever possible, it is best to substitute unsaturated fat for saturated fat. Unsaturated fat is usually liquid at room temperature and can be either mono-unsaturated or polyunsaturated. Examples of foods high in monounsaturated fat are olive and canola oils. Those high in polyunsaturated fat include safflower, sunflower, corn, and soybean oils. Experts advise limiting trans-fatty acids in the diet. These fats raise total cholesterol and LDL cholesterol. Trans-fatty acids are produced when oils are partially hydrogenated (partially solidified) to make margarine. They appear in many types of stick margarines, and are also ingredients in some commercial baked goods. New FDA labeling regulations require manufacturers to show trans-fatty acid content on Nutrition Facts Labels.

Foods high in starch and fiber are excellent substitutes for foods high in saturated fat. These foods—breads, cereals, pasta, grain, fruits, and vegetables—are low in saturated fat and cholesterol. They are also usually lower in calories. In addition, research indicates that some forms of fiber may help reduce blood cholesterol (LDL) levels. Specifically using plant-based sources for much of the dietary protein is beneficial in reducing (LDL) cholesterol. In addition, some research indicates that meat-based protein, even aside from its fat content, may stimulate (LDL) cholesterol levels. So, reducing meat-based protein is a good idea. Other nutritional factors that can favorably influence blood cholesterol include omega-3 fatty acids (found primarily in fish), garlic, and green tea.

Relationship between Cholesterol and Cardio Vascular Disease (CVD). Decreasing saturated fat and trans-fatty acids has been shown to be more effective in combating CVD than decreasing cholesterol intake. Throughout the past forty years, there has been much information published about the risk of increasing cholesterol from eating foods high in cholesterol, specifically eggs. *The Report of the DGAC on the Dietary Guidelines for Americans, 2010* indicates that consuming one egg per day does not increase serum cholesterol or triglycerides. However, for people with Type 2 Diabetes, consuming one egg per day does have a detrimental effect on serum cholesterol and increases the risk for CVD. Figure 5.5 offers suggestions for choosing foods low in saturated fat and cholesterol.

Dietary cholesterol can raise blood cholesterol levels, although usually not as much as saturated fat. High cholesterol foods include egg yolks, liver, the fat in meats and poultry, shellfish, and dairy fat (cream, whole milk, regular cheeses, etc.). (Cholesterol is found only in foods of animal origin.) Cholesterol intake of less than 300 mg per day is recommended.

Experts also advise maintaining a healthy weight. People who are overweight tend to have higher blood cholesterol levels than people of a healthy weight. Overweight adults with an "apple" shape—bigger (pot) belly—tend to have a higher risk for heart disease than those with a "pear" shape—bigger hips and thighs. For anyone who is overweight, losing even a little weight can help to lower LDL and raise HDL. Being physically active and controlling caloric intake helps with weight management, while lowering LDL.

Drug Treatment. Drug treatment is considered appropriate for adults who have a high LDL level, especially if they also have other CAD risk factors. Drugs referred to as bile acid sequestrants, such as cholestyramine, are approved for use in clients with high LDL levels who don't respond to dietary changes alone. Constipation is the most common side effect. Niacin-containing drugs are also used to bring down cholesterol levels. Side effects, which may include flushing, itching, and upset stomach, limit its use for some people. Another drug category, used in addition to Medical Nutrition Therapy, that is effective in lowering your total and LDL cholesterol is called statins. Examples of statin drugs are atorvastatin (Lipitor®), simvastatin (Zocor®), lovastatin (Mevacor®), pravastatin (Pravachol®), and rosuvastatin (Crestor®). The most common side effect is muscle or joint pain although nausea, constipation, and diarrhea may

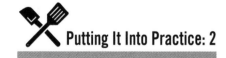

Putting It Into Practice: 2

How would you adjust the following recipe to lower the saturated fat grams?

Baked Custard

- 3 slightly beaten eggs
- ¼ cup sugar
- ¼ tsp. salt
- 2 cups milk
- 1 tsp. vanilla

(Check your answer at the end of this chapter)

Figure 5.5   Choosing Foods Low in Saturated Fat and Cholesterol

MEAT, POULTRY, FISH, AND SHELLFISH

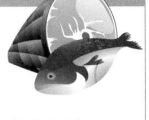

Buying Tips

- Choose lean cuts of meat. Look for meats labeled "lean" or "extra lean." Eat moderate portions— no more than about 6 ounces a day (a 3 ounce portion is about the size of a deck of cards).

- Limit organ meats like liver, sweetbreads, and kidneys. Organ meats are high in cholesterol, even though they are fairly low in fat.

- Limit high-fat processed meats like bacon, bologna, salami, hot dogs, and sausage. Some chicken and turkey hot dogs are lower in saturated fat and total fat than pork and beef hot dogs. There are also "lean" beef hot dogs that are low in fat and saturated fat. Usually, processed poultry products have more fat and cholesterol than fresh poultry. To be sure, check the nutrition label on deli products to find those that are lowest in fat and saturated fat.

- Try fresh ground turkey or chicken made from white meat, like the breast.

- Limit use of goose and duck. They are higher in saturated fat, even with the skin removed.

- Choose shellfish only occasionally. Squid, shrimp, and oysters are fairly high in cholesterol; scallops, mussels, and clams are low in cholesterol.

- Buy canned fish packed in water, not oil.

Preparation Tips

- Trim fat from meat and remove skin from poultry before eating.

- Bake, broil, microwave, poach, or roast instead of frying. If frying, use a nonstick pan and nonstick cooking spray or a small amount of vegetable oil to reduce the fat.

- When roasting meat, place the meat on a rack so the fat can drip away.

- Brown ground meat and drain well before adding other ingredients.

- Use fat free ingredients like fruit juice, wine, or defatted broth to baste meats and poultry.

DAIRY FOODS

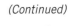

Buying Tips

- Choose skim or 1% milk, rather than 2% or whole milk.

- When looking for hard cheese, select versions that are labeled fat-free, reduced-fat, low-fat, light, or part skim.

- When shopping for soft cheeses, choose low-fat (1%) or nonfat cottage cheese, farmer cheese, pot cheese, or part skim or light ricotta.

- Use low-fat or nonfat yogurt; try it in recipes or as a topping.

- Try low-fat or fat-free sour cream or cream cheese blends for spreads, toppings, or in recipes.

Preparation Tips

- Try low-fat cheese in casseroles, or try a sharp-flavored regular cheese and use less than the recipe calls for. Save most of the cheese for the top.

- Use skim, 1% or evaporated skim milk for cream soups or white sauces.

(Continued)

| Figure 5.5 | Choosing Foods Low in Saturated Fat and Cholesterol *(Continued)* |

EGGS

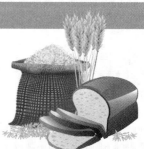

Buying Tips

- Eggs are included in many processed foods and baked goods. Look at the nutrition label to check the cholesterol content.

- Try egg substitutes.

Preparation Tips

- Substitute two egg whites for one whole egg in recipes. (Egg whites are cholesterol-free.) Or, use egg substitutes.

FRUITS AND VEGETABLES

Buying Tips

- Buy fruits and vegetables often—fresh, frozen, or canned. They have no cholesterol and most are low in saturated fat. Also, most fruits and vegetables, except avocados, coconut, and olives, are low in total fat.

Preparation Tips

- Use fruits as a snack or dessert.

- Prepare vegetables as snacks, side dishes, and salads. Season with herbs, spices, lemon juice, or fat-free or low-fat mayonnaise. Limit use of regular mayonnaise, salad dressings, and cream, cheese, or other fatty sauces.

BREADS, CEREALS, PASTA, RICE, AND DRY PEAS AND BEANS

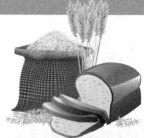

Buying Tips

- Use whole grain breads, rolls, and cereals often.

- Limit baked goods made with large amounts of fat, especially saturated fat, such as: croissants, biscuits, doughnuts, butter rolls, muffins, coffee cake, Danish pastry. Avoid baked goods listing palm, palm kernel, and coconut oils as ingredients. These oils are high in saturated fats, even though they are vegetable oils.

- Choose ready-to-eat cereals often. Most are low in saturated fat, except for granola, muesli, or oat-bran types made with coconut or coconut oil.

- Buy dry peas and beans often.

Preparation Tips

- Try pasta or rice in soups, or with low-fat sauces as main dishes or casseroles.

- Stretch meat dishes with pasta or vegetables for hearty meals.

- Bake homemade muffins and quick breads using unsaturated vegetable oils; substitute two egg whites for each egg yolk, or use egg substitutes. Experiment with substituting applesauce for oil or cut back the amount of oil in the recipe. For each two cups of flour, only ¼ cup of vegetable oil is necessary.

- Use dry peas and beans as the main ingredient in casseroles, soups, or other one-dish meals.

occur. There may be potentially serious side effects if you have liver or kidney disease. If statins are effective at lowering your LDL cholesterol, you may be on it for your lifetime.

Stroke

Stroke is the third leading cause of death in the U.S., after heart disease and cancer. About 500,000 Americans have a stroke each year. Of these, 150,000 people die while another 200,000 are left with some disability. A **stroke** occurs when blood vessels bringing oxygen to the brain burst or become clogged. The interruption of blood flow to the brain stops body functions and damages nerve cells. The brain must have a continuous supply of blood rich in oxygen and nutrients for energy. If deprived of blood flow for more than a few minutes, brains cells die. The functions these cells control—such as speech, muscle movement, or comprehension—die with them.

The majority of strokes are caused by blockages in the arteries that supply blood to the brain. The blockages may be caused by a clot, also called thrombus, that forms on the inner lining of a brain or neck artery already partly clogged by atherosclerotic plaque. A blood clot formed in another part of the body may also cause a stroke. Usually a wandering clot like this—called an embolus—breaks off from plaque in an artery wall, or originates in the heart. The most serious kinds of stroke occur not from blockage, but from hemorrhage. A hemorrhage occurs when a spot in a brain artery weakened by disease—usually high blood pressure or atherosclerosis—ruptures and leaks blood. If an artery inside the brain ruptures, it is called a cerebral hemorrhage. Sometimes, hemorrhage may be caused by an aneurysm, a section of the artery wall so thin that it may balloon out and burst, especially when high blood pressure is present.

Relationship Between Stroke and Diet. As you have read, a stroke can occur because of a blockage caused by atherosclerosis. Following the Medical Nutrition Therapy for atherosclerosis may improve your risk of a stroke. If a stroke occurs, the effects can range in severity from a slight one-sided facial sagging that disappears within two weeks, to inability to walk, inability to talk, or loss of control of bodily functions. Some stroke victims have trouble chewing and/or swallowing foods. In addition, some experience poor orientation, e.g. inability to find food on the plate. Both factors can place individuals at risk for malnutrition. The kind of disability a stroke victim is left with depends on the location and extent of brain damage. The brain is resourceful. After brain swelling goes down following a stroke, small blood vessels around the blocked area enlarge to allow more blood flow to the damaged section. Some incapacitated cells may recover partially or completely. In many cases, other brain cells can assume the functions of the damaged ones.

An incident involving physical symptoms that lasts less than 24 hours and leaves no permanent disability is called a transient ischemic attack (TIA) or "mini-stroke." Some individuals have repeated attacks of TIAs without any serious consequences, but these symptoms should not be ignored and need immediate medical attention.

High Blood Pressure

Hypertension is a medical condition involving chronic high blood pressure. High blood pressure means that the heart has to pump harder than it should to get blood to all the parts of the body. Because high blood pressure usually doesn't give early warning signs, it is known as the "silent killer." Hypertension raises chances of experiencing a stroke, a heart attack, and kidney problems. The higher the blood pressure, the greater the risk. An estimated 60 million people, more than a third of the adult population, have hypertension. Each year, half a million strokes and over a million heart attacks result from hypertension.

With the Dietary Guidelines for Americans, 2010, comes a heightened concern about increasing blood pressure levels in children and teens. Studies have shown that high blood pressure in youth increases the development of atherosclerosis. Blood pressure rises with age as a normal part of growth. With the increase in blood pressure levels in children, an increase in the number of adults with hypertension is probable.

Blood pressure is expressed as a fraction, such as 120/80 millimeters of mercury (abbreviated as "mmHg"). The numerator (120) is called the **systolic pressure**—the pressure of blood within arteries when the heart is pumping. The denominator (80) is called the **diastolic pressure**—the pressure in the arteries when the heart is resting between beats. A typical blood pressure for a young adult might be 120/80 mmHg. Hypertension Stage 1 (see Figure 5.6) is the most common form of high blood pressure. To be diagnosed as hypertensive, a person has had at least two to three readings performed on each of three separate visits.

When persistently elevated blood pressure is due to a medical problem, such as hormonal abnormality or an inherited narrowing of the aorta (the largest artery leading from the heart), it's called secondary hypertension. This means the high blood pressure is secondary to another condition. The causes of most cases of hypertension are unknown, however. These cases are known as essential hypertension. Because the cause remains a mystery, essential hypertension cannot be cured. But it can be controlled. Treatment of clients with

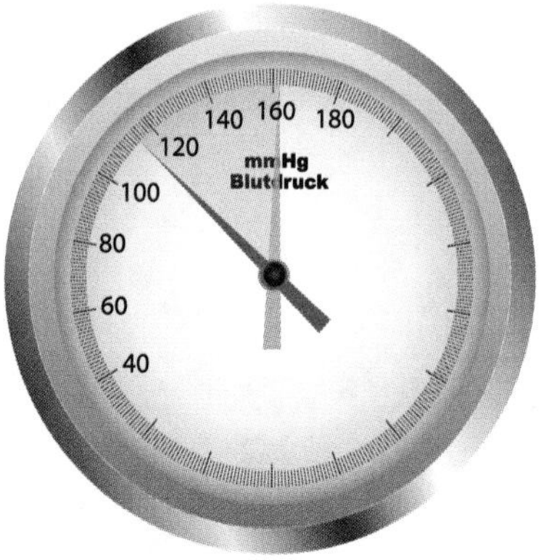

Figure 5.6 Categories for Blood Pressure Levels in Adults (in mmHg, or millimeters of mercury)

Category	Systolic (top number)		Diastolic (bottom number)
Normal	Less than 120	*And*	Less than 80
Prehypertension	120-139	*Or*	80-89
High blood pressure			
Stage 1	140-159	*Or*	90-99
Stage 2	160 or higher	*Or*	100 or higher

Source: National Heart, Lung, and Blood Institute, 2008

hypertension is long-term and includes lifestyle modifications and possibly medications. Lifestyle modifications include weight reduction, increased physical activity, medical nutrition therapy, moderation of alcohol intake, and tobacco avoidance.

When lifestyle modifications do not succeed in lowering blood pressure enough, drugs are the next step. Reducing blood pressure with drugs clearly decreases the incidence of cardiovascular death and disease. Two classes of antihypertensive drugs—diuretics and beta blockers—are common for initial drug therapy. **Diuretics** are a class of blood pressure medications that cause increased urine output. Some cause an increased excretion of potassium in the urine, and a client may need to eat high potassium foods. Beta blockers reduce the heart rate so that the heart puts out less blood.

Medical Nutrition Therapy. Often, nutritional advice for hypertension includes suggestions about sodium intake. Sodium is the main mineral in salt. The current recommendation is to reduce sodium intake to less than 1,500 mg of sodium daily. Interestingly, reducing dietary sodium is not effective for everyone who has hypertension. Scientists estimate that about half of people with hypertension are sensitive to sodium. For them, reducing dietary sodium may be very effective. See Figure 5.7 for sodium recommendations.

One level teaspoon of salt provides about 2,300 milligrams of sodium. However, most people do not obtain the majority of their sodium by adding salt to foods. In fact, about 75 percent of our dietary sodium is added to food during processing and manufacturing. Figure 5.8 illustrates sodium content of many foods. Besides salt, common sources of sodium in the diet are:

✓ Processed foods with salt or other sodium-containing compounds added

✓ Other sodium-containing compounds, such as baking soda, baking powder, monosodium glutamate (MSG), and soy sauce

✓ Foods in which sodium is naturally present. Milk and milk products are somewhat high in sodium.

✓ In some areas, the water supply supplies 10 percent of an individual's daily sodium consumption. Sodium is often present in water that has gone through a water softening device.

✓ Some medications, such as some antacids

With the Dietary Guidelines for Americans, 2010, comes a significant change in the recommendation for dietary sodium. In the past, a typical sodium restricted diet was described as a No Added Salt diet or a 4 gram (4000 mg) Sodium diet. This typically eliminated adding salt at the table and some very high-sodium foods. Another type of therapeutic diet was a 2 Gram (2000mg) Sodium diet or Sodium Controlled Diet, which added limiting milk, regular bread, and starch foods to the previous limitations. The Report of the DGAC on the Dietary Guidelines for Americans, 2010, suggests that besides individuals controlling their sodium intake, the efforts "must be accompanied by an overall reduction of the level of sodium in the food supply." Current nutrient label claims for sodium is shown in Figure 5.11. Both sodium and potassium

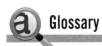

Glossary

Hypertension
Medical condition involving chronic high blood pressure

Systolic Pressure
The top number of the blood pressure reading

Diastolic Pressure
The bottom number or the denominator of the blood pressure reading. A tip to remember is that both diastolic and denominator begin with a "d."

Diuretics
A class of blood pressure medications that cause increased urine output

Stroke
When blood vessels bringing oxygen to the brain burst or become clogged

Figure 5.7	Recent Sodium Recommendations of Scientific and Public Health Agencies and Organizations	
Organizations	Date Published	Sodium Recommendation
U.S. ADULTS		
American Heart Association	2010	**Sodium:** <1,500 mg per day for adults. The recommendation for 1,500 mg/d does not apply to individuals who lose large volumes of sodium in sweat, such as competitive athletes and workers exposed to extreme heat stress (e.g., foundry workers and firefighters), or to those directed otherwise by their healthcare provider (Lloyd-Jones, 2010). Web reference (accessed 23 March 2010): http://circ.ahajournals.org/cgi/content/full/112/13/2061
American Society of Hypertension	2009	Lower sodium intake as much as possible, with a goal of no more than 2,300 mg/d in the general population and no more than 1,500 mg/d in Blacks, middle- and older-aged persons, and individuals with hypertension, diabetes, or chronic kidney disease (Appel, 2009). Web reference (accessed 23 March 2010): http://www.ash-us.org/assets-new/pub/pdf_files/DietaryApproachesLowerBP.pdf
U.S. CHILDREN		
American Academy of Pediatrics	2006	Adopted American Heart Association Position. Sodium recommendation by age: 1-3 yrs <1,500 mg; 4-8 yrs <1,900 mg; 9-13 yrs <2,200 mg; 14-18 yrs <2,300 mg (AHA/Gidding et al., 2006). Web reference (accessed 9 March 2010): http://pediatrics.aappublications.org/cgi/content/full/117/2/544
Academy of Nutrition And Dietetics (AND) formerly known as American Dietetic Association (ADA)	2008	The current recommendation for adequate daily sodium intake for children 4-8 yrs is 1,200 mg/day, and for older children 1,500 mg/day (ADA, 2008). http://www.adajournal.org/article/S0002-8223(08)00496-3/abstract

Adapted from the Report of the DGAC Dietary Guidelines for Americans, 2010, Part D, Section 6, pg. 5 http://www.cnpp.usda.gov/DGAs2010-DGACReport.htm. Accessed August 8, 2010.

are frequently listed as NA or K on a diet order. A 2 gram sodium diet might also be a 2 gram NA diet. An increased potassium diet might be listed as increased K diet. See Figure 5.10 for tips on reducing sodium intake.

Another factor that may impact Medical Nutrition Therapy is potassium intake. Today, average intake of dietary potassium is below the recommended levels of 4700 mg per day. Because increasing dietary potassium has been shown to lower blood pressure, therapeutic diets should emphasize both a lower sodium intake and an increased potassium intake. Figure 5.9 shows a few good to excellent food sources of potassium. For a more extensive food list, see Appendix E.

One diet that addresses both reduced sodium and increased potassium is the DASH diet. The DASH diet stands for Dietary Approaches to Stop Hypertension and was designed to treat hypertension. The DASH diet is part of the National High Blood Pressure Education Program stemming from the National Institute of Health. There are several versions of the DASH diet. The version selected for this chapter is the one that best addresses the Dietary Guidelines for Americans, 2010. Figure 5.12 shows a comparison of the DASH diet guidelines to the usual U.S. intake and the USDA Base Pattern. As you can see, the

Figure 5.8 Food Sources of Sodium

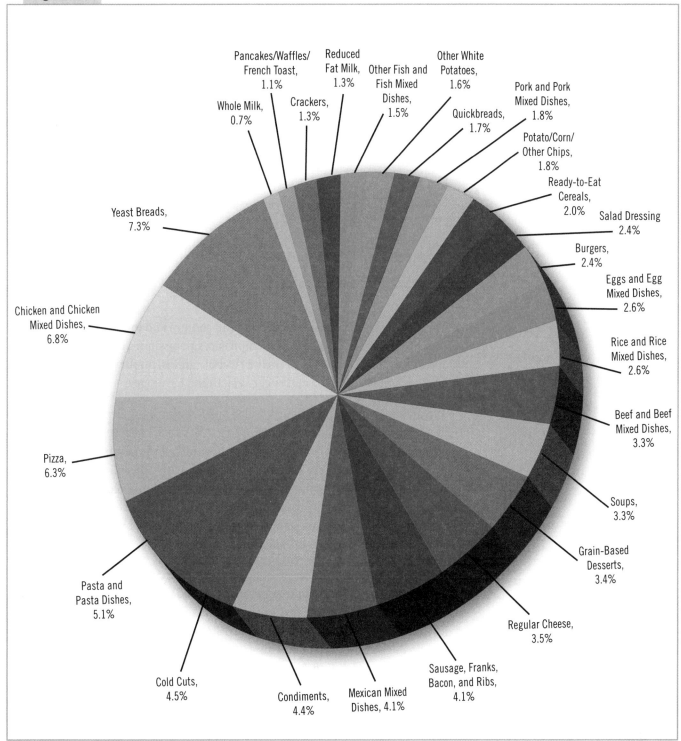

Pancakes/Waffles/French Toast, 1.1%
Reduced Fat Milk, 1.3%
Other Fish and Fish Mixed Dishes, 1.5%
Other White Potatoes, 1.6%
Whole Milk, 0.7%
Crackers, 1.3%
Quickbreads, 1.7%
Pork and Pork Mixed Dishes, 1.8%
Potato/Corn/Other Chips, 1.8%
Ready-to-Eat Cereals, 2.0%
Salad Dressing 2.4%
Yeast Breads, 7.3%
Burgers, 2.4%
Eggs and Egg Mixed Dishes, 2.6%
Chicken and Chicken Mixed Dishes, 6.8%
Rice and Rice Mixed Dishes, 2.6%
Beef and Beef Mixed Dishes, 3.3%
Pizza, 6.3%
Soups, 3.3%
Grain-Based Desserts, 3.4%
Pasta and Pasta Dishes, 5.1%
Regular Cheese, 3.5%
Cold Cuts, 4.5%
Condiments, 4.4%
Mexican Mixed Dishes, 4.1%
Sausage, Franks, Bacon, and Ribs, 4.1%

Sources of Sodium Among the US Population, 2005-2006. Risk Factor Monitoring and Methods Branch. Applied Research Program. National Cancer Institute. Printed in the Report of the DGAC Dietary Guidelines for Americans, 2010, Part D. Section 6, pg. 19 http://www.cnpp.usda.gov/DGAs2010-DGACReport.htm Accessed August 8, 2010.

Figure 5.9	Food Sources of Potassium
Measurement	Food Source
738	Baked Potato, 1 small
595	White Beans, ½ cup
556	Tomato Juice, 1 cup
531	Plain Low-Fat Yogurt, 8 oz.
542	Sweet Potato, 1 medium
496	Fresh Orange Juice, 1 cup
425	Low-Fat Chocolate Milk, 1 cup
422	Banana, 1 medium
400	Spinach, cooked, ½ cup
371	Pork Loin, 3 oz.

usual U.S. intake is considerably higher in sodium and lower in potassium than the DASH diet. The DASH diet emphasizes potassium-rich vegetables, fruits, and low-fat milk products. It includes whole grains, poultry, fish, and nuts, and limits red meats, sweets, and sugar-containing beverages.

The National Institutes of Health also suggests limiting alcohol consumption to no more than 1 ounce of ethanol (e.g., 24 ounce beer, 10 ounce wine, or 2 ounce 100-proof whiskey) per day for most men and no more than 0.5 ounce per day for women. Very much in accordance with other dietary guidance for health, a DASH diet includes plenty of fresh fruits and vegetables, as well as low-fat or fat-free dairy products. Note that dairy products are rich sources of calcium. Calcium appears to have a protective role in managing hypertension, so maintaining adequate calcium intake is important.

Note that limiting sodium does not mean sacrificing flavor. Often, reducing sodium intake requires some adjustment and adaptation. People who have become accustomed to reduced sodium intake may find that they begin to enjoy other flavors in foods more. Figure 5.13 lists some ideas for creating herb blends useful as replacements for salt. In addition, many excellent cookbooks provide advice for seasoning foods with herbs and spices.

Congestive Heart Failure. Another common disease of the circulatory system is called **congestive heart failure (CHF)**. Atherosclerosis and hypertension can both lead to this condition, in which the heart itself weakens. In an effort to provide adequate circulation throughout the body, the heart works harder and harder, but is not highly effective. The heart beats faster and becomes enlarged. This can lead to fluid retention in the body, as well as a certain degree of malnutrition. Malnutrition occurs as the blood fails to deliver adequate oxygen and nutrients to body tissues. Due to excess fluid, however, an individual with CHF may not look malnourished. Experts estimate that at least 5 million Americans have CHF, and the National Institutes of Health project that this

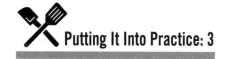

Putting It Into Practice: 3

If a diet order is written as 2 gm NA, what does this mean?

(Check your answer at the end of this chapter)

Figure 5.10 Tips for Reducing Sodium Intake

- Choose low or reduced sodium, or no-salt-added versions of foods and condiments when available.

- Buy vegetables fresh, frozen, or canned with no salt added.

- Use fresh poultry, fish, and lean meat, rather than canned, smoked, or processed types.

- Choose ready-to-eat breakfast cereals that are lower in sodium.

- Limit cured foods (such as bacon and ham), foods packed in brine (such as pickles, pickled vegetables, olives, and sauerkraut), and condiments (such as MSG, mustard, horseradish, catsup, and barbecue sauce). Limit even lower sodium versions of soy sauce and teriyaki sauce. Treat these condiments like table salt. Replace pickles and olives with fresh lettuce, greens, or tomatoes.

- Replace high-sodium cheeses and peanut butter with low-sodium varieties.

- Use spices instead of salt. In cooking and at the table, flavor foods with herbs, spices, lemon, lime, vinegar, or salt-free seasoning blends. Start by cutting salt in half.

- Cook rice, pasta, and hot cereals without salt. Cut back on instant or flavored rice, pasta, and cereal mixes, which usually have added salt.

- Choose convenience foods that are lower in sodium. Cut back on frozen dinners, mixed dishes such as pizza, packaged mixes, canned soups or broths, and salad dressings, as these often have a lot of sodium.

- Rinse canned foods, such as tuna, to remove some sodium.

- Use unsalted pretzels or crackers, or fresh fruits and vegetables to replace salty snack foods.

- Use fresh or frozen vegetables instead of canned, or choose low-sodium canned foods.

Compiled from National Heart, Lung, and Blood Institute and other sources.

Figure 5.11 Nutrient Label Claims for Sodium

Label	Claim
Sodium Free	Less than 5 mg of sodium
Very Low Sodium	35 mg or less of sodium
Low sodium	140 mg or less of sodium
Reduced or Less Sodium	At least 25% less sodium than the usual food product
Light in Sodium	At least 50% less sodium than the usual food product

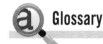 **Glossary**

Congestive Heart Failure (CHF)
Inability of the heart to effectively pump blood to the body's organs—can be due to coronary artery disease

Chronic Obstructive Pulmonary Disease (COPD)
A group of lung diseases that includes chornic bronchitis, emphysema, and asmatic bronchitis

condition may become a new epidemic. Dietary treatment typically includes a sodium restricted diet, e.g. 2 Gram Sodium diet. This is because the body may not be able to rid itself of extra sodium, and sodium can contribute to fluid retention. A fluid restriction may also be necessary. Dietary treatments for underlying conditions, such as atherosclerosis and hypertension, are also recommended. If a client is overweight, effective weight management may also reduce the burden on the heart.

Dietary Pattern Comparison, Current U.S. Intake, DASH-Sodium Diet, and USDA Food Patterns
Figure 5.12 **(adjusted to 2000 Calories)**

Dietary Pattern	Usual US Intake: Adults	DASH with Reduced Sodium	USDA Base Pattern
Citation	NHANES 2001-04; 2005-06; Ages 19+	Karanja et al, 1999 and Lin et al., 2003	Britten et al., 2006
NUTRIENTS			
Calories	2000	2000	2000
Carbohydrates (% total kcal)	48.4%	58%	56.7%
Protein (% total kcal)	15.2%	18%	15.2%
Total Fat (% total kcal)	33.5%	27%	32%
Saturated Fat (% total kcal)	10.9%	6%	8.4%
Monounsaturated (% total kcal)	12.5%	10%	12.0%
Polyunsaturated (% total kcal)	6.8%	8%	9.0%
Cholesterol (mg)	269	143	229
Fiber (g)	15	29	30
Potassium (mg)	2909	4371	3478
Sodium (mg)	2846	1095	1722
FOOD GROUPS			
Vegetables total (cup)	1.6	2.1	2.5
Fruits and Juices (cup)	1.0	2.5	2
Grains total (oz.)	6.4	7.3	6
Whole Grains (oz.)	0.6	3.9	3
Milk and Milk Products (cup)	1.5	0.7	—
Low-Fat Milk (cup)	Not Described	1.9	3
ANIMAL PROTEINS			
Meat (oz.)	2.5	1.4	2.5
Poultry (oz.)	1.2	1.7	1.5
Eggs (oz.)	0.4	Not Described	0.4
Fish (total oz.)	0.5	1.4	0.5
PLANT PROTEINS			
Legumes (oz.)	Not Described	0.4	See Vegetables
Nuts and Seeds (oz.)	0.5	0.9	0.6
Oils (g)	17.7	24.8	27
Solid Fats (g)	43.2	Not Described	16
Added Sugar (g)	79.0	12 (Snacks/Sweets)	32
Alcohol (g)	9.9	No Recommendation	No Recommendation

Usual US Intakes – WWEIA, NHANES 2001-2004 and WWEIA, NHANES 2005-2006, one-day mean intakes consumed per individual. Male and female intakes adjusted to 2000 calories, averaged, and rounded to one decimal point. Adapted from the Report of the DGAC on the Dietary Guidelines, 2010, Section B, Table B2.4, pg. B2-22

Figure 5.13   Herb Blends to Replace Salt

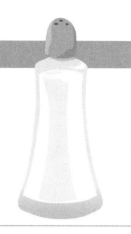

These can be placed in shakers and used instead of salt:

- Saltless Surprise: 2 tsp. garlic powder and 1 tsp. each of basil, oregano, and powdered lemon rind (or dehydrated lemon juice). Put ingredients into a blender and mix well. Store in glass container, label well, and add rice to prevent caking.
- Pungent Salt Substitute: 3 tsp. basil, 2 tsp. each of savory (summer savory is best), celery seed, ground cumin seed, sage, marjoram, and 1 tsp. lemon thyme. Mix well, then powder with a mortar and pestle.
- Spicy Saltless Seasoning: 1 tsp. each of cloves, pepper, and coriander seed (crushed), 1 tsp. paprika, and 1 Tbsp. rosemary. Mix ingredients in a blender. Store in airtight container.

Chronic Obstructive Pulmonary Disease (COPD)

Chronic obstructive pulmonary disease (COPD) is group of diseases that includes chronic bronchitis, emphysema and asthmatic bronchitis. These afflictions reduce the airflow out of the lungs. The most common symptom is shortness of breath. COPD is a leading cause of disability and death in the U.S., and 90 percent of cases result from smoking. COPD can cause malnutrition due to loss of appetite, changes in taste, or gastrointestinal distress. In addition, COPD can make the body work harder to breathe. This increases energy (calorie) needs from day-to-day. In some cases, protein-calorie malnutrition occurs as the body breaks down muscle to provide energy. Body wasting and decreased resistance to infection can result.

Nutritional care for a client with COPD targets maintaining adequate nutritional status without overfeeding. Too much food makes the body produce excess carbon dioxide, which can be difficult for lungs to exhale. In acute breathing problems, or when a client is on a ventilator (breathing machine), Registered Dietitians sometimes increase the percentage of calories from fat. When the body uses fat, it needs less oxygen and produces less carbon dioxide, as compared with a high carbohydrate diet. Thus, a high-fat diet (e.g. 50 percent of calories from fat) reduces the load on the lungs. For a client with COPD, it is also important to maintain adequate intake of nutrients such as vitamins A and C to help guard against infection. Fluid retention around the lungs may be a problem. If so, dietary fluid restriction may be needed. Clients who experience difficulties in eating comfortably require common-sense support, which may include small, frequent meals and a diet planned around foods the client enjoys and tolerates well.

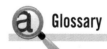

Glossary

Diabetes Mellitus
A metabolic disorder marked by high levels of blood glucose resulting from defects in insulin production, insulin action, or both

Hyperglycemia
High blood sugar

Hypoglycemia
Low blood sugar

Type 1 Diabetes (T1D)
When the body's immune system destroys pancreatic beta cells and insulin cannot be made

Type 2 Diabetes (T2D)
Begins as insulin resistance where the cells do not use insulin properly. Gradually the pancreas loses the ability to produce any insulin.

SECTION B | Diabetes and Weight Management

Diabetes Mellitus

Diabetes mellitus is a metabolic disorder in which the body cannot use glucose properly. Either there is an insufficient level of insulin, or the insulin is ineffective. Insulin is a hormone (a chemical messenger) made by the pancreas, an organ located near the liver. Insulin enables glucose in the blood to enter the body's cells, where it is burned for energy. Without glucose, the cells are deprived of energy. In diabetes, too much glucose accumulates in the blood. This condition is called **hyperglycemia**, which means high blood sugar. Ironically, with all this excess "food" in the bloodstream, body cells are starved for energy. The kidneys remove the extra glucose by dumping it into the urine, a condition called **glycosuria**. When not treated, diabetes can result in weight loss, insatiable hunger (called polyphagia), unquenchable thirst (called polydipsia), frequent urination (called polyuria), dehydration, weakness, and fatigue. Although diabetes is popularly called "sugar diabetes," it is not caused by sugar. High sugar levels in the blood and urine are a result, not a cause, of diabetes.

Diabetes is a serious disease. It is the seventh leading cause of death in the U.S., and prevalence is on the rise. More than 8 percent of the U.S. population has diabetes. That's about 236 million people. The American Diabetes Association estimates that about one-third of people with diabetes have not had the condition diagnosed. The life expectancy for people with diabetes is only two-thirds that of the general population. Poorly controlled diabetes can, over time, result in extensive damage throughout the body, affecting kidneys, heart, blood vessels, nerves, and vision. Diabetes is the nation's leading cause of kidney failure and adult blindness. And, because of its damaging effect on blood vessels and nerves of the lower limbs, it can require amputations of toes, feet, or legs. Having diabetes increases the risk of having a stroke or heart disease by two to four times. It is hardly surprising that this is a very expensive disease that costs the nation over $174 billion each year in healthcare costs, time lost from work, and Social Security disability payments (see Figure 5.15).

Diagnosis and Classification of Diabetes

Diagnosis of diabetes is generally dependent upon a laboratory test called a fasting blood glucose (FBS). In this test, the glucose concentration in the blood is measured after an eight to twelve-hour overnight fast. A normal fasting blood glucose is less than 120 mg/dl (milligrams per deciliter). A diagnosis of diabetes is generally made after testing on two occasions has revealed

Figure 5.14 Plasma Glucose Levels

Plasma Glucose Result (mg/dL)	Diagnosis
99 or below	Normal
100 to 125	Pre-diabetes (impaired fasting glucose)
126 or above	Diabetes*

* Confirmed by repeating the test on a different day.

Figure 5.15 2007 Age-Adjusted Estimates of Percentages of Adults* with Diagnosed Diabetes

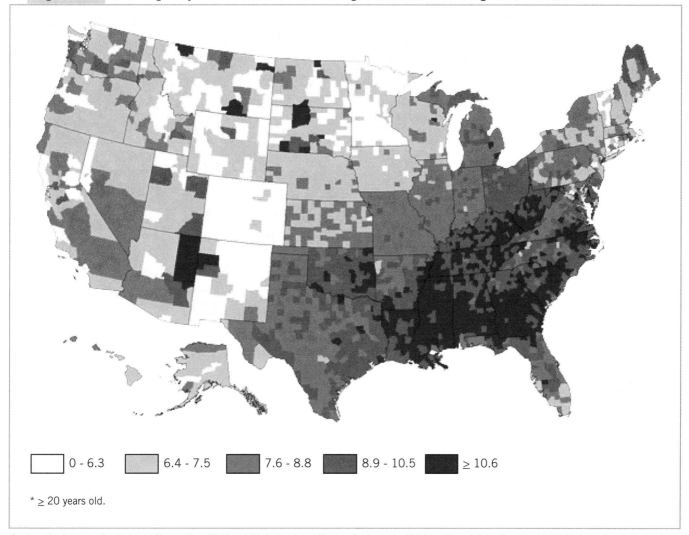

| | 0 - 6.3 | | 6.4 - 7.5 | | 7.6 - 8.8 | | 8.9 - 10.5 | | ≥ 10.6 |

* ≥ 20 years old.

Centers for Disease Control and Prevention: National Diabetes Surveillance System. Available online at: http://www.cdc.gov/diabetes/statistics/index. htm. Retrieved 9/17/2010.

concentrations over 126 mg/dl (see Figure 5.14). Physicians may also perform an oral glucose tolerance test (GTT) to better understand how the body handles glucose. This begins with a fasting blood glucose measurement. Next, a patient receives a concentrated glucose drink. At intervals afterwards, a technician keeps re-testing blood glucose. This provides a pattern of glucose levels that demonstrates the body's response.

There are three categories of diabetes: Type 1, Type 2, and gestational diabetes. Each one will be discussed in this section as well as a condition called prediabetes.

Type 1 diabetes occurs when a group of cells in the pancreas, called the beta cells, is unable to make insulin. Clients with Type 1 diabetes must depend on insulin injections to control their disease. Researchers say that Type 1 is actually an auto-immune illness. This means that special cells in the body whose job is to fight disease go awry. They destroy cells in the pancreas that make insulin. This is determined by genetics or may occur from an illness. Type 1 diabetes and other auto-immune illnesses tend to run in families. The National

Institutes of Health is already testing a vaccine that may prevent this disorder. Only five to ten percent of Americans with diabetes have Type 1. Type 1 usually begins in childhood. Classic symptoms of Type 1 diabetes appear abruptly and include excessive thirst and urination, hunger, and weight loss.

The most immediately life-threatening aspect of Type 1 diabetes is called *ketosis*, or the presence of dangerous chemicals called ketones in the blood. Because the cells don't have enough glucose to burn for energy, they start burning fat. In the process of burning fat for energy, they produce ketones. Presence of ketones in the blood is unnatural, and begins to disturb the delicate chemical balance of the bloodstream. If not managed, this condition can lead to coma or even death.

Most cases of diabetes, from 90 to 95 percent, are classified as **Type 2 diabetes**. Some clients with Type 2 require insulin, but most do not. In this form of the disease, an individual's pancreas does make insulin, but the cells are not as sensitive to it; the body cells don't use the insulin. Type 2 tends to strike adults over 30. As the population gets older, the percentage of people with diabetes increases. At least 80 percent of those with Type 2 diabetes are obese. Obesity is a risk factor for Type 2 diabetes, as is advanced age and family history. Symptoms of Type 2 match the symptoms for Type 1, but they are often overlooked because they tend to come on gradually and are less pronounced. Other symptoms that may signal the presence of Type 2 diabetes are tingling or numbness in the lower legs, feet or hands; skin or genital itching; and gum, skin, or bladder infections that recur and are slow to clear up.

Gestational diabetes is a condition characterized by abnormal glucose tolerance during pregnancy. It begins during the second half of pregnancy and ends after delivery. Most women are tested between the 24th and 28th week of gestation for diabetes. Some individuals with gestational diabetes require insulin, but most can use diet alone as a control.

Prediabetes is a condition when people have higher blood glucose levels after fasting but not high enough to be classified as diabetes. It is still important because people with prediabetes have an increased risk of developing Type 2 diabetes, heart disease, and stroke. In 2007, 26 percent of adults over age 20 had prediabetes, and 35 percent of adults over age 60. Studies have shown that this population can prevent or delay diabetes with weight loss and increased physical activity.

Diabetes Management

Diabetes is not curable; it has to be managed. Treatment is designed to maintain as near-normal blood glucose levels as possible (referred to as glycemic control). Studies show that control of the blood sugar levels slow the progression of the complications of diabetes. People with diabetes juggle three factors to maintain near-normal blood glucose levels:

✓ Insulin or oral glucose-lowering medications

✓ Food

✓ Exercise

Putting It Into Practice: 4

If a client's medical chart shows a fasting blood sugar of 300, what type of diagnosis might you expect to see?

(Check your answer at the end of this chapter)

The guiding principle is that food (especially carbohydrate) increases blood glucose levels, while insulin and exercise lower them. When these three factors are not balanced properly, **hyperglycemia** can result, with uncomfortable symptoms and the ongoing risk of complications. Occasionally, these three factors become unbalanced in the other direction, causing low blood sugar, or **hypoglycemia**. Characterized by dizziness and weakness, hypoglycemia may occur when medications or exercise are in excess and/or there is not enough food consumed. In other words, factors at play are reducing blood sugar levels too well. Treatment for hypoglycemia is quick administration of foods containing glucose that is absorbed quickly, such as orange juice or corn syrup.

In some healthcare facilities, a diabetes management team may provide care for clients. This team usually includes a Registered Dietitian, a registered nurse, a physician, and other healthcare professionals, along with the client. Together, team members perform an assessment, set goals, implement a nutrition intervention, and evaluate and monitor results. Client education for individuals with diabetes is termed diabetes self-management education (DSME). Many clients are taught conventional or intensive management, including the proper use of insulin or hypoglycemic agents, diet, exercise, and other aspects of self-care.

Insulin and Oral Hypoglycemic Agents

When the body is not producing enough insulin, a physician may prescribe insulin. Insulin is a hormone, and like many hormones, insulin is a protein. It is normally injected several times each day. It can't be taken by mouth because the digestive enzymes will digest it. People with diabetes normally give themselves insulin by subcutaneous injection (below the skin) at different sites. Insulin may also be administered through an insulin pump, which delivers small doses to the body on a continual basis. The pump is surgically inserted through the abdomen. Sometimes, insulin preparations are combined in a drug regimen. Preparations of insulin vary by how quickly they act and for how long. Types of insulin include:

✓ Rapid-acting insulin: starts working in 5-20 minutes and finishes working in 3-5 hours. Examples include Humalog and Novolog.

✓ Short-acting insulin: starts working in 30 minutes and finishes working in 5-8 hours. Examples include Regular (R) insulin.

✓ Intermediate-acting insulin: starts working in 1-3 hours and finishes working in 16-24 hours. Examples include NPH (N) and Lente (L) insulin.

✓ Long-acting insulin: starts working in 4-6 hours and finishes working in 24-28 hours. Examples include Ultralente (U) insulin.

✓ Very long-acting insulin: starts working in 1 hour and finishes working in 24 hours. This type provides even control of blood glucose for 24 hours at a time. Examples include Lantus.

Oral hypoglycemic agents are drugs taken by mouth to lower blood glucose levels in individuals with Type 2 diabetes. See Figure 5.16 for the incidence of treatment with insulin or oral medication. Some oral agents stimulate the body to produce more of its own insulin. Oral hypoglycemic agents are used

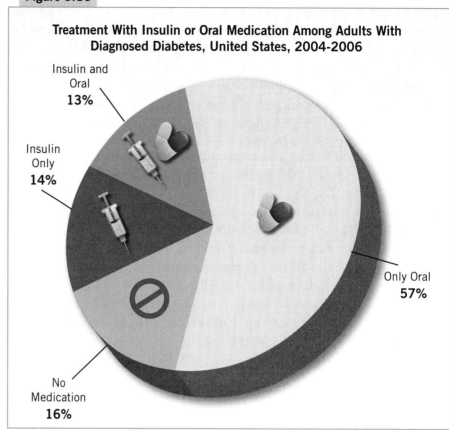

Figure 5.16

Treatment With Insulin or Oral Medication Among Adults With Diagnosed Diabetes, United States, 2004-2006

Insulin and Oral **13%**

Insulin Only **14%**

No Medication **16%**

Only Oral **57%**

Source: 2004-2006 National Health Interview Survey

only for Type 2 diabetes. Examples include: Glucophage®, Metformin®, Glyset®, Precose®, Prandin®, Starlix®, and Glucovance®. How these medicines work varies; each is a little bit different. Some need to be taken with meals, while others do not. With some, it is important to avoid alcohol, which may cause stomach upset. Some varieties of oral hypoglycemic medicines come in an extended release form, which provides fairly even control of blood sugar over a long period of time. Typically, these are taken once per day. Other medicines may be prescribed for two or three doses per day, taken at specific times. With insulin, as well as with oral medicines, meals must be planned in conjunction with a medication schedule to optimize control and prevent hypoglycemia. For example, a dose of medicine that has fairly rapid action on blood glucose could lead to hypoglycemia for a client who does not eat a meal shortly afterwards.

Medical Nutrition Therapy

Medical Nutrition Therapy for diabetes is often complicated because it may be accompanied by other chronic diseases. Those complications might be one or more of the following: heart disease and stroke, high blood pressure, blindness, kidney disease, nervous system disease, amputations, and dental disease. People with diabetes over age 60 are two to three times less likely to walk one-quarter of a mile, climb stairs, or do housework. In all of these chronic disease cases, blood glucose control is the foundation of treatment for diabetes.

The goals of medical nutrition therapy are as follows:

✓ Maintain as near-normal blood glucose levels as possible

✓ Achieve optimal blood lipid levels

✓ Provide enough calories to maintain or attain reasonable weight

✓ Prevent and treat short-term and long-term complications of diabetes

✓ Improve overall health through proper nutrition

A diabetic diet needs to be custom-tailored to the individual based on type of diabetes, medication(s), nutritional status and needs, weight management objectives, medical treatment goals, food preferences, culture, age, ability to understand the diet, and lifestyle. Meal planning approaches include myPyramid, Exchange Lists, and Carbohydrate Counting. In any plan, recommendations are to provide a caloric breakdown as follows:

✓ 50-60 percent of total calories from carbohydrate, with a maximum of 10 percent of total calories being from sugar (the remainder should come from high starch foods, which are more nutrient-dense).

✓ 30 percent of total calories from fat, with no more than 10 percent of total calories from saturated fat

✓ 15-20 percent of total calories from protein

MyPyramid or Choose MyPlate

The myPyramid model can provide an excellent resource for meal planning. In addition to following MyPyramid or Choose MyPlate guidelines, individuals with diabetes should:

✓ Eat meals and snacks at regular times every day

✓ Eat about the same amount of food each day

✓ Try not to skip meals or snacks

✓ Check blood sugar about 1.5-2 hours after eating to be sure they are not overdoing carbohydrates. The American Diabetes Association suggests 180 mg/dl as a good upper limit for this.

The American Diabetes Association also offers a list of tips and suggestions for managing diabetes using myPyramid.

Exchange System

The exchange system classifies foods into groups according to how much protein, fat, and carbohydrate they contain. Serving sizes are specified, too. These groups are called **exchange lists.** The Exchange System is being phased out and is still found in healthcare today. This creates a system in which foods within any given group can be swapped or exchanged for others in the same group. Any of these trades provides about the same amount of protein, fat, and carbohydrate. Of course, with these three macronutrients being equal, calories are about equal, too. The exchange system is a tool for managing a diet that has a controlled amount of each macronutrient, in controlled proportions, such as 15 percent protein, 30 percent fat, and 55 percent carbohydrate. Detailed Exchange Lists for Meal Planning appear in Appendix C. There are seven exchange lists: starch, fruit, milk, other carbohydrates, vegetables, meat and meat substitutes, and fat. A nutrition caregiver sets up an appropriate meal plan in consultation with the client. A typical plan lists how many exchanges of each food group may be eaten at each meal and snack. An exchange plan requires education for the client and others involved in meals. It requires a client to keep careful track of food at every sitting, and to measure food—at least until serving sizes become familiar. As with myPyramid, this system does not require one exchange or serving per meal. For example, an individualized exchange diet may call for two servings from the starch group, one serving from the fruit group, and one-half serving from the milk group at breakfast. Translated into food, this might be:

✓ 1 whole English muffin (2 bread exchanges)

✓ 1/2 cup of orange juice (1 fruit exchange)

✓ 1/2 cup of skim milk (1/2 milk exchange)

One challenge of using the exchange system is that many people do not eat single foods. Instead, they mix and combine foods into stews, casseroles, fajitas, pizza, and much more. Learning to count combination dishes requires education and sometimes nutritional analysis. The American Diabetes Association provides references for counting combination foods in an exchange system. In an exchange system, some basic advice still holds true: It's important to choose a variety of foods to provide needed nutrients.

Carbohydrate Counting

For clients who want more freedom and more flexibility than the exchange system, Carbohydrate Counting may work well. The total amount of carbohydrate is more important than where it comes from. The key is keeping the total carbohydrate content of the meal consistent each day. See Appendix D for Chart of Carbohydrate Servings Choices.

Carbohydrate grams can be counted by reading nutrition labels (see Figure 5.17), using tables of nutrient content of foods, or using the exchange lists. In the exchange lists, one exchange of starch, fruit, or milk each has about 15 grams of carbohydrate. One exchange of each of these foods is called one

Figure 5.17   Nutrition Facts of a Granola Bar

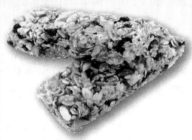

Ingredients: Rolled oats, high maltose corn syrup, sugar, high fructose corn syrup, crisp rice, palm kernel oil, yellow corn meal, fructose, canola oil, yogurt powder, corn bran, nonfat milk, soy lecithin, salt, honey, sunflower meal, peanut flour, almond flour.

Nutrition Facts

Serving Size: 2 Bars (42 g)

Amount Per Serving

Calories 180   *Calories from Fat 50*

	% Daily Value*
Total Fat 6g	9%
Saturated Fat 0.5g	3%
Trans Fat 0.5g	
Cholesterol 0mg	0%
Sodium 160mg	7%
Total Carbohydrates 29g	10%
Dietary Fiber 2g	15%
Sugars 11g	
Protein 4g	

Vitamin A 0%	Vitamin C 0%
Calcium 0%	Iron. 6%

* Percent Daily Values are based on a 2,000 calorie diet. Your daily values may be higher or lower depending on your calorie needs.

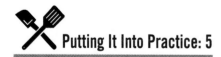

Putting It Into Practice: 5

What medical conditions are commonly managed using a carbohydrate counting diet?

(Check your answer at the end of this chapter)

carbohydrate choice. A meal plan can then be worked out that sets a specific number of carbohydrate choices at each meal or snack for the day.

For an individual who needs 1,800 calories, 225-270 grams of carbohydrate would be needed to meet the 50-60 percent of daily caloric intake from carbohydrate. This would mean 15-18 carbohydrate choices per day would be divided for the meals and snacks needed. The total number of meals and snacks, as well as the timing, is based on the individual's nutritional needs, lifestyle, and type of medication. Anyone counting carbohydrates needs to recognize that this is only a part of a healthful eating scheme. By focusing on carbohydrate alone, some clients may forget about limiting fat, or consuming adequate vitamins, minerals, and fiber. The Choose MyPlate, Dietary Guidelines for Americans, or similar guidance helps address overall wisdom in developing a healthy diet.

Exercise

A physician needs to approve an exercise program before a person with diabetes starts the program. This is because when an individual with uncontrolled diabetes (indicated by blood glucose levels of 240 to 300 mg/dl) exercises, the liver releases additional glucose and the hyperglycemia worsens. On the other hand, individuals with good blood glucose control (under 150 to 180 mg/dl) can benefit in many ways from exercising. Exercise lowers blood glucose levels because muscle cells use more glucose. Regular exercise results in greater sensitivity of the body to insulin and increases glucose tolerance. Exercise is especially helpful in decreasing cardiovascular risk factors and promoting weight loss. Some individuals with Type 2 diabetes gradually achieve better blood glucose control through weight loss. Individuals using conventional management are usually advised to eat a snack with 10-15 grams of carbohydrate before moderate exercise of an hour or less.

Monitoring

In order to keep an eye on how well the client is maintaining glycemic control, caregivers monitor the following variables:

✓ Blood sugar levels: People with diabetes routinely do self-monitoring of blood glucose (SMBG) by pricking the skin and then applying a drop of blood to a reagent strip. A glucose meter will read the sugar in the blood and display the blood glucose level. How often a person with diabetes does SMBG depends on the type of diabetes, the degree of glycemic control, and the treatment regimen (medication, diet, exercise). Some people use insulin pumps.

✓ Blood lipid levels to include total cholesterol, LDL, HDL, and triglycerides.

✓ Glycosylated hemoglobin: Hemoglobin is the part of the red blood cell that carries oxygen. During the life span of a red blood cell, glucose in the blood binds to hemoglobin A, the major form of hemoglobin in the red blood cell. When glucose binds to hemoglobin A, the hemoglobin is said to be glycosylated. Glycosylated hemoglobin values reflect average blood glucose levels during the past six to twelve weeks, and they are a useful indicator of how well a client is controlling his/her blood glucose level. Normal values for the laboratory used by your facility should be consulted.

✓ Body weight.

Follow-up is needed at least every six to twelve months for adults and every three to six months for children to assure good control of blood sugar, to evaluate any changes or complications, and to reinforce education.

Medical Nutrition Therapy of Overweight and Obesity

Obesity is posing a major health problem with children and teens. There is no single cause for obesity, and therefore no single cure. It occurs when energy intake exceeds the amount of energy expended. Over time, every 3500 excess calories become one extra pound of body weight. Figure 5.18 shows how energy intake has increased over time and where those added calories are coming from. According to the American Journal of Clinical Nutrition, the primary source of added sugars in the American diet is carbonated drinks. Besides carbonated beverages, the increase in calories is partly due to the increase in all high-calorie beverages: sport drinks, juice drinks, smoothies, shakes, and creamy coffee drinks.

There is a trend to more dining out and consequently, less eating right. According to the *Report of the DGAC on the Dietary Guidelines of Americans 2010,* the number of restaurants increased from 1972 to 1998 by 89 percent and the number of fast food restaurants by 147 percent. At the same time, the amount of time spent in food preparation at home decreased from 91 minutes to 51 minutes per day, meaning we're using more prepared food products. It is no wonder that tens of millions of Americans are dieting at any given time and that overweight and obesity are among the most prevalent health problems in the U.S. today.

Glycemic Index

There is some research evidence to suggest that body fatness is determined by glycemic index of food. The glycemic index is a measure of how quickly a food containing 50 g of carbohydrate affects blood sugar after eating. Foods higher in simple sugar are converted to glucose more quickly so they would have a higher glycemic index. One research study showed that obese children lost weight more quickly when consuming a low glycemic index diet.

Research also suggests that the location of body fat is an important factor in health risks for adults. Excess fat around the waistline, along with low HDL, high blood triglycerides, high blood pressure, and high fasting blood sugar, are linked to Type 2 diabetes and heart disease. This condition is called metabolic syndrome. Smoking and too much alcohol increase abdominal fat and the risk for diseases related to obesity. Vigorous exercise helps to reduce abdominal fat and decrease the risk for these diseases. Waist-to-hip ratio can be calculated by dividing the number of inches around the waistline by the circumference of the hips. For example, someone who has a 27-inch waist and 38-inch hips would have a ratio of 0.71. A woman whose ratio is 0.8 or higher would be at high risk of weight-related health problems (such as heart disease, hypertension, and diabetes), as would a man whose ratio is 0.95 or above.

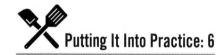

Putting It Into Practice: 6

In Figure 5.17, where do the 29 grams of carbohydrate come from in the granola bar?

(Check your answer at the end of this chapter)

Figure 5.18

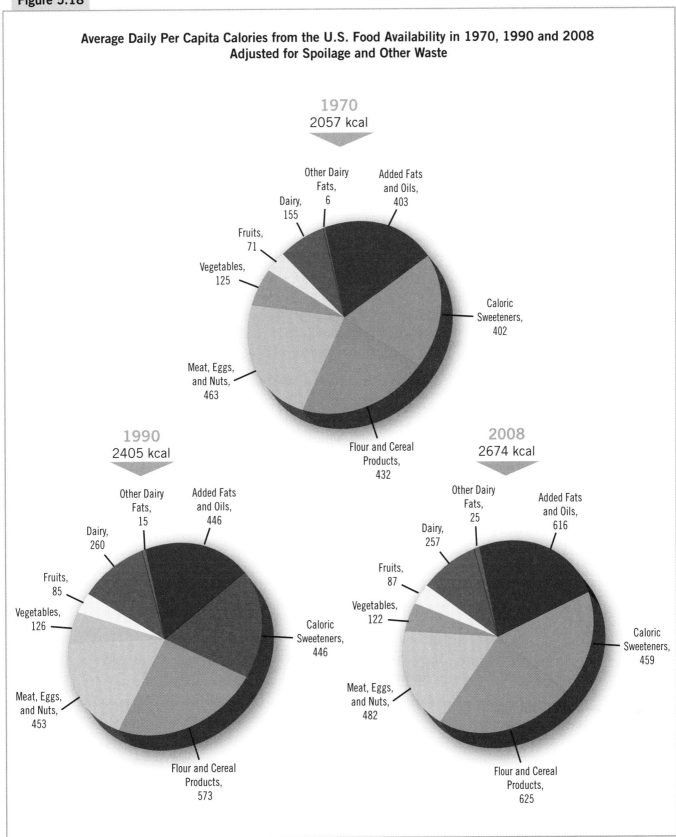

Average Daily Per Capita Calories from the U.S. Food Availability in 1970, 1990 and 2008
Adjusted for Spoilage and Other Waste

1970
2057 kcal

Other Dairy Fats, 6
Dairy, 155
Fruits, 71
Vegetables, 125
Added Fats and Oils, 403
Caloric Sweeteners, 402
Meat, Eggs, and Nuts, 463
Flour and Cereal Products, 432

1990
2405 kcal

Other Dairy Fats, 15
Dairy, 260
Fruits, 85
Vegetables, 126
Added Fats and Oils, 446
Caloric Sweeteners, 446
Meat, Eggs, and Nuts, 453
Flour and Cereal Products, 573

2008
2674 kcal

Other Dairy Fats, 25
Dairy, 257
Fruits, 87
Vegetables, 122
Added Fats and Oils, 616
Caloric Sweeteners, 459
Meat, Eggs, and Nuts, 482
Flour and Cereal Products, 625

*ERS Food Availability (Per Capita) Data System , Report of the DGAC on the Dietary Guidelines for Americans, 2010, D-1, pg. 10. http://www.cnpp.
usda.gov/Publications/DietaryGuidelines/2010/DGAC/Report/D-1-EnergyBalance.pdf Accessed August 11, 2010.*

Overweight people who lose even relatively small amounts of weight are likely to:

✓ Lower their blood pressure

✓ Reduce abnormally high levels of blood glucose

✓ Bring blood levels of cholesterol and triglycerides down to more desirable levels

✓ Reduce sleep apnea or irregular breathing during sleep

✓ Decrease the risk of osteoarthritis

✓ Decrease depression

✓ Improve appearance and self-esteem

Treatment of Obesity

Obesity has been and continues to be resistant to treatment. The prospect of attaining and maintaining normal weight is very low—about 5 percent. Because many factors affect how much or how little food a person eats and how that food is used, losing weight is not simple. A comprehensive approach to treating obesity focuses on the whole person. Treatment success is measured not only by the number of pounds lost, but also by other factors, such as improved self-image. Components of this approach typically include nutrition education, exercise, behavior modification, attitude modification, social support, maintenance support, and sometimes drugs or surgery.

More and more health professionals are adopting a non-dieting approach to obesity. This approach emphasizes helping clients adopt a healthier lifestyle. In many cases, diets simply don't work. By restricting food intake, diets can lead to unmanageable hunger and obsession with food, which may lead to binge eating. Those who follow extremely low-calorie regimens essentially starve their bodies. The body may also respond by reducing basal energy expenditure. The result is that the body begins to require fewer calories. Anyone who follows an extremely restrictive diet or a low carbohydrate diet is likely to lose lean body mass (e.g. muscle) as well as fluid. This may look great on the scales, but it doesn't last, and isn't a healthy condition. A realistic weight loss plan avoids this yo-yo syndrome by targeting one to two pounds of weight loss per week. Eating fewer fat calories and exercising can help many obese people to lose some weight—and keep it off, too.

Nutrition Education

Anyone who wants to lose weight needs to understand several basic concepts of nutrition before planning a diet:

✓ Calories should not be overly restricted because this practice decreases the likelihood of success. A progressive weight loss of one to two pounds a week is considered safe.

✓ No foods should be forbidden, as that only makes them more attractive.

✓ Eating regularly (not skipping meals including breakfast) is crucial to minimize the possibility of getting overly hungry. People tend to overeat when hungry.

✓ Portion control is vital. Measuring and weighing foods is helpful because "eyeballing" is not always accurate.

✓ Variety, balance, and moderation are key to satisfying all nutrient needs.

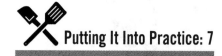

Putting It Into Practice: 7

If 3500 calories are equivalent to one pound of fat, how many calories would you need to decrease every day to lose one pound of fat in one week?

(Check your answer at the end of this chapter)

✓ Weighing oneself is important but should not be done every day because minor weight gains and losses can occur on a daily basis due to fluid shifts. Weekly weigh-ins are more meaningful and less likely to cause disappointment.

Exercise

Exercise is a vital component of any weight loss program. It may be more effective in reducing fat stores than dieting alone, and can result in significant weight loss even without eating less. Regular physical activity:

✓ Burns off calories to help lose extra pounds or maintain desirable weight

✓ Tones muscles

✓ Helps control appetite

✓ Helps in coping with stress

✓ Improves self-image

✓ Increases resistance to fatigue; energizes

✓ Helps counter anxiety and depression

✓ Promotes relaxation

Besides burning calories, an added bonus of a regular exercise regimen is that it helps shift the body's balance to include proportionally more muscle and less fat. In turn, this change in body composition increases the basal energy expenditure. Even at rest, a person with more muscle needs more calories. In short, exercise can help an overweight person feel and look better. See Figure 5.19 for calories burned with exercise.

Behavior Modification

Behavior modification deals with identifying and changing behaviors that affect weight gain. Keeping a food diary helps to identify eating habits. A food diary is a daily record of types and amounts of foods and beverages consumed, as well as time and place of eating, with whom a person eats a meal, mood at the time, and degree of hunger. A diary can increase awareness about how and why a person eats. Once harmful patterns that encourage overeating are identified, the behavior can be changed to become more positive.

Figure 5.19   Calories and Exercise

Activity	Calories Burned Per Hour	Activity	Calories Burned Per Hour
Bicycling, 6 mph	240	Swimming, 25 yards/minute	275
Bicycling, 12 mph	410	Swimming, 50 yards/minute	500
Jogging, 5½ mph	740	Tennis, Singles	400
Jogging, 7 mph	920	Walking, 2 mph	240
Jumping Rope	750	Walking, 3 mph	320
Running in Place	650	Walking, 4½ mph	440
Running, 10 mph	1,280		

These are calories expended by a 150-pound person. For a 100-pound person, reduce the calories by ⅓; for a 200-pound person, multiply by 1⅓.

Source: National Heart, Lung, and Blood Institute

For example, overeating may occur in reaction to stressful situations, emotions, or cravings. A client can learn to handle these situations in new ways. Solutions may include exercising or using relaxation techniques to relieve stress; or switching to a new activity—such as taking a walk, knitting, or reading. Delay can also be effective. A client simply decides to wait five minutes before eating. A craving may dissipate during this time. Positive self-talk is important for good control. Instead of saying to oneself, "I cannot resist that cookie," a client can say, "I will resist that cookie." An understanding of causes of unhealthy eating, if applicable, forms a crucial basis for long-term weight management. Clients can use behavior modification to make long-lasting lifestyle changes.

Attitude Modification

The most common attitude problem obese people have is thinking they are either on or off a diet. Being "on a diet" implies that at some point the diet will be over, resulting in weight gain if old habits are resumed. Dieting should not be so restrictive and with such unrealistic goals that the person cannot wait to get "off the diet." Remember, the original Greek meaning of "diet" is "manner of living." When combined with exercise, behavior and attitude modification, social support, and a maintenance plan, dieting is really a plan of sensible eating that allows for periodic indulgences.

Setting realistic goals, followed by monitoring and self-reward when appropriate, is critical to the success of any weight loss program. Through goal setting, goals involving complex behavior changes can be broken down into a series of small, successive steps. Goals need to be reasonable and stated in a positive, behavioral manner. For example, if a problem behavior is buying a chocolate bar every afternoon at work, a goal may be to bring an appropriate afternoon snack in from home. If this goal is not truly attainable, perhaps one chocolate bar per week should be allowed and worked into the diet.

Even with reasonable goals, occasional lapses in behavior occur. A constructive attitude is critical. After eating and drinking too much at a party one night, for example, feelings of guilt and failure are not uncommon. The solution is to accept the situation and simply continue as planned.

Two other attitudes concern hunger and foods that are "bad for you." Hunger is a physiological need for food, whereas appetite is a psychological need. Eating should be in response to hunger, not to appetite. Obese people frequently think certain foods are good for them and certain foods are bad. No food is inherently good or bad. Some foods do contain more nutrients per calorie, and some are empty calories with few nutrients. However, no food is so bad that it can never be eaten.

Social Support

In general, obese people are more likely to lose weight when their families and friends are supportive and involved in their weight loss plans. When possible, clients need to enlist the help of someone who is easy to talk to, understanding, and genuinely interested in helping. Partners can model good eating habits and give praise and encouragement. The client needs to tell the partner exactly how

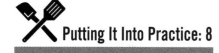

Putting It Into Practice: 8

What factors would you need to consider when an elderly widow is leaving your healthcare facility to return home? She has been successful so far on a weight loss diet.

(Check your answer at the end of this chapter)

to be supportive by, for example, not offering high-calorie snacks. Requests of the partner need to be specific and positive. For their help, partners should be rewarded. Something new in the past two years is using social media as a means of providing social support. Many physicians, exercise professionals, Registered Dietitians, and weight loss companies are taking advantage of popular social networking sites to connect with individuals who are interested in dieting. One popular Website, http://www.sparkpeople.com/, encourages realistic goal setting, with both weight loss and exercise. You can personalize your diet and fitness plan, connect with Registered Dietitians and trainers, and join a support group of people like you. So far, little research has been done to determine the long-term effect of these activities in maintaining weight loss.

Drugs and Surgery

In some situations, obesity becomes so severe that it threatens health, even in the immediate short-term. Or, it may be so difficult to manage that a physician feels more aggressive treatment is in order. A physician may prescribe drugs for weight loss. Researchers have developed some drugs that may alter appetite, feelings of fullness, and body metabolism. So far, experts agree there is no perfect diet drug. People who use two drugs approved for long-term use, orlistat (Xenical®) and sibutramine (Meridia®), have been successful in losing five to eleven pounds above and beyond that produced by diet and exercise alone after one year. Orlistat cuts down on the action of lipase. Lipase is an enzyme that helps the body digest fat. Reduced action from lipase results in less fat absorption. In 2007, the FDA approved an over-the-counter version of Orlistat for weight loss. It can cause side effects, such as diarrhea. Drugs in this category may reduce absorption of fat-soluble vitamins (A, E, and K), so supplementation may be warranted. Also, if taken along with a high-fat diet (>30 percent of calories), they may cause diarrhea.

Surgery for obesity is an increasingly popular treatment for individuals who are obese. Gastric bypass surgery actually reduces the size of the stomach. It makes eating very much food at one time difficult, because the smaller stomach becomes full easily. After surgery, some patients experience gastric upset and/or vomiting. Most lose about ten pounds per month. Due to poor absorption, patients may require supplementation with calcium, iron, and/or vitamin B12. About 80 percent of patients lose weight following gastric bypass, but only 30 percent attain a desirable weight. Over time, many patients re-gain weight. This dramatic procedure requires long-term behavior change, and a team approach to weight management.

Two other types of weight loss surgery are gastroplasty and gastric banding. Both of these restrict the amount of food that can be taken into the stomach. Like gastric bypass surgery, the success of the surgery depends upon personal motivation, a commitment to a new lifestyle and healthy eating habits.

Menu Planning for Weight Loss and Maintenance

Without drugs, surgery, or non-existent miracle cures, an individual who wishes to lose weight is back to commonsense nutrition. While it's not as exciting—or expensive—as many approaches in the marketplace, a gradual approach to dietary change can have lasting effects on weight control. This is a big advantage over dramatic treatments, many of which tend to produce only temporary results. A commonsense approach combines regular exercise with reduced caloric intake to shift the balance of calories and achieve weight loss. There are many diet options where one or more macronutrients are restricted (ie. low-fat, low-carbohydrate). The *Report of the DGAC on the Dietary Guidelines for Americans, 2010*, revealed that none of these were successful for "enhancing weight loss or weight maintenance." They did find that decreasing caloric intake led to increased weight loss and improved weight maintenance. Their report recommended the following:

✓ Protein: 10-35 percent of total calories

✓ Carbohydrate: 45-65 percent of total calories

✓ Fat: 20-35 percent of total calories

Specifically, the report states, "Diets that are less than 45 percent carbohydrate or more than 35 percent protein are difficult to adhere to, are not more effective than other calorie-controlled diets for weight loss and weight maintenance, and may pose health risks, and are therefore not recommended for weight loss or maintenance." One tool for nutritional planning is the weight loss pyramid described in Chapter 2. The following advice can be useful:

✓ Eat a variety of foods that are low in calories and high in nutrients.

✓ Eat less fat and fewer high-fat foods.

✓ Eat smaller portions and limit second helpings of foods high in fat and calories.

✓ Eat more vegetables and fruits without fats and sugars added in preparation or at the table.

✓ Eat whole-grain pasta, rice, breads, and cereals without fats and sugars added in preparation or at the table.

✓ Eat less sugar and fewer sweets (like candy, cookies, cake, soda).

✓ Drink less or no alcohol.

Maintenance Support

Only recently has weight maintenance started to receive the attention it deserves as a crucial component of a weight loss program. Unfortunately, little is known about factors associated with weight maintenance success or what support is needed during the first few months of weight maintenance, when a majority of dieters begin to relapse. Being at a normal, or more normal, weight can bring about stress, as adjustments are needed. Food is no longer a focal point, and old friends and activities may not fit very well into the new lifestyle. Support and encouragement from significant others may diminish. A formal maintenance program can help deal with those issues as well as others.

SECTION C | Gastrointestinal and Modified Consistency

As you already know, the gastrointestinal tract (GI) involves several organs and runs through the center of our bodies. A number of dietary disorders, chronic illnesses, or simple GI upsets can affect the GI tract. This chapter provides a brief introduction to the most common GI conditions and Medical Nutrition Therapy, starting with the mouth. Review Figure 4.2 to see the GI tract organs.

Tooth Decay

The major health problems caused by eating sugary foods, and also starchy foods, are tooth decay and cavities (*dental caries*). The more often these foods—even small amounts—are eaten and the longer they are in the mouth before teeth are brushed, the greater the risk for tooth decay. This is because every time we eat something containing sugar or starch, the bacteria that naturally live on teeth produce acid for 20 to 30 minutes. This acid eats away at the teeth, and cavities may eventually develop. Eating sugary or starchy foods as frequent between-meal snacks may be more harmful to teeth than having them at meals. Foods such as dried fruits, candies, soda pop, breads, cereals, cookies, and crackers increase chances of dental caries when eaten frequently. Fruit chews and chewy candies are particularly troublesome. Foods that do not seem to cause cavities include some vegetables, meats, fish, aged cheeses, and nuts. To prevent cavities, it is important to brush teeth frequently and thoroughly, floss daily, and avoid chewy sweets (Figure 5.20).

Tooth decay leads to tooth loss and dentures or dental bridges later in life. Approximately 50 percent of Americans have lost their teeth by age 65. Despite widespread use of dentures, chewing still presents problems for many elderly people who may require a modified consistency diet. Another concern, according to the American Heart Association, is that "poor oral health is linked to coronary heart disease."

Figure 5.20 How to Keep Teeth and Gums Healthy

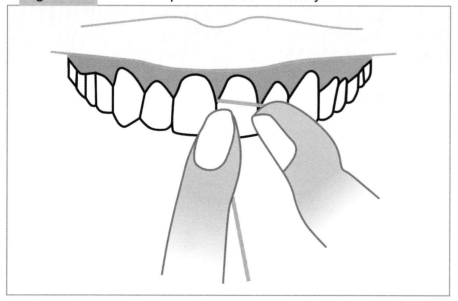

Modified Consistency Diets

Some clients have difficulty chewing or swallowing due to surgery, loosely-fitting dentures, missing teeth, inadequate saliva production (this commonly occurs in aging), mouth injury or infection, surgery of the head and neck, or stroke. Depending on the nature and severity of the problem, any of the following diets that are modified in consistency may be needed: full liquid diet, puree diet, mechanical soft diet, or dysphagia diet. Each is described below.

Puree Diet

The puree diet includes foods that require very little, if any, chewing. It may be recommended for alert clients with impaired ability to chew or swallow. Because pureed foods do not look very appetizing, many hospital and nursing home cooks and managers are making efforts to improve the appearance of pureed diets. For example, some cooks use thickeners to make pureed foods cohesive and then shape them to look like the original foods. Although there are several commercial thickeners available, some cooks use thickeners such as cornstarch or instant mashed potato flakes. Many of the commercial food thickeners are powdered and can be mixed directly with liquids and pureed foods.

Mechanical Soft Diet

The mechanical soft diet is a modification of the regular diet, and consists of foods that are easy to chew. Figure 5.21 lists guidelines for a mechanical soft diet. It includes many of the foods on the regular diet simply modified for consistency. Because each client's need for chopped or ground foods will vary, this diet must be individualized to each client.

Dysphagia Diets

Dysphagia means difficulty swallowing. A number of signs may suggest a problem with dysphagia:

Figure 5.21   Guidelines for a Mechanical Soft Diet

- Meat and poultry must be ground, chopped, or moist and tender. Ground meats can be used in soups, stews, and casseroles. Cooked dried beans and peas, soft cheeses, and eggs are additional softer protein sources. Fish must be flaked.
- Cook vegetables thoroughly, without skins, and dice or chop by hand, if necessary, before or after cooking.
- Serve mashed potatoes or rice with gravy, if desired.
- Salads are possible if chopped.
- Soft fruits such as fresh bananas, berries, or melon; canned peaches, pears, or applesauce are some possible choices.
- Soft breads can be made even softer by removing the crust.
- Puddings and custard are good dessert choices.
- Many foods that are not soft can be easily chopped by hand or blended in a blender or food processor to allow a wider variety of foods.
- No nuts or seeds are allowed, as they are hard to chew.

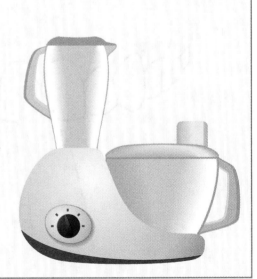

✓ Oral leaking or drooling

✓ Choking or gagging

✓ Pocketing food (capturing it in the cheeks)

✓ Taking longer than two to ten seconds to swallow

✓ Weakness, poor motivation

✓ Poor chewing ability, which may lead to choking on food

If any of these signs occurs, the client may need further evaluation to avoid severe choking or aspiration. This information should be referred to the Registered Dietitian or nursing supervisor so the speech pathologist can be notified. In all, up to 14 percent of hospitalized patients and up to 50 percent of residents in nursing homes may be experiencing a form of dysphagia. Dysphagia may be caused by stroke, neurological disease, dementia, or other factors. It poses the danger of aspiration and choking, while also increasing the likelihood of dehydration and malnutrition over time. There are many variations of dysphagia; it's a very individualized condition. A speech pathologist can perform an in-depth evaluation of swallowing, and recommend the type of dietary treatment required.

There is no universal diet for clients with dysphagia. One misconception about dysphagia clients is that foods need to be thin and liquid in order to be swallowed. On the contrary, liquids (especially thin liquids) are usually harder to swallow than solid foods. As needed, liquids can be thickened to nectar, honey, or pudding consistency. Pre-thickened liquids or thickening products on the market can help in providing appropriate foods.

The National Dysphagia Diet (NDD), now the national standard for dietary treatment of dysphagia, accounts for modifications in food textures, as well as liquids. Based on evaluation, a customized dysphagia diet recommendation contains two specifications: one for food texture, and a second one for liquids. Thus, a dysphagia diet may be specified as: NDD 3 or Dysphagia Advanced with thin liquids, or NDD Level 1 or Dysphagia Pureed with honey-like liquids. Figure 5.22 describes NDD guidelines.

When clients have swallowing problems, the speech pathologist may encourage special positioning and other suggestions to help ease swallowing during meals. In general, positioning residents as close to a 90-degree angle as possible makes swallowing easier and safer. If clients are in bed, you may need to support their heads, backs, necks, and sides. It may also be helpful to wait for the client to swallow prior to placing any more food in the mouth, and alternate solids and liquids.

Gastroesophageal Reflux Disease (GERD)

Gastroesophageal reflux disease (GERD) or reflux esophagitis is the medical term for what many people call acid indigestion or heartburn. A muscle called the lower esophageal sphincter relaxes to let food into the stomach, and then closes immediately so the acidic stomach contents won't go back up the esophagus. When this muscle doesn't close tightly, the acidic stomach contents splash up into the esophagus, causing irritation. This irritation is described as

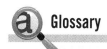

Glossary

Gastroesophageal Reflux Disease (GERD)
Where stomach acid comes up into the esophagus and causes acid indigestion or heartburn

Gastritis
Inflammation of the stomach lining

Dysphagia
Difficulty swallowing

acid indigestion or heartburn. Reflux esophagitis frequently develops due to aging. It can also be caused by a condition called a hiatal hernia. Normally, the lower esophageal sphincter sits right in the diaphragm, a strong muscle that separates the abdominal cavity from the chest cavity. The esophagus is above the diaphragm and the stomach is below it. In the case of a hiatal hernia, part of the stomach extends up through the diaphragm into the chest cavity. Because the diaphragm no longer reinforces the esophageal sphincter, stomach contents reflux into the esophagus.

Unfortunately, reflux esophagitis can do much more harm than just causing a burning sensation. Chronic heartburn can result in inflamed and scarred tissue in the esophagus, which can reduce its inner diameter. This is known as esophageal stricture. Cells that line the esophagus can eventually become cancerous.

Nutritional care goals include reducing gastric acidity and preventing esophageal reflux. Treatment for reflux esophagitis often includes the following:

- ✓ Avoid/limit foods that irritate the esophagus: citrus fruits and juice, tomatoes, spicy foods (especially chili powder and black pepper), and coffee.
- ✓ Avoid/limit foods that decrease pressure: alcohol; caffeine-containing drinks such as coffee, tea, and cola soft drinks; chocolate, peppermint, spearmint, and fat.
- ✓ Eat smaller amounts of food at meals. Drink most fluids between meals.
- ✓ Reduce fat intake. High-fat meals empty from the stomach slowly.
- ✓ Wait two to three hours after eating a meal to lie down or exercise.
- ✓ Wear clothing that does not constrict the waist or abdomen, so as not to increase the upward pressure on the lower esophageal sphincter.
- ✓ Refrain from stooping over; instead bend from the knees.
- ✓ Elevate the head of the bed.
- ✓ Reduce weight if overweight because obesity increases pressure within the stomach.
- ✓ Avoid smoking.

In addition, physicians may prescribe any of a variety of medications to help control GERD, including antacids and drugs that prevent acid production in the stomach.

Gastritis and Peptic Ulcer Disease

Gastritis is a painful inflammation of the mucosal lining of the stomach. The top layer of cells lining the stomach, called the mucosa, protects the stomach lining from the acidic gastric juices. Gastritis symptoms may include nausea, vomiting, anorexia, pain, bleeding, and belching.

Gastritis may be either acute (meaning it has a relatively short duration) or chronic (meaning it lasts a long time). Food allergies, overeating, chronic doses of aspirin or nonsteroidal anti-inflammatory drugs (such as ibuprofen), radiation therapy, stress, and/or infections can cause acute gastritis. Nutritional care generally includes withholding food for one to two days to let the stomach rest and heal.

Stomach

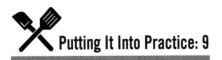

Putting It Into Practice: 9

When a client is coughing during their meals, to whom should he/she be referred?

(Check your answer at the end of this chapter)

Figure 5.22 **National Dysphagia Diet (NDD)**

NDD Food Texture Levels: NDD Level 1 • Dysphagia Pureed

Smooth, pureed, homogenous, very cohesive, pudding-like foods that require very little chewing ability.

General Guidelines

- Bread should be pre-gelled through the entire thickness, pureed or pureed into other foods in accordance with recipes.
- Fruits and vegetables should be pureed with no pulp, seeds or chunks.
- Mashed potatoes should be served with gravy, sauce, butter or margarine to moisten.
- Soups should be pureed smooth.
- Avoid scrambled, fried or hard-boiled eggs. Souffles are allowed.
- Avoid fruited yogurt, un-blenderized cottage cheese, peanut butter, and any food with lumps, including soups and hot cereal.

NDD Food Texture Levels: NDD Level 2 • Dysphagia Mechanically-Altered

Cohesive, moist, semisolid foods that require some chewing ability. Included in this level are fork-mashable fruits and vegetables. Excluded are most bread products, crackers, and other dry foods.

General Guidelines

- Bread should be pre-gelled through the entire thickness or pureed according to recipe.
- Fruits should be soft, canned or cooked. Soft, ripe bananas are allowed. Avoid canned pineapple.
- Vegetables should be soft, well-cooked, easily mashed with a fork, and in pieces smaller than 1/2 inch.
- Meat should be tender and moist, ground, or cubed smaller than 1/4 inch. Moisten with gravy.
- Avoid dry whole grain cereal with nuts, seeds and coconut.
- Avoid items that are difficult to chew, including large chunks or nuts.

NDD Food Texture Levels: NDD Level 3 • Dysphagia Advanced

Soft-solid foods which require more chewing ability. This level is near regular textures. Included are easy-to-cut whole meats, fruits, and vegetables. Excluded are hard, crunchy fruits and vegetables, sticky foods, and very dry foods.

General Guidelines

- Breads and cereals should be well moistened.
- Fruits such as bananas or soft, peeled fruits such as peaches, berries, nectarines, kiwi or melon without seeds may be tolerated.
- Avoid potato skins, corn, and raw vegetables.
- Meat must be very tender, small pieces, or ground, and well moistened.
- Avoid items that are difficult to chew: nuts, seeds, popcorn, potato chips, coconut, etc.

NDD Food Texture Levels: NDD Level 4 • Regular

Any solid food texture

NDD Liquid Levels: Thin

Thin liquids include clear liquids, milk, commercial nutritional supplements, water, tea, coffee, soda, beer, wine, broth, and clear juice. Individuals tolerating thin liquids will also be able to tolerate foods containing thin liquids, such as watermelon, grapefruit or oranges. Foods like ice cream, frozen yogurt, or plain gelatin which turn to liquid in the mouth are also considered thin liquids.

(Continued)

Figure 5.22   National Dysphagia Diet (NDD) *(Continued)*

NDD Liquid Levels: Nectar-Like

Medium thickness liquids include nectars, vegetable juices, and handmade milkshakes or shakes made with thickeners. Thin liquids can be thickened with commercial thickeners or purchased pre-thickened to nectar-like thickness.

NDD Liquid Levels: Honey-Like

Honey-like is thicker than the nectar-like level and resembles the consistency of honey at room temperature. Commercial thickeners can be added using package instructions to bring any liquids to this level of thickness or purchased commercially pre-thickened to honey-like thickness.

NDD Liquid Levels: Spoon-Thick

This includes high viscosity liquids too thick for a straw. Commercial thickeners can be added to any beverage to obtain this level of thickness or purchased commercially pre-thickened to spoon-thick.

Reprinted from Dining with Dysphagia, by Carlene Russell, MS, RD, LD, FADA. The Master Track Series, Association of Nutrition & Foodservice Professionals, 2003.

Chronic gastritis is often Ulcerative colitis seen in elderly populations. As this type of gastritis progresses, stomach cells become smaller in size, stomach secretions decrease, and production of intrinsic factor (needed for vitamin B12 absorption) falls. Nutritional care for chronic gastritis involves an individualized diet that avoids foods causing discomfort.

Ulcers affect more than 25 million Americans at some point in their lives, according to the National Institutes of Health. Ulcer sufferers describe an ulcer as a burning, cramping, gnawing, or aching in the abdomen that comes in waves, for three to four days at a time, but may subside completely for weeks or months. Pain is worst before meals and at bedtime, when the stomach is usually empty.

Mention "ulcer" and most people envision a stressed-out, workaholic, junk food-gobbling worrier. But that image is substantially incorrect. Now, the medical community views painful ulcers in a new light—as an easily treatable bacterial infection. The name of the bacteria is Helicobacter pylori. The ulcer itself in an open sore in the lining of the stomach (called a gastric ulcer) or in the first few centimeters of the duodenum (called a duodenal ulcer). The mucosa is eroded away, exposing the underlying submucosa, which is rich in nerves and blood vessels. Ulcers therefore cause pain and possibly bleeding. Both types of ulcers are termed peptic ulcer disease (PUD), which means chronic inflammation of the stomach and duodenum.

Treatment for peptic ulcers generally includes anti-secretory drugs (drugs that reduce the amount of acid secreted in the stomach), antibiotics, antacids, and nutritional care. Examples of anti-secretory drugs used in peptic ulcer disease include Tagamet® (cimetidine), Pepcid® (famotidine), and Zantac® (ranitidine hydrochloride). The use of antibiotics to remove Helicobacter pylori prevents most peptic ulcers from recurring.

The nutritional care goals for PUD revolve around reducing and neutralizing stomach acid secretion and limiting discomfort. These goals can be met by:

✓ Avoiding any foods or beverages that cause indigestion (in medical terms, indigestion is called dyspepsia)

✓ Eating small, frequent meals and avoiding large meals that cause stomach distention

✓ Following a bland diet

The foods allowed on the bland diet have changed over the years, and now the diet is much more liberal. Because of the success of drugs and antacids in reducing gastric acid levels, this diet is not recommended often, and may be nearly obsolete. A bland diet usually excludes the following gastric stimulants:

✓ Alcohol

✓ Regular and decaffeinated coffee

✓ Red and black pepper

Like many other diets, the bland diet needs to be individualized to meet each client's needs.

Gastroparesis

Gastroparesis means gastro (stomach) paresis (paralysis). For diabetic clients, it may also be called diabetic enteropathy. Gastroparesis is seen more frequently in diabetic clients and occurs when the vargus nerve in the stomach ceases to function. There are two types of digestion action in the stomach: chemical, from the hydrochloric acid; and mechanical, from the stomach pulsing to break up the food. That pulsing action is driven by the vargus nerve. When the vargus nerve is damaged from diabetes, the pulsing, churning action in the stomach does not occur. The food is not broken down and the stomach empties too slowly into the small intestine.

Medical Nutrition Therapy for gastroparesis revolves around reducing the amount of food eaten at one time and limiting those foods that are harder to digest such as high-fiber and high-fat foods. It may also mean consuming more foods in a liquid form:

✓ Smaller, more frequent meals (6-8 or more if necessary).

✓ Consume solid food early in the day and switch to liquids for the evening meal.

✓ Restrict high fiber and high-fat foods.

✓ Chew foods extremely well so some mechanical breakdown of the food occurs before it enters the stomach.

Nausea and Vomiting

Nausea is an unpleasant feeling in the stomach, accompanied by an urge to vomit. A number of medical conditions and medications can prompt nausea. Because nauseous clients do not feel like eating, nausea that lasts for more than a few days can create nutritional concerns.

Whereas a muscular process called peristalsis normally moves foods down the gastrointestinal tract, vomiting occurs when the waves of peristalsis reverse direction. Vomiting is often seen as a symptom of a disease or of the body's equilibrium being upset, such as on a ship. Vomiting is the body's way to get rid of an irritating substance, and is not dangerous unless large amounts of fluids are lost. The best advice for simple cases of vomiting includes at least four hours of no food or water, followed by drinking small amounts of fluid as tolerated and resting. When vomiting is more prolonged and therefore serious, medical care to replace lost fluids and restore electrolyte balance is essential.

Medical Nutrition Therapy for nausea and vomiting frequently calls for using the BRAT diet. **BRAT** is an acronym for:

✓ Bananas

✓ Rice

✓ Applesauce

✓ Toast

Consuming these more bland foods may give the stomach a rest because they are easier to digest. In the past, the BRAT diet was often given to children when they had nausea and vomiting. The research now suggests that children should return to a normal diet as quickly as possible in order to assure adequate nutrition.

Inflammatory Bowel Disease

Inflammatory bowel disease (IBD) includes two conditions with similar symptoms and clinical management: Crohn's disease and ulcerative colitis. The causes for either disease are not known, and there is no cure. They often first show up between 15 and 30 years of age, but may continue for a lifetime.

Crohn's disease, also called regional enteritis, is characterized by longterm, progressive inflammation of sections of the intestinal tract and lesions in the mucosal wall of the small intestine, large intestine, and/or rectum. The lesions often go through the entire intestinal wall. Chronic inflammation can cause fistulas (abnormal passages from an internal organ to a body surface or to another internal organ), abscesses (localized inflammation), and obstruction. Symptoms include persistent diarrhea, abdominal pain, fatigue, malabsorption, weight loss, anemia, fever, and anorexia.

During acute phases of Crohn's disease, enteral and parenteral nutrition may be used, particularly if the client has part of the intestines surgically removed. Once the acute phase closes, medical nutrition therapy often includes a diet high in protein (due to the protein losses from the mucosal lesions and poor dietary intake) and calories (due to weight loss commonly seen). Fiber is generally limited if intestines are inflamed, and fat is limited if it is not being absorbed properly. Any other offending foods, such as milk in the case of lactose intolerance, should be omitted. Supplemental vitamins and minerals are often used.

Ulcerative colitis is a disease that causes inflammation and sores, called ulcers, in the lining of the large intestine. Ulcerative colitis usually affects the lower part of the colon. Inflammation destroys intestinal cells, resulting in ulcers. Intestinal mucosa become so fragile that they bleed easily. Symptoms include painful diarrhea (often bloody), rectal bleeding, dehydration, anorexia, and malnutrition.

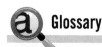

Glossary

BRAT Diet
Used to help the stomach rest after nausea, vomiting, or diarrhea. The diet is comprised of bananas, rice, applesauce, and toast.

Inflammatory Bowel Disease (IBD)
A disease that can cause ulceration of the mucosa lining in both the large and small intestine. Two types of IBD are ulcerative colitis and Crohn's disease.

During active phases of ulcerative colitis, bowel rest is often necessary, meaning the client cannot eat or drink anything by mouth. Once the client resumes eating, the same guidelines are used for ulcerative colitis as for Crohn's disease.

A high-protein diet is one in which high-protein snacks or supplements, such as from the dairy and meat groups, are given in addition to the regular diet. The diet consists of approximately 1.5 grams of protein/kilogram of body weight per day for an adult. An effective diet is also high in calories.

Diverticular Disease

Diverticulosis is a disease of the intestine in which the intestinal walls become weakened and bulge out into pockets called *diverticula*. (A single one of these pockets is called a *diverticulum*.) About 10 percent of Americans over 40, and half of Americans over 60 have diverticula. Most don't know it. There are no symptoms unless these pouches become infected or inflamed due to fecal matter collecting in the pockets. This condition develops in about one or two out of every ten people who have diverticula, and is called **diverticulitis**. If the terminology seems confusing, consider this rule of medical terminology:

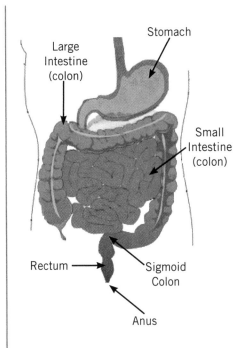

✓ The word ending osis or asis means "presence of"

✓ Diverticulosis means "presence of diverticula"

✓ The word ending itis means "inflammation of"

✓ Diverticulitis means "inflammation of diverticula"

This trick can help you understand and remember many other medical terms, such as gastritis (inflammation of the stomach), arthritis (inflammation of the joints), and others.

A low-fiber diet, along with decreased strength of intestinal muscle walls that occurs during aging, probably explain why diverticula develop. Increased fiber is recommended to decrease the pressure in the intestine that causes the pockets to form. A high-fiber diet (20-35 grams per day) is often prescribed.

While an individual with diverticulosis will benefit from a high-fiber diet, this is not true for the acute, temporary condition of diverticulitis. Dietary treatment of diverticulitis often restricts fiber so that it doesn't add to the inflammation. Typically, this diet eliminates most fresh fruit (except ripe bananas) and raisins, substituting canned or cooked fruits without seeds. Fruit juices are allowed. Nuts, crunchy peanut butter, popcorn, wild rice, bran, whole grains, coconut, and other foods with small particles that could become trapped in diverticula are also omitted. Cooked or canned vegetables without skins or seeds are permitted. Dried beans (legumes), peas, sauerkraut, and winter squash are not permitted. During this treatment, a patient may receive antibiotics. When the problem has resolved, an individual can usually return to a high-fiber diet.

Diarrhea and Irritable Bowel Syndrome

Diarrhea, frequent watery bowel movements, may be the result of emotional upset, food allergies, lactose intolerance, foodborne illness, gastrointestinal disease, medications, radiation therapy, or other conditions. Prolonged diarrhea can be serious, causing dehydration, weight loss, and malnutrition.

Diarrhea is often treated with a mixture of water, salts, and sugar, called oral rehydration therapy (ORT). In serious cases of diarrhea, bowel rest may be necessary. This allows the gastrointestinal tract to heal. Fluid and electrolytes are given intravenously in these cases. After adequate bowel rest, the client may start on a clear liquid diet and slowly progress back to a regular diet. Lactose and any irritating foods are omitted from the diet.

Diarrhea alternating with constipation may be a sign of **irritable bowel syndrome (IBS)**, a condition of unknown cause that first presents itself around age 20. Other symptoms of irritable bowel syndrome are abdominal pain, bloating, gas, indigestion, nausea, and rectal pain. According to the National Institute of Diabetes & Digestive & Kidney Diseases, a whopping one in five adults suffers from irritable bowel syndrome. The good news, though, is that this condition does not lead to any serious harm. It really describes a cluster of gastrointestinal symptoms that are, unfortunately, common.

The National Institute of Diabetes & Digestive & Kidney Diseases says that the following have been associated with a worsening of IBS symptoms:

✓ Large meals

✓ Bloating from gas in the colon

✓ Medicines

✓ Wheat, rye, barley, chocolate, milk products, or alcohol

✓ Drinks with caffeine, such as coffee, tea, or colas

✓ Stress, conflict, or emotional upsets

Symptoms may respond to stress, and for women, to phases in the menstrual cycle. Dietary recommendations include a high-fiber diet (unless diarrhea is present), adequate fluid intake, and smaller meals.

Constipation

Constipation is among the most common gastrointestinal problems in the U.S., and it accounts for two million visits to the doctor every year, according to the National Institutes of Health. **Constipation** is passage of small amounts of hard, dry bowel movements, usually fewer than three times a week. Bowel movements may be difficult and/or painful. Some people also experience a feeling of being bloated.

Because the gastrointestinal system tends to slow down with aging, occurrence of constipation is common in older Americans. It is also more common among individuals who have limited mobility, as imposed by an injury, disability, or medical condition. Constipation can be an after effect of stroke, or a side effect of various neurological disorders. It may also occur in certain hormonal disorders, gastrointestinal disorders, and other conditions. In addition, lifestyle habits can influence constipation. Infrequent exercise, low intake of dietary fiber, high intake of fat, and low intake of fluids can all contribute to constipation. Laxative abuse can also trigger constipation. Laxatives are considered habit-forming, and can damage nerve cells in the colon and interfere with the colon's natural ability to contract. Likewise, frequent use of enemas

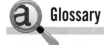

Glossary

Diverticulosis
A disease of the intestine where the intestinal walls become weakened and bulge into pockets called diverticula

Diverticulitis
A disease where the diverticula described above become inflamed or infected

Irritable Bowel Syndrome (IBS)
Common disorder that affects the large intestine that can cause abdominal pain, bloating, nausea, and diarrhea

Constipation
Passage of small amounts of hard, dry bowel movements— usually fewer than three times a week

can diminish normal bowel functioning. Furthermore, many medications can cause constipation; it's a common side effect of drugs such as narcotics, antacids, antidepressants, blood pressure medications, antispasmodics, and even dietary iron supplements. Individuals who change the consistency of their diets because of chewing or swallowing problems may inadvertently reduce dietary fiber intake, too.

Treatments for constipation include diet, laxatives, stool softeners, and drugs that stimulate bowel contractions, such as Correctol®, Dulcolax®, Purge®, and Senokot®. Exercise may also be a component of treatment. A diet that helps to correct constipation includes 20-35 grams of fiber daily and adequate fluid intake.

Food Allergies and Adverse Food Reactions/Intolerance

Food allergies, adverse food reactions/intolerance, and food sensitivity is addressed in this section because they frequently present symptoms in the gastrointestinal tract.

Food allergy is diagnosed when an abnormal immunologic response to a dietary protein occurs. There are two types of food allergies, immunoglobulin E (IgE)-mediated and non-IgE or cell mediated. Nearly five percent of Americans have a confirmed diagnosis of food allergies, 3.7 percent of adults and 6 percent of children younger than three years of age. Many others self-report a food allergy. There are eight major food allergens that cause more than 90 percent of all food allergies. They are:

✓ Milk

✓ Eggs

✓ Peanuts

✓ Tree nuts (such as almonds, macadamia nuts, pecans, walnuts, pine nuts)

✓ Soy

✓ Wheat

✓ Fish

✓ Crustacean shellfish (such as shrimp, crab, lobster)

Children who are allergic to cow's milk, eggs, soy, and wheat may outgrow their allergy by the time they reach ten years. Peanut, tree nut, fish, and shellfish allergies are usually not outgrown. Food allergies are increasing among children and the percentage of young children with a peanut allergy doubled from 1997 to 2002. As you can see, food allergies are becoming a serious problem.

An IgE-mediated food allergy may present symptoms that involve the respiratory tract and include congested, runny, and/or itchy nose, sneezing, raspy cough, and/or wheezing. A life-threatening allergic reaction that involves the respiratory system is called anaphylaxis. **Anaphylaxis** comes on rapidly, usually from food, and involves hives, swelling of the throat, difficulty breathing and eventually, loss of consciousness. The treatment is an epinephrine (adrenaline) shot. Most people who are at risk carry epinephrine with them, as it must be administered promptly to be effective. For people, including young children, who are risk of anaphylaxis, a Food Allergy Action Plan should be provided to schools, places of work, healthcare facilities, and any extended family members to help communicate specific dietary needs.

Food allergy symptoms that involve the gastrointestinal tract are swelling or itching of the lips, mouth and/or throat, nausea, vomiting, cramping and/or diarrhea. Allergic reactions to foods that affect the GI tract are usually cell-mediated. In addition, esophagitis and gastroenteritis can be caused by chronic response to food allergens. These may require trial elimination diets to determine the exact allergen. An elimination diet requires eliminating the suspected food from the diet for a period of time. If the client improves, then suspected foods may be reintroduced one at a time, under medical supervision. The Certified Dietary Manager can play a role in helping clients complete a food diary when trying to determine food allergies.

The most well-known cell-mediated allergic reaction is **Celiac Disease**, also known as Gluten-Sensitive Enteropathy (GSE), and Celiac Sprue. In 2004, interest in celiac disease heightened after a National Institutes of Health Conference reported research suggesting that celiac disease was more common than originally thought. Now, according to the Celiac Sprue Association, only three percent of people with celiac disease know they have the condition, while 2.1 million people are undiagnosed. Interest in celiac disease has also caught the attention of food retailers. More than 27,000 food and beverage products with the "gluten-free" claim have hit the markets worldwide since 2006, and predictions are for many more in the next five years.

Celiac disease is a hypersensitivity to the protein called gluten present in wheat, barley, rye, and a few other grains. With celiac disease, gluten is not absorbed properly. As the disease progresses, the villi of the intestinal mucosa are damaged. The end result of this damage is that the surface area for absorption of nutrient decreases by as much as 95 percent. Symptoms include diarrhea, weight loss, anemia, and other nutrient deficiencies.

Figure 5.23   Food Recommendations for a Gluten-Free Diet

Foods to Avoid	Foods to Use Caution (Read the Labels)	Foods that are Allowed
• Foods made with wheat flour, wheat starch, wheat germ, cracked wheat • Foods made from rye flour • Foods made with barley • Foods made with Triticale (a grain that is a cross between wheat and rye)	• Many candies • Gravy mixes • Most processed meats (bologna, salami, other cold cuts) • Sauce mixes and foods prepared in sauces • Seasoned tortilla chips • Soy sauce • Oats—should be labeled gluten-free	• Foods made with corn starch • Buckwheat flour, rice flour, tapioca flour, soy flour, quinoa, millet • Wild rice, rice • Nuts, legumes • Flax seed, flax seed meal • Amaranth, quinoa, millet • Potatoes

The primary treatment for GSE is a gluten-free diet (see Figure 5.23). A gluten-free diet often brings quick, dramatic results within days, followed by weight gain in about one week. It will take two to three months before the intestine regains its normal appearance.

In cell-mediated food allergies, avoidance is the best treatment. With celiac disease, nutrition counseling is the cornerstone of treatment as it requires a life-long avoidance of foods containing gluten.

Non-Allergic Food Reactions

Other food items that people report as food allergies such as strawberries, mushrooms, chocolate, tomatoes and peppers, may actually be **food intolerances**. Unlike food allergies that can be life threatening, food intolerances do not cause an immune response in the body. The most common food intolerance is lactose intolerance.

Lactose intolerance is a condition caused by inadequate amount of lactase in the body. Lactase is an enzyme needed by the intestine to digest lactose, the form of sugar in milk and other dairy products. Symptoms of lactose intolerance include abdominal cramps, bloating, and diarrhea, which can start about 30 minutes to two hours after ingesting milk products. Symptoms stem from the activity of intestinal bacteria that digest the lactose and produce gas and acid. The symptoms normally clear up within two to five hours.

Certain groups of people are more susceptible to lactose intolerance than others, e.g. Asian Americans, Native Americans, Latinos, and African Americans. Individuals suffering from lactose intolerance vary tremendously as to severity of symptoms. Most can drink small amounts of milk without any symptoms, especially if eaten with other foods. Chocolate milk and whole milk may be better tolerated than skim or 2 percent milk, due to variations in fat content and the presence of other sugars, which may delay emptying of the stomach. Lactose-reduced milk and other modified dairy products are available, as is the enzyme lactase, which can be added to milk to reduce the lactose content. Eight fluid ounces of lactose-reduced milk contain only three grams of lactose compared with 12 grams in regular milk.

Although most dairy foods (such as milk, ice cream, cottage cheese, eggnog, and cream) contain much lactose, some contain less. Yogurt is often well tolerated because it is cultured with live bacteria that digest lactose. This is not always the case with frozen yogurt, because most of it does not contain enough of the yogurt culture. Aged hard cheeses contain very little lactose and usually do not cause symptoms because most of the lactose is removed during processing or is digested by the bacteria used in making certain cheeses. Anyone who suffers lactose intolerance may be at risk for consuming inadequate calcium, as milk and dairy products are the chief sources in most diets. Without a comfortable alternative, many lactose-intolerant individuals may need to take calcium supplements.

Other non-allergic food reactions that may resemble food allergies are reactions to food additives such as sulfites, monosodium glutamate (MSG), and

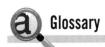

Glossary

Food Allergies
An immune response to dietary protein that is either cell-mediated or non-cell mediated

Food Intolerance
Does not produce an immune response but may not be tolerated for various reasons such as lactose intolerance where one cannot digest the milk, sugar, or lactose

Anaphylaxis
A life-threatening allergic reaction that usually shuts down the respiratory system

Celiac Disease
Caused by a cell-mediated hypersensitivity to gluten, the protein found in wheat, rye, and barley

food colorings such as FD & C Yellow No. 5. A more in-depth discussion of sulfites and food toxins causing illnesses is included in the *Management of Foodservice & Food Safety* textbook.

Gastrointestinal Progression Diets

Often, before or after surgery, testing, or various stresses and disorders affecting the gastrointestinal system, physicians will prescribe special diets such as a clear liquid diet, a full liquid diet, a soft diet, or a fiber restricted diet. Typically, these therapeutic diets are used temporarily.

Clear Liquid Diet

The clear liquid diet allows foods that are clear liquid foods or become clear liquid at room temperatures. Figure 5.24 lists foods included in a clear liquid diet, and Figure 5.25 shows a sample menu. The clear liquid diet may be used:

✓ After surgery (Usually it's the first diet because it is easily digested and absorbed.)

✓ Before surgery (starting about eight hours before surgery, all foods and fluids are usually withheld. This is to prevent vomiting while under anesthesia, which could lead to aspiration—when food, vomit, or other foreign substances accidentally enter the lungs.)

✓ Before various diagnostic tests (such as tests involving the intestinal tract, because the clear liquid diet helps keep the intestines clear)

✓ Following periods of vomiting, diarrhea, or other upset of the digestive tract

✓ In the acute stages of many illnesses, such as fever, when only the clear liquid diet may be tolerated

✓ To test the ability to tolerate oral feedings

The clear liquid diet is intended to provide fluids, electrolytes, and some energy, with minimal stimulation of the digestive tract and minimal development of fecal material (also called residue). It is useful in preventing dehydration and relieving thirst. This diet is inadequate in all nutrients except vitamin C and should not be used for more than three days without supplementation.

Full Liquid Diet

The full liquid diet contains foods that are either liquid at room temperature or become liquid at room temperature. It differs from the clear liquid diet mostly by the addition of cereals and milk products. Figure 5.26 lists foods included in a full liquid diet, and Figure 5.27 shows a sample menu.

Figure 5.24	Foods Included in a Clear Liquid Diet
• Apple, grape, cranberry, or cranapple juice	• Clear broth, bouillon, consommé
• Strained orange or grapefruit juice	• Flavored gelatin
• Fruit punch, lemonade, limeade	• Fruit ice, popsicle
• Carbonated beverages	• Tea and coffee
	• Sugar and salt

Putting It Into Practice: 10

You have several clients with food allergies in your facility. Which of the following Worcestershire sauce products should you purchase for your facility and why?

(Check your answer at the end of this chapter)

Worcestershire Sauce #1

Ingredients: Distilled white vinegar, water, molasses, high fructose corn syrup, salt, soy sauce, natural flavorings, caramel coloring, anchovies, soy flour, polysorbate 80, garlic extract

Worcestershire Sauce #2

Ingredients: Distilled vinegar, water, molasses, corn syrup, salt, anchovies, tamarind extract, sugar, spices, garlic powder, xanthan gum, natural flavors

The full liquid diet is indicated in postoperative situations when the client has not fully recovered the ability to consume and tolerate solid food. In this case, a full liquid diet often acts as a transition between a clear liquid and soft or regular diet. It may also be indicated for clients who have esophageal or stomach disorders that interfere with the normal handling of solid foods.

The full liquid diet is adequate in calories, protein, vitamin C, calcium, sodium, and potassium. It is inadequate in iron, niacin, and folacin, and other nutrients. However, due to the limited selection of foods, a multivitamin and mineral supplement may be necessary if this diet is to be used for more than two weeks and a commercial liquid formula is not used.

Soft Diet (or "GI Soft Diet")

The soft diet is designed for use during transition from liquid to regular diet after surgery. It provides a modified consistency, but is also intended to be easy on the gastrointestinal tract during a sensitive time. Foods in a soft diet are:

✓ Soft in consistency (but not ground or chopped)

✓ Mildly spiced

✓ Moderately low in fiber content

Cooked vegetables and fruits without seeds or peels are allowed. Raw vegetables, highly seasoned or fried foods, and nuts and seeds are not allowed. This diet must be individualized to each client.

Finger Food Diet

The Finger Food Diet has existed for many years. However, the increased attention to this diet is due to the emphasis on maintaining quality of life by providing additional rehabilitation services. Finger foods are useful for clients with physical or functional impairments who have lost their ability to eat with utensils. They allow a client to maintain independent eating ability, e.g. in the case of Alzheimer's disease.

The biggest obstacle with this diet may be family members who feel it is socially unacceptable to eat with fingers and beneath the dignity of the client. If the family is not aware of the need to maintain independence in eating, they may believe it is more acceptable to eat with a spoon and/or be fed by staff. A team effort among the client, family, foodservice staff, speech therapy, and nursing staff will help make this diet a successful intervention.

The characteristics of finger foods include:

✓ Bite-size pieces—not too large or too small

✓ Not too soft, squishy, slippery, or crumbly

✓ No thick, gooey sauces or gravy poured on the food

A finger food diet may include foods such as: pudding in an ice cream cone, chicken nuggets, sandwiches cut into quarters, cold cereals formed in large pieces (e.g. shredded wheat), bar cookies, donuts, turnovers, peanut butter on crackers, tater tots or baked potatoes cut into pieces, batter-dipped vegetables, corn on the cob, thin soup served in a mug, popcorn, bite-sized fruit or vegetable pieces.

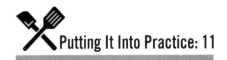

Putting It Into Practice: 11

You are working with a client who just transferred in from the hospital. In her medical record you read where she was started on a Clear Liquid Diet on 8-10-11. Today's date is 8-15-11 and she is still on the Clear Liquid Diet. What should you do?

(Check your answer at the end of this chapter)

Figure 5.25 Sample Menu for a Clear Liquid Diet

Breakfast

1 cup strained orange juice

½ cup gelatin

2 tsp. sugar

1 cup coffee

12 oz. ginger ale

Lunch

1 cup apple juice

¾ cup clear broth

½ cup fruit ice

2 tsp. sugar

1 cup tea

12 oz. lemon-lime flavored soda

Dinner

1 cup cranberry juice

¾ cup consommé

½ cup gelatin

1 cup tea

12 oz. lemon-lime flavored soda

Figure 5.26 Foods Included in a Full Liquid Diet

- Carbonated beverages, coffee and tea (regular and decaffeinated), fruit drinks

- Milk and milk drinks, yogurt without seeds or nuts

- Pureed meat added to broth or cream soup

- Custard, gelatin desserts, smooth ice cream, sherbet, puddings, popsicle

- Cooked, refined cereal; mashed potatoes in cream soup

- All vegetable juices, pureed vegetables in soup

- All fruit juices

- Sugar, honey, syrup, clear hard candy

- Butter, margarine, cream, vegetable oils

- Consommé, broth, bouillon, strained soup made from allowed foods

- Salt

- Commercial liquid formulas that are nutritionally complete

      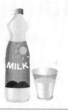 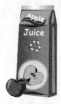

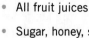

Figure 5.27 **Sample Menu for a Full Liquid Diet**

Breakfast

1 cup whole milk	non-dairy creamer
1 cup eggnog	2 tsp. sugar
1 cup orange juice	1 Tbsp. honey
½ cup cooked strained oatmeal	salt
	coffee

Lunch

1 cup whole milk	1 tsp. sugar
1 cup vanilla milkshake	½ cup sherbet
1 cup apple juice	salt, pepper
non-dairy creamer	tea
¾ cup strained cream of potato soup	

Dinner

1 cup whole milk	¾ cup strained vegetable
1 cup chocolate milkshake	beef soup
½ cup egg custard	1 tsp. sugar
1 cup cranberry juice	salt, pepper
non-dairy creamer	tea

Fatty Liver, Hepatitis, and Cirrhosis

Organs that Impact Digestion

In our discussion about gastrointestinal progression diets, it is important to consider the organs involved with digestion: the liver, the gallbladder, and the pancreas.

The liver, the largest organ in the body, has many important roles. Following are some of its functions:

✓ The liver converts blood glucose to fat and glycogen. The liver can also make glucose. The liver has an important role in regulating blood glucose levels.

✓ The liver makes triglycerides and cholesterol. It also excretes cholesterol in bile.

✓ The liver makes many of the proteins found in the blood, such as the proteins necessary for blood to clot after an injury.

✓ The liver removes drugs, hormones, and other molecules by excreting them in the bile.

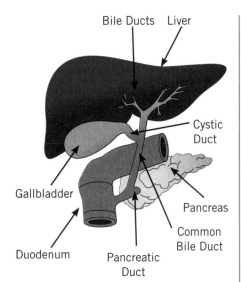

Bile Ducts   Liver

Cystic Duct

Gallbladder

Pancreas

Common Bile Duct

Duodenum   Pancreatic Duct

Fatty liver, a condition in which triglycerides build up in the liver and cause it to swell, is often an early sign of more liver problems to come. Fatty liver most often occurs due to excessive alcohol intake, infection, or malignant disease. It can also be caused by certain drugs or by extremely low protein intake (to the point of protein malnutrition). Treatment for fatty liver centers on removing its cause, whether it be alcohol, drugs, or a poor diet. The effects of fatty liver can be reversed when the cause is eliminated.

Hepatitis is more serious than fatty liver, and refers to inflammation of the liver due to alcohol, viruses, drugs, toxins, or viral infection. Symptoms include low fever, fatigue, nausea, anorexia, vomiting, constipation or diarrhea. Symptoms cause malnutrition in some instances, particularly in cases of alcohol abuse. A high-calorie, high-protein diet is appropriate for malnourished clients, and fat soluble vitamins in water soluble form are often prescribed.

Cirrhosis is a term used for advanced stages of liver disease that occurs when fatty liver or hepatitis are not reversed. At this point, liver cells harden and die. The damage can't be reversed. The liver shrinks and is not able to complete all of its vital functions. Cirrhosis due to alcohol abuse is called Laennec's cirrhosis. It is the most common type of cirrhosis.

Symptoms of cirrhosis include nausea, anorexia, weight loss, weakness, iron-deficiency anemia, stomach pain, esophageal varices (blood vessels that project into the esophagus), steatorrhea (fat is malabsorbed and is found in the stool), and ascites. **Ascites** is the abnormal accumulation of fluid in the abdomen. The level of ammonia in the blood, which is toxic to the brain and nervous system, also increases. **Edema** is the overall term for abnormal water retention.

When cirrhosis progresses to the point where the liver function has decreased to 25 percent or less, **hepatic** failure occurs. Liver failure is characterized by **jaundice**, a yellowing of the skin. Over time, liver failure results in portal ystemic encephalopathy (PSE), which affects the brain and is a life-threatening complication of liver failure. Symptoms range from confusion and poor coordination to flapping of the hands (called asterixis), and finally to loss of consciousness and coma.

Several laboratory tests help in evaluation of liver function. Elevated liver enzymes mean the liver cells are being destroyed and the enzymes are released into the blood. This suggests liver failure. Blood ammonia tests are also used as a measurement of the degree of liver failure. The liver converts proteins into amino acids. Ammonia is a byproduct. The liver converts ammonia into urea. Urea is excreted by the kidneys. When the liver is failing, it cannot convert ammonia to urea. Thus, high blood ammonia level is an early sign of liver failure. It may be accompanied by symptoms of confusion. A low protein diet may be part of the therapy at this point, because this minimizes the production of ammonia. In cases of hepatic coma, hepatic formulas that are low in a type of amino acid called aromatic amino acids, and high in branched-chain amino acids may be used. Figure 5.28 shows the MNT for cirrhosis.

Figure 5.28 Medical Nutrition Therapy for Cirrhosis

- High calories, 35-45 cal/kg body weight
- High protein 1.0-1.5g/kg body weight
- Moderate fat
- Vitamin and mineral supplementation
- Fluid and sodium restrictions if ascites and edema are present

Gallbladder Disease

The liver also makes and secretes bile, a substance that aids in the digestion and absorption of fats. Bile is carried by ducts from the liver to the gallbladder. The gallbladder stores and concentrates bile until food is in the stomach and duodenum. Then the gallbladder contracts and bile travels to the duodenum.

There are various diseases of the gallbladder, such as gallstones (cholelithiasis), or inflammation of the gallbladder (cholecystitis), which is usually caused by gallstones. A low-fat diet, usually interpreted to mean 40 grams of fat per day, may be used to treat these diseases in the hospital. Clients with chronic cholecystitis may need a long-term diet with 25 to 30 percent of calories from fat. Less fat in the diet results in fewer gallbladder contractions and less pain. A client who has the gallbladder removed can progress as tolerated to a regular diet.

Pancreatitis

Pancreatitis is an inflammation of the pancreas in which pancreatic enzymes are blocked from emptying, causing some of these strong enzymes to digest the pancreas itself. Pancreatitis can be either acute or chronic. Gallstones are the most common cause of acute pancreatitis, while alcohol abuse is a common cause of chronic pancreatitis. Symptoms include tender abdomen, nausea, vomiting, fever, and rapid pulse. Pancreatitis causes fat malabsorption and steatorrhea. When fat is lost in the stool, so are calories and fat-soluble vitamins.

During acute pancreatitis, oral feedings are usually withheld until the acute phase subsides to give the pancreas a rest, at which time the client may slowly progress as tolerated to a low-fat diet. For clients with chronic pancreatitis, dietary treatment includes pancreatic enzyme replacements (taken orally with meals), a low-fat diet, vitamin and mineral supplements, and MCT oil if steatorrhea is present.

Renal Disease

The kidneys perform the vital function of maintaining the proper balance of water, electrolytes (sodium, potassium, and chloride), and acids in body fluids. This is done by secreting some substances into the urine and holding back others in the bloodstream for use in the body. In addition to forming urine, the kidneys also have an endocrine function, meaning they produce hormones. The kidneys secrete rennin (a substance that is important in maintaining normal blood pressure), erythropoietin (a hormone that regulates the production of red blood cells), and a form of vitamin D.

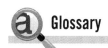 **Glossary**

Edema
Unhealthy water retention

Ascites
Abnormal accumulation of fluid in the abdomen

Hepatic
Relating to the liver

Jaundice
Yellowing of the skin associated with liver disease

Renal Failure
When kidneys fail to function normally

SECTION D | Renal and Additional Therapeutic Needs

Certain conditions damage the cells of the kidneys, making it difficult for the kidneys to perform their jobs. **Renal failure** occurs when the kidneys fail to maintain normal fluid and electrolyte balance and to excrete waste products within normal limits. It may strike at any age, due to a variety of causes. Renal failure may occur over a period of time (chronic renal failure) or suddenly (acute renal failure). Acute renal failure may result from shock, burns, or severe injuries. It is often reversible.

Chronic renal failure (CRF) is not reversible, due to the progressive destruction of kidney tissue. Many diseases can damage the kidneys, such as nephritis (inflammation of the kidneys), high blood pressure, and complications of diabetes. Clients who suffer from chronic renal failure may eventually require dialysis, in which waste materials such as urea (a byproduct of protein metabolism that can be toxic at high levels) are separated from the bloodstream. Dialysis removes excess wastes and fluids but can't perform any of the hormonal functions of the kidney. When the client is to the point of requiring dialysis or a kidney transplant, the disease is referred to as end-stage renal disease (ESRD).

Part of the treatment for ESRD may be dialysis, a mechanical process that removes wastes. There are two types of dialysis: hemodialysis and peritoneal dialysis. In hemodialysis, the client's blood is routed through a dialysis machine, which performs many of the kidney's functions. Then, the blood is returned to the body. In peritoneal dialysis, fluid is introduced into the abdominal cavity by a catheter or tube permanently placed into the abdomen.

The goals of the renal diet are as follows:

✓ To provide normal growth in children

✓ To achieve and maintain an optimal nutritional status through adequate protein, energy, vitamin, and mineral intake

✓ To attain and maintain a desirable body weight

✓ To lighten the work of a diseased kidney by reducing the amount of waste products, such as urea made from protein, that have to be excreted

✓ To control edema and electrolyte imbalance by controlling sodium, potassium, and fluid intake

✓ To replace proteins that are lost in hemodialysis

✓ To prevent or slow down the development of bone disease (called renal osteodystrophy) by controlling phosphorus (the blood level of which increases during renal failure, leading to bone disease) and increasing calcium intak.

✓ To provide a palatable diet

Of all the modified diets, the renal diet is probably the most complex. The intake of protein, sodium, potassium, phosphorus, and fluid are carefully regulated from day-to-day. Actual nutrient restrictions vary based on many factors, such as:

✓ Degree of kidney failure

Glossary

Cancer
When cells grow at an unrestricted rate or there is excessive multiplication of cells

Tumors
Growths of cancerous cells

Malignant
A tumor that is likely to spread

Benign
A tumor that is not likely to spread

Metastasis
Transfer of cancer from one part of the body to another organ or part of the body

Cancer Cachexia
Extreme weight loss or body wasting that may not be reversed

✓ Age of the client

✓ Mode of treatment and/or dialysis

✓ Need to maintain or achieve an ideal or desired weight

✓ Other medical conditions: diabetes, high blood pressure, hyperlipidemia, or malnutrition

The National Kidney Foundation has established Dietary Guidelines for Adults Starting on Hemodialysis. As stated before, the renal diet looks at protein, sodium, potassium, phosphorus, and fluid. In general, adults on hemodialysis should:

✓ Eat more high-protein foods

✓ Eat less high-salt, high-potassium and high-phosphorus foods

✓ Lean how much fluid to safely drink (including coffee, tea, and water)

See Figure 5.29 for the Dietary Guidelines for Adults Starting on Hemodialysis and additional information for chronic kidney disease. Figure 5.30 shows a sample menu for a client on hemodialysis.

Cancer

Cancer is the second leading cause of death. In 2006, over 11 million people in the U.S. had cancer of some type. **Cancer** is a disease characterized by unrestricted and excessive multiplication of body cells. **Tumors** are growths of cancerous cells and may be either **malignant** (meaning cancerous growth is continuing and may be life-threatening) or **benign** (meaning not cancerous). Cancerous cells can also leave their original site of growth and travel through the blood and lymph to spread throughout the body, referred to as **metastasis**.

Sometimes the first signs of cancer are weight loss and anorexia, and diet is an important part of cancer treatment. Cancer cells require calories and nutrients to grow, and basal energy use is increased in cancer clients. This helps explain part of the weight loss. Cancer clients may need 35 to 50 calories per kilogram of body weight simply to maintain their current weight. To complicate matters more, cancer clients often have little interest in eating. They experience nausea and vomiting, feel full quickly, and do not taste many foods normally. These symptoms may be caused by the cancer or by the treatment, which may include radiation, chemotherapy, and surgery. Good nutritional status is important to withstand the effects of treatment.

The traditional cancer therapies, radiation therapy and chemotherapy, interfere with nutritional status. In radiation therapy, high-energy rays are used to destroy cancerous tissues and stop the growth of cancer cells. Chemotherapy is the treatment of cancer with drugs. Some effects of radiation therapy and chemotherapy include nausea, vomiting, taste alterations, diarrhea, malabsorption, and reduced salivary secretions in the case of radiation treatment of the head and neck. The result can be **cancer cachexia** (malnutrition).

Surgery is another major approach to treating cancer. Surgery removes cancerous tissue. In these situations, providing proper nutrition will require dietary modifications such as small, frequent meals for clients who have had part of

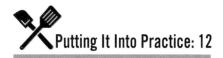

Putting It Into Practice: 12

What should you look for on a nutrition label for a client with chronic kidney disease?

(Check your answer at the end of this chapter)

the stomach removed. About half of cancer clients experience an extreme state of malnutrition and wasting of the body called cancer cachexia. Symptoms include significant weight loss, loss of appetite, feeling full early, abnormal taste and smell abilities, anemia, and other nutritional deficiencies.

Following are approaches to overcome some of the nutritional problems that present in cancer clients.

Figure 5.29 Dietary Guidelines for Adults Starting on Hemodialysis

Nutrient	Dietary Guidelines for Adults Starting on Hemodialysis[1]	Nutrition for Chronic Kidney Disease in Adults[2]
Salt & Sodium	• Use less salt and eat fewer salty foods • Use herbs, spices, and low-salt flavor enhancers • Avoid salt substitutes made with potassium	• Limit sodium intake to 1500 mg per day • Choose sodium-free or low-sodium food products • Use lemon juice, salt-free seasoning mixes, or hot pepper sauce • Avoid salt substitutes that use potassium
Meat/Protein	• Eat a high protein food at every meal or 8-10 oz. every day • 3 oz. = size of a deck of cards: a medium pork chop, a ¼ lb. hamburger, ½ chicken breast, a medium fish fillet • 1 oz. = 1 egg or ¼ cup egg substitute, ¼ cup tuna, ¼ cup ricotta cheese, 1 slice of low-sodium lunchmeat • Note: Peanut butter, nuts, seeds, dried beans, peas, and lentils have protein but are not recommended because they are high in both potassium and phosphorus	• Reduce daily protein intake by 0.2 g/kg of body weight (e.g. a 154 lb. man would reduce protein from 56 grams to 42 grams/day) • Limit meat to two 3-oz. servings daily
Grains, Cereals, and Breads	• Unless you need to limit your calorie intake for weight loss and/or manage carbohydrate intake for Diabetes, you may eat 6-11 servings from this group each day • Avoid "whole grain" and "high fiber" foods to help you limit your intake of phosphorus	• No specific recommendation
Milk, Yogurt, and Cheese	• Limit your intake of milk, yogurt, and cheese to ½ cup milk or ½ cup yogurt or 1 oz. cheese per day • The phosphorus content is the same for all types of milk—skim, low-fat, and whole • If you do eat any high phosphorus foods, take a phosphate binder with that meal • Certain brands of non-dairy creams and "milk" (such as rice milk) are low in phosphorus and potassium • Dairy foods "low" in phosphorus	• Limit your intake of high-phosphorus foods, including dairy foods

(Continued)

Figure 5.29 Dietary Guidelines for Adults Starting on Hemodialysis *(Continued)*

Nutrient	Dietary Guidelines for Adults Starting on Hemodialysis[1]	Nutrition for Chronic Kidney Disease in Adults[2]
Fruit and Juice	• Eat 2-3 servings of low potassium fruits each day • Always AVOID star fruit (carambols) • Limit oranges, orange juice, kiwis, nectarines, prune, prune juice, raisins, and dried fruit, bananas, melons (cantaloupe and honeydew) • Fruits low in potassium (see Appendix E)	• Limit high-potassium foods including oranges, orange juice, melons, apricots, bananas, and kiwi
Vegetables and Salads	• Eat 2-3 servings of low-potassium vegetables each day • Avoid potatoes, tomatoes, winter squash, pumpkin, asparagus, avocado, beets, beet greens, cooked spinach, parsnips, and rutabaga • Vegetables low in potassium (see Appendix E)	• Limit high-potassium foods including potatoes, tomatoes, sweet potatoes, cooked spinach, beans (baked, kidney, lima, pinto)
Dessert	• Depending upon your calorie needs, your Registered Dietitian may recommend high-calorie desserts • Limit dairy-based desserts and those made with chocolate, nuts, and bananas • If you are a diabetic, discuss low carbohydrate dessert choices with your Registered Dietitian	• No specific recommendation

1. Source: National Kidney Foundation. 2. Source: National Institute of Diabetes and Digestive and Kidney Diseases.

Figure 5.30 Sample Menu for a Client on Hemodialysis

This meal plan provides 2150 calories, 91 grams protein, 2300 mg sodium, 18 mg (46 mEq) potassium, 950 mg phosphorus, 38 oz. of oral fluid.

Breakfast

• Cranberry Juice, 4 oz.
• Eggs (2) or ½ cup egg substitute
• Toasted white bread, 2 slices with butter or tub margarine or fruit spread

Lunch

• Tuna salad sandwich made with 3 oz. tuna on a hard roll with lettuce and mayonnaise (other choices for sandwiches include egg and chicken salad, lean roast beef, low salt ham and turkey breast)
• Coleslaw, ½ cup
• Pretzels (low salt)
• Canned and drained peaches, ½ cup
• Lemon-lime beverage, 8 oz. (cola drinks are high in phosphorus)

Dinner

• Hamburger patty, 4 oz. on a bun; ½ tsp. ketchup
• Salad, 1 cup (lettuce, cucumber, radishes, peppers, with olive oil and vinegar dressing).
• Lemonade, 8 oz.
• Aim for at least 2-3 "fish" meals each week. Many fish are rich in heart-healthy "omega-3" fats. Tuna and salmon (rinsed or canned without salt) and shellfish are excellent heart-healthy protein choices

Snack

• Milk, 4 oz.
• Slice of apple pie

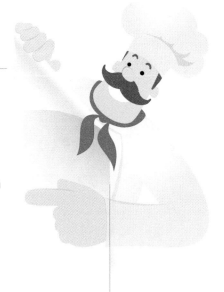

Source: National Kidney Foundation

Loss of Appetite

Causes of anorexia and weight loss include emotional stress and depression, chemotherapy, radiation treatment, and the cancer itself, especially if it is in the gastrointestinal tract. These strategies may help stimulate appetite:

✓ Ask the physician and nursing staff about effective medications to control nausea and pain. Give these one hour before meals to promote better intake.

✓ Large amounts of food tend to overwhelm a reluctant eater. Try smaller portions of nutrient-dense food every one to two hours.

✓ Update food preferences and dislikes often, since these may change during the course of the illness.

✓ Cater to special requests, even if this means purchasing food not normally stocked.

✓ Offer high-calorie, high-protein foods (described in Chapter 16).

✓ Avoid foods with strong odors: use boiling bag and outdoor grill or fans.

Even though many high-calorie foods are high in fat, and in some cases also saturated fat, keep in mind that there are situations where taking in adequate calories is more important than worrying about fat content.

Early Satiety

Feeling full midway through the meal is a common occurrence. These tips may be useful:

✓ Encourage five or six mini-meals throughout the day.

✓ Serve a well-balanced, nutrient-dense breakfast since many clients feel good in the morning.

✓ Instruct the client to save high-fat foods until the end of the meal because these promote satiety.

✓ Have high-calorie snacks available at the bedside.

Nausea and Vomiting

In addition to medications, the following tactics may help control nausea and vomiting:

✓ Allow the client to eat when less nauseated; be flexible with mealtimes.

✓ Eat before cancer treatments.

✓ Encourage nutrient-dense fluids between meals to prevent dehydration. Use fruit juice, milkshakes, and liquid medical nutritional products.

✓ Avoid food with strong odors and flavors if these are offensive.

✓ Offer cold meals rather than hot foods, as this minimizes aromas.

✓ Bland or dry food like toast or crackers may be well tolerated.

Dry or Sore Mouth

Changes in saliva make the client more prone to dental problems. Encourage good oral hygiene and frequent saline (saltwater) rinses. These nutrition tips will help bring relief during meals:

✓ Drink plenty of liquids at meals; use straws.

✓ Eat foods that are easy to chew such as cottage cheese, soft fruits, custards, milkshakes.

✓ Use sugarless gum to stimulate salivation.

✓ Analgesics may relieve pain while eating.

✓ Avoid crisp and raw food, which may scratch the mouth and throat, causing discomfort. Also, acidic and salty food may irritate these areas.

✓ Soft foods are better tolerated; a pureed texture may be needed temporarily.

✓ Add liquid, gravy, and sauces to moisten food.

✓ Drink fruit nectar instead of juice

Swallowing Difficulties

Swallowing problems occur when the esophagus is exposed to radiation, usually two to three weeks after treatment begins.

✓ Soft and pureed consistencies are better tolerated.

✓ Serve food at room temperature or very cold.

✓ Liquids may be easier to manage; consider liquid medical nutritional products.

✓ Request an evaluation from the speech pathologist.

Changes in Taste and Smell

Sensations may be decreased or may just be different from normal. Check with the client often to inquire about food aversions, and then make appropriate substitutions for the offending foods.

✓ Highly seasoned food may be appreciated.

✓ Meat may be better accepted cold or with something sweet like jelly or applesauce.

✓ Try soybean-based tofu and dairy products as protein alternatives if meats are refused.

✓ Plastic disposable utensils may reduce complaints of altered/metallic taste.

✓ Pay particular attention to the presentation of food on the plate and to mealtime ambiance.

✓ Rinse mouth before eating.

✓ Use sugar-free mints, gum, or lemon drops.

Diarrhea

A temporary lactose intolerance may develop, causing diarrhea. Eliminate milk and milk products to determine whether the diarrhea is from lactose intolerance.

✓ Try low-lactose milk or a lactose-free medical nutritional product.

✓ Encourage potassium-rich food to replace losses. Good sources are bananas, apricots, raisins, citrus fruits, and potatoes.

✓ Avoid high-fat food, which may aggravate the situation.

✓ Eat soups, broth, sport drinks, and canned fruits to help replace sodium and potassium.

AIDS

Acquired Immunodeficiency Syndrome (AIDS) is a serious illness that affects the body's ability to fight infection. The human immunodeficiency virus (HIV) causes AIDS. HIV is spread primarily through sexual intercourse with an HIV-infected person, contaminated needles or blood, or from mother to infant during pregnancy or lactation. When first infected with HIV, a client generally has no symptoms. As time progresses, symptoms appear and often include exhaustion, fever, diarrhea, weight loss, muscle pain, and mouth infections. AIDS actually refers to the final stage of HIV infection, when health problems such as recurrent pneumonia, cancers, severe diarrhea, and malabsorption are the most serious.

The wasting and malnutrition just discussed with regard to cancer cachexia are commonly seen in HIV-infected clients. There are many possible reasons for this, such as anorexia, inadequate diet, increased metabolic rate, GI tract infections, drugs, reduced gastric acid secretion, diarrhea, and malabsorption.

As you can imagine, early nutrition support is important to build up nutrient stores and body weight. As long as possible, an oral diet is generally preferable, using high-protein, high-calorie foods and supplements as necessary. A concern for HIV-infected and AIDS clients is making sure food is safe to eat. The body ordinarily is well-equipped to deal with bacteria that cause foodborne illness, but these clients are at far greater risk of serious illness. Because of weakened immune systems, these individuals are more susceptible to contracting a foodborne illness. Once contracted, these infections, with their severe vomiting and diarrhea, can be difficult to treat and they can come back again and again. This can further weaken the immune system and hasten the progression of HIV infection, and be fatal for persons with AIDS.

Individuals with AIDS may lose up to 34 percent of their ideal body weight in the four to five months before death. They have inadequate nutrient intakes for reasons similar to those of people with cancer—altered perceptions, drug therapy, dry mouth, lack of energy to eat, depression, nausea/vomiting, etc. Accelerated nutrient losses may occur because of diarrhea, drug therapy, infections, or malabsorption. Sound nutritional status may improve a person's response to drug therapy, reduce duration of hospital stays, and promote physical independence. For dietary considerations, follow the same nutritional approaches as cancer patients.

Alzheimer's Disease

Alzheimer's Disease is the most common form of dementia (impairment of mental functioning), although it is not part of normal aging. It proceeds in stages over months or years and gradually destroys memory, reason, judgment, language, and eventually the ability to carry out even simple tasks. About half of individuals over age 85 have Alzheimer's disease, but it can also appear as early as middle age. It accounts for 60 percent of admissions to nursing homes. Managing the nutritional well-being of a resident with Alzheimer's disease is challenging and ever-changing, as no two individuals' needs and abilities are the same. Techniques that successfully maintain food intake and weight in some residents may not work for others. Nutrition management of a resident with Alzheimer's must be individualized according to the person's ability and current stage of the disease.

Understanding the progression of the disease is the first step toward nutrition management. There are basically three stages of Alzheimer's:

✓ **Early Stage.** This stage is characterized by forgetfulness, a tendency to misplace things, and some withdrawal from usual interests. Individuals may have trouble finding the right words to communicate their thoughts. Initially, they may not have problems eating their meals, but environmental surroundings may cause a problem. They may not want to eat in public or in a noisy environment. This stage of Alzheimer's may go unnoticed.

✓ **Intermediate Stage.** Persons with Alzheimer's usually cannot initiate a specific movement or course of action without assistance during this stage. There is confusion and difficulty carrying out usual routines. Individuals may begin to need re-direction at mealtime as they forget how to use flatware or are unaware of what to do with the food in front of them. Some individuals also wander at mealtimes and therefore require constant supervision. Partial to total feeding is usually required. At times, they may refuse to open their mouths, making the dining experience a conflict situation between client and caregiver. Situations like this can promote violent behavior in some individuals. Also, clients become disoriented with respect to their surroundings, time, and place. This may explain why they become lost walking to the dining room or forget if they have eaten meals. Losing the ability to remember whether they have eaten not only can lead to weight loss, but also to weight gain.

✓ **Late Stage.** At this stage, the person's motor skills deteriorate. Patients lose the ability to chew and swallow, and often to speak. Their sensitivity to seizures, aspiration, and pneumonia increases, making it difficult for caregivers to provide them with fluids and food orally. Food and fluid textures have to be modified to promote oral intake as long as possible. Correct feeding and positioning techniques must be exhibited by the caregiver during mealtimes. Decisions by families and medical staff must be made regarding enteral nutrition support.

Compiling a comprehensive nutrition assessment upon admission of each client with Alzheimer's is a key aspect in nutritional management. Continuous assessment is necessary due to the disease progression. During the initial three to five days after admission, the client must be closely monitored at mealtimes for changes in eating/feeding ability. Depending on the severity of the eating skill deficiency, close monitoring should be done weekly to monthly.

Nutritional care strategies must be individualized to patients and their current stages of the disease. All techniques do not work for all clients with Alzheimer's. The old saying, "If at first you don't succeed, try, try again," is never more true than for this population. Nutritional management of persons with Alzheimer's requires implementing techniques appropriate for specific problems, as outlined on the next page.

To maintain weight and appetite:

✓ Serve the larger meals at breakfast when the resident is more alert and his/her appetite is larger. Even clients with good appetites will consume smaller evening meals due in part to the **"sundowning"** effect (increased restlessness and anxiety as evening approaches).

✓ Provide nutrient-dense foods routinely in the diet, such as whole milk with meals, fortified cereal at breakfast, and additional juices and whole grain breads.

✓ Offer nutritious snacks between meals, such as juice and graham crackers, sandwich halves, fruit, and cheese.

✓ Implement a weekly weight program for all clients. Close monitoring is a must.

✓ Involve all facility staff during mealtimes to assist residents in the dining rooms and those who receive room service.

Observe for changes in a client's eating habits, such as decreased use of utensils, playing with food, or using fingers. If observed, make appropriate changes in meal service to maintain their independence. To maintain feeding independence:

✓ If there is a decreased use of utensils: offer utensils only as needed, use "hand-over-hand" techniques in promoting self-feeding, and provide verbal cues for client, e.g., "Mrs. Jones, pick up your fork."

✓ If the client is playing with or mixing food: offer one food at a time, place foods in individual bowls, put condiments on food before serving, and have staff provide constant redirection and verbal cues at mealtimes.

✓ If the client is using fingers to eat, maximize the situation. Offer finger foods to allow resident to maintain independence, yet eat in a dignified manner.

If the client experiences confusion at meal times:

✓ Offer meals at the same time, same place, and same seating arrangement every day.

✓ Serve the meal immediately after the resident is in the dining room.

✓ Allow adequate time for meals.

✓ Make the physical environment pleasant and calming.

✓ Limit the use of intercoms.

✓ Play soft background music.

✓ Seat residents in groups of four to six.

✓ Use square rather than round tables.

✓ Set the table with solid, contrasting colors between the china and the tablecloth.

✓ Limit the centerpieces at mealtimes.

✓ Maintain a high staff-to-resident ratio at mealtime.

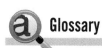

Glossary

Alzheimer's Disease
Most common form of dementia marked by loss of cognitive ability

Sundowning Effect
When confusion or disorientation worsens at the end of the day

If the client has difficulty chewing and/or swallowing:

✓ Check fit of dentures, if applicable.

✓ Position the resident correctly (at 90-degree angle) in chair, wheelchair, or bed.

✓ Provide verbal cues in a soft, gentle manner to remind residents to chew food, eat slowly, and swallow.

✓ Evaluate for need of a texture-modified diet. Offer soft or ground meat first, then go to soft scoop pureed consistency.

✓ Use gravies and sauces to moisten food.

✓ Ensure that food temperatures are safe.

✓ Avoid offering a food with a combination of textures, e.g. vegetable soup.

✓ Consult a speech therapist for swallowing evaluation.

✓ Learn techniques to overcome problems of refusing to open mouth or of pocketing food.

According to Dr. Glenn Smith at the Mayo Clinic, the Mediterranean Diet may benefit the brain. People who follow the Mediterranean Diet are less likely to decline mentally. Research has found the following benefits of the Mediterranean Diet:

✓ Slows mental decline in older adults

✓ Reduces the chance of mild cognitive impairment (MCI) that occurs prior to more serious mental impairment and Alzheimer's

✓ If MCI occurs, the diet reduces the chance of MCI progressing into Alzheimer's

Immobilization

Long periods of immobilization, such as following an injury or simply being bedridden, can result in development of pressure ulcers. **Pressure ulcers**, pressure sores, or **decubitus ulcers** are lesions caused by unrelieved pressure resulting in damage to underlying tissue. Over one million patients in hospitals and nursing homes suffer from pressure ulcers. The first preventive step is to identify clients at high risk for pressure ulcers, explained in Figure 5.31. Clients with pressure ulcers need to be followed closely, using a staging system (see Figure 5.32).

Nutrition plays a vital role in preventing and treating pressure ulcers. Clients who are malnourished and/or eating and drinking poorly have a greater chance of developing pressure ulcers. Medical Nutrition Therapy for this condition commonly includes a high-calorie, high-protein diet along with adequate fluids.

The nutritional needs for calories, protein, and fluid increase with the stage of the ulcer, as shown in Figure 5.32. Multivitamin/mineral supplements are frequently given for Stages II-IV. Additional vitamin C and zinc may be given for Stage IV but the research to support this is not substantiated. More aggressive calorie, protein, and vitamin/mineral supplementation is needed for a client with multiple pressure ulcers.

Figure 5.31   Risk Factors for Pressure Ulcers

- Impaired transfer or bed mobility
- Bedridden, hemiplegia, quadriplegia
- Loss of bowel or bladder control
- Peripheral vascular disease
- Diabetes mellitus
- Hip fracture
- Weight loss/poor nutrition
- Pressure ulcer history
- Impaired tactile sensory perception
- Medications
- Restraints
- Severe chronic pulmonary obstructive disease
- Sepsis
- Terminal cancer
- Chronic or end-stage renal, liver, and/or heart disease
- Disease or drug related immunosuppression
- Full-body cast
- Steroid, radiation or chemotherapy
- Renal dialysis
- Head of bed elevated the majority of the day

Figure 5.32   Pressure Ulcer Staging and Nutritional Needs

A staging system describes the extent of tissue damage in pressure ulcers. Stages also influence nutritional recommendations. The stages and related nutritional advice follow:

Stage/Needs	Calories	Protein	Fluid
Stage I: Intact skin with non-blanchable redness of a localized area usually over a bony prominence. Darkly pigmented skin may not have visible blanching; its color may differ from the surrounding area.	30 cal/kg	1.0-1.1 gm/kg	30 ml/kg
Stage II: Partial thickness, loss of dermis presenting as a shallow open ulcer with a red/pink wound bed, without slough. May also present as an intact or open/ruptured serum-filled blister.	30 cal/kg	1.2 gm/kg	30 ml/kg
Stage III: Full thickness tissue loss. Subcutaneous fat may be visible but bone, tendon or muscle are not exposed. Slough may be present but does not obscure the depth of tissue loss. May include undermining and tunneling.	35 cal/kg	1.3-1.4 gm/kg	30-35 ml/kg
Stage IV: Full thickness tissue loss with exposed bone, tendon or muscle. Slough or eschar may be present on some parts of the wound bed. Often includes undermining and tunneling.	35 cal/kg	1.5-1.6 gm/kg	35 ml/kg

Source: National Pressure Ulcer Advisory Panel, 2007

Developmentally Disabled and Handicapped Clients

The term developmental disability refers to a severe, chronic disability that:

✓ Is attributable to a mental or physical impairment, or a combination of mental and physical impairments

✓ Is manifested before the person reaches the age of 22 years

✓ Is likely to continue indefinitely

✓ Results in substantial functional limitations in three or more of the following areas of major life activity: self-care, receptive and expressive language, learning, mobility, self-direction, capacity for independent living, and economic self-sufficiency.

✓ Reflects the person's need for a combination and sequence of special interdisciplinary or generic care, treatment, or other services that are lifelong or of extended duration and individually planned and coordinated (Developmental Disabilities Assistance and Bill of Rights Act, 1978).

Examples of developmental disabilities are mental retardation, cerebral palsy (partial paralysis and lack of muscular coordination), muscular dystrophy (progressive weakness and deterioration of muscles), epilepsy (sudden, passing disturbances of brain function), and autism (withdrawal and lack of responsiveness to others). Developmentally disabled children are at high risk for nutritional problems and deficiencies. Frequent nutrition-related problems that contribute to nutritional risk include the following:

✓ Feeding problems. There may be either physical or psychological factors that cause feeding problems. For example, in children with cerebral palsy, the muscles involved in chewing and swallowing may not function normally. In change.

✓ **Drug-nutrient interactions.** Many individuals with developmental disabilities are on long-term medications to treat chronic problems such as epilepsy and infections. Nutrition counseling may be needed as well as vitamin or mineral supplements.

✓ Obesity. Some developmentally disabled are more prone to obesity due to limited activity, poor muscle tone, small stature, and/or overeating. Nutrition counseling and exercise may be useful.

✓ Constipation. Constipation is common due to decreased activity and certain medications.

✓ Dehydration. Some developmentally disabled individuals are not able to feel or express thirst. Others need extra fluids because of drooling or to prevent frequent urinary infections. Fluid intake should be encouraged and individuals assisted when necessary.

Nutrition intervention is more effective with an interdisciplinary team approach that includes other professionals such as nurses, occupational therapists, physical therapists, social workers, and dentists. Nutrition intervention is also more effective when the traditional nutrition assessment process has been modified for this population. For example, it is necessary to overcome difficulties in weighing and measuring clients and in selecting appropriate standards (such as weight) for comparison. Nutrition programs for the

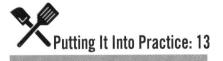

Putting It Into Practice: 13

What are the three most important dietary interventions for pressure ulcers?

(Check your answer at the end of this chapter)

developmentally disabled can greatly benefit these individuals by improving their health and their capacity to socialize and function in an educational, work, or home environment.

A physical handicap can be caused by a variety of illnesses or accidents. Some of the common causes are arthritis, amputations, spinal cord injuries, stroke, Parkinson's disease, or multiple sclerosis. These illnesses can result in feeding problems for either emotional or physical reasons. Depression, which can occur with any illness, can result in a loss of appetite leading to weight loss, or in increased consumption of high-calorie, easily consumed foods, leading to obesity. Depressed clients may be extremely demanding and very selective in their food preferences. Demands requiring many substitutions can be very frustrating to the foodservice staff. Tremors or paralysis may make it difficult for a client to use utensils. Dysphagia may make eating certain consistencies of food difficult. Figure 5.33 addresses feeding problems and adaptations.

Figure 5.33 **Feeding Problems and Adaptations**

Problem/Challenge	Possible Adaptation
One handedness; difficulty cutting meat	Rocker knife or roller knife
Poor hand coordination	Weighted utensils, scoop dish, plate guard, covered cups with slotted opening
Hand deformity, difficulty grasping	Built-up handles on eating utensils
Limited neck motion—unable to tilt head back	Cut-out plastic cup (nose cup)
Muscle weakness	Utensil holder, two-handled cups, clamp-on handles
Visual problems	Clock method for locating food on tray, plate guard, scoop dish
Shakiness	Sippy cup, swivel utensils

Source: *Becky Dorner. 1996. Dignity in dining: feeding techniques for elderly and disabled clients. Dietary Manager Magazine.*

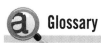

Glossary

Pressure Ulcers, aka Pressure Sores, Decubitus Ulcers
Lesions caused by pressure

Drug-Nutrient Interaction
Can lead to nutrient malabsorption or the drug not working effectively

END OF CHAPTER

 Putting It Into Practice Questions & Answers

1. Can you guess (a) how many, and, (b) which of the leading causes of death are directly related to diet?

    A. *Seven out of the nine leading causes of death have a relationship to diet: Heart Disease: #1, Cancer: #2, Stroke: #3, Alzheimer's: #6, Diabetes: #7, and Kidney Disease: #9.*

2. How would you adjust the following recipe to lower the saturated fat grams?

    - 3 slightly beaten eggs *(use ¾ cup egg substitute)*
    - ¼ cup sugar
    - ¼ tsp. salt
    - 2 cups milk *(use non-fat milk or for a more creamy consistency, non-fat evaporated milk)*
    - 1 tsp. vanilla

3. If a diet order is written as 2 gm NA, what does this mean?

    A. *2000 mg of sodium per day*

4. If a client's medical chart shows a fasting blood sugar of 300, what type of diagnosis might you expect to see?

    A. *Diabetes*

5. What medical conditions are commonly managed using a carbohydrate counting diet?

    A. *Obesity and Diabetes*

6. In Figure 5.17 food Label, where do the 29 grams of carbohydrate come from in the granola bar?

    ## Nutrition Facts

    Serving Size: 2 Bars (42 g)

    Amount Per Serving

    Calories 180   *Calories from Fat 50*

	% Daily Value*
Total Fat 6g	9%
Saturated Fat 0.5g	3%
Trans Fat 0.5g	
Cholesterol 0mg	0%
Sodium 160mg	7%
Total Carbohydrates 29g	10%
Dietary Fiber 2g	15%
Sugars 11g	
Protein 4g	

Vitamin A	0%	Vitamin C	0%
Calcium	0%	Iron	6%

    * Percent Daily Values are based on a 2,000 calorie diet. Your daily values may be higher or lower depending on your calorie needs.

    Ingredients: Rolled oats, high maltose corn syrup, sugar, high fructose corn syrup, crisp rise, palm kernel oil, yellow corn meal, fructose, canola oil, yogurt powder, corn bran, nonfat milk, soy lecithin, salt, honey, sunflower meal, peanut flour, almond flour.

    A. *There are 209 grams of total carbohydrates. Of those 29 grams, 2 grams are dietary fiber (rolled oats, crisp rice, yellow corn meal, corn bran); and 11 grams are sugar (high maltose corn syrup, high fructose corn syrup, fructose, honey). The remaining 16 grams come from the oat and flours (sunflower meal, peanut flour, almond flour). You would need the ingredient listing to determine the other carbohydrate sources.*

    Note: Sugar content on food labels include fruit and milk sugars so the sugar content includes the yogurt powder and the nonfat milk.

    (Continued)

Putting It Into Practice Questions & Answers *(Continued)*

7. If 3500 calories are equivalent to one pound of fat, how many calories would you need to decrease every day to lose one pound of fat in one week?

    A. *To lose one pound in one week, divide 3500 by 7 days. You would have to decrease your caloric intake by 500 each day in order to lose one pound of fat in one week.*

8. What factors would you need to consider when an elderly widow is leaving your healthcare facility to return home? She has been successful so far on a weight loss diet.

    A. *Remember there are many factors that impact weight control. Does this person have a good attitude regarding her diet? Does she have social support at home or a close circle of friends? What drugs is she taking? Does she prepare her own meals or does she eat out frequently? Can she exercise regularly? Would/could she consider keeping a food diary for a few weeks to help her change behaviors at home?*

9. When a client is coughing during their meals, to whom should he/she be referred?

    A. *The Speech or Occupational Therapist. Coughing during meals could mean a swallowing problem and he/she should be assessed by a Speech or Occupational Therapist.*

10. You have several clients with food allergies in your facility. Which of the following Worcestershire sauce products should you purchase for your facility and why?

    Worcestershire Sauce #1

    Ingredients: Distilled white vinegar, water, molasses, high fructose corn syrup, salt, soy sauce, natural flavorings, caramel coloring, anchovies, soy flour, polysorbate 80, garlic extract

    Worcestershire Sauce #2

    Ingredients: Distilled vinegar, water, molasses, corn syrup, salt, anchovies, tamarind extract, sugar, spices, garlic power, xanthan gum, natural flavors

    A. *Choose Worcestershire Sauce #2 because it does not contain soy products. For people with allergies, soy products may be a concern. As an added note, both of these contain anchovies so neither could be used for a strict vegan client.*

11. You are working with a client who just transferred in from the hospital. In her medical record you read where she was started on a Clear Liquid Diet on 8-10-11. Today's date is 8-15-11 and she is still on the Clear Liquid Diet. What should you do?

    A. *Contact your Registered Dietitian regarding a diet order change. A Clear Liquid Diet should only be prescribed for three or less days.*

12. What should you look for on a nutrition label for a client with chronic kidney disease?

    A. *Sodium and protein are listed on the actual label so make a note of the grams of sodium and protein. Then, read the ingredient label to locate sources of potassium or phosphorus., e.g. meat products may have potassium chloride, potassium lactate, sodium phosphate, and sodium aluminum phosphate.*

13. What are the three most important dietary interventions for pressure ulcers?

    A. *Calories, protein, and fluid.*

Explore Complementary and Alternative Therapies

Overview and Objectives

Alternative therapies often come up during the provision of nutritional care. A Certified Dietary Manager needs to understand alternative therapies and know how to assess them to promote optimum nutrition for clients.

After completing this chapter, you should be able to:

✓ Define alternative therapies

✓ Identify risks and benefits of alternative therapies

✓ Classify use of alternative therapies in long-term and acute care

✓ List questions to ask in evaluating dietary supplements and other complementary and alternative treatments

✓ Identify the role of basic nutrition concepts in assessment and implementation of complementary and alternative therapies

✓ Explain the role of the Certified Dietary Manager for assisting clients in alternative therapies

Have you ever been to a chiropractor, a naturopath, or a homeopath? How does their treatment fit into what you have been studying? Alternative practices often come up during the provision of nutritional care. You will want to understand complementary and alternative approaches to medical care and how to assess them in order to promote optimum nutrition for your clients. Both terms describe practices that fall outside of conventional medicine in the U.S.

The National Center for Complementary and Alternative Medicine (NCCAM) of the National Institutes of Health provides this definition:

Complementary and alternative medicine is a group of diverse medical and healthcare systems, practices, and products that are not presently considered to be part of conventional medicine.

What do we mean by **conventional medicine**? This is the science used by physicians (Medical Doctors—MDs, and Doctors of Osteopathy—DOs), as well as allied health professionals, as they are trained in the U.S. Sometimes, conventional medicine is also called mainstream medicine, orthodox medicine, biomedicine, or allopathy.

Anything that does not fall within this broadly accepted group of practices is **Complementary and Alternative Medicine (CAM)**. **Complementary medicine** is an unconventional medical practice that is used to complement or *add to* conventional medical practice. **Alternative medicine** is an unconventional medical practice that is used *instead of* conventional medicine. CAM therapies may also be called unconventional medicine, simply meaning they are not part of the routine therapeutic approach to treatment.

Integrative medicine is medical practice that combines conventional practice with CAM practices. For example, a physician treating anxiety who prescribes both a drug regimen and meditation is practicing integrative medicine.

NCCAM explains: "While scientific evidence exists regarding some CAM therapies, for most there are key questions that are yet to be answered through well-designed scientific studies—questions such as whether these therapies are safe and whether they work for the purposes for which they are used." Figure 6.1 provides information about the more common CAM therapies among adults in the 2007 NCCAM survey. Check the following Website for updated information about the safety and effectiveness of CAM therapies: http://nccam.nih.gov/news/alerts/

The number of people seeking complementary or alternative medicines has increased dramatically from 2002 to 2007. A NCCAM report, *The Use of Complementary and Alternative Medicine in the United States*, 2008, states, "In the U.S., approximately 38 percent of adults (about 4 in 10) and approximately 12 percent of children (about 1 in 9) are using some form of CAM." Figure 6.2 shows the most common CAM therapies among adults from the NCCAM 2007 survey. From the NCCAM report, "The most popular natural products are fish oil/omega-3, glucosamine, Echinacea, and flaxseed. Glucosamine is a substance found in the fluid around joints and used by the body to make and repair cartilage. Glucosamine in dietary supplements is made in the laboratory or from the shells of shrimp, lobster, and crabs."

People are willing to pay 11.2 percent of total out-of-pocket expenditures on CAM healthcare in the U.S. Compare that to the total healthcare expenditures in Figure 6.3.

Types of CAM

NCCAM identifies five types of CAM: alternative medical systems, mind-body interventions, biologically based therapies, manipulative and body-based methods, and energy therapies. Here is a closer look at types of CAM.

Alternative Medical Systems (See Figure 6.1 for explanations of examples)
Represent complete and separate systems for understanding health and illness. Examples include:

✓ Acupuncture

✓ Ayureda

✓ Homeopathic

✓ Naturopathic

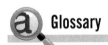

Glossary

Conventional Medicine
Medicine practiced by physicians (Medical Doctors—MDs, and Doctors of Osteopathy—Dos) as well as allied health professionals

CAM
Complementary and alternative medicines that do not fall within conventional medicine practices

Complementary Medicine
Using an unconventional medical practice in addition to conventional medicine

Alternative Medicine
Using an unconventional medicinal practice in place of conventional medicine

Integrative Medicine
Combines conventional practices with CAM practices

Figure 6.1   CAM Therapy Included in the 2007 National Health Interview Survey (NHIS)

CAM Therapy	Definition
Acupuncture* (AK-you-punk-shur)	Involves inserting thin needles into specific points on the body to relieve pain or other symptoms
Ayurveda* (ah-yur-VAY-dah)	A system of medicine from India over 5,000 years old. The chief aim is to cleanse the body of substances that can cause disease and to balance the body, mind, and spirit.
Biofeedback*	Uses electronic devices to teach clients how to consciously regulate bodily functions such as breathing, heart rate, and blood pressure. It is used to reduce stress, eliminate headaches, relieve pain, and recondition injured muscles.
Chelation (Key-LAY-shun) **Therapy***	A chemical process used to bind molecules, such as metals or minerals. It has been scientifically proven to rid the body of excess or toxic metals such as lead.
Chiropractic (ki-roh-PRAC-tic) or **Osteopathic** (ash-tee-ph-PATH-ic) **Manipulation***	Both are systems of hands-on techniques or adjustments to alleviate pain, restore function, and promote health and well-being.
Deep Breathing Exercises	Involves slow and deep inhalation through the nose followed by slow and complete exhalation.
Diet-Based Therapies	Examples are the South Beach Diet, a vegetarian diet, and the Ornish diet (a high-fiber, low-fat, vegetarian diet. Oils, avocados, nuts and seeds, and meats of all kinds are avoided).
Energy Healing Therapy/Reiki* (RAY-kee)	A Japanese word meaning universal life energy. Reiki is based on the belief that when spiritual energy is channeled through a Reiki practitioner, the patient's spirit is healed, which in turn heals the physical body.
Guided Imagery	Involves relaxation techniques followed by visualizing calm and peaceful images.
Homeopathic (home-ee-oh-PATH-ic) **Treatment**	A belief where "like cures like," meaning that small, highly diluted quantities of medicinal substances are given to cure symptoms. Homeopathic remedies are derived from many natural sources including plants, metals, and minerals.
Hypnosis*	An altered state of consciousness used to treat many health conditions including ulcers, chronic pain, respiratory ailments, stress, and headaches.
Massage Therapy*	Therapists manipulate muscle and connective tissue to enhance functions of those tissues and promote relaxation and well-being.
Meditation	Involves techniques from Eastern religious or spiritual traditions where a person learns to focus attention and suspend the stream of thoughts that normally occupy the mind.
Natural Products	Non-vitamin and non-mineral, such as herbs and other products from plants, and enzymes.
Naturopathy* (nay-chur-o-PATH-e)	Focuses on the healing power in the body that establishes, maintains, and restores health. Treatments include nutrition and lifestyle counseling, dietary supplements, medicinal plants, exercise, homeopathy, and traditional Chinese medicine.
Progressive Relaxation	A system of tensing and relaxing successive muscle groups to relieve tension and stress
Qi Gong (chee-Gung)	An ancient Chinese discipline using gentle physical movements, mental focus, and deep breathing directed toward specific parts of the body.
Tai Chi (TY-chee)	A mind-body practice that was originally a martial art. A person moves his body slowly and gently while breathing deeply and meditating. It is believed to enhance the flow qi (an ancient term given to what is believed to be vital energy) in the body.
Traditional Healers*	Someone who uses an ancient medical practice handed down from generation to generation.
Yoga	An ancient East Indian practice where, in order to be in harmony with oneself and the environment, he has to integrate the body, the mind, and the spirit. This occurs through deep breathing, meditation, and physical postures or poses.

* Indicates a practitioner-based therapy

Source: National Center for Complementary and Alternative Medicine (NCCAM), National Institutes of Health

Figure 6.2   Ten Most Common CAM Therapies Among Adults: 2007

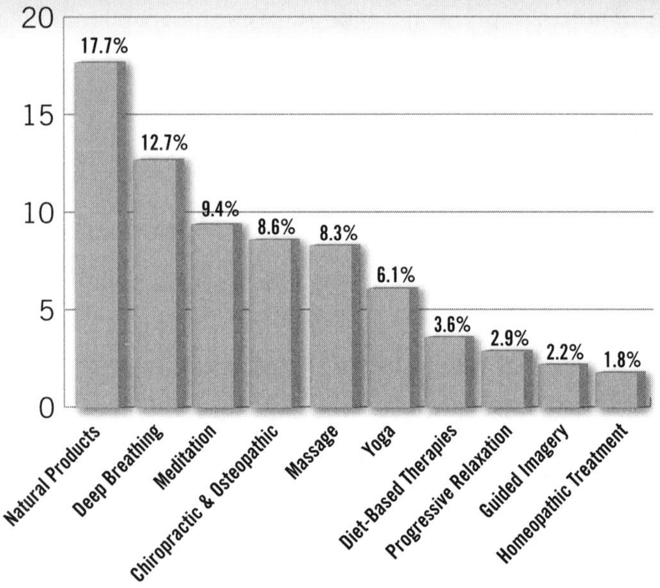

Therapies with significant increases between 2002 and 2007

	2002	2007
Deep Breathing	11.6 percent	12.7 percent
Meditation	7.6 percent	9.4 percent
Massage	5.6 percent	8.3 percent
Yoga	5.1 percent	6.1 percent

National Center for Complementary and Alternative Medicine, http://nccam.nih.gov/news/camstats/2007/graphics.htm. Data accessed August 20, 2010.

Mind-Body Interventions (See Figure 6.1 for explanations of examples)

Uses the influence of the mind on the body or "mind over matter"

✓ Biofeedback

✓ Guided imagery

✓ Hypnosis

✓ Traditional healers

Biologically Based Therapies (See Figure 6.1 for explanations of examples)

Uses biological agents, such as herbs, special foods, or nutritional supplements to produce therapeutic results

✓ Chelation therapy

✓ Natural products

✓ Naturapathy

✓ Probiotics

Manipulative and Body-Based Methods (See Figure 6.1 for explanations of examples)

Involves moving or manipulating parts of the body to promote healing

✓ Chiropractic

✓ Massage therapy

✓ Tai Chi

✓ Yoga

Uses energy fields believed to surround and penetrate the body

✓ Reiki

✓ Qi Gong

Figure 6.3   CAM Out of Pocket Spending

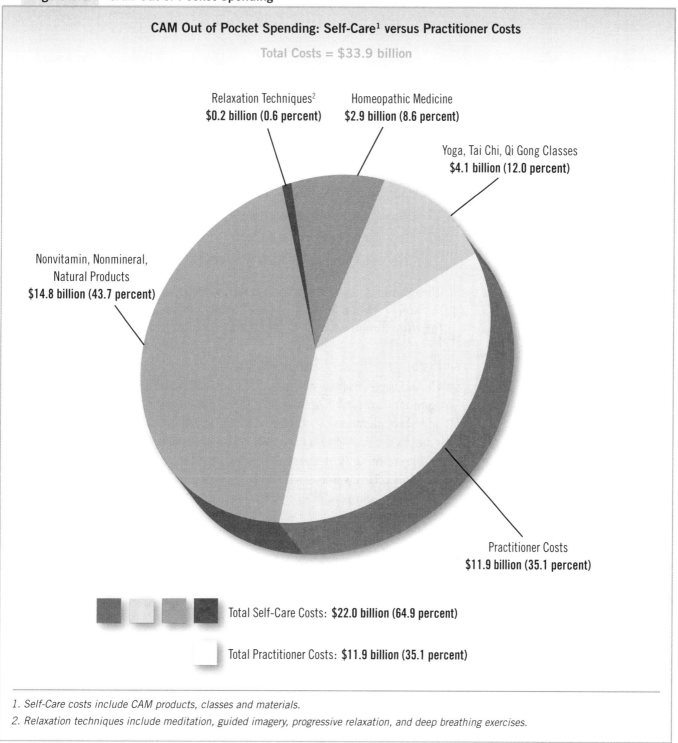

1. Self-Care costs include CAM products, classes and materials.
2. Relaxation techniques include meditation, guided imagery, progressive relaxation, and deep breathing exercises.

National Center for Complimentary and Alternative Medicine, nccam.nih.gov/news/camstats/costs/graphics.htm. Data accessed August 29, 2010

Evolving Research on CAM Therapies

✓ Hot spices, specifically turmeric, have been shown in lab studies to fight breast cancer by limiting the growth of stem cells.

✓ Ginko Biloba, taken to improve cognitive health or memory function, *did not* lesson cognitive decline in recent NCCAM studies.

✓ Phytonutrients lutein and zeaxanthin have been found to help prevent age-related macular degeneration, the number one cause of irreversible blindness in the U.S.

✓ Glucosamine—taken for relief of arthritis symptoms. In a 2010 study, glucosamine was *not* more effective than a **placebo**.

✓ Probiotics for digestive health is an industry on the rise. Probiotics or "friendly bacteria" are thought to improve digestive health. The greatest use of probiotics today is fermented dairy products such as yogurt, kefir, and cheese. In the *Environmental Nutrition* newsletter, October, 2009, author Virginia Shanta Retely promoted using the guidelines from the U.S.robiotics.org Website when evaluating probiotic products:

  • "They must be alive when consumed

  • They should be documented to have a health benefit

  • They must be given at levels to result in a health benefit."

The examples above are just a few of the emerging research evidence on CAM therapies. Logon to this Website to follow the advances in CAM therapies http://nccam.nih.gov.

Herbs and Dietary Supplements

Herbs, large doses of vitamins and minerals, and other food components are common forms of CAM. In fact, sales of dietary supplements and foods with added supplements or functional food ingredients total billions of dollars each year. As the role of nutrition in health gains increasing attention from the scientific community, it is easy to believe there is a dietary solution to nearly every condition. This is not exactly true. Dietary practices can become an important component of overall healthcare, however.

When it comes to herbs and other nutritional supplements, it's important to understand that "natural" does not necessarily mean "safe." Many of nature's poisons are entirely natural—but deadly. Arsenic is an example. Meanwhile, some of today's drug therapies have been derived from plants. An example is digitalis, a medicine for regulating heartbeat. Digitalis comes from the Foxfire plant and was a Native American medicine. Thus, the key point is that any chemical compound that has biological activity—whether derived from natural sources or created in a laboratory—must be evaluated scientifically. It needs to be proven safe and effective. In addition, the manufacture and dosage need to be controlled.

According to the FDA, a **dietary supplement**:

✓ is a product (other than tobacco) that is intended to supplement the diet that bears or contains one or more of the following dietary ingredients: a vitamin, a mineral, an herb or other botanical, an amino acid, a dietary substance for use by man to supplement the diet by increasing the total daily intake, or a concentrate, metabolite, constituent, extract, or combination of these ingredients

✓ is intended for ingestion in pill, capsule, tablet, or liquid form

✓ is not represented for use as a conventional food or as the sole item of a meal or diet

✓ is labeled as a "dietary supplement"

Under the Dietary Supplement Health and Education Act passed by Congress in 1994, dietary supplements are considered foods, not drugs. It is a manufacturer's responsibility to ensure that their products are safe and properly labeled prior to marketing. This means that dietary supplements are not subject to the same controls as prescription and over-the-counter drugs. For a drug to reach the market, the manufacturer must first prove safety and effectiveness to the FDA. Dietary supplements, in contrast, must be proven unsafe by the FDA to be removed from the market.

In addition, the regulation prohibits dietary supplement manufacturers from making health claims on product labels. For example, a label cannot state that this supplement will "cure cancer" or "treat arthritis." However, manufacturers are allowed to describe the supplement's effects on "structure or function" of the body or "well-being." To use these claims, manufacturers must have substantiation that the statements are truthful and not misleading. A product label must bear the note: "This statement has not been evaluated by the Food and Drug Administration. This product is not intended to diagnose, treat, cure, or prevent any disease." A dietary supplement must have a label identifying its ingredients and must provide nutrition labeling. See *Nutrition in the News* at the end of this chapter.

Clearly, a dietary supplement package can imply health benefits that may not be well substantiated. What else is not regulated? Controls on product composition, purity and quality, and quantities are minimal. In 2003, the FDA proposed a new rule to control these issues. In short, the contents of a dietary supplement preparation may not be exactly what a consumer thinks. For example, the FDA evaluated a group of soy products on the market and found that some contained as little as half the amount of isoflavones (active ingredients) claimed. Another review found that a supplement of folic acid contained only 35 percent of its declared dose. Conversely, a supplement may contain much larger doses of active ingredients than the label indicates. This can pose risks related to overdosage. In addition, a dietary supplement may contain contaminants such as lead, pesticides, bacteria, or undeclared ingredients. Among other things, the proposed new rule would establish good manufacturing practices for dietary supplements.

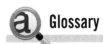 **Glossary**

Placebo
A substance given in clinical trials that contain no medication or active ingredient

Dietary Supplement
A product intended to supplement the diet

Meanwhile, in 2001, the **U.S. Pharmacopeia (USP)**, which is a research group that is not a part of the government, announced a certification program for dietary supplements. Based on testing, a supplement can contain a USP certification mark to indicate that ingredients are as claimed. Of course, this mark does not verify that the supplements are effective treatments for specific health conditions.

In 2003, the Medicare Prescription Drug Improvement and Modernization Act of 2003 (MMA) was signed into law. As part of that law, U.S. Pharmacopeia (USP) has submitted model guidelines for drug categories and classes that may be used by prescription drug plans to the **Centers for Medicare and Medicaid Services (CMS)**. Those guidelines are in effect through benefit year 2011. The USP will form a new Model Guidelines Expert Panel for the 2010-2015 cycle and submit it to CMS in January, 2011.

It's important to note that safe and effective dosages for herbs and other dietary supplements may not be well established. At least for recognized vitamins and minerals, we have reference standards. Thus, even for an herb that may have beneficial effects, a consumer might not take a dosage that proves beneficial. Or, a consumer may easily overdose. Meanwhile, consumers may mistakenly assume that "more is better" when it comes to supplementation. This can be dangerous. Even a vitamin or mineral known to be essential for life can become toxic in excessive doses. Figure 6.4 identifies overdose risks of several dietary supplements.

To avoid overdose of vitamins and minerals, it's helpful to return to basic nutrition science. The body has basic requirements for nutrients. Excesses of many of the water-soluble vitamins are simply excreted in urine. Fat-soluble vitamins and minerals can, in some cases, accumulate in the body. Generally, dietetic professionals recommend that supplementation of vitamins and minerals be used to correct deficiencies, based on an assessment of nutritional status and nutritional needs. A tolerable upper intake level (UL) is the highest level of daily nutrient intake that is likely to pose no risk of adverse health effects for most people. This is different from a recommended level of intake. It provides a reference for evaluating the safety of supplementation.

Drug Interactions

Among the risks of using dietary supplements can be the interactions they present. Herbs, for example, may interact with each other to cause dangerous effects. Herbs may also interact with conventional drugs to modify their action. For instance, the herbal supplement gingko has many potential drug interactions. Gingko can increase blood levels of antidepressant drugs, accidentally building high drug levels. Used with an antipsychotic medication, gingko can cause seizures. Both gingko and coenzyme Q10 are supplements that can interfere with the action of anticoagulant medications, such as warfarin or coumadin. The result can be excessive bleeding. Both ginseng and coenzyme Q10 can enhance the action of a drug designed to lower blood sugar. The result can be a crisis with hypoglycemia (very low blood sugar). St. John's Wort may eliminate a number of drugs from the body very quickly. There is concern that tak-

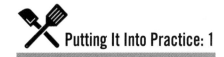

Putting It Into Practice: 1

A client reports that they are taking single supplements of Vitamin B6 and vitamin A. What other information will you need about the supplements?

(Check your answer at the end of this chapter)

Figure 6.4   Risks of Overdose

Dietary Supplement	Common Uses of the Supplement	Effects of Overdose
Vitamin B6 > 100 mg/day	A once-popular remedy for carpal tunnel syndrome and premenstrual syndrome (PMS)	Neurological toxicity, nerve injury
Niacin > 500 mg/day	Recommended to help reduce blood cholesterol levels	Gastrointestinal distress, liver damage, very low blood pressure, occasionally life-threatening conditions
Vitamin A > 25,000 International Units (IU)/day	Taken to slow the development of macular degeneration	Liver damage, birth defects, damage to bones and cartilage
Selenium > 800 micrograms/day	Some people believe it prevents cancer	Tissue damage
Germander	Believed to aid in the treatment for gout	Liver disease
Comfrey	Used historically to treat gastrointestinal distress; the oral supplement was banned by the FDA in 2001; may be used topically for sprains, strained muscles	Liver damage/cirrhosis, sometimes life-threatening
Chaparral	Often consumed as a tea for anti-cancer or reducing the effects of radiation or sun damage; listed by the FDA as a supplement to avoid	Liver damage

Note: > is the symbol for more than.

ing this supplement may reduce the effectiveness of oral contraceptives. It can also interact with antidepressant drugs to cause headache, upset stomach, and restlessness. Before surgery, it can be dangerous to take certain herbal supplements, including ginseng or goldenseal, which may raise blood pressure. Other herbs can slow down blood clotting and increase the risk of excessive bleeding. These include garlic, ginger, gingko, and feverfew.

Because many consumers use dietary supplements as complementary or alternative therapies, they may not choose to discuss these therapies with physicians. Typically, an individual using dietary supplements considers this treatment "separate" from a physician's care. However, it is actually important for a physician to know the complete picture. A Certified Dietary Manager can facilitate this process by asking patients questions about what dietary supplements they use, reporting this information in the diet history, and discussing it with other members of the healthcare team.

Evaluating CAM Therapies

The following questions can help you evaluate any type of medical therapy.

✓ What research supports the safety of this treatment?

✓ What are the possible risks and side effects?

✓ What research indicates this treatment is effective?

✓ Has research been published in a medical journal that is reviewed by trained medical scientists?

✓ Has the research been well-controlled, or is the therapy based on anecdotal reports?

 Glossary

CMS
Centers for Medicare and Medicaid Services

USP
U.S. Pharmacopeia provides model guidelines for prescription drugs

✓ What will the treatment involve?

✓ What will it cost?

✓ Is this treatment intended to complement other therapies or replace them (alternative medicine)?

✓ Has this treatment been discussed with a physician?

✓ What are the other options, and how does this treatment compare?

Figure 6.5 identifies red flags that may indicate fad or fraud in proposed treatments. In addition, the FDA notes that four key assumptions often come into play when consumers are making decisions about therapies. These appear in Figure 6.6.

Healthcare Policy

In 2003, the White House Commission on CAM Policy issued policy suggestions for the healthcare industry. They recommended ten principles for healthcare policy:

1. A wholeness orientation in healthcare delivery. Health involves all aspects of life—mind, body, spirit, environment—and high-quality healthcare must support care of the whole person.

2. Evidence of safety and efficacy. The Commission is committed to promoting the use of science and appropriate scientific methods to help identify safe and effective CAM services and products and to generate evidence that will protect and promote the public health.

3. The healing capacity of the person. The person has a remarkable capacity for recovery and self-healing, and a major focus of healthcare is to support and promote this capacity.

4. Respect for individuality. Every person is unique and has the right to healthcare that is appropriately responsive to him or her, respecting preferences and preserving dignity.

5. The right to choose treatment. Every person has the right to choose freely among safe and effective care or approaches, as well as among qualified practitioners who are accountable for their claims and actions and responsive to the person's needs.

6. An emphasis on health promotion and self-care. Good healthcare emphasizes self-care and early intervention for maintaining and promoting health.

7. Partnerships are essential for integrated healthcare. Good healthcare requires teamwork among clients, healthcare practitioners (conventional and CAM), and researchers committed to creating optimal healing environments and to respecting the diversity of all healthcare traditions.

8. Education as a fundamental healthcare service. Education about prevention, healthful lifestyles, and the power of self-healing should be made an integral part of the curricula of all healthcare professionals and should be made available to the public.

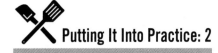

Putting It Into Practice: 2

A client reports that they are using natural products to treat a skin lesion. What would you do with this information?

(Check your answer at the end of this chapter)

Figure 6.5 Fads, Frauds, and Quackery

 The following claims are cause for caution. Each is a red flag suggesting that the scientific basis for safety and effectiveness may be missing. Based on these red flags, a treatment could be a fad, fraud, or form of quackery. Quackery is a medical treatment that does not perform as claimed and is offered by an untrained or uniformed individual.

Medical Cure	The treatment is described as a miracle, breakthrough, or cure-all. Few treatments are actually this effective!
Anecdotal Evidence *(Reported Observations)*	Descriptions of the treatment use stories about individual success, rather than citing controlled medical research.
Shaky Terminology	Some unfounded treatments may claim to purify, energize, or detoxify the body. These terms have little scientific meaning.
Too Good to Be True	A claim tells only the good, without identifying possible risks or side effects.

Source: FDA

Figure 6.6 Four Questionable Assumptions

Questionable Assumption #1

"Even if a product may not help me, at least it won't hurt me."

It's best not to assume that this will always be true. When consumed in high enough amounts, for a long enough time, or in combination with certain other substances, all chemicals can be toxic, including nutrients, plant components, and other biologically active ingredients.

Questionable Assumption #2

"When I see the term 'natural,' it means that a product is healthful and safe."

Consumers can be misled if they assume this term assures wholesomeness, or that these food-like substances necessarily have milder effects, which makes them safer to use than drugs. The term "natural" on labels is not well-defined and is sometimes used ambiguously to imply unsubstantiated benefits or safety. For example, many weight-loss products claim to be "natural" or "herbal" but this doesn't necessarily make them safe. Their ingredients may interact with drugs or may be dangerous for people with certain medical conditions.

Questionable Assumption #3

"A product is safe when there is no cautionary information on the product label."

Dietary supplement manufacturers may not necessarily include warnings about potential adverse effects on the labels of their products. If consumers want to know about the safety of a specific dietary supplement, they should contact the manufacturer of that brand directly. It is the manufacturer's responsibility to determine that the supplement it produces or distributes is safe and that there is substantiated evidence that the label claims are truthful and not misleading.

Questionable Assumption #4

"A recall of a harmful product guarantees that all such harmful products will be immediately and completely removed from the marketplace."

A product recall of a dietary supplement is voluntary and while many manufacturers do their best, a recall does not necessarily remove all harmful products from the marketplace.

Source: FDA

9. Dissemination of comprehensive and timely information. The quality of healthcare can be enhanced by promoting efforts that thoroughly and thoughtfully examine the evidence on which CAM systems, practices, and products are based and making this evidence widely, rapidly, and easily available.

10. Integral public involvement. The input of informed consumers and other members of the public must be incorporated in setting priorities for healthcare, healthcare research, and in reaching policy decisions, including those related to CAM, within the public and private sectors.

In its report, the White House Commission on CAM Policy also offered more perspective that is helpful to Certified Dietary Managers in evaluating CAM:

> Although most CAM modalities have not yet been proven to be safe and effective, it is likely that some of them eventually will be proven to be safe and effective, whereas others will not...

> The question is not, *Should Americans be using complementary and alternative medicine modalities?* as many—perhaps most—already are doing so. For the most part, however, they are making these choices in the absence of valid scientific information to guide them in making informed and intelligent choices.

> Many of the commissioners agree with the editors of *The New England Journal of Medicine* who stated in 1998: 'There cannot be two kinds of medicine—conventional and alternative. There is only medicine that has been adequately tested and medicine that has not, medicine that works and medicine that may or may not work. Once a treatment has been tested rigorously, it no longer matters whether it was considered alternative at the outset. If it is found to be reasonably safe and effective, it will be accepted.

A Certified Dietary Manager's Role

In line with recommended healthcare policy and the state of knowledge on CAM therapies today, Certified Dietary Managers and others involved in providing healthcare can take several approaches to CAM:

✓ Recognize the individual rights of healthcare consumers to choose their own care

✓ Respect individual preferences

✓ Facilitate communications with clients about CAM therapies, particularly use of dietary supplements

✓ Help communicate information about individuals' CAM therapy choices to the entire healthcare team

✓ Inform clients of possible risks; help to educate

✓ Keep an open mind, and continue to keep abreast of new findings in this fast-growing area of medical science

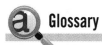

Glossary

Quackery
A medical treatment that does not perform as claimed and is offered by an untrained or uninformed individual

Nutrition in the News

Dietary Supplements: What You Need to Know

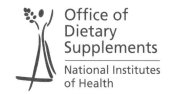

Office of
Dietary
Supplements
National Institutes
of Health

The majority of adults in the United States take one or more dietary supplements either every day or occasionally. Today's dietary supplements include vitamins, minerals, herbals and botanicals, amino acids, enzymes, and many other products. Dietary supplements come in a variety of forms: traditional tablets, capsules, and powders, as well as drinks and energy bars. Popular supplements include vitamins D and E; minerals like calcium and iron; herbs such as echinacea and garlic; and specialty products like glucosamine, probiotics, and fish oils.

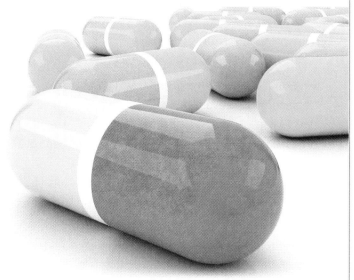

The Dietary Supplement Label

All products labeled as a dietary supplement carry a Supplement Facts panel that lists the contents, amount of active ingredients per serving, and other added ingredients (like fillers, binders, and flavorings). The manufacturer suggests the serving size, but you or your health care provider might decide that a different amount is more appropriate for you.

Effectiveness

If you don't eat a nutritious variety of foods, some supplements might help you get adequate amounts of essential nutrients. However, supplements can't take the place of the variety of foods that are important to a healthy diet. Good sources of information on eating well include the Finding Your Way to a Healthier You (http://www.health.gov/dietaryguidelines/dga2005/document/html/brochure.htm) and My Pyramid (http://www.MyPyramid.gov). Scientific evidence shows that some dietary supplements are beneficial for overall health and for managing some health conditions. For example, calcium and vitamin D are important for keeping bones strong and reducing bone loss; folic acid decreases the risk of certain birth defects; and omega-3 fatty acids

from fish oils might help some people with heart disease. Other supplements need more study to determine their value. The U.S.Food and Drug Administration (FDA) does not determine whether dietary supplements are effective before they are marketed.

Safety and Risk

Many supplements contain active ingredients that can have strong effects in the body. Always be alert to the possibility of unexpected side effects, especially when taking a new product.

(Continued)

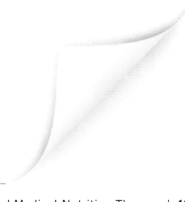

Dietary Supplements: What You Need to Know *(Continued)*

Supplements are most likely to cause side effects or harm when people take them instead of prescribed medicines or when people take many supplements in combination. Some supplements can increase the risk of bleeding or, if a person takes them before or after surgery, they can affect the person's response to anesthesia. Dietary supplements can also interact with certain prescription drugs in ways that might cause problems. Here are just a few examples:

- Vitamin K can reduce the ability of the blood thinner Coumadin® to prevent blood from clotting.
- St. John's wort can speed the breakdown of many drugs (including antidepressants and birth control pills) and thereby reduce these drugs' effect.
- Antioxidant supplements, like vitamins C and E, might reduce the effectiveness of some types of cancer chemotherapy.

Keep in mind that some ingredients found in dietary supplements are added to a growing number of foods, including breakfast cereals and beverages. As a result, you may be getting more of these ingredients than you think, and more might not be better. Taking more than you need is always more expensive and can also raise your risk of experiencing side effects. For example, getting too much vitamin A can cause headaches and liver damage, reduce bone strength, and cause birth defects. Excess iron causes nausea and vomiting and may damage the liver and other organs.

Be cautious about taking dietary supplements if you are pregnant or nursing. Also, be careful about giving them (beyond a basic multivitamin/mineral product) to a child. Most dietary supplements have not been well tested for safety in pregnant women, nursing mothers, or children.

If you suspect that you have had a serious reaction from a dietary supplement, let your health care provider know. He or she may report your experience to the FDA. You may also submit a report to the FDA by calling 800-FDA-1088 or completing a form at http://www.fda.gov/Safety/MedWatch/HowToReport. In addition, report your reaction to the dietary supplement company by using the contact information on the product label.

Quality

Dietary supplements are complex products. The FDA has established quality standards for dietary supplements to help ensure their identity, purity, strength, and composition. These standards are designed to prevent the inclusion of the wrong ingredient, the addition of too much or too little of an ingredient, the possibility of contamination, and the improper packaging and labeling of a product. The FDA periodically inspects facilities that manufacture dietary supplements.

In addition, several independent organizations offer quality testing and allow products that pass these tests to display their seals of approval. These seals of approval provide assurance that the product was properly manufactured, contains the ingredients listed on the label, and does not contain harmful levels of contaminants. These seals of approval do not guarantee that a product is safe or effective. Organizations that offer this quality testing include:

- U.S. Pharmacopeia
- ConsumerLab.com
- NSF International
- Natural Products Association

Keep in Mind

Don't decide to take dietary supplements to treat a health condition that you have diagnosed yourself, without consulting a health care provider.

- Don't take supplements in place of, or in combination with, prescribed medications without your health care provider's approval.
- Check with your healthcare provider about the supplements you take if you are scheduled to have any type of surgical procedure.

(Continued)

6 CHAPTER

Federal Government Information Sources on Dietary Supplements

NATIONAL INSTITUTES OF HEALTH
The National Institutes of Health supports research on dietary supplements.

Office of Dietary Supplements
http://ods.od.nih.gov

The Office of Dietary Supplements provides accurate and up-to-date scientific information about dietary supplements.

National Center for Complementary and Alternative Medicine http://nccam.nih.gov

National Center for Complementary and Alternative Medicine Clearinghouse: 1-888-644-6226

National Library of Medicine
http://www.nlm.nih.gov

Medline Plus http://medlineplus.gov
PubMed http://www.pubmed.gov

NIH Health Information
http://health.nih.gov

U.S.FOOD AND DRUG ADMINISTRATION
http://www.fda.gov/Food/DietarySupplements

The Food and Drug Administration issues rules and regulations and provides oversight of dietary supplement labeling, marketing, and safety.

FEDERAL TRADE COMMISSION
http://www.ftc.gov

The Federal Trade Commission polices health and safety claims made in advertising for dietary supplements.

U.S.DEPARTMENT OF AGRICULTURE
http://www.nutrition.gov http://fnic.nal.usda.gov

The U.S.Department of Agriculture provides information on a variety of food and nutrition topics.

U.S.DEPARTMENT OF HEALTH AND HUMAN SERVICES
http://www.healthfinder.gov

The U.S.Department of Health and Human Services provides an encyclopedia of health topics, personal health tools, and health news.

- The term "natural" doesn't always mean safe. A supplement's safety depends on many things, such as its chemical makeup, how it works in the body, how it is prepared, and the dose used. Certain herbs (for example, comfrey and kava) can harm the liver.
- Before taking a dietary supplement, ask yourself these questions:
  > What are the potential health benefits of this dietary supplement product?
  > What are its potential benefits for me?
  > Does this product have any safety risks?
  > What is the proper dose to take?
  > How, when, and for how long should I take it?

If you don't know the answers to these questions, use the information sources listed in this brochure and talk to your health care providers.

Talk with Your Healthcare Provider

Let your healthcare providers (including doctors, pharmacists, and Registered Dietitians) know which dietary supplements you're taking so that you can discuss what's best for your overall health. Your healthcare provider can help you determine which supplements, if any, might be valuable for you.

Keep a record of the supplements you take in one place, just as you should be doing for all of your medicines. Note the specific product name, the dose you take, how often you take it, and the reason why you use each one. You can also bring the products you use with you when you see your healthcare provider.

(Continued)

Dietary Supplements: What You Need to Know *(Continued)*

Federal Regulation of Dietary Supplements

Dietary supplements are products intended to supplement the diet. They are not drugs and, therefore, are not intended to treat, diagnose, mitigate, prevent, or cure diseases. The FDA is the federal agency that oversees both dietary supplements and medicines.

In general, the FDA regulations for dietary supplements are different from those for prescription or over-the-counter drugs. Unlike drugs, which must be approved by the FDA before they can be marketed, dietary supplements do not require premarket review or approval by the FDA. While the supplement company is responsible for having evidence that their products are safe and the label claims are truthful and not misleading, they do not have to provide that evidence to the FDA before the product is marketed.

Dietary supplement labels may carry certain types of health-related claims. Manufacturers are permitted to say, for example, that a dietary supplement addresses a nutrient deficiency, supports health, or is linked to a particular body function (like immunity or heart health). Such a claim must be followed by the words, "This statement has not been evaluated by the Food and Drug Administration. This product is not intended to diagnose, treat, cure, or prevent any disease."

Manufacturers must follow certain good manufacturing practices to ensure the identity, purity, strength, and composition of their products. If the FDA finds a product to be unsafe or otherwise unfit for human consumption, it may take enforcement action to remove the product from the marketplace or work with the manufacturer to voluntarily recall the product.

Also, once a dietary supplement is on the market, the FDA monitors information on the product's label and package insert to make sure that information about the supplements content is accurate and that any claims made for the product are truthful and not misleading. The Federal Trade Commission, which polices product advertising, also requires all information about a dietary supplement product to be truthful and not misleading.

The federal government can take legal action against companies and Websites that sell dietary supplements when the companies make false or deceptive statements about their products, if they promote them as treatments or cures for diseases, or if their products are unsafe.

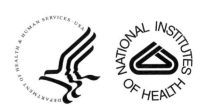

Reprinted with permission: Office of Dietary Supplements: http://ods.od.nih.gov

END OF CHAPTER

 Putting It Into Practice Questions & Answers

1. A client reports that they are taking single supplements of vitamin B6 and vitamin A. What other information will you need about the supplements?

   A. *You will need to know how many milligrams per day they are taking for each of these supplements. Both of these can cause a health risk if taken in an overdose amount. See Figure 6.4. Ask questions such as:*

   - *How often are you taking the supplement?*
   - *Are you taking them in conjunction with a multi-vitamin?*

2. A client reports that they are using natural products to treat a skin lesion. What would you do with this information?

   A. *Ask the client for additional information such as:*

   - *Can you tell me what products you are taking?*
   - *How often are you taking the supplement?*
   - *Have you informed your physician that you are taking these products?*
   - *Can you tell me the brand name?*

   Also, make sure to document the answers to your questions in the medical record.

Document Nutritional Information in Medical Records

7

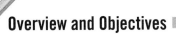

Overview and Objectives

Documentation of nutritional data and using standardized language are critical tools for medical management as well as regulatory compliance.

After completing this chapter, you should be able to:

✓ Explain the uses of common documents, including a diet manual, medical record, and an MDS form

✓ Chart in medical records using appropriate forms and formats

✓ Translate commonly used abbreviations into medical terms

✓ Enter and retrieve data using a computer

✓ Describe the impact of HIPAA regulations on medical documentation

✓ Use current nutritional information forms

In a healthcare environment, it is not enough to provide excellent care. It is also crucial to document all medical care, including nutrition-related care. Why? Documentation serves a number of purposes. Among them:

✓ Documentation provides a standardized reference that you and other caregivers can use on an ongoing basis as you provide care. It helps you focus details about how you are implementing a plan of care. It also helps you compare information from one time to another, and to track changes in nutritional status.

✓ Documentation becomes a communication tool with other members of the healthcare team. This is important because you need to work together to accomplish high-quality care for any individual.

✓ Documentation is required by government agencies, and is mandatory for healthcare facilities to obtain key information about the client, the facility, type of provider and the reason for assessment.

✓ Documentation lays groundwork for a healthcare facility to receive reimbursement for the services it provides (e.g. from insurance companies and Medicare).

✓ Documentation is a legal record.

✓ Documentation is part of quality standards for healthcare facilities.

✓ Documentation is also a resource for monitoring quality of services.

186 | Nutrition Concepts and Medical Nutrition Therapy

As you can see, documentation has a multi-faceted rationale. The need to document care applies not only to Certified Dietary Managers, but also to all members of the healthcare team. In fact, most care documents are shared by members of the team. It is also apparent that when you write down what you do, you are not writing just for yourself. Much of what you document will be read and used by others. Thus, you need to follow certain guidelines that are universally used and understood in the healthcare professions. Furthermore, documentation is guided by policies and procedures in your own place of employment. While the principles are universal, details about how, where, and what to document vary. Wherever you work, it is an excellent idea to become familiar with all policies and procedures about documentation and to follow them closely.

What types of standardized documents does a Certified Dietary Manager use and maintain? Among the most common are: **diet manual**, a medical record, a dietary reference card, and an MDS form (used in long-term care).

Diet Manuals

A diet manual specifies therapeutic diets and their application. Usually, a diet manual is used like a reference book. Today, diet manuals such as AND's Nutrition Care Manual, are available for purchase online. The manual standardizes names for diets, which is important. When a physician orders a diet, standard terminology allows communication among the physician, dietary caregivers, and the entire healthcare team. For example, if a physician were to order a "diabetic diet," what would you do to implement this order? Now that you know the range of dietary interventions for diabetes, you know that this term doesn't specify enough. But perhaps your facility develops a diet for diabetes centered on myPyramid. Perhaps your diet manual will describe a diet such as: "Diabetes Pyramid Diet." Your diet manual will outline in detail about how each food group is used in developing menus and serving meals. For some diets, the manual may specify foods to be used and foods to omit. In some ways, a diet manual may resemble an expanded version of this chapter, minus the background on medical conditions. It will also give more information about how to dictate an order. A carbohydrate counting diet, for instance, must include a level of carbohydrate or daily goal. It may read: "Carbohydrate Counting—210 grams per day." This form of control is helpful so that a physician's intent and the actual result coincide.

Most healthcare facilities adopt or adapt a diet manual from an outside source. The The Academy of Nutrition and Dietetics (AND) [formerly known as The American Dietetic Association (ADA)], as well as many state and local chapters of dietetic associations, develop diet manuals and offer them in the professional marketplace. Usually, very large healthcare facilities develop their own manuals—a massive undertaking. Whatever your source, as a Certified Dietary Manager in healthcare, you will need to identify this standard for dietary planning. Deciding on a diet manual and nutritional care specifications is done in communication with physicians and other members of the healthcare team. In a large facility, a formal approval process may be required. In a small facility, the medical director alone may approve the diet manual. A diet manual should be readily available for reference by all caregivers, and should form the basis for

 Glossary

Diet Manual
Standardized document that specifies therapeutic diets and their application; each facility will specify the diet manual they intend to use

Medical Record
Formal, legal account of a client's health and disease

Problem Oriented Medical Record (POMR)
A medical record that utilizes a system of collecting, planning data and client care focused on a client's problems

Progress Note
A notation in the medical record by a health professional

menu planning and meal service. The diet manual also dictates what information must be relayed in nutrition education.

Medical Record

A **medical record** is a formal, legal account of a client's health and disease, intended to promote continuity of care among healthcare providers. It contains information to:

✓ Identify the client

✓ Support the diagnosis (findings)

✓ Justify the treatment (test results)

✓ Document the diagnosis and treatment

A medical record may also be called a medical chart or a chart. Today's medical record may be a hybrid consisting of both paper and electronic documents. Each facility has its own procedures and guidelines for recording in the medical record. By 2014, all medical records are to be in electronic format.

There are a variety of formats for recording information in the medical record. Many facilities use the **problem-oriented medical record (POMR)**. The POMR is a system of collecting data and planning client care that focuses on the client's problems. The POMR promotes standardization and organization of the client record and gives a clear view of the care provider's line of reasoning. Much of the information in a POMR is organized according to problems. The POMR includes:

✓ Collection of data

  • Information from an interview with client, family, and caregiver

  • Health assessment or physical exam information of the client

  • Results from various laboratory and radiologic tests

✓ A problem list

  • Chronologic list of problems that the healthcare team will need to treat

  • Date of each problem's onset

  • The action taken

  • The treatment or resolution

  • Date of the treatment

✓ Plans for addressing each problem/progress notes (Nutrition Care Process)

✓ Evaluation summary including plans for follow-up or referral

The problem list is continually updated. Physicians and professionals from various disciplines (nursing, nutrition, physical therapy, etc) write progress notes in the chart. A **progress note** summarizes a client's progress related to a specific problem. For example, imagine a client has a problem identified as poor nutritional status (protein and calories). A progress note will review this problem, evaluate effectiveness of the plan for improving nutritional status, and state how the condition has changed. Progress notes are written at key intervals during the course of a client's stay or anytime a client's condition changes.

The The Academy of Nutrition and Dietetics (AND) [formerly known as The American Dietetic Association (ADA)] has implemented a Nutrition Care Process (NCP) that will impact documenting nutritional data. The purpose of this new process is to standardize the process for providing care and standardize the language so that communication among team members is more uniform. This will be especially advantageous with electronic health records.

The **Nutrition Care Process** has five steps known as ADIME:

1. Nutrition Assessment—this step includes nutrition screening
2. Nutrition Diagnosis
3. Nutrition Intervention
4. Monitoring
5. Evaluation

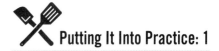

Putting It Into Practice: 1

The client tells you that they are allergic to peanuts. Which component of SOAP data would this be?

(Check your answer at the end of this chapter)

Figure 7.1   **Nutrition-Related Components of SOAP Data**

Subjective Information	Objective Information	Assessment	Plan
• Eating habits and patterns	• Height	• Evaluation of weight as it compares to standards and usual past weight	• Weight goal
• Food preferences	• Actual weight	• Evaluation of appropriateness of prescribed diet	• Initiate/recommend supplemental feedings
• Appetite	• Ideal body weight	• Evaluation of nutrient and drug interactions	• Initiate/recommend vitamin/mineral supplements
• Reaction/adherence to diet	• Percent weight change	• Evaluation of laboratory values	• Initiate/recommend diet instruction prior to discharge
• Problems chewing or swallowing	• Diet order	• Evaluation of diet history	• Initiate/recommend calorie counts (intake records)
• Food allergies	• Pertinent laboratory values	• Evaluation of eating/feeding ability	• Request more laboratory tests
• Usual weight	• Nutritional needs (calories and protein)	• Evaluation of client's compliance with diet	• Request daily weights
• Changes in eating habits	• Calorie count or food intake information	• Evaluation of any other problems that are nutritionally related	• Referral to other health team members
• Changes in weight	• Medications (as they pertain to nutrition)	Examples:	Examples:
• Previous diets and instructions	• Observed feeding or eating ability	• Client is able to make menu selections consistent with 4 gram sodium diet.	• Will provide liquid, complete nutritional supplement between meals.
• Habits—activity, sleep, bowel	• Diet history taken	• Diet history shows client's daily intake of sodium is over 10 grams due to frequent consumption of high sodium foods.	• Will design 1,800 calorie diabetic diet with client.
• Use of vitamin/mineral supplements	• Diet instruction given	• Client's low albumin indicates significant malnutrition.	• Start calorie count tomorrow AM.
• Use of medications	Examples:		
Examples:	• Client is blind.		
• Client reports feeling nauseated and wants less food.	• Diet order is 1,800 cal AND.		
• Client reports feeling better and is requesting more food.	• Client given diet instruction on fat-controlled diet.		
• Client reports difficulty swallowing due to sore mouth. Has requested liquids or soft foods only.			

The first step, nutrition assessment, consists of five areas:

✓ Food/Nutrition-Related History

✓ Anthropometric Measurements

✓ Biochemical Data, Medical Tests, and Procedures

✓ Nutrition-Focused Physical Findings

✓ Client History

Nutrition assessment begins after nutrition screening data indicates that the client may benefit from nutrition care. These five areas include information that Certified Dietary Managers can collect and document.

Historically, using the POMR method, notes in the client's chart were structured according to the SOAP format. **SOAP** is an acronym for information types. It stands for: Subjective, Objective, Assessment, and Plan. While this method is considered out-dated for recording in the medical record, it is still useful as a way to organize nutrition screening data for Step 1 of the Nutrition Care Process. Figure 7.1 gives examples of each type of information in SOAP.

With the implementation of the electronic health record, most of the documentation will be done electronically. It is very important that you work with the **Interdisciplinary Team (IDT)** at your facility to determine who is going to enter what data in the electronic health record. Each department may have data to enter under separate tabs. It may look similar to your hard copy medical record; it may have many more sections. You will also need to discuss with your Registered Dietitian what information you should collect and enter. You may enter nutrition data into an electronic screen (see Figure 7.2a - 7.2c) per your discussion with your Registered Dietitian.

The first determination, using the nutrition screening information, will be whether the client is at nutritional risk. Depending upon the process in your facility, a referral may come from nursing. The Registered Dietitian, using the screening information you have entered, will complete the NCP Assessment Step 1. From there, the Registered Dietitian will determine the diagnosis. With the new NCP, there are many diagnoses (identified by number) to choose. The diagnosis should be a specific nutrition problem that can be addressed through nutrition intervention. An example of a nutrition diagnosis is: N1-5.3 Inadequate Protein Intake. This is not the medical diagnosis but it is a problem that can be addressed through nutrition intervention. The Registered Dietitian will also write what is called a PES statement. PES stands for Problem, Etiology, Signs and Symptoms and is written to describe the nutrition problem, identify the root cause "as evidenced by," and the evidence "related to" from the assessment data to support the diagnosis. For instance, a PES statement for a client in a nursing home who has difficulty feeding himself might read:

✓ Problem: Self-feeding difficulty, related to decreased dexterity, as evidenced by unable to feed himself with regular dishes and utensils.

✓ Interventions: Scoop plate, large handled utensils, spill-proof drinking cups

✓ Monitoring & Evaluation: Meal intake 95 percent

(Continued on pg. 194)

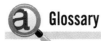

Glossary

SOAP

A structured type of collecting data—stands for Subjective, Objective, Assessment, and Plan

Subjective

Data from the client's point of view or as told by the client or family members

Objective

Data that is acquired by inspection, examination with a stethoscope, from a laboratory, and radiologic tests

Assessment

Analysis based on the subjective and objective data

Plan

Recommended actions of the caregiver's to further information, therapy, education or counseling

Nutrition Care Process

New method of documenting nutritional data with five steps: ADIME

IDT

Interdisciplinary team of health professionals that collaborate in the completion of the RAI

Figure 7.2a   Sample Electronic Health Record

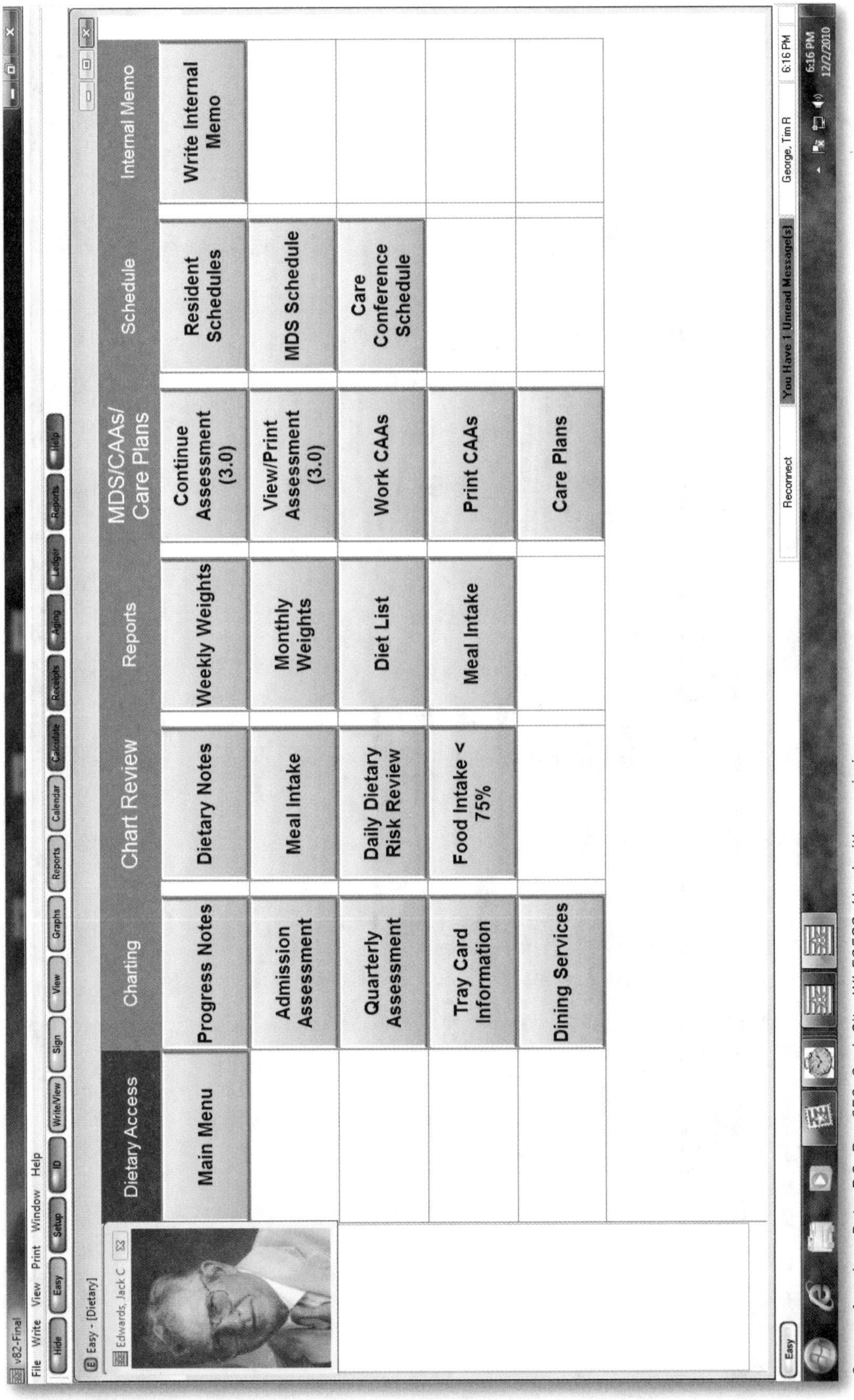

Source: American Data, P.O. Box 650, Sauk City, WI 53583. Used with permission.

Figure 7.2b **Sample Electronic Health Record**

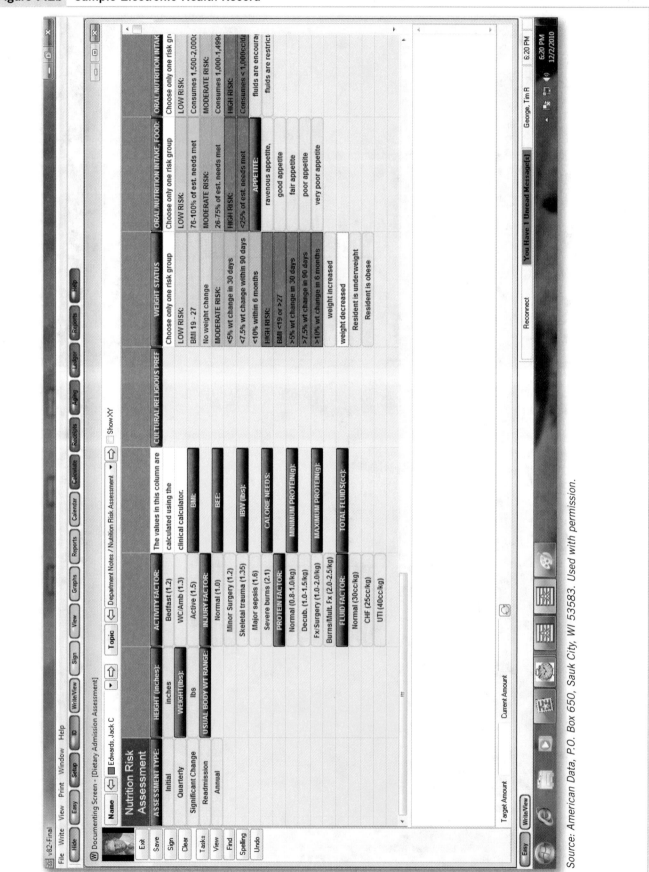

Source: *American Data, P.O. Box 650, Sauk City, WI 53583. Used with permission.*

Figure 7.2c   Sample Electronic Health Record

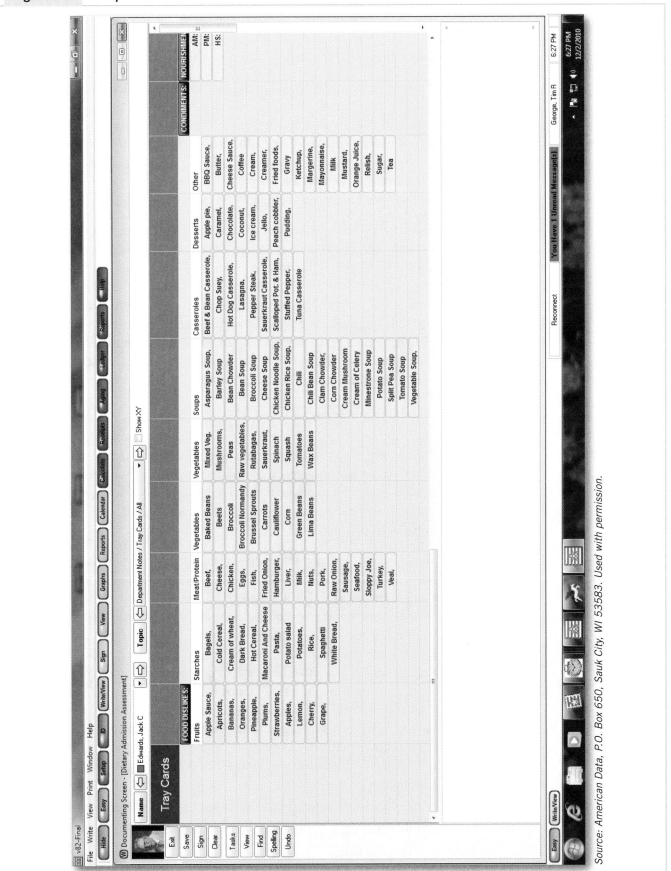

Source: American Data, P.O. Box 650, Sauk City, WI 53583. Used with permission.

A client may have several PES statements if he/she has several nutritional problems.

The Drake Center of Cincinnati, Ohio, has developed a manual form to document information for the Nutrition Care Process (see Figure 7.3). Notice that each step of the Nutrition Care Process is addressed.

Another charting format is the narrative format, in which the caregiver simply writes a narration or description of all relevant data, findings, and care in a logical format. A narrative note should be brief and concise. The narrative format may be what the Certified Dietary Manager uses in preparation for the Nutrition Care Process information. Figure 7.4 shows an electronic narrative chart note that includes a narrative note from both the Certified Dietary Manager and the Registered Dietitian.

No matter which charting format a facility uses, the total content of the chart notes should be very similar. In long-term care facilities, care plans are written separately. The care plan form is used by all disciplines, such as nursing and physical therapy. Writing in the progress notes and in the care plan is often the responsibility of the Registered Dietitian. State regulations vary as to who is responsible for writing progress notes and care plans. In some states, the Certified Dietary Manager may update care plans and chart in the medical record. State regulations also vary as to how often the progress notes and care plans must be updated. It may be 30 days, 60 days, or another interval of time.

Charting Standards

There are some standard rules to be used in charting, along with specific guidelines for the type of progress notes you should use in your facility. Always sign your entries in the medical record, and include your credentials. Keep in mind that if you do not document something, it has—for legal and regulatory purposes—not occurred. Figure 7.5 lists some standard rules for keeping good nutrition-related records.

You should also document to show what information you have reviewed and researched. For example, a sample note might indicate that you have tried to find out the usual weight for a client and were not able to do so. It may also show that you have reviewed a list of the client's medications to see if any might be affecting the patient's nutritional status. These notations are important to demonstrate that you did not simply forget or overlook important aspects of nutrition care. As a shortcut, healthcare professionals use many abbreviations for medical and clinical terms in medical records. Figure 7.6 lists some common abbreviations. In any facility, accepted standards for abbreviations may vary slightly. It is important to remember that the medical record is a legal document that will be read by many people. Do not criticize others or appear to be assuming a role you are not qualified for in a progress note. For example, you would not want to write:

Client did not receive her lunch tray because nurse forgot to pass it **OR**

I think this client has diabetes—please check **OR**

Client is a jerk

Figure 7.3 Nutrition Care Process Form

The Drake Center Nutrition Assessment

Developed by Clinical Nutrition Staff, Drake Center,
Cincinnati, Ohio, used with permission

Date/Time Initiated: _____

Assessment

DIAGNOSIS / PMH:

DIET:

Intake:

Chewing / Swallowing:

Allergies / Religious / Ethnic Food Preferences:

Use of Herbals / Supplements:	Bowels:
Mental Status:	Feeding Ability:
HT	WT:	Usual WT:	Goal WT:
Ideal WT:	% IBW:	Adjusted WT:	BMI below 19 above 30:
WT History:			

LAB VALUES

Date	RBC	HGB	HTT	MCV	MCH	TLC	NA	K	BUN	CR	GLU	CA	ALB	PAB	Mg	PO4

MEDICATIONS:

SKIN CONDITION:

ESTIMATED NEEDS: Kcal: Protein: Fluid:

Diagnosis

NUTRITION DIAGNOSIS AND PROBLEMS

related to:

as evidenced by: related to:

as evidenced by:

⋏ No nutrition diagnosis identified at this time.

Intervention

NUTRITION PRESCRIPTION:

⋏ Food and/or nutrient delivery:

⋏ Nutrition Education:

⋏ Coordination of Nutrition Care:

Monitoring

Follow up:	⋏ 5-7 days	⋏ 10-12 days	⋏ 12-14 days	⋏ Quarterly
⋏ Other:	⋏ Monitor with MDS	⋏ Plan of care initiated		
Signature:				

Form # MR 601
Revised 12/09   ORIGINAL TO CHART   COPY TO DIETITIAN

Figure 7.4   Electronic Chart Note in Narrative Format Using Nutrition Care Process Standardized Language

Date	Narrative
11/19/2010	New Resident Admission
Recorded by the Certified Dietary Manager	What did you eat on a typical day prior to admission; resident was having a hard time re-membering question I was asking him from the past. As to foods he had at home he stated whatever was around to eat he ate. Updated meal card choices with the resident. Stated he enjoys the food. Also stated he enjoys the activities he has been attending. Explained the guest try policy to him, happy hours, and monthly birthday parties. Resident has been coming to the dining room for meals. Talked about his carbohydrate counting diet and he does like to use the clothing protector with meals. • Do you have trouble swallowing? *No* • Do you have trouble chewing? *No* • Do you like to drink liquids? *Yes, like juices and milk, states he's not been drinking coffee.* • How would you rate your appetite? *Good* • Do you use/need any assistive devices to help with eating? *Yes, has been using Kennedy cups, large handled utensils and a scoop plate.* • Do you drink nutritional supplement at home prior to admission? *No* • Do you take any vitamin, minerals, or herbal products at home *No* • Do you prefer any dietary bowel aides? *No* • Do you drink alcoholic beverages? *No* • Do you have any religious, cultural, or ethical beliefs that affect what you eat? *Yes, stated Methodist* The following teaching was completed: Diet order, Guest tray policy, Happy Hour.
11/23/20 **Recorded by the Interdisciplinary Team**	**Dietary Progress Note:** Other purpose: care conference **Family /Resident Visit:** met with resident, discussed: meals, no trouble eating per resident, food is good and he gets enough to eat. **Assessment:** Same as previous note dated 11/18/10 was 155.5# so weight is stable. Intakes are good. Medications: Lantus Insulin was decreased to 12 units at HS from 20 units D-stix; since insulin change = 70-76 mg/dl in the a.m., 183-261 at noon, 96-320 mg/dl in the after-noon, and 219-279 at HS. Skin condition: B=18 **POC Recommendations:** See Care Plan and CAAs
11/24/2010 **Recorded by the Registered Dietitian**	**Dietary Progress Note:** PPS: 14 day: Assessment dates: 11/19/10 - 11/24/10 **Assessment:** Diet Order: carbohydrate counting diet; Supplement: note, Dietary Bowel Aides: None; Chewing/Swallowing Difficult: none; Adaptive Eating Devices: Special Utensils: large handles utensils, Scoop Plate, Other: Kennedy cups; Weights: 11/19/10: 155.6# - no wt change; Usual Body7 Weight: current wt; Height: 73"; BMI: 20.5 – normal; Dining Area: Wil-low dining room; Medications: include: simvastatin, dyazide, Lantus, Humalog; Labs: none; D-stix: (11/18-24/10) AM range: 60-92 mg/dl – improved after ASSESSMENT: Diet Order: carbohydrate counting diet; Supplement: note, Dietary Bowel Aides: None; Chewing/Swal-lowing Difficult: none; Adaptive Eating Devices: Special Utensils: large handles utensils, Scoop Plate, Other: Kennedy cups; Weights: 11/19/10: 155.6# - no wt change; Usual Body7 Weight: current wt; Height: 73"; BMI: 20.5 – normal; Dining Area: Willow dining room; Medi-cations: include: simvastatin, dyazide, Lantus, Humalog; Labs: none; D-stix: (11/18-24/10) AM range: 60-92 mg/dl – improved aftr change in Lantus to 12 units at hs on 11/19/10; noon range: 146-302 mg/dl; supper range: 96-320 mg/dl; hs range: 130-315 mg/dl. Receives humalog sliding scale at meals and separate humalog sliding scale at hs. Meal Intake: 95% - 18 meals; Self Feeding Ability7: set up; Fluid: 1080 ml/3 meals; Dehydration Risk: 0, Skin Condition: intact; Braden: 18 Stable nutritionally as evidenced by good meal intake, feeds self with adaptive devices, wt is stable for resident, and skin is intact. Continue wto work with blood sugars and insulin orders.

(Continued)

Date	Narrative
11/24/2010 **Recorded by the Registered Dietitian**	**Estimated Needs** :Kcalorie: 1440 x 1.3 = 1873; Protein: 84 grams per day; Fluids: 2100 ml/24 hours. **Goal:** Maintain wt at 155 +/- 5# x three months. Achieve and maintain A1c< or = 7% x three months. **Progress to Goals:** Met goal re: wt; unable to assess A1c – no new orders at this time. Detail Goal Changes: Goal will be retained. **PES Statement:** Problem altered nutrition labs – glucose/A1C Related to: Diabetes, recent CVA Manifested by: elected d-stix and A1C **Interventions:** Carb counting diet, insulin as ordered, collaboration with MD re: suggested insulin changes **Monitoring and Evaluation:** labs/d-stix – improving.

Figure 7.4 Electronic Chart Note in Narrative Format Using Nutrition Care Process Standardized Language *(Continued)*

Thank you to Joan Bahr, MS, RD, Director of Nutrition Services at Southwest Health Center, Platteville, WI and to Cindy Morrissey, CDM, CFPP for sharing nutrition documentation from their long-term care center electronic records for the narrative notes

Meal-Related Documents

In a healthcare facility, a designated dietary team member reviews the diet order. A **diet order** is the diet prescribed by the physician for an individual client. This is usually a written order in the medical record. Often, it is the responsibility of a nurse or someone on the nursing staff to notify the foodservice department of a diet order. Although diet orders most often are transmitted via an internal document called a diet sheet, sometimes they are transmitted by phone, in what is called a verbal order. Verbal orders from the nursing units should be discouraged, because they do not provide solid documentation. Both nursing and foodservice need to develop and jointly approve a policy and procedure for communicating and documenting diet order transmission. If policies and procedures where you work permit verbal orders, the name of the person transmitting and receiving the diet order and the time it is received should be written down. Such orders should be verified in writing before the next meal to confirm accuracy. If you are using electronic health records, diet orders will be transmitted electronically.

In almost all healthcare facilities, diet orders are written by the physician, although sometimes the Registered Dietitian can change an order. As explained earlier in this chapter, a physician should order only diets listed in the facility's approved diet manual. In a typical healthcare facility, the diet manual is reviewed and/or updated on a regular basis and approved by the Registered Dietitian and the medical director of the facility.

Now that the diet order has been sent to dietary services, it must be recorded in foodservice department records. Within a foodservice department, nutrition caregivers used to maintain an internal record of the meal-related information. This is a card in a kardex system (a small, portable file system). Today it may be part of a diet office software and maintained on a computer system. Typically, a kardex card computerized format lists food preferences, allergies or intolerances, and meal planning patterns used in meal service. It also lists the diet order as copied from the physician's order in the medical record. It may also

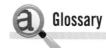

Glossary

Diet Order
The diet prescribed by the physician for an individual client

Figure 7.5   Rules for Keeping Good Client Records

- Use the color ink your facility requires (usually, this is black).

- Include direct quotes from clients (marked with quotation marks) as appropriate in the *Subjective* portion of a SOAP note.

- Aside from documenting subjective information obtained from a client, place only facts in the medical record. Do not speculate.

- Complete all blocks and spaces on forms.

- Use facilty-approved abbreviations; do not invent your own.

- Date all entries accurately.

- Refer to days of the week as dates.

- Write legibly and spell words correctly.

- Do not erase anything. If you need to make a correction, just cross through it and write "error" above it.

- Document missed appointments or any other acts of poor compliance.

- Do not be uncomplimentary in remarks about the client or client's family.

- Do not record anything in the record that does not pertain to the client.

- Do not use the medical record to criticize others.

- Be complete and accurate.

- Be as brief as possible. Remember that others have to read your notes, and everyone is busy. Complete sentences are not necessary.

- Do not make (or appear to make) a diagnosis of a medical condition, as this is the physician's role.

- Always sign your entries with your name and your credentials.

- Document all relevant information. If you don't document something, it is presumed it did not occur.

Adapted from a presentation by James G. Zimmerly at 1984 American Dietetic Association Annual Meeting, Washington, DC.

contain other information about the plan of care and relevant clinical data used in monitoring nutritional status. A sample of a manual card appears in Figure 7.7.

Alternately, some long-term care operations maintain tray cards or meal cards indicating preferences and diet-related guidelines for individual client meals. Tray cards and menus may be color-coded to indicate a specific diet. The color-coding helps foodservice workers assemble trays quickly, as they can glance ahead at the color and anticipate which foods are needed. Documents such as these exist primarily as a convenience for carrying out meal service. Maintaining a kardex card or tray card does not substitute for formal, legal documentation as required of the entire healthcare team. Maintaining a kardex card or tray does not substitute for formal, legal documentation as required of the entire healthcare system.

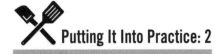

Putting It Into Practice: 2

What do the abbreviations stand for in this chart note?

Chart Note: *Patient is sob. Implemented nutritional supplement bid.*

(Check your answer at the end of this chapter)

Figure 7.6   **Common Abbreviations for Medical Records**

ABC	Ambulatory/Bed/Chair	**FBS**	Fasting Blood Sugar	**prn**	As necessary
A/C	Alert/Confused	**fl**	Fluid	**PT**	Physical Therapy
ac	Before food or meals	**g/c**	Geriatric chair	**pt**	Patient
ADL	Activities of Daily Living	**gd**	Good	**qAM**	Every morning
ADR	Adverse Drug Reaction	**GI**	Gastrointestinal	**qd***	Every day
ad lib	As desired	**gm**	Gram	**qh**	Every hour
AHD or	Arteriosclerotic	**GTT**	Glucose Tolerance Test	**qid**	Four times a day
ASHD	Heart Disease	**hb/Hg/**	Hemoglobin	**resp**	Resiration
alb	Albumin	**Hgb**		**ROM**	Range of Motion
bid	Two times daily	**Hct**	Hematocrit	**Rx**	Treatment
BM	Bowel Movement	**hs***	Bedtime	**s̄**	without
BP	Blood Pressure	**IU**	International Unit	**sob**	Shortness of breath
BUN	Blood Urea Nitrogen	**IV**	Intravenous	**stat**	Immediately
c̄	with	**K**	Potassium	**supp**	Suppository
CBC	Complete Blood Count	**liq**	Liquid	**tab**	Tablet
cc*	Cubic centimeter	**mg**	Milligram	**tid**	Three times a day
CHF	Congestive Heart Failure	**ml**	Milliliter	**Tx**	Treatment
co, c/o	Complains of	**Na**	Sodium	**URI**	Upper Respiratory Infection
CRF	Chronic Renal Failure	**noc**	At night	**UTI**	Urinary Tract infection
CV	Cardiovasular	**NPO**	Nothing by Mouth	**via**	By way of
Dx	Diagnosis	**OOB**	Out of Bed	**WBC**	White Blood Count
ECG,	Electrocardiogram	**OT**	Occupational Therapy	**WNL**	Within Normal Limits
EKG		**OTC**	Over-the-Counter Medication	**wt**	Weight
eg	For example	**PH**	Hematocrit		
et	and	**po**	By mouth		

* Avoid these if subject to Joint Commission standards.

Federal Regulations Concerning Nutrition and Documentation in Nursing Facilities

Nursing homes (NH) and non-critical access hospital swing beds (SBs) participating in the Medicare and Medicaid programs must follow federal regulations developed by the Centers for Medicare & Medicaid Services (CMS). Regulations address quality of care. CMS requires certain documentation in a standardized format. Both institutional licensure and reimbursement for services depend on proper documentation. Individual states enforce the regulations, and sometimes adapt them. States also enforce regulations controlling licensure for the facilities. Thus, in any state where you work, you need to become familiar with the standards.

A centerpiece of the CMS regulations is the **Resident Assessment Instrument (RAI)**. This is a specialized form of medical documentation required of every healthcare facility that is receiving funding from Medicare and/or Medicaid. The RAI helps healthcare team members assess and plan high-quality care. The documentation process is a tool to help clinicians; the documentation is

Document Nutritional Information in Medical Records

Figure 7.7   Sample Dietary Kardex Card

Diet Order		
Physician	_____	
Diagnosis	_____	
	_____	
Allergies	_____	

DATE	INT	DIET ORDERED
8/1/07	RM	Mechanical Soft, NAS

Beverage   **Room**
B _____   Dining Room
L _____   Usual Servings
D _____   Small ☐
                            Medium ☐
                            Large ☐

Room No.	Name:
306	H.K. Smith

Nourishments	
AM	_____
PM	_____
HS	_____
	_____

	Carb.	Dairy	Fruit	Meat	Veg.
Likes					
Dislikes					

Current Diet Order:
Mechanical Soft, no added salt

required above and beyond the medical record that is already being maintained. The RAI includes three basic components: the **Minimum Data Set (MDS)** and **Care Area Assessment (CAA)** process and RAI Utilization Guidelines.

Minimum Data Set (MDS)

The MDS is a standardized reporting form used by members of the healthcare team to do an assessment of each resident. MDS 3.0 is new in 2010 and "has been designed to improve reliability, accuracy and usefulness of the MDS." MDS 3.0 actively engages the client in interviews and conversations. Members of the healthcare team work together to complete the form, which may be maintained on paper or in a computerized system. Regulations require a facility to transmit MDS forms to CMS on a regular basis. By current regulations, this transmission is an electronic (not paper) process.

The **Minimum Data Set (MDS)** form outlines a minimum amount of data (information) that caregivers must collect and use. It is designed for use by a number of healthcare professionals as an interdisciplinary care tool. The MDS includes a fact sheet and a full assessment form that is used upon admission and once a year, or more often if there is a significant change in the client's condition. A shortened version of the MDS, called the MDS Quarterly Assessment Form, is filled out every three months. The MDS form collects basic information such as:

✓ Disease diagnoses

✓ Health conditions

✓ Physical and mental functional status

✓ Sensory and physical impairments

✓ Nutritional status and requirements

✓ Special treatments or procedures

Glossary

RAI
Resident Assessment Instrument consists of three components and is utilized to assess each client's functional capacity and needs

MDS
Minimum Data Set is the starting point of the RAI and is a standardized tool for collecting information that is the core of the RAI

CAA
Care Area Assessment is the second component of the RAI and is used to make decisions about areas suggested by the MDS

CAT
Care Area Triggers are related to one or more items in the MDS and are the flags for the interdisciplinary team member

✓ Mental and psychosocial status

✓ Discharge potential

✓ Dental condition

✓ Activities potential

✓ Drug therapy

The Registered Dietitian/Certified Dietary Manager may complete Section K, "Oral/Nutritional Status," on the MDS 3.0, and become involved in helping with nutrition-related components in other sections of the MDS form as well. A sample page from the MDS form appears in Figure 7.8.

Figure 7.8 **A Sample from the MDS 3.0 Form: Section K**

K0100. Swallowing Disorder	
Signs and symptoms of possible swallowing disorder	
↓ Check all that apply	
☐	A. Loss of liquids/solids from mouth when eating or drinking
☐	B. Holding food in mouth/cheeks or residual food in mouth after meals
☐	C. Coughing or choking during meals or when swallowing medications
☐	D. Complaints of difficulty or pain with swallowing
☐	Z. None of the above

Section K asks for information on the following:

1. Swallowing disorder

2. Height and weight

3. Weight loss

4. Nutritional approaches

5. Percent Intake by artificial route

The client's assessment must be coordinated by a registered nurse. Every facility should assign MDS items or portions to a specific health professional such as the Registered Dietitian or Certified Dietary Manager for Section K. Linda Handy, MS, RD, a retired specialty surveyor/trainer, CDPH, and dietary consultant, has recommended the following information if the Certified Dietary Manager fills out Section K.

Role of the Certified Dietary Manager in Completing Section K

✓ To ensure accurate information

✓ To communicate with Registered Dietitian and team

✓ To facilitate and follow up on recommendations by team (Registered Dietitian and speech, OT, physician, medical director, nursing)

✓ To participate in the RAI Process, including ongoing evaluation, progress, decline, trends

The intent of this section is to prevent malnutrition and dehydration, and to ensure the appropriate use of feeding tubes. See Figure 7.12: CMS Guidelines for Section K. Note that in CMS forms, "cc" is the standard unit of measure for fluids.

Care Area Assessment (CAA) Process and Care Planning

CAA is the second part of the Resident Assessment Instrument (RAI). The CMS's RAI Version 3.0 Manual, Chapter 4, has a great diagram, shown below in Figure 7.9, that illustrates the RAI process. As you can see from this figure, the CAA process is the decision making process. The interdisciplinary team (IDT) reviews the responses to items coded on the MDS and then interprets and addresses specific care areas to provide additional information that can be used for the care plan. There are 20 areas of care that must be addressed and they are listed in Figure 7.10. There are no specific tools or forms for the additional assessment of the triggered areas. Teams are encouraged to use clinical practice guidelines and critical thinking skills. Since the RAI must be completed within 14 days, the CAAs, as part of the RAI, must also be completed and documented within the same 14 days. See Figure 7.11 for the timeline to complete an RAI.

Figure 7.9	Overview of the Resident Assessment Instrument (RAI) and Care Area Assessments (CAAs)

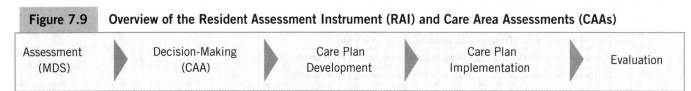

Assessment (MDS) → Decision-Making (CAA) → Care Plan Development → Care Plan Implementation → Evaluation

Utilization Guidelines

Utilization Guidelines are instructions concerning when and how to use the RAI. As an example, if the MDS identifies dehydration that is a Care Area Trigger (CAT), further evaluation through the Care Area Assessment (CAA) is warranted. For each CAT, there is "CAT logic" to be used as you review the trigger in the Care Area Assessment process. (See Figure 7.13 for an actual "CAT" logic for Swallowing/Nutritional Status.) Dehydration may have an impact on specific issues, the risk of issues, or conditions for the client. As you assess the dehydration, your interdisciplinary team may identify the cause, any risk factors, and the complications associated with dehydration. Once you have completed the Care Area Assessment, you can then decide whether or not to develop a care plan. Not every **Care Area Trigger (CAT)** needs a care plan, but you must assess every Care Area Trigger (CAT).

A significant change is defined as a major change in the client's status that is not self-limiting, has an impact on more than one area of the client's health status, and requires interdisciplinary review or revision of the care plan. Examples include unplanned weight loss of 5 percent or more in 30 days or 10 percent in 180 days; emergence of a pressure ulcer at Stage II or higher (where no ulcers were previously present at Stage II or higher); a need for extensive assistance or total dependence in eating; or a condition in which the resident is judged to be unstable.

Documentation should support your decision-making regarding whether to proceed with a care plan for a triggered CAA and if so, the type(s) of care plan interventions that are appropriate for a particular client. Documentation may appear anywhere in the clinical record (e.g. progress notes, consults, flowsheets, etc.), as dictated by the charting policies and procedures of your own facility.

(Continued on pg. 213)

Figure 7.10 CAA in the Resident Assessment Instrument (RAI)

1. Delirium
2. Cognitive Loss/Dementia
3. Visual Function
4. Communication
5. Activity of Daily Living (ADL) Functional/Rehabilitation Potential
6. Urinary Incontinence and Indwelling Catheter
7. Psychosocial Well-Being
8. Mood State
9. Behavioral Symptoms
10. Activities
11. Falls
12. Nutritional Status
13. Feeding Tubes
14. Dehydration/Fluid Maintenance
15. Dental Care
16. Pressure Ulcer
17. Psychotropic Medication Use
18. Physical Restraints
19. Pain
20. Return to Community Referral

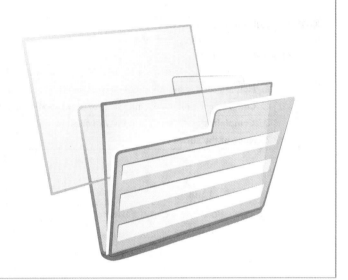

Figure 7.11 Timeline for RAI

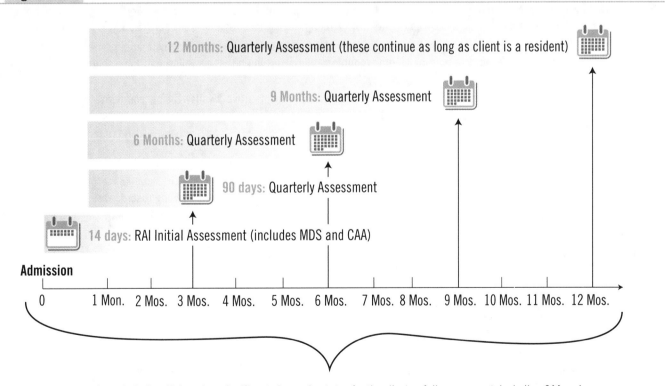

12 Months: Quarterly Assessment (these continue as long as client is a resident)

9 Months: Quarterly Assessment

6 Months: Quarterly Assessment

90 days: Quarterly Assessment

14 days: RAI Initial Assessment (includes MDS and CAA)

Admission

0   1 Mon.   2 Mos.   3 Mos.   4 Mos.   5 Mos.   6 Mos.   7 Mos.   8 Mos.   9 Mos.   10 Mos. 11 Mos. 12 Mos.

Anytime after admission, if there is a significant change in status for the client, a full assessment, including CAA and care planning must be conducted. This is true for both a decline or improvement.

Figure 7.12   CMS Guidelines for Completing the MDS—Section K

Intent: The items in this section are intended to assess the many conditions that could affect the resident's ability to maintain adequate nutrition and hydration. This section covers swallowing disorders, height and weight, weight loss, and nutritional approaches. Nurse assessors should collaborate with the Registered Dietitian and foodservice staff to ensure that items in this section have been assessed and calculated accurately.

K0100: Swallowing Disorder

K0100. Swallowing Disorder	
Signs and symptoms of possible swallowing disorder	
↓ Check all that apply	
☐	A. Loss of liquids/solids from mouth when eating or drinking
☐	B. Holding food in mouth/cheeks or residual food in mouth after meals
☐	C. Coughing or choking during meals or when swallowing medications
☐	D. Complaints of difficulty or pain with swallowing
☐	Z. None of the above

Item Rationale

Health-related Quality of Life

- The ability to swallow safely can be affected by many disease processes and functional decline.
- Alterations in the ability to swallow can result in choking and aspiration, which can increase the resident's risk for malnutrition, dehydration, and aspiration pneumonia.

Planning for Care

- Care planning should include provisions for monitoring the resident during mealtimes and during functions/activities that include the consumption of food and liquids.
- When necessary, the resident should be evaluated by the physician, speech language pathologist and/or occupational therapist to assess for any need for swallowing therapy and/or to provide recommendations regarding the consistency of food and liquids.
- Assess for signs and symptoms that suggest a swallowing disorder that has not been successfully treated or managed with diet modifications or other interventions (e.g., tube feeding, double swallow, turning head to swallow, etc.) and therefore represents a functional problem for the resident.
- Care plan should be developed to assist resident to maintain safe and effective swallow using compensatory techniques, alteration in diet consistency, and positioning during and following meals.

Steps for Assessment

1. Ask the resident if he or she has had any difficulty swallowing during the 7-day look-back period. Ask about each of the symptoms in K0100A through K0100D. Observe the resident during meals or at other times when he or she is eating, drinking, or swallowing to determine whether any of the listed symptoms of possible swallowing disorder are exhibited.

2. Interview staff members on all shifts who work with the resident and ask if any of the four listed symptoms were evident during the 7-day look-back period.

3. Review the medical record, including nursing, physician, dietician, and speech language pathologist notes, and any available information on dental history or problems. Dental problems may include poor fitting dentures, dental caries, edentulous, mouth sores, tumors and/or pain with food consumption.

Coding Instructions Check all that apply.

- **K0100A, loss of liquids/solids from mouth when eating or drinking.** When the resident has food or liquid in his or her mouth, the food or liquid dribbles down chin or falls out of the mouth.
- **K0100B, holding food in mouth/cheeks or residual food in mouth after meals.** Holding food in mouth or cheeks for prolonged periods of time (sometimes labeled pocketing) or food left in mouth because resident failed to empty mouth completely.

(Continued)

Figure 7.12 CMS Guidelines for Completing the MDS—Section K *(Continued)*

- **K0100C, coughing or choking during meals or when swallowing medications.** The resident may cough or gag, turn red, have more labored breathing, or have difficulty speaking when eating, drinking, or taking medications. The resident may frequently complain of food or medications "going down the wrong way."

- **K0100D, complaints of difficulty or pain with swallowing.** Resident may refuse food because it is painful or difficult to swallow.

- **K0100Z, none of the above:** if none of the K0100A through K0100D signs or symptoms were present during the look-back.

Coding Tips

- Do not code a swallowing problem when interventions have been successful in treating the problem and therefore the signs/symptoms of the problem (K0100A through K0100D) did not occur during the 7-day look-back period.

- Code even if the symptom occurred only once in the 7-day look-back period.

K0200: Height and Weight

K0200. Height and Weight - While measuring, if the number is X.1 - X.4 round down; X.5 or greater round up	
☐☐ inches	**A. Height** (in inches). Record most recent height measure since admission
☐☐☐ pounds	**B. Weight** (in pounds). Base weight on most recent measure in last 30 days; measure weight consistently, according to standard facility practice (e.g., in a.m. after voiding, before meal, with shoes off, etc.)

Item Rationale

Health-related Quality of Life

- Diminished nutritional and hydration status can lead to debility that can adversely affect health and safety as well as quality of life.

Planning for Care

- Height and weight measurements assist staff with assessing the resident's nutrition and hydration status by providing a mechanism for monitoring stability of weight over a period of time. The measurement of weight is one guide for determining nutritional status.

Steps for Assessment for K0200A, Height

1. On admission, measure and record height in inches.

2. Measure height consistently over time in accordance with the facility policy and procedure, which should reflect current standards of practice (shoes off, etc.).

3. For subsequent assessments, check the medical record. If the last height recorded was more than one year ago, measure and record the resident's height again.

Coding Instructions for K0200A, Height

- Record height to the nearest whole inch.

- Use mathematical rounding (i.e., if height measurement is X.5 inches or greater, round height upward to the nearest whole inch. If height measurement number is X.1 to X.4 inches, round down to the nearest whole inch). For example, a height of 62.5 inches would be rounded to 63 inches and a height of 62.4 inches would be rounded to 62 inches.

Steps for Assessment for K0200B, Weight

1. On admission, weigh the resident and record results.

2. Measure weight consistently over time in accordance with standard nursing home practice including time of day or scale (e.g., after voiding, before meal).

(Continued)

Figure 7.12   CMS Guidelines for Completing the MDS—Section K *(Continued)*

3. For subsequent assessments, check the medical record and enter the weight taken within 30 days of the ARD of this assessment.

4. If the last recorded weight was taken more than 30 days prior to the ARD of this assessment or previous weight is not available, weigh the resident again.

5. If the resident's weight was taken more than once during the preceding month, record the most recent weight.

Coding Instructions for K0200B, Weight

• Use mathematical rounding (i.e., If weight is X.5 pounds [lbs] or more, round weight upward to the nearest whole pound. If weight is X.1 to X.4 lbs, round down to the nearest whole pound). For example, a weight of 152.5 lbs would be rounded to 153 lbs and a weight of 152.4 lbs would be rounded to 152 lbs.

• If a resident cannot be weighed, for example because of extreme pain, immobility, or risk of pathological fractures, use the standard no-information code (-) and document rationale on the resident's medical record.

K0300: Weight Loss

K0300. Weight Loss	
Enter Code ☐	**Loss of 5% or more in the last month or loss of 10% or more in last 6 months** 0. **No** or unknown 1. **Yes, on** physician-prescribed weight-loss regimen 2. **Yes, not on** physician-prescribed weight-loss regimen

Item Rationale

Health-related Quality of Life

• Weight loss can result in debility and adversely affect health, safety, and quality of life.

• For persons with morbid obesity, controlled and careful weight loss can improve mobility and health status.

• For persons with a large volume (fluid) overload, controlled and careful diuresis can improve health status.

Planning for Care

• Weight loss may be an important indicator of a change in the resident's health status or environment.

• If significant weight loss is noted, the interdisciplinary team should review for possible causes of changed intake, changed caloric need, change in medication (e.g., diuretics), or changed fluid volume status.

• Weight loss should be monitored on a continuing basis; weight loss should be assessed and care planned at the time of detection and not delayed until the next MDS assessment.

Steps for Assessment

This item compares the resident's weight in the current observation period with his or her weight at two snapshots in time:

• At a point closest to 30-days preceding the current weight.

• At a point closest to 180-days preceding the current weight.

This item does not consider weight fluctuation outside of these two time points, although the resident's weight should be monitored on a continual basis and weight gain or loss assessed and addressed on the care plan as necessary.

> **DEFINITIONS**
>
> **5% weight loss in 30 days**
>
> Start with the resident's weight closest to 30 days ago and multiply it by .95 (or 95%). The resulting figure represents a 5% loss from the weight 30 days ago. if the resident's current weight is equal to or less than the resulting figure, the resident has lost more than 5% body weight.

> **DEFINITIONS**
>
> **10% weight loss in 30 days**
>
> Start with the resident's weight closest to 180 days ago and multiply it by .90 (or 90%). The resulting figure represents a 10% loss from the weight 180 days ago. If the resident's current weight is equal to or less than the resulting figure, the resident has lost 10% or more body weight.

(Continued)

Figure 7.12 CMS Guidelines for Completing the MDS—Section K *(Continued)*

For a New Admission

1. Ask the resident, family, or significant other about weight loss over the past 30 and 180 days.
2. Consult the resident's physician, review transfer documentation, and compare with admission weight.
3. If the admission weight is less than the previous weight, calculate the percentage of weight loss.
4. Complete the same process to determine and calculate weight loss comparing the admission weight to the weight 30 and 180 days ago.

For Subsequent Assessments

1. From the medical record, compare the resident's weight in the current observation period to his or her weight in the observation period 30 days ago.
2. If the current weight is less than the weight in the observation period 30 days ago, calculate the percentage of weight loss.
3. From the medical record, compare the resident's weight in the current observation period to his or her weight in the observation period 180 days ago.
4. If the current weight is less than the weight in the observation period 180 days ago, calculate the percentage of weight loss.

> ### DEFINITIONS
>
> **Physician-Prescribed Weight-loss Regimen**
>
> A weight reduction plan ordered by the resident's physician with the care plan goal of weight reduction. May employ a calorie-restricted diet or other weight loss diets and exercise. Also includes planned diuresis. It is important that weight loss is intentional.
>
> **Body Mass Index (BMI)**
>
> number calculated from a person's weight and height. BMI is used as a screening tool to identify possible weight problems for adults. Visit http://www.cdc.gov/healthyweight/assessing/bmi/adult_bmi/index.html

Coding Instructions

Mathematically round weights as described in Section K0200B before completing the weight loss calculation.

- **Code 0, no or unknown:** if the resident has not experienced weight loss of 5% or more in the past 30 days or 10% or more in the last 180 days or if information about prior weight is not available.
- **Code 1, yes on physician-prescribed weight loss regimen:** if the resident has experienced a weight loss of 5% or more in the past 30 days or 10% or more in the last 180 days, and the weight loss was planned and pursuant to a physician's order.
- **Code 2, yes, not on physician-prescribed weight-loss regimen:** if the resident has experienced a weight loss of 5% or more in the past 30 days or 10% or more in the last 180 days, and the weight loss was not planned and prescribed by a physician.

Coding Tips

- A resident may experience weight variances in between the snapshot time periods. Although these require follow up at the time, they are not captured on the MDS.
- If the resident is losing/gaining a significant amount of weight, the facility should not wait for the 30- or 180-day time frame to address the problem. Weight changes of 5% in 1 month, 7.5% in 3 months, or 10% in 6 months should prompt a thorough assessment of the resident's nutritional status.
- To code K0300 as 1, yes, the expressed goal of the diet must be inducing weight loss.
- On occasion, a resident with normal BMI or even low BMI is placed on a diabetic or otherwise calorie-restricted diet. In this instance, the intent of the diet is not to induce weight loss, and it would not be considered a physician-ordered weight-loss regimen.

Examples

1. Mrs. J has been on a physician ordered calorie-restricted diet for the past year. She and her physician agreed to a plan of weight reduction. Her current weight is 169 lbs. Her weight 30 days ago was 172 lbs. Her weight 180 days ago was 192 lbs.

   Coding: K0300 would be coded 1, yes, on physician-prescribed weight-loss regimen.

(Continued)

Figure 7.12 **CMS Guidelines for Completing the MDS—Section K** *(Continued)*

Rationale:

- 30-day calculation: 172 x 0.95 = 163.4. Since the resident's current weight of 169 lbs is more than 163.4 lbs, which is the 5% point, she has not lost 5% body weight in the last 30 days.
- 180-day calculation: 192 x .90 = 172.8. Since the resident's current weight of 169 lbs is less than 172.8 lbs, which is the 10% point, she has lost 10% or more of body weight in the last 180 days.

2. Mr. S has had increasing need for assistance with eating over the past 6 months. His current weight is 195 lbs. His weight 30 days ago was 197 lbs. His weight 180 days ago was 185 lbs.

   Coding: K0300 would be coded 0, No.

   Rationale:

   - 30-day calculation: 197 x 0.95 = 187.15. Because the resident's current weight of 195 lbs is more than 187.15 lbs, which is the 5% point, he has not lost 5% body weight in the last 30 days.
   - 180-day calculation: Mr. S's current weight of 195 lbs is greater than his weight 180 days ago, so there is no need to calculate his weight loss. He has gained weight over this time period.

3. Ms. K underwent a BKA (below the knee amputation). Her preoperative weight 30 days ago was 130 lbs. Her most recent postoperative weight is 102 lbs. The amputated leg weighed 8 lbs. Her weight 180 days ago was 125 lbs.

   Was the change in weight significant? Calculation of change in weight must take into account the weight of the amputated limb (which in this case is 6% of 130 lbs = 7.8 lbs).

   30-day calculation:

   - **Step 1:** Add the weight of the amputated limb to the current weight to obtain the weight if no amputation occurred: 102 lbs (current weight) + 8 lbs (weight of leg) = 110 lbs (current body weight taking the amputated leg into account)
   - **Step 2:** Calculate the difference between the most recent weight (including weight of the limb) and the previous weight (at 30 days) 130 lbs (preoperative weight) - 110 lbs (present weight if had two legs) = 20 lbs (weight lost)
   - **Step 3:** Calculate the percent weight change relative to the initial weight: 20 lbs (weight change) /130 lbs (preoperative weight) = 15% weight loss
   - **Step 4:** The percent weight change is significant if >5% at 30 days. Therefore, the most recent postoperative weight of 102 lbs (110 lbs, taking the amputated limb into account) is >5% weight loss (significant at 30 days).

   180-day calculation:

   - **Step 1:** Add the weight of the amputated limb to the current weight to obtain the weight if no amputation occurred: 102 lbs (current weight) + 8 lbs (weight of leg) = 110 lbs (current body weight taking the amputated leg into account)
   - **Step 2:** Calculate the difference between the most recent weight (including weight of the limb) and the previous weight (at 180 days): 125 lbs (preoperative weight 180 days ago) - 110 lbs (present weight if had two legs) = 15 lbs (weight lost)
   - **Step 3:** Calculate the percent weight change relative to the initial weight: 15 lbs (weight change) / 130 lbs (preoperative weight) = 12% weight loss
   - **Step 4:** The percent weight change is significant if >10% at 180 days. The most recent postoperative weight of 110 lbs (110 lbs, taking the amputated limb into account) is >10% weight loss (significant at 180 days). Present weight of 110 lbs >10% weight loss (significant at 180 days).

   Coding: K0300 would be coded 2, yes, weight change is significant; not on physician-prescribed weight-loss regimen.

   Rationale: The resident had a significant weight loss of >5% in 30 days and did have a weight loss of >10% in 180 days, the item would be coded as 2, yes weight change is significant; not on physician-prescribed weight–loss regime, with one of the items being triggered. This item is coded for either a 5% 30-day weight loss or a 10% 180-day weight loss. In this example both items, the criteria are met but the coding does not change as long as one of them are met.

(Continued)

Figure 7.12   CMS Guidelines for Completing the MDS—Section K *(Continued)*

K0500: Nutritional Approaches

K0500. Nutritional Approaches		
↓ **Check all that apply**		
☐	**A. Parenteral/IV feeding**	
☐	**B. Feeding tube** - nasogastric or abdominal (PEG)	
☐	**C. Mechanically altered diet** - require change in texture of food or liquids (e.g., pureed food, thickened liquids)	
☐	**D. Therapeutic diet** (e.g., low salt, diabetic, low cholesterol)	
☐	**Z. None of the above**	

Item Rationale

Health-related Quality of Life

- Nutritional approaches that vary from the normal (e.g., mechanically altered food) or that rely on alternative methods (e.g., parenteral/IV or feeding tubes) can diminish an individual's sense of dignity and self-worth as well as diminish pleasure from eating.
- The resident's clinical condition may potentially benefit from the various nutritional approaches included here. It is important to work with the resident and family members to establish nutritional support goals that balance the resident's preferences and overall clinical goals.

Planning for Care

- Alternative nutritional approaches should be monitored to validate effectiveness.
- Care planning should include periodic reevaluation of the appropriateness of the approach.

Steps for Assessment

Review the medical record to determine if any of the listed nutritional approaches were received by the resident during the 7-day look-back period.

Coding Instructions

Check all that apply. If none apply, check K0500Z. None of the above.

- **K0500A**, parenteral/IV feeding
- **K0500B**, feeding tube
- **K0500C**, mechanically altered diet
- **K0500D**, therapeutic diet
- **K0500Z**, none of the above

Coding Tips

> **DEFINITIONS**
>
> **Parenteral/IV Feeding**
>
> Introduction of a nutritive substance into the body by means other than the intestinal tract (e.g., subcutaneous, intravenous).
>
> **Feeding Tube**
>
> Presence of any type of tube that can deliver food/nutritional substances/fluids/medications directly into the gastrointestinal system. Examples include, but are not limited to nasogastric tubes, gastrostomy tubes, jejunostomy tubes, percutaneous endoscopic gastrotomy (PEG) tubes.

K0500 includes any and all nutrition and hydration received by the nursing home resident in the last 7 days either at the nursing home, at the hospital as an outpatient or an inpatient, provided they were administered for nutrition or hydration.

- Parenteral/IV feeding—The following fluids may be included when there is supporting documentation that reflects the need for additional fluid intake specifically addressing a nutrition or hydration need. This supporting documentation should be noted in the resident's medical record according to State and/or internal facility policy:
  - > IV fluids or hyperalimentation, including total parenteral nutrition (TPN), administered continuously or intermittently
  - > IV fluids running at KVO (Keep Vein Open)

(Continued)

Figure 7.12   CMS Guidelines for Completing the MDS—Section K *(Continued)*

> IV fluids contained in IV Piggybacks

> Hypodermoclysis and subcutaneous ports in hydration therapy

- The following items are NOT to be coded in K0500A:

  > IV Medications—Code these when appropriate in O0100H, IV Medications.

  > IV fluids administered solely for the purpose of "prevention" of dehydration. Active diagnosis of dehydration must be present in order to code this fluid in K0500A.

  > IV fluids used to reconstitute and/or dilute medications for IV administration.

  > IV fluids administered as a routine part of an operative or diagnostic procedure or recovery room stay.

  > IV fluids administered solely as flushes.

  > Parenteral/IV fluids administered in conjunction with chemotherapy or dialysis.

- Guidelines on basic fluid and electrolyte replacement can be found online at http://www.merck.com/mmpe/sec19/ch276/ch276b.html.

- Enteral feeding formulas:

  - Should not be coded as a mechanically altered diet.

  - Should only be coded as **K0400D, Therapeutic Diet** when the enteral formula is to manage problematic health conditions, e.g. enteral formulas specific to diabetics.

DEFINITIONS

Mechanically Altered Diet

A diet specifically prepared to alter the texture or consistency of food to facilitate oral intake. Examples include soft solids, puréed foods, ground meat, and thickened liquids. A mechanically altered diet should not automatically be considered a therapeutic diet.

Therapeutic Diet

A diet ordered to manage problematic health conditions. Therapeutic refers to the nutritional content of the food. Examples include calorie-specific, low-salt, low-fat, lactose free, no added sugar, and supplements during meals.

Examples

1. Mrs. H is receiving an antibiotic in 100 cc of normal saline via IV. She has a urinary tract infection (UTI), fever, abnormal lab results (e.g., new pyuria, microscopic hematuria, urine culture with growth >100,000 colony forming units of a urinary pathogen), and documented inadequate fluid intake (i.e., output of fluids far exceeds fluid intake) with signs and symptoms of dehydration. She is placed on the nursing home's hydration plan to ensure adequate hydration. Documentation shows IV fluids are being administered as part of the already identified need for additional hydration.

   Coding: K0500A would **be checked**. The IV medication would be coded at IV Medications item (O0100H).

   Rationale: The resident received 100 cc of IV fluid and there is supporting documentation that reflected an identified need for additional fluid intake for hydration.

2. Mr. J is receiving an antibiotic in 100 cc of normal saline via IV. He has a UTI, no fever, and documented adequate fluid intake. He is placed on the nursing home's hydration plan to ensure adequate hydration.

   Coding: K0500A would **NOT be checked**. The IV medication would be coded at IV Medications item (O0100H).

   Rationale: Although the resident received the additional fluid, there is no documentation to support a need for additional fluid intake.

K0700: Percent Intake by Artificial Route

Complete only if K0500A or K0500B is checked. Skip to Section L, Oral/Dental Status, if neither is checked.

K0700. Percent Intake by Artificial Route - Complete K0700 only if K0500A or K0500B is checked	
Enter Code ☐	**A. Proportion of total calories the resident received through parenteral or tube feeding** 1. 25% or less 2. 26-50% 3. 51% or more
Enter Code ☐	**B. Average fluid intake per day by IV or tube feeding** 1. 500 cc/day or less 2. 501 cc/day or more

(Continued)

Figure 7.12 CMS Guidelines for Completing the MDS—Section K *(Continued)*

Item Rationale

Health-related Quality of Life

Nutritional approaches that vary from the normal, such as parenteral/IV or feeding tubes, can diminish an individual's sense of dignity and self-worth as well as diminish pleasure from eating.

Planning for Care

- The proportion of calories received through artificial routes should be monitored with periodic reassessment to ensure adequate nutrition and hydration.
- Periodic reassessment is necessary to facilitate transition to increased oral intake as indicated by the resident's condition.

K0700A: Proportion of Total Calories the Resident Received through Parental or Tube Feedings in the Last 7 Days

Steps for Assessment

1. Review intake records to determine actual intake through parenteral or tube feeding routes.
2. Calculate proportion of total calories received through these routes.
   > If the resident took no food or fluids by mouth or took just sips of fluid, stop here and **code 3, 51% or more.**
   > If the resident had more substantial oral intake than this, consult with the dietician.

Coding Instructions

Select the best response:

1. 25% or less
2. 26% to 50%
3. 51% or more

Example

Calculation for Proportion of Total Calories from IV or Tube Feeding:

Mr. H has had a feeding tube since his surgery. He is currently more alert and feeling much better. He is very motivated to have the tube removed. He has been taking soft solids by mouth, but only in small to medium amounts. For the past 7 days, he has been receiving tube feedings for nutritional supplementation. The Registered Dietitian has totaled his calories per day as follows:

Oral and Tube Feeding Intake		
	Oral	**Tube**
Sun.	500	2,000
Mon.	250	2,250
Tues.	250	2,250
Wed.	350	2,250
Thurs.	500	2,000
Fri	250	2,250
Sat.	350	2,000
Total	2,450	15,000

Coding: K0700A would be coded 3, 51% or more.

(Continued)

Figure 7.12   CMS Guidelines for Completing the MDS—Section K *(Continued)*

Rationale:

- Total Oral intake is 2,400 calories.
- Total Tube intake is 15,000 calories
- Total calories is 2,450 + 15,000 = 17,450
- Calculation of the percentage of total calories by tube feeding: 15,000/17,450 = 859 x 100 = 85.9%
- Mr. H received 85.9% of his calories by tube feeding, therefore K0700A code 3, 51% or more is correct

K0700B: Average Fluid Intake per Day by IV or Tube Feeding in the Last 7 Days

Steps for Assessment

1. Review intake records from the last 7 days.
2. Add up the total amount of fluid received each day by IV and/or tube feedings only.
3. Divide the week's total fluid intake by 7 to calculate the average of fluid intake per day.
4. Divide by 7 even if the resident did not receive IV fluids and/or tube feeding on each of the 7 days.

Coding Instructions

Code for the average number of cc's of fluid the resident received per day by IV or tube feeding. Record what was actually received by the resident, not what was ordered.

- **Code 1:** 500 cc/day or less
- **Code 2:** 501 cc/day or more

Examples

1. **Calculation for Average Daily Fluid Intake:** Ms. A has swallowing difficulties secondary to Huntington's disease. She is able to take oral fluids by mouth with supervision, but not enough to maintain hydration. She received the following daily fluid totals by supplemental tube feedings (including water, prepared nutritional supplements, juices) during the last 7 days.

IV Fluid Intake	
Sun.	1,250 cc
Mon.	775 cc
Tues.	925 cc
Wed.	1,200 cc
Thurs.	1,200 cc
Fri	500 cc
Sat.	450 cc
Total	6,300 cc

Coding: K0700B would be coded 2,501 cc/day or more.

Rationale: The total fluid intake by supplemental tube feedings = 1,000 cc divided by 7 days = 142.9 cc/day 142.9 cc is less than 500 cc, therefore code 1, 500 cc/day or less is correct.

For each triggered CAT, indicate whether a new care plan, care plan revision, or continuation of current care plan is necessary to address the problem(s) identified in your assessments. The Care Planning Decision column must be completed within seven days of completing the Resident Assessment Instrument (MDS and RAPs).

To summarize, when a CAA is triggered, the Registered Dietitian/Certified Dietary Manager must participate in an additional assessment using the CAA process. Some facilities use computer-based systems that automatically identify triggers based on the MDS data. The Registered Dietitian/Certified Dietary Manager must still document the nature of the condition, risk factors, factors to consider in care planning, referrals, and the reasons to proceed or not proceed with care planning.

Excerpts from the CAA/CATs for Nutritional Status, Feeding Tubes, and Dehydration/Fluid Maintenance appear in Figure 7.13. It tells healthcare team members what information to look for.

There are several other CATs that may require dietary services interventions.

✓ Cognitive Loss or Dementia. Cognitive loss may put residents at risk for eating problems.

✓ ADL Function Rehabilitation Potential. A resident may have difficulties feeding himself or herself.

✓ Mood State. A mood state problem may cause loss of appetite and weight.

✓ Activities. Offering nutrition supplements can be part of an activity program.

✓ Dental Care. A client's teeth/dentures affect his or her ability to eat.

✓ Pressure Ulcer. Pressure ulcers have nutritional implications.

✓ Psychotropic Drugs. Drugs can decrease appetite or change a client's ability to taste and smell foods.

Assessments On Return Stay/Readmission

If a facility has discharged a client without the expectation that the client would return, then the returning client is considered a new admission (return stay) and would require an initial admission RAI comprehensive assessment within 14 days of admission. This typically occurs when a client bed has not been held while they are out of the facility.

If a client returns to a facility following a temporary absence for hospitalization or therapeutic leave, it is considered a readmission. Facilities are not required to assess a client who is readmitted, unless a significant change in the client's condition has occurred. In these situations, follow the procedures for significant change assessments.

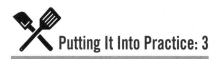

Putting It Into Practice: 3

You have just admitted an elderly woman from the hospital an elderly woman who has a severe UTI. She is in good spirits, very aware, alert, communicative, and eating well. Your IDT completes the RAI by the end of 14 days. On day 16, she is confused, unable to communicate verbally, and refusing to eat or drink. When would you need to complete another RAI?

(Check your answer at the end of this chapter)

(Contintiued on pg. 217)

Figure 7.13   CAA Process and Care Planning

Nutritional Status

Undernutrition is not a response to normal aging, but it can arise from many diverse causes, often acting together. It may cause or reflect acute or chronic illness, and it represents a risk factor for subsequent decline.

The Nutritional Status CAA process reflects the need for an in-depth analysis of residents with impaired nutrition and those who are at nutritional risk. This CAA triggers when a resident has or is at risk for a nutrition issue/condition. Some residents who are triggered for follow-up will already be significantly underweight and thus undernourished, while other persons will be at risk of undernutrition. This CAA may also trigger based on loss of appetite with little or no accompanying weight loss and despite the absence of obvious, outward signs of impaired nutrition.

Nutritional Status CAT Logic Table

Triggering Conditions (any of the following):

1. Dehydration is selected as a problem health condition as indicated by: **J1500C = 1**

2. Body mass index (BMI) is too low or too high as indicated by: **BMI < 18.5 OR BMI > 24.9**

3. Any weight loss as indicated by a value of 1 or 2 as follows: **K0300 = 1 OR K0300 = 2**

4. Parenteral/IV feeding is used as nutritional approach as indicated by: **K0500A = 1**

5. Mechanically altered diet is used as nutritional approach as indicated by: **K0500C = 1**

6. Therapeutic diet is used as nutritional approach as indicated by: **K0500D = 1**

7. Resident has one or more unhealed pressure ulcer(s) at Stage 2 or higher, or one or more likely pressure ulcers that are unstageable at this time as indicated by:

   ((M0300B1 > 0 AND M0300B1 <= 9) OR

   (M0300C1 > 0 AND M0300C1 <= 9) OR

   (M0300D1 > 0 AND M0300D1 <= 9) OR

   (M0300E1 > 0 AND M0300E1 <= 9) OR

   (M0300F1 > 0 AND M0300F1 <= 9) OR

   (M0300G1 > 0 AND M0300G1 <= 9))

Feeding Tubes

This CAA focuses on the long-term (greater than 1 month) use of feeding tubes. It is important to balance the benefits and risks of feeding tubes in individual residents in deciding whether to make such an intervention a part of the plan of care. In some acute and longer term situations, feeding tubes may provide adequate nutrition that cannot be obtained by other means. In other circumstances (for example, in individuals with advanced dementia), feeding tubes may not enhance survival or improve quality of life. Also, feeding tubes can be associated with diverse complications that may further impair quality of life or adversely impact survival. For example, tube feedings will not prevent aspiration of gastric contents or oral secretions and feeding tubes may irritate or perforate the stomach or intestines.

When this CAA is triggered, nursing home staff should follow their facility's chosen protocol or policy for performing the CAA.

Feeding Tubes CAT Logic Table

Triggering Conditions (any of the following):

1. Feeding tube is used as nutritional approach as indicated by: **K0500B = 1**

The information gleaned from the assessment should be used to identify and address the resident's status and underlying issues/conditions that necessitated the use of a feeding tube. In addition, the CAA information should be used to identify any related risk factors. The next step is to develop an individualized care plan based directly on these conclusions. The focus of the care plan should be to address the underlying cause(s), including any reversible issues and conditions that led to using a feeding tube.

(Continued...)

Figure 7.13 CAA Process and Care Planning *(Continued)*

Dehydration/Fluid Maintenance

Dehydration is a condition in which there is an imbalance of water and related electrolytes in the body. As a result, the body may become less able to maintain adequate blood pressure and electrolyte balance, deliver sufficient oxygen and nutrients to the cells, and rid itself of wastes. In older persons, diagnosing dehydration is accomplished primarily by a detailed history, laboratory testing (e.g., electrolytes, BUN, creatinine, serum osmolality, urinary sodium), and to a lesser degree by a physical examination. Abnormal vital signs, such as falling blood pressure and an increase in the pulse rate, may sometimes be meaningful symptoms of dehydration in the elderly.

When this CAA is triggered, nursing home staff should follow their facility's chosen protocol or policy for performing the CAA.

Dehydration/Fluid Maintenance CAT Logic Table

Triggering Conditions (any of the following):

1. Fever is selected as a problem health condition as indicated by: **1550A = 1**
2. Vomiting is selected as a problem health condition as indicated by: **J1550B = 1**
3. Dehydration is selected as a problem health condition as indicated by: **1550C = 1**
4. Internal bleeding is selected as a problem health condition as indicated by: **J1550D = 1**
5. Infection present as indicated by:

   (I1700 = 1) OR

   (I2000 = 1) OR

   (I2100 = 1) OR

   (I2200 = 1) OR

   (I2300 = 1) OR

   (I2400 = 1) OR

   (I2500 = 1) OR

   ((M1040A = 1))

6. Constipation present as indicated by: **H0600 = 1**
7. Parenteral/IV feeding is used as nutritional approach as indicated by: **K0500A = 1**
8. Feeding tube is used as nutritional approach as indicated by: **K0500B = 1**

The information gleaned from the assessment should be used to identify whether the resident is dehydrated or at risk for dehydration, as well as to identify any related possible causes and contributing and/or risk factors. The next step is to develop an individualized care plan based directly on these conclusions. The focus of the care plan should be to prevent dehydration by addressing risk factors, to maintain or restore fluid and electrolyte balance, and to address the underlying cause or causes of any current dehydration.

Dental Care

The ability to chew food is important for adequate oral nutrition. Having clean and attractive teeth or dentures can promote a resident's positive self-image and personal appearance, thereby enhancing social interactions. Medical illnesses and medication-related adverse consequences may increase a resident's risk for related complications such as impaired nutrition and communication deficits. The dental care CAA addresses a resident's risk of oral disease, discomfort, and complications.

When this CAA is triggered, nursing home staff should follow their facility's chosen protocol or policy for performing the CAA. This CAA is triggered when a resident has indicators of an oral/dental issue/condition.

Dental Care CAT Logic Table

Triggering Conditions (any of the following):

1. Any dental problem indicated by:

   (L0200A = 1) OR

(Continued...)

Figure 7.13 **CAA Process and Care Planning** (Continued)

(L0200B = 1) OR

(L0200C = 1) OR

(L0200D = 1) OR

(L0200E = 1) OR

(L0200F = 1)

The information gleaned from the assessment should be used to identify the oral/dental issues and/or conditions and to identify any related possible causes and contributing and/or risk factors. The next step is to develop an individualized care plan based directly on these conclusions. The focus of the care plan should be to address the underlying cause or causes of the resident's issues and/or conditions.

Pressure Ulcer

A pressure ulcer can be defined as a localized injury to the skin and/or underlying tissue, usually over a bony prominence, as a result of pressure or pressure in combination with shear and/or friction. Pressure ulcers can have serious consequences for the elderly and are costly and time consuming to treat. They are a common preventable and treatable condition among elderly people with restricted mobility.

When this CAA is triggered, nursing home staff should follow their facility's chosen protocol or policy for performing the CAA.

Pressure Ulcer CAT Logic Table

Triggering Conditions (any of the following):

1. ADL assistance for bed mobility was needed, or activity did not occur, or activity only occurred once or twice as indicated by:

   (G0110A1 >= 1 AND G0110A1 <= 4) OR

   (G0110A1 = 7 OR G0110A1 = 8)

2. Frequent urinary incontinence as indicated by: **H0300 = 2 OR H0300 = 3**

3. Frequent bowel continence as indicated by: **H0400 = 2 OR H0400 = 3**

4. Weight loss in the absence of physician-prescribed regimen as indicated by: **K0300 = 2**

5. Resident at risk for developing pressure ulcers as indicated by: **M0150 = 1**

6. Resident has one or more unhealed pressure ulcer(s) at Stage 2 or higher, or one or more likely pressure ulcers that are unstageable at this time as indicated by:

   (M0300B1 > 0 AND M0300B1 <= 9) OR

   (M0300C1 > 0 AND M0300C1 <= 9) OR

   (M0300D1 > 0 AND M0300D1 <= 9) OR

   (M0300E1 > 0 AND M0300E1 <= 9) OR

   (M0300F1 > 0 AND M0300F1 <= 9) OR

   (M0300G1 > 0 AND M0300G1 <= 9))

7. Resident has one or more unhealed pressure ulcer(s) at Stage 1 as indicated by: **M0300A > 0 AND M0300A <= 9**

8. Resident has one or more pressure ulcer(s) that has gotten worse since prior assessment as indicated by:

   (M0800A > 0 AND M0800A <= 9) OR

   (M0800B > 0 AND M0800B <= 9) OR

   (M0800C > 0 AND M0800C <= 9)

9. Trunk restraint used in bed has value of 1 or 2 as indicated by: **P0100B = 1 OR P0100B = 2**

10. Trunk restraint used in chair or out of bed has value of 1 or 2 as indicated by: **P0100E = 1 OR P0100E = 2**

The information gleaned from the assessment should be used to draw conclusions about the status of a resident's pressure ulcers(s) and to identify any related causes and contributing and/or risk factors. The next step is to develop an individualized care

(Continued...)

Figure 7.13   CAA Process and Care Planning *(Continued)*

plan based directly on these conclusions. If a pressure ulcer is not present, the goal is to prevent them by identifying the resident's risks and implementing preventive measures. If a pressure ulcer is present, the goal is to heal or close it.

Psychotropic Medication Use CAT Logic Table

Triggering Conditions (any of the following):

1. Antipsychotic medication administered to resident in last 7 days or since admission as indicated by: **N0400A = 1**
2. Antianxiety medication administered to resident in last 7 days or since admission as indicated by: **N0400B = 1**
3. Antidepressant medication administered to resident in last 7 days or since admission as indicated by: **N0400C = 1**
4. Hypnotic medication administered to resident in last 7 days or since admission as indicated by: **N0400D = 1**

The information gleaned from the assessment should be used to draw conclusions about the appropriateness of the resident's medication (in consultation with the physician and the consultant pharmacist) and to identify any adverse consequences, as well as any related possible causes and contributing and/or risk factors. The next step is to develop an individualized care plan based directly on these conclusions. Important goals of therapy include maximizing the resident's functional potential and well-being, while minimizing the hazards associated with medication side effects.

HIPAA

In April 2003, a new security regulation called HIPAA took effect. HIPAA stands for **Health Insurance Portability and Accountability Act,** a federal law intended to protect the privacy of healthcare clients, while also standardizing exchange of healthcare information. If you work in a healthcare facility, the manner in which you handle medical records and related documents will be guided, in part, by HIPAA.

HIPAA dictates that client information and health-related data will be kept secure. "Secure" as defined in the law refers to two key ideas:

✓ Patient privacy and the right to keep personal and medical information confidential

✓ Safeguarding information, such as computer files, from physical and technical hazards

Thus, if you maintain a computer system that holds clients' nutrition care records, you need to be sure that access is limited and protected, and be sure the system itself is safely maintained. Here are some examples of how you might accomplish these tasks:

✓ Control access to computers by requiring a login with user names and passwords. Do not keep a written record of these (or keep one in a highly secured location).

✓ Control availability of user names and passwords, and delete access if, for example, someone leaves employment.

✓ If client information is held on laptops, personal digital assistants (PDA), camera phones, or other portable computers, make sure these computers are secured and locked to prevent unauthorized use.

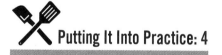

Putting It Into Practice: 4

As a Certified Dietary Manager, it is your responsibility to visit all new hospital clients to discuss their options for food. You are just coming out of Sue Smith's room when you encounter a friend who is visiting another patient. You know she is also a friend of Sue's so you ask her if she knows that Sue Smith was just admitted to the hospital because of her diabetes. Is this a violation of HIPAA?

(Check your answer at the end of this Chapter)

✓ Maintain routine back-ups of computer data. Use virus and worm protection, as well as other safeguards, to prevent data destruction.

✓ Check your insurance coverage; some companies will not cover you for a violation.

The Centers for Medicare and Medicaid Services (CMS) has a plan to establish a national **Electronic Health Record (EHR)**. Many hospitals have already adopted part of the plan by establishing shared electronic health records. The national plan will make patient information from multiple providers readily available in order to improve patient outcomes and safety. Diet Office Software that integrates with the EHR will become more fully implemented in the effort to fulfill a national EHR.

On a more general level, you and every employee of a healthcare facility must adhere to an established policy addressing privacy. You will need to refrain from discussing client information in public areas where others could overhear it. If you destroy client records, you may need to shred them. If you carry a kardex, you may need to keep it under your direct supervision at all times, and secure it when it is not in use. You will also need to handle all documents in such a way that individual records, care plans, MDS forms, etc., cannot be seen by others (except authorized members of the healthcare team). For example, you cannot lay a printout with patient names and diagnoses on a chair while you are chatting with a patient and a family member.

Another fundamental HIPAA concept is called chain of trust. Healthcare facilities and related organizations have to exchange data in order to accomplish many tasks, such as insurance reimbursement. An organization must establish a chain of trust with others, meaning that it transmits data only to other organizations who have committed to following HIPAA regulations.

To develop a plan for complying with HIPAA, you can first examine where security of information is vulnerable. Then, you develop procedures for protecting information at each of these points. HIPAA compliance strategies and policies are still fairly new in the industry, and are evolving rapidly. If you work in a healthcare facility, you will want to become familiar with HIPAA-related policies and procedures and follow them carefully. You may be called upon to help develop policies and procedures related to records in the foodservice department. Any time there is a change in the way you handle health information, you will need to re-evaluate and possibly revise the HIPAA policies and procedures.

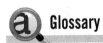

Glossary

Health Insurance Portability and Accountability Act (HIPAA)
Standardizes the exchange of healthcare information and assures client/patient privacy and the right to keep information confidential

Electronic Health Record (EHR)
One of the methods to adopt the full exchange of healthcare information where all records are updated and maintained electronically

END OF CHAPTER

Putting It Into Practice Questions & Answers

1. The client tells you that they are allergic to peanuts. Which component of SOAP data would this be?

   A. *Information that the client tells you is considered subjective information (S).*

2. What do the abbreviations stand for in this chart note?

   Chart Note: Patient is sob. Implemented nutritional supplement bid.

   A. *The patient is "short of breath" or sob. Usually this is written: "The Patient has sob" and then it means shortness of breath. The supplement was given twice a day or bid.*

3. You have just admitted an elderly woman from the hospital who has a severe UTI. She is in good spirits, very aware, alert, communicative, and eating well. Your IDT completes the RAI by the end of 14 days. On day 16, she is confused, unable to communicate verbally, and refusing to eat or drink. When would you need to complete another RAI?

   A. *The physician should be called as soon as possible and a new RAI done right away.*

4. As a Certified Dietary Manager, it is your responsibility to visit all new hospital clients to discuss their options for food. You are just coming out of Sue Smith's room when you encounter a friend who is visiting another patient. You know she is also a friend of Sue's so you ask her if she knows that Sue Smith was just admitted to the hospital because of her diabetes. Is this a violation of HIPAA?

   A. *Yes, this is a HIPAA violation. You are not allowed to discuss the names or the diagnoses of any client/patient with a non-healthcare professional.*

CHAPTER 8

Interview Clients for Nutrition Related Information

![pencil icon]

Overview and Objectives

After documenting nutritional data, the next step is to interview clients. You determine who your clients are and will use at least one technique to gather information about client needs. You will use this information to examine how clients' needs influence the foodservice operation.

After completing this chapter, you should be able to:

✓ Identify different types of clients

✓ Plan and ask appropriate questions of clients

✓ Gather information from client and/or family member(s)

✓ Identify significant information and problems

✓ Recognize nonverbal responses and communication cues

✓ Record information systematically and carefully

✓ Utilize ethical and confidentiality principles and practices

✓ Gather client information from other multi-disciplinary team members

✓ Address food customs and nutritional needs of various racial, cultural, and religious groups

Who Are Your Customers/Clients?

If you were asked to describe your customers/clients, what would you say? If you started describing the hospital patients or nursing home clients, you would be partially correct. They are a very important part of your clientele. Another part of your clientele is the staff that work and eat at your facility. If you prepare meals for members of the community, such as "meals on wheels", they are also your customers/clients. Do you prepare meals for family members on special occasions? Are there other groups you serve that aren't mentioned here? Everyone you provide meal service to is considered a client. Each of them has different needs and different expectations. A successful foodservice department knows who their clients are and routinely surveys each group. This chapter will discuss interviewing patients/clients/caregivers for nutrition related information.

Interviewing Clients Begins With Good Communication Techniques

As we begin this discussion about interviewing clients, let's start with some basics about communication. Communicating clearly is the key to success when working with clients. Communication is a two-way process (see Figure 8.1). Yes, you will have to speak clearly and you will have to make sure your client hears and understands what you are saying. There are five basic steps in communication that are important in interviewing clients:

✓ Prepare for the communication
  - Know why you are interviewing the client
  - Plan what you intend to ask before you interview the client
  - Anticipate how your client might be feeling

✓ Conduct the interview
  - Explain why you are interviewing the client
  - Speak slowly and clearly
  - Speak confidently
  - Explain clearly what you expect
  - Ask the client to relate back to you the purpose of your visit

✓ Receive the message
  - Don't judge what they are telling you or judge the person
  - Look for the key points or specific answers to your questions
  - Give feedback to acknowledge your understanding

✓ Evaluate the effectiveness of your communication
  - Communication can break down due to some common communication barriers:
    > Message quality: Have you used words the client understands? Were the instructions clear? Did you ask enough questions to get all of the information you need?
    > Noise: Did the client have a television/radio/other multimedia on while you were trying to communicate? Were other people in the room talking? Is there equipment running in the room?
    > Time: Were you in a hurry? Was the client in a hurry? Is the interview tool too long for one session?
    > Conflict: Is the client angry? Are you having a bad day?

✓ Overcome the communication barriers
  - Message quality: If you use technical terms, make sure to explain them (even the word diet history might seem foreign or they may not understand the word "fat" in food). Continue to seek feedback in your interview by asking questions such as, "Would you like me to go through that again?" Focus clearly on what you need and why you are there.
  - Noise: Ask, if appropriate, that they minimize their multimedia equipment so you can conduct the interview. If other people or equipment in the room contribute to distracting noise, ask if you can go somewhere else to conduct the interview.

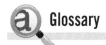

Glossary

Communication
The exchange of information by writing, speaking, or gestures

Nonverbal Communication
The form of communication without speaking or writing that includes gestures, facial expressions, and body language

Verbal Communication
Communicating thoughts, messages, or information by speaking

Written Communication
Communicating thoughts, messages, or information by writing

• Time: Before you begin the interview, make sure both you and your client have enough time to complete the questions.

• Conflict: Don't take it personally and remain patient and professional.

There are three types of **communication**; **written**, **verbal**, and **nonverbal**. The steps above can be used with both verbal and written communication. Nonverbal communication is the communication that occurs without language such as gestures, facial expressions, or the way we use our voices—speaking softly or loudly. Nonverbal communication is just as important as verbal and written communication because it gives you clues as to how well you are communicating. If your client won't look at you during an interview, that tells you something about how interested they are, or in this case, aren't. Let's review the common types of nonverbal communication:

✓ Facial Expressions: smiling, frowning, sneering, rolling the eyes, raising the eyebrows all convey how they are receiving the message. As the sender, you need to watch for changes in facial expression to make sure you are communicating clearly.

✓ Eye-contact: Are your clients looking you directly in the eye? That can mean they are interested and being attentive to what you are saying. It is important to know that in some cultures, direct eye contact can only be used between certain people.

✓ Gestures: If you are interviewing people of different cultures, be aware that they may have a different meaning for some gestures. Become aware of how you gesture when you talk so you will use appropriate hand gestures.

✓ Physical contact: Shaking hands is a typical American greeting. Touching, holding, embracing, patting on the back all convey messages, and those messages may be different in different cultures. Be careful about how you use physical contact with clients.

✓ Distance: How close you stand to a client while interviewing is another form of nonverbal communication. If you stand too close, it may violate the client's 'personal space.'

✓ Posture: If your client is sitting up and looking at you, you can conclude they are interested. If they are slouching or leaning away from you, you might conclude that they are not interested.

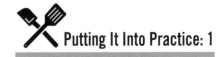

Putting It Into Practice: 1

You are interviewing a client in their room. What type of communication is this? You notice that they are wrinkling their eyebrows during one of the questions. What type of nonverbal communication is this?

(Check your answer at the end of this chapter)

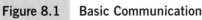

Figure 8.1   Basic Communication

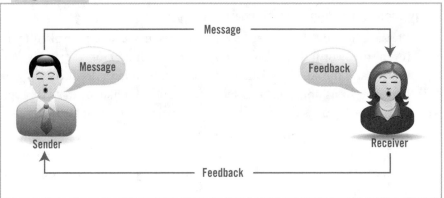

As you begin your career as a Certified Dietary Manager, consider developing a checklist that will remind you of the basics needed for good communication. This can be part of any interview or survey instrument you use. See Figure 8.2 for an example.

Figure 8.2   Checklist for Good Communication Skills

- I care about how clients respond to my messages.
- I don't use jargon in my messages.
- I don't judge people.
- I watch for nonverbal communication clues.
- I try to make each person feel important by listening to their messages.
- I am sensitive to feedback.
- My message is simple, direct, and clear.

Interviews for Nutrition Information

Each facility will have its own process for when the Certified Dietary Manager and/or Registered Dietitian first visits a new admission. Some facilities have an immediate visit to gather food preferences. Some facilities visit after the first week to gather diet information and assess the quality of their foodservice (see Figure 8.3 for an example). Long-term care facilities conduct a diet history within the first 14 days as part of nutrition screening.

Diet History. A diet history is a unique assessment of the client's food intake patterns. A diet history has two features: it describes actual intake, and it gives information about why the client makes certain food choices. It also includes a review of many factors that may have an impact on nutrition, such as lifestyle, social factors, medical conditions, and more.

A diet history usually begins with a series of questions. A Registered Dietitian or Certified Dietary Manager may ask:

✓ Where do you usually eat?

✓ How often do you usually eat

✓ When do you usually eat?

✓ Do you eat by yourself or with others?

✓ Who does the food shopping in your household?

✓ How is your appetite?

✓ Have you had any appetite changes in last month? 6 months?

✓ Do you have hunger or cravings during the day?

✓ Are you having any problems or concerns with eating?

✓ Are you having any problems in chewing?

✓ Are you having any problems in swallowing?

✓ Are you experiencing any digestive concerns, such as nausea, vomiting, constipation, or acid indigestion?

✓ Have you experienced any weight changes within the past 30 days/180 days?

✓ Who does the cooking?

✓ Do you have any food allergies or intolerances?

✓ Do you currently follow a special diet?

✓ Do you currently take any nutritional supplements?

✓ Are there any foods you avoid? If so, why?

Questions such as these and many others begin to build a picture of a person's overall dietary situation. A diet history may include one or more tools designed to develop a snapshot of a client's eating habits. Additional methods of collecting food records will be covered in Chapter 9, Nutrition Screening. As you are conducting the interview, remember to focus on the checklist for good communication. The diet history may be your first opportunity to make a great impression.

Figure 8.3   Patient Comment Card

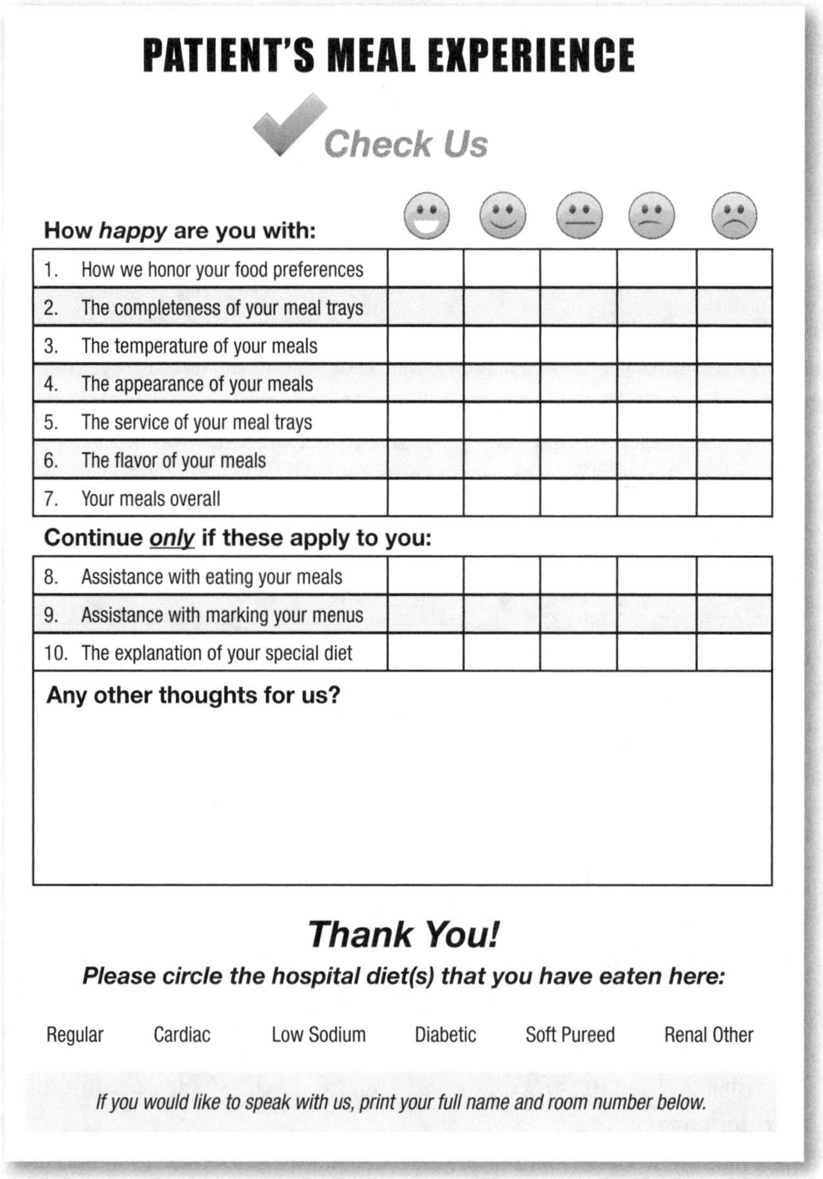

PATIENT'S MEAL EXPERIENCE

Check Us

How *happy* are you with:	😀	🙂	😐	🙁	😞
1. How we honor your food preferences					
2. The completeness of your meal trays					
3. The temperature of your meals					
4. The appearance of your meals					
5. The service of your meal trays					
6. The flavor of your meals					
7. Your meals overall					

Continue _only_ if these apply to you:

	😀	🙂	😐	🙁	😞
8. Assistance with eating your meals					
9. Assistance with marking your menus					
10. The explanation of your special diet					

Any other thoughts for us?

Thank You!

Please circle the hospital diet(s) that you have eaten here:

Regular   Cardiac   Low Sodium   Diabetic   Soft Pureed   Renal Other

If you would like to speak with us, print your full name and room number below.

Source: Larry Robers, et al, Adventist health, 1999.

Some facilities have adopted electronic means of collecting diet history information. See Figure 8.4 for a sample page from an electronic diet history questionnaire. This questionnaire and the software to analyze it, the Diet*Calc version 1.4.3, are available from the National Institute of Health, http://riskfactor. cancer.gov/DHQ/dietcalc/. The advantages of the electronic questionnaire are the ability to:

✓ electronically compute calorie information

✓ document more detailed information

✓ expedite the analysis of the data for problems

What happens if the client is unable to communicate because they cannot speak or are not cognitive? If they are unable to speak, you can use pictures or food models and ask them to respond in writing to your questions. If they are not cognitive, ask close family members to assist you in completing the diet history. If there are no family members available, observe them during several meal times to collect diet information and review transfer information in the medical record.

Some of your clients may not speak English. Speak slowly and use gestures and facial expressions. Use pictures or draw it. Be patient. You may need to use an interpreter.

Conducting Effective Interviews

In addition to the checklist for good communication, there are other tips for conducting effective interviews that will help you be successful (see Figure 8.5—Tips for Conducting Effective Interview). A function of a diet history is to gather information about why a client eats what they do. During the interview, it is important to address food customs that are cultural, racial, or religious in origin. If you work in an area with a large minority population, your interview should have specific questions relating to their culture. Figure 8.6 provides questions to ask a Hispanic client. If your client will be staying with you over a religious holiday, will he/she expect certain foods to be served, such as roast turkey at Christmas? Addressing food customs by serving preferred foods will encourage your client to maintain adequate health. Another tool that may help you in addressing cultural food choices are the food pyramids for different cultures, such as the Mediterranean Pyramid, the Asian Pyramid, and the Latin-American Pyramid (www.oldwayspt.org). Figure 8.7 lists common and uncommon foods and flavors of the Asian Diet Pyramid. If you serve an Asian population, try incorporating these foods into your diet history form.

All of us have biases when working with a diverse client base. If you follow the checklist for good communication skills in Figure 8.2, you will stay open and engaged with your client. If your client is hostile regarding his diet, you can deflate that hostility by acknowledging their feelings. If you listen, you can find something to agree with them.

Figure 8.4   **Sample Page From an Electronic Diet History Questionnaire**

Over the <u>past 12 months</u>...

85. How often did you eat **liver** (all kinds) or **liverwurst**?

☐ NEVER (GO TO QUESTION 86)

☐ 1–6 times per year   ☐ 2 times per week
☐ 7–11 times per year   ☐ 3–4 times per week
☐ 1 time per month   ☐ 5–6 times per week
☐ 2–3 times per month   ☐ 1 time per day
☐ 1 time per week   ☐ 2 or more times per day

85a. Each time you ate **liver** or **liverwurst**, how much did you usually eat?

☐ Less than 1 ounce
☐ 1 to 4 ounces
☐ More than 4 ounces

86. How often did you eat **bacon** (including low-fat)?

☐ NEVER (GO TO QUESTION 87)

☐ 1–6 times per year   ☐ 2 times per week
☐ 7–11 times per year   ☐ 3–4 times per week
☐ 1 time per month   ☐ 5–6 times per week
☐ 2–3 times per month   ☐ 1 time per day
☐ 1 time per week   ☐ 2 or more times per day

86a. Each time you ate **bacon**, how much did you usually eat?

☐ Fewer than 2 slices
☐ 2 to 3 slices
☐ More than 3 slices

86b. How often was the bacon you ate **light, low-fat,** or **lean bacon**?

☐ Almost never or never
☐ About ¼ of the time
☐ About ½ of the time
☐ About ¾ of the time
☐ Almost always or always

87. How often did you eat **sausage** (including low-fat)?

☐ NEVER (GO TO QUESTION 88)

☐ 1–6 times per year   ☐ 2 times per week
☐ 7–11 times per year   ☐ 3–4 times per week
☐ 1 time per month   ☐ 5–6 times per week
☐ 2–3 times per month   ☐ 1 time per day
☐ 1 time per week   ☐ 2 or more times per day

87a. Each time you ate **sausage**, how much did you usually eat?

☐ Less than 1 patty or 2 links
☐ 1 to 3 patties or 2 to 5 links
☐ More than 3 patties or 5 links

87b. How often was the sausage you ate **light, low-fat,** or **lean sausage**?

☐ Almost never or never
☐ About ¼ of the time
☐ About ½ of the time
☐ About ¾ of the time
☐ Almost always or always

88. How often did you eat **fish sticks** or **fried fish** (including fried seafood or shellfish)?

☐ NEVER (GO TO QUESTION 89)

☐ 1–6 times per year   ☐ 2 times per week
☐ 7–11 times per year   ☐ 3–4 times per week
☐ 1 time per month   ☐ 5–6 times per week
☐ 2–3 times per month   ☐ 1 time per day
☐ 1 time per week   ☐ 2 or more times per day

88a. Each time you ate **fish sticks** or **fried fish**, how much did you usually eat?

☐ Less than 2 ounces or less than 1 fillet
☐ 2 to 7 ounces or 1 fillet
☐ More than 7 ounces or more than 1 fillet

89. How often did you eat **fish** or **seafood that was NOT FRIED** (including shellfish)?

☐ NEVER (GO TO INTRODUCTION TO QUESTION 90)

☐ 1–6 times per year   ☐ 2 times per week
☐ 7–11 times per year   ☐ 3–4 times per week
☐ 1 time per month   ☐ 5–6 times per week
☐ 2–3 times per month   ☐ 1 time per day
☐ 1 time per week   ☐ 2 or more times per day

89a. Each time you ate eat **fish** or **seafood that was NOT FRIED**, how much did you usually eat?

☐ Less than 2 ounces or less than 1 fillet
☐ 2 to 5 ounces or 1 fillet
☐ More than 5 ounces or more than 1 fillet

Source: National Institute of Health, 2007

Figure 8.5   Tips for Conducting Effective Interviews

- Plan questions in advance and use a form to keep track.
- Introduce yourself by name and title.
- Avoid yes-or-no questions. Instead, use open-ended questions, such as: "Tell me more about..."
- Ask for more information or clarification when needed. This can be done by paraphrasing (summarizing and rephrasing what has been said).
- Allow the client time to give an answer. Silence can be helpful.
- Use nonverbal language to show the client you are listening. For example, maintain good eye contact and lean slightly toward the client to demonstrate your attention.
- Avoid leading questions which give the client the answer you expect. For example, do not ask, "You don't eat pizza often, do you?"
- When closing the interview, express your appreciation to the client and review the next steps, if appropriate.

Supplementing the Diet History

Once you have completed the diet history, you will gather client information from other multi-disciplinary team members. Who is on the Interdisciplinary Team (IDT)? Generally, it is the director of nursing, Registered Dietitian and/or Certified Dietary Manager, occupational and/or speech therapist, social worker, client, and/or family members. So far you have only gathered information from the client and/or family members. You may want to contact the personal physician if you need information on usual body weight. The occupational or speech therapist may know if they have a swallowing disorder or need adaptive equipment. The social worker can provide information on how the client is adjusting to their new environment. Nursing staff may provide information about the amount of food consumed from trays and information on medicines that might have food-drug interactions.

Talking with others to gather information is one method of gathering additional diet history information and also requires good communication skills. Solid working relationships building on mutual respect are essential. In the course of a work day, a Certified Dietary Manager interacts with many members of the team. This provides an opportunity to ask questions and relate observations. Information communication can play a strong role in client care. However, these interactions must be managed professionally. Team members need to exert care to protect client confidentiality at all times. They need to avoid discussing client needs in public areas.

Each facility has its own policies regarding sharing client information. In addition, it will be critical to know and follow HIPAA guidelines (Health Insurance Portability and Accountability Act). This act requires the provision for security and privacy of client data.

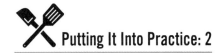

Putting It Into Practice: 2

You have just completed a diet history of a new admission, a male, age 88. He likes most foods as long as they are seasoned with butter and salt. He has a few broken teeth and eats mostly soft foods. His wife recently passed away and in the past month he thinks he has lost weight. He is not happy to be in the facility. What other IDT members would you consult with for follow-up information?

(Check your answer at the end of this chapter)

Figure 8.6   Questions Asked to a Hispanic Client

Over the past 12 months...

51. How often did you eat **chili**?

☐ NEVER (GO TO QUESTION 52)

☐ 1–6 times per year   ☐ 2 times per week
☐ 7–11 times per year   ☐ 3–4 times per week
☐ 1 time per month   ☐ 5–6 times per week
☐ 2–3 times per month   ☐ 1 time per day
☐ 1 time per week   ☐ 2 or more times per day

51a. Each time you ate **chili**, how much did you usually eat?

☐ Less than ½ cup
☐ ½ to 1¾ cups
☐ More than 1¾ cups

52. How often did you eat **Mexican foods** (such as tacos, tostados, burritos, tamales, fajitas, enchiladas, quesadillas, and chimichangas)?

☐ NEVER (GO TO QUESTION 53)

☐ 1–6 times per year   ☐ 2 times per week
☐ 7–11 times per year   ☐ 3–4 times per week
☐ 1 time per month   ☐ 5–6 times per week
☐ 2–3 times per month   ☐ 1 time per day
☐ 1 time per week   ☐ 2 or more times per day

52a. Each time you ate **Mexican foods**, how much did you usually eat?

☐ Less than 1 taco, burrito, etc.
☐ 1 to 2 tacos, burritos, etc.
☐ More than 2 tacos, burritos, etc.

53. How often did you eat **cooked dried beans** (such as baked beans, pintos, kidney, blackeyed peas, lima, lentils, soybeans, or refried beans)? *(Please don't include bean soups or chili.)*

☐ NEVER (GO TO QUESTION 54)

☐ 1–6 times per year   ☐ 2 times per week
☐ 7–11 times per year   ☐ 3–4 times per week
☐ 1 time per month   ☐ 5–6 times per week
☐ 2–3 times per month   ☐ 1 time per day
☐ 1 time per week   ☐ 2 or more times per day

53a. Each time you ate **beans**, how much did you usually eat?

☐ Less than ½ cup
☐ ½ to 1 cup
☐ More than 1 cup

53b. How often were the beans you ate **refried beans, beans prepared with any type of fat**, or **with meat added**?

☐ Almost never or never
☐ About ¼ of the time
☐ About ½ of the time
☐ About ¾ of the time
☐ Almost always or always

54. How often did you eat **other kinds of vegetables**?

☐ NEVER (GO TO QUESTION 55)

☐ 1–6 times per year   ☐ 2 times per week
☐ 7–11 times per year   ☐ 3–4 times per week
☐ 1 time per month   ☐ 5–6 times per week
☐ 2–3 times per month   ☐ 1 time per day
☐ 1 time per week   ☐ 2 or more times per day

54a. Each time you ate **other kinds of vegetables**, how much did you usually eat?

☐ Less than ¼ cup
☐ ¼ to ½ cup
☐ More than ½ cup

55. How often did you eat **rice** or **other cooked grains** (such as bulgur, cracked wheat, or millet)?

☐ NEVER (GO TO QUESTION 56)

☐ 1–6 times per year   ☐ 2 times per week
☐ 7–11 times per year   ☐ 3–4 times per week
☐ 1 time per month   ☐ 5–6 times per week
☐ 2–3 times per month   ☐ 1 time per day
☐ 1 time per week   ☐ 2 or more times per day

55a. Each time you ate **rice** or **other cooked grains**, how much did you usually eat?

☐ Less than ½ cup
☐ ½ to 1½ cups
☐ More than 1½ cups

55b. How often was **butter, margarine**, or **oil** added to your rice **IN COOKING OR AT THE TABLE**?

☐ Almost never or never
☐ About ¼ of the time
☐ About ½ of the time
☐ About ¾ of the time
☐ Almost always or always

Source: National Institute of Health, 2007

Figure 8.7 Common Foods and Flavors of the Asian Diet Pyramid

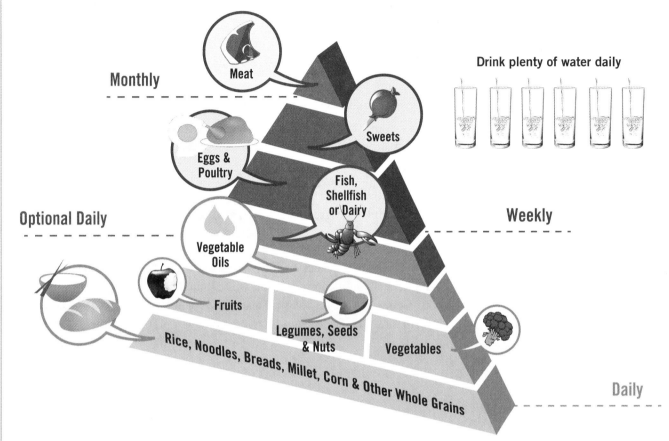

© 2000 Oldways Preservation & Exchange Trust www.oldwayspt.org

Vegetables & Tubers
Bamboo Shoots, Bean Sprouts, Bitter Melon, Bok Choy, Broccoli, Cabbage, Carrots, Chiles, Daikon, Eggplant, Galangal, Kumquats, Leeks, Lemons, Lemongrass, Lettuce, Lime, Lotus Root, Peppers, Kale, Kombu, Mushrooms, Mustard Greens, Peppers, Pineapple, Pumpkin, Scallions, Seaweed, Snow Peas, Spinach, Sweet Potatoes, Taro Root, Turnips, Water Chestnuts, Yams

Fruits
Apricots, Bananas, Cherries, Coconut, Dates, Dragon Fruit, Grapes, Kiwifruit, Longan, Lychee, Mandarins, Mangoes, Melon, Mangosteen, Milk Fruit, Oranges, Papaya, Pears, Pineapple, Rambutan, Tangerines

Grains
Barley, Breads (Examples include: Dumplings, Chapatis, Mantou, Naan, Roti), Buckwheat, Rice, Millet, Noodles (Examples include: Soba, Somen, Rice, Udon)

Fish & Seafood
Abalone, Clams, Cockles, Crab, Eel, King Fish, Mussels, Octopus, Oysters, Roe, Scallops, Sea Bass, Shrimp, Squid, Tuna, Whelk, Yellowtail

Poultry, Eggs, Cheese, and Yogurt
Chicken, Duck, Eggs (Chicken, Quail, and Duck), Cheeses and Butter (Ghee, Paneer), Yogurt (Chaas, Lassi)

Nuts, Seeds, and Legumes
Almonds, Beans (Adzuki, Edamame, Mung, Soy), Cashews, Hazelnuts, Lentils, Miso, Peanuts, Seasame Seeds, Tofu, Tempeh

Herbs and Spices
Amchoor, Asafoetida, Basil (Thai), Cardamom, Chiles, Clove, Coriander, Curry Leaves, Fennel, Fenugreek, Garlic, Ginger, Ginseng, Kafir Lime Leaves, Masala, Mint, Parsley, Pepper, Scallion, Star Anise, Tumeric, Wasabi

Meats and Sweets
Pork, Beef, Sweets (Examples include: Chinese mooncakes, Indian Rice Pudding, Japanese sugared sweet potatoes, Thai mango-coconut pudding)

Water and Alcohol
Drink plenty of water. All alcohol in moderation.

Another method of team members sharing information is through the medical record. To gather information from a medical record, you must first become acquainted with how records are organized in your facility. As you read in Chapter 7, some facilities maintain records electronically on a computer system. Many small healthcare facilities use paper-based systems. A typical medical record includes the following components:

✓ An admission sheet listing patient information, admission date, reason for admission, and names and contact details for family members

✓ A section for physicians' orders, including diet, medications, tests, and treatments

✓ A page listing problems

✓ A section for test results

✓ A section for progress notes from all disciplines

Documenting Interview Information

Every time you conduct an interview, it is import to record the information systematically and carefully. You will create a note in the medical record per your facility's process. You may also create paper or electronic food preference information to assist the foodservice staff when preparing trays.

END OF CHAPTER

Putting It Into Practice Questions & Answers

1. You are interviewing a client in their room. What type of communication is this? You notice that they are wrinkling their eyebrows during one of the questions. What type of non-verbal communication is this?

   A. *An interview is a type of verbal communication. Wrinkling eyebrows is a facial expression and a type of non-verbal communication.*

2. You have just completed a diet history of a new admission, a male, age 88. He likes most foods as long as they are seasoned with butter and salt. He has a few broken teeth and prefers soft foods. His wife recently passed away and in the past month he thinks he has lost weight. He is not happy to be in the facility. What other IDT members would you consult with for follow-up information?

   A. *Because he prefers soft foods, you might follow-up with a speech therapist just to make sure his swallowing isn't also a concern. With the death of his wife and suggested weight loss, follow-up with the social worker to see about possible depression. You will also want to check the medical record to see his lab values since he wants all foods to be seasoned with butter and salt.*

Conduct Routine Nutrition Screening

Overview and Objectives

Nutrition screening helps a Certified Dietary Manager identify healthcare clients in need of nutrition intervention. It is also required for compliance with regulations and standards.

After completing this chapter, you should be able to:

✓ Identify the goal of nutrition screening

✓ Explain the difference between nutrition screening and nutrition assessment

✓ Recognize routine versus at-risk clients using established guidelines

✓ Identify appropriate data to be gathered

✓ Explain the term body mass index (BMI)

✓ Differentiate between ideal body weight (%IBW), usual body weight (UBW), current body weight

✓ Utilize appropriate data-gathering format/approach for specific client types(s)

✓ Complete client forms efficiently

✓ Review examples of common food-drug interactions

✓ Calculate BEE and total energy needs

✓ Identify federal regulations related to evaluating patient status and care

✓ Collect client information from medical record

For the first half of the 21st century, Americans will see an unprecedented increase in the number of elderly. As baby boomers grow older, people 85 and over are expected to be the fastest-growing group of elderly persons. Combine that with the fact that elderly persons are at increased risk for nutritional problems, and we see an increased need to identify those who are most at risk. During the 1990's, the American Academy of Family Physicians, the The Academy of Nutrition and Dietetics (AND) [formerly known as The American Dietetic Association (ADA)], and the National Council on Aging promoted a Nutritional Screening Initiative. The purpose of the initiative was to use a simple screening tool to discover nutrition concerns before serious illnesses occurred. The tool has been useful in educating the public but not as beneficial at identifying those who needed immediate intervention.

In 2002, the The Academy of Nutrition and Dietetics (AND) [formerly known as The American Dietetic Association (ADA)] developed a Nutrition Care Process and Model to clarify how dietetics professionals provide care to clients. In 2008, the AND redesigned the nutrition care process to aid healthcare facilities, as well as legislators, in recognizing and providing appropriate medical nutrition therapy for clients in hospitals and long-term care facilities.

Nutrition Care Process

The **nutrition care process** is intended to provide a standardized process of providing care to clients. The The Academy of Nutrition and Dietetics (AND) [formerly known as The American Dietetic Association (ADA)] defines the nutrition care process in four steps. This chapter focuses on Step 1.

1. Nutrition Assessment includes collecting information to identify nutrition problems, verify the data, and evaluate that information. This step has two components: nutrition screening and nutrition assessment.

2. Nutrition Diagnosis involves defining all nutrition-related problems, using standardized terminology defined by the AND. AND identified 62 diagnosis/problems.

3. Nutrition Intervention the actions taken to correct a nutrition problem. This step involves both planning and implementing and begins with a plan of care followed by a team approach to implement the plan.

4. Nutrition Monitoring and Evaluation involves follow-up to determine how well the interventions are working. Further definition of this step is in progress.

Nutrition Screening

Nutrition screening is a systematic method for identifying individuals at risk for nutrition problems. It is part of the first step in the Nutrition Care Process—Nutrition Assessment. It is a process applied to an entire group in order to select members of that group who are candidates for further intervention. Nutrition screening can be done in public healthcare settings, such as health fairs, or outpatient clinics. In a healthcare facility such as a nursing home or hospital, every individual who is admitted should undergo a routine nutrition screening. We know who may need nutrition therapy by performing nutrition screening.

One of the responsibilities of many Certified Dietary Managers who happen to work in healthcare facilities is to conduct routine nutrition screening. Screening is typically a fairly simple process, based on indicators. **Indicators** are pieces of information that might suggest a concern or risk. Many are numbers or measurements. They are built upon statistics. For example, we might discover that many individuals found to be less than 90 percent of their ideal body weight turn out to have significantly higher rates of complications from surgery. Based on that, we might set an indicator for nutrition screening as less than 90 percent of ideal body weight. In fact, there is a huge body of research on this idea. Through research, experts have been able to identity findings and figures that can help to predict the level of nutrition risk. Other indicators might be based on diagnosis, usual food intake, or laboratory data.

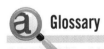 **Glossary**

Nutrition Care Process
Four steps to provide a standardized care process: Nutrition Assessment, Nutrition Diagnosis, Nutrition Intervention, Nutrition Monitoring and Evaluation

Nutrition Screening
A component of Nutrition Assessment meant to identify potential nutrition problems

Indicators
Pieces of information, such as weight measurement, that might suggest a concern or risk

If we determine that some of the indicators for risk are present, what happens next? There are several approaches to determining the level of risk based on indicators. One method is simply to count the risk factors. A screening policy may specify: *If three or more indicators of nutrition risk are present, this patient will be flagged for a complete nutrition assessment.*

In another scheme, each risk factor receives a point value. Factors judged to increase nutrition risk receive more points. In a nutrition risk scoring system, each risk indicator has a point value, and the total point value identifies the level of nutrition risk. Some systems even define risk levels based on the score. One system may have two levels of risk, such as: moderate risk and high risk. Another may have three levels, or even five.

Figure 9.1 (Mini-Nutritional Assessment MNA®) provides a nutrition screening and assessment tool from Nestle Clinical Nutrition. Note that this example uses a scoring system. In some tools, more points equal greater risk. In the Nestle example, fewer points mean greater risk. Whether to use high scores or low scores for expressing a risk is not important. However, it is important to understand any tool you happen to be applying in your place of employment, and to use and interpret it accurately.

Even a nutrition risk scoring system may incorporate certain overrides or automatic flags. Let's say you work with a system that specifies 20 points or higher as indicating risk. The system might also say that any individual who has been diagnosed with a pressure ulcer is automatically classified as being at nutrition risk. Even a resident who scores only 16 on the nutrition risk score would be "flagged" for nutrition assessment based on the presence of a pressure ulcer. Overrides or automatic flags can be helpful to be certain that individuals who might benefit from medical nutrition therapy receive appropriate assessment.

Also, note that the example in Figure 9.1 combines screening and assessment into one document. This can be a simple method of keeping important information together. A nutrition screening result usually becomes part of a permanent medical record. Screening information is thus available to other caregivers. For example, a Certified Dietary Manager may complete a nutrition screening and place it into the formal record. In follow-up, a Registered Dietitian may gather and evaluate more information to develop a nutrition assessment.

Nutrition Screening Indicators

There are many factors that may suggest nutrition risk. By no means is it necessary to use all possible criteria to identify risk. Criteria used in screening are usually representative of a cluster of related findings. In other words, a key indicator used for nutrition screening may represent the tip of an iceberg. If this factor exists, we consider it likely that other risk factors exist along with it. Indicators used in screening (and in nutrition assessment) fall into four basic categories. It may be helpful if you remember it as A-B-C-D.

✓ **A**nthropometric measurements

✓ **B**iochemical tests

✓ **C**linical information

✓ **D**iet history

Conduct Routine Nutrition Screening

| Figure 9.1 | Mini Nutritional Assessment MNA® |

Nestlé Nutrition Institute

Mini Nutritional Assessment
MNA®

Last name: _____ First name: _____

Sex: _____ Age: _____ Weight, kg: _____ Height, cm: _____ Date: _____

Complete the screen by filling in the boxes with the appropriate numbers. Total the numbers for the final screening score.

Screening

A Has food intake declined over the past 3 months due to loss of appetite, digestive problems, chewing or swallowing difficulties?
0 = severe decrease in food intake
1 = moderate decrease in food intake
2 = no decrease in food intake ☐

B Weight loss during the last 3 months
0 = weight loss greater than 3 kg (6.6 lbs)
1 = does not know
2 = weight loss between 1 and 3 kg (2.2 and 6.6 lbs)
3 = no weight loss ☐

C Mobility
0 = bed or chair bound
1 = able to get out of bed / chair but does not go out
2 = goes out ☐

D Has suffered psychological stress or acute disease in the past 3 months?
0 = yes   2 = no ☐

E Neuropsychological problems
0 = severe dementia or depression
1 = mild dementia
2 = no psychological problems ☐

F1 Body Mass Index (BMI) (weight in kg) / (height in m^2)
0 = BMI less than 19
1 = BMI 19 to less than 21
2 = BMI 21 to less than 23
3 = BMI 23 or greater ☐

IF BMI IS NOT AVAILABLE, REPLACE QUESTION F1 WITH QUESTION F2.
DO NOT ANSWER QUESTION F2 IF QUESTION F1 IS ALREADY COMPLETED.

F2 Calf circumference (CC) in cm
0 = CC less than 31
3 = CC 31 or greater ☐

Screening score
(max. 14 points) ☐☐

12-14 points:	Normal nutritional status
8-11 points:	At risk of malnutrition
0-7 points:	Malnourished

For a more in-depth assessment, complete the full MNA® which is available at **www.mna-elderly.com**

Ref.   Vellas B, Villars H, Abellan G, et al. *Overview of the MNA® - Its History and Challenges.* J Nutr Health Aging 2006;10:456-465.
Rubenstein LZ, Harker JO, Salva A, Guigoz Y, Vellas B. *Screening for Undernutrition in Geriatric Practice: Developing the Short-Form Mini Nutritional Assessment (MNA-SF).* J. Geront 2001;56A: M366-377.
Guigoz Y. *The Mini-Nutritional Assessment (MNA®) Review of the Literature - What does it tell us?* J Nutr Health Aging 2006; 10:466-487.
® Société des Produits Nestlé, S.A., Vevey, Switzerland, Trademark Owners
© Nestlé, 1994, Revision 2009. N67200 12/99 10M
For more information: www.mna-elderly.com

© Nestle 1994. Revision 2009. Reprinted with permission.

Clearly, there are many types of information that can suggest nutritional risk. A nutrition screening process will use only a few pieces of information as indicators or predictors. However, a nutrition assessment uses most or all of the relevant information available.

Nutritional status is a person's state of nutritional health. We focus the most attention on information that reflects overall nutritional status, or protein-calorie status. Basically, this is a measurement of status for the macronutrients. If a person is in negative energy balance and losing weight rapidly, we assume some protein has been lost from the body. Weight loss and protein loss are associated with negative health outcomes. If we examine whether a person is in a deficiency state for iron, we are looking at iron status. Nutritional status can describe any nutrient or groups of nutrients. Most screening focuses on calories and protein in the body. In some environments, a Certified Dietary Manager may assist in screening, and/or in gathering some of the nutrition-related information. Here is a closer look at the information involved:

Anthropometric Measurements. Anthropometric measurements are measurements of the human body and should be where nutrition screening begins. The most common examples are height and weight. These two figures are actually very useful, provided that accurate measurements are made. Adults should be weighed on a beam balance scale that is calibrated regularly to ensure accuracy. The best time to weigh a client is in the morning before breakfast and after the bladder has been emptied. For consistency, clients should always be weighed at the same time of day, and on the same scale, wearing the same amount of clothing. This makes comparisons of weight from one date to another most meaningful. There are specialized scales available for clients who are unable to stand. Even when weights are taken correctly, factors such as fluid retention, adaptive equipment on wheelchairs, and wedges or pillows may adversely affect a weight reading. It is important to obtain a weight upon admission and regularly thereafter. Do not simply rely on a weight recorded at a different facility.

An accurate measurement of height is also important. Relying upon the client's self-reported height or a visual estimate is not adequate. Whenever possible, height should be measured with the client standing straight against a measuring tape or stick on a vertical wall or instrument. If this is not possible, using a tape measure to check height from feet to head is an option. Another alternative is to measure the distance from the fingertip to the midpoint of the chest, and then double that number. Usually, this gives a reasonable estimate of actual height. However, it is not highly accurate.

There are many guidelines and standards that may be used for evaluating body weight. Standards are generally based on height. In general, a good standard also accounts for differences between males and females, as well as differences in body frame size. For example, a person with a small frame (small bones) should ideally weigh less than a person of the same height who has a larger frame size. Weight alone doesn't tell all, however. Another consideration is what that weight consists of. A person who exercises regularly, and in

Glossary

Ideal Body Weight (IBW)
An estimate of what would be a healthy weight for an individual according to a standard

Actual Weight
An individual's current weight

Percent of IBW
A comparison of the actual weight to the ideal body weight

Frame Size
Calculated from the ratio of height to wrist circumference

particular, someone who does strength training, may accumulate a great deal of muscle mass. This may translate into a high body weight, but it may be a healthy condition. Some experts use various methods to evaluate percent body fat.

Using weight and height, we can determine ideal body weight. **Ideal body weight (IBW)** is an estimate of what would be a healthy weight for an individual. It is based on height, sex, and frame size. You may check reference tables to determine ideal body weight, or use a simple formula (Figure 9.2) to calculate IBW. A common formula used today was created by Dr. GJ Hamwi. Here is an example for a 5-foot, 11-inch male with a large frame:

106 pounds + (11 x 6) = 172 pounds

172 pounds x 0.10 = 17 pounds

172 pounds + 17 pounds = 189 pounds IBW

Figure 9.2   Hamwi Formula to Calculate Ideal Body Weight (IBW)

Woman

IBW = 100 lbs for first 5 feet in height + 5 lbs for each inch over 5 feet.

Men

IBW = 106 lbs for first 5 feet + 6 lbs for each inch over 5 feet.

Frame Adjustments (Men and Women)

For a small frame, subtract 10% of the total

For a large frame, add 10% to the total

For heights less than 60", subtract 2.5 lbs for each inch below 60".

Did you notice in the Hamwi formula for ideal body weight an adjustment for frame size? **Frame size** refers to the thickness of bones, or underlying body build and height. To determine your own frame size, there is a quick and simple measurement. Wrap your hand around your dominant wrist (if you are right handed, wrap your left hand around your right wrist), closing your middle finger and thumb together around the smallest part of the wrist. Then use this gauge:

✓ If your thumb and finger overlap, you have a small frame size.

✓ If your thumb and finger meet, you have a medium frame size.

✓ If your thumb and finger do not meet, you have a large frame size.

There are more exact measurements of frame size that can be done with a tape measure (see Figure 9.3). It is important is to adjust for a person's frame size as your determine ideal body weight.

Once we know a person's ideal body weight, we can compare this with actual weight. **Actual weight** is what a person weighs right now. When we compare the two figures, we examine percent of IBW. **Percent of IBW** describes how closely a person's actual weight resembles the ideal. Figure 9.4 shows how to calculate percent of IBW. Figure 9.5 shows how to calculate percent of weight change.

Figure 9.3   Determining Frame Size

Frame Size from Height-Wrist Circumference Ratios (r)[a]

Frame Size	Male r Values	Female r Values
Small	>10.4	>11.0
Medium	9.6-10.4	10.1-11.0
Large	<9.6	<10.1

[a] $r = \dfrac{\text{height (cm)}}{\text{wrist circumference (cm)}}$

The wrist is measured where it bends (distal to the st[...]loid process) on the right arm (see illustration)

[a.] *For the most accurate measurement, measure elbow breadth with a caliper.*

Place tape here

Styloid process ("wristbone")

How to Determine Body Frame by Elbow Breadth

To make a simple approximation of frame size, do the following: Extend the arm, and bend the forearm upward at a 90° angle. Keep the fingers straight, and turn the inside of the wrist away from the body. Place the thumb and index finger on the two prominent bones on either side of the elbow. Measure the space between the fingers against a ruler or a tape measure.[a] Compare the measurements with the following standards. These standards represent the elbow measurements for medium-framed men and women of various heights. Measurements smaller than those listed include a small frame, and larger measurements include a large frame.

Men		Women	
Height in 1-Inch Heels	Elbow Breadth	Height in 1-Inch Heels	Elbow Breadth
5 ft. 2 in. to 5 ft. 3 in.	2-1/2 to 2-7/8 in.	4 ft. 10 in. to 4 ft. 11 in.	2-1/4 to 2-1/2 in.
5 ft. 4 in. to 5 ft. 7 in.	2-5/8 to 2-7/8 in.	5 ft. 0 in. to 5 ft. 3 in.	2-1/4 to 2-1/2 in.
5 ft. 8 in. to 5 ft. 11 in.	2-3/4 to 3 in.	5 ft 4 in to 5 ft. 7 in.	2-3/8 to 2-5/8 in.
6 ft. 0 in. to 6 ft. 3 in.	2-3/4 to 3-1/8 in.	5 ft. 8 in. to 5 ft. 11 in.	2-3/8 to 2-5/8 in.
6 ft. 4 in. and over	2-7/8 to 3-1/4 in.	6 ft 0 in. and over	2-1/2 to 2-3/4 in.

Source: Metropolitan Life Insurance Company

Figure 9.4   How to Calculate Percent of IBW

Percent of IBW = (Actual Weight ÷ IBW) x 100

Figure 9.5   How to Calculate Percent of Weight Change

Percent weight change = [(Usual weight - Actual weight) ÷ usual weight] x 100

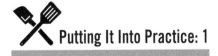 Putting It Into Practice: 1

Can you name the anthropometric measurements commonly used in nutrition screening?

(Check your answer at the end of the chapter)

Here are two examples of calculating percent of IBW:

1. Marla weighs 156 pounds. Her IBW is 115 pounds.
   Percent of IBW = (156 pounds ÷ 115 pounds) x 100
       = 1.36 x 100
       = 136
   Marla is at 136 percent of her IBW.

2. Jacob weighs 137 pounds. His IBW is 148 pounds.
   Percent of IBW = (137 pounds ÷ 148 pounds) x 100
       = 0.93 x 100
       = 93
   Jacob is at 93 percent of his IBW.

Note that in these examples, we are rounding calculations to the nearest whole number. IBW and related calculations are only estimates, so it is not necessary to extend decimal places. Roughly speaking, percent of ideal body weight gives an indication of whether a person is potentially undernourished or overweight. For example, one rule of thumb says that a person at or below 90 percent of IBW may be a nutritional risk. However, this measurement alone does not tell all. Imagine Jacob from the example above. Currently, he is below his IBW. To better understand his nutritional state, what we really need to know is what the recent trend has been. Jacob weighs 137 pounds right now. We have to wonder: Has he always been a thin man? If so, maybe there is not a concern here. On the other hand, what if Jacob weighed 159 pounds just six months ago and is now down to this weight? This should concern us greatly because it indicates a severe downward trend in his weight. We can guess his weight will continue to fall without intervention. This rapid weight loss may be due to health conditions such as cancer, dysphagia, or depression. Furthermore, if he is losing weight at a rapid clip, he may be losing some of his lean body mass. **Lean body mass** describes the weight of all parts of the body that are NOT fat, e.g. muscle, bones, and organs. If Jacob is losing lean body mass, his body systems may not be functioning at their best. He is likely at risk.

A final way to measure body mass is to examine the percentage of body weight that is fat. Obviously, as body fat percentage increases, so does the health risk. Figure 9.7 shows BMI classifications and desirable body fat percentage.

How can we determine what is really going on here? The answer is by calculating percent weight change. **Percent weight change** indicates by what proportion the body weight has changed over a certain period of time. Here is an example:

Jacob weighs 137 pounds now. He weighed 159 pounds six months ago.
Percent weight change = [(159 pounds - 137 pounds) ÷ usual weight] x 100
       = [22 ÷ usual weight] x 100
       = [22 ÷ 159] x 100
       = 0.14 x 100
       = 14 percent

Jacob has experienced a 14 percent weight change over six months. Another way to say this is: He has lost 14 percent of his body weight over the past six months.

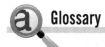
Glossary

Lean Body Mass
The weight of all parts of the body not counting the fat (e.g. muscle, bones, and organs)

Percent Weight Change
A proportion of current body weight to usual body weight or weight change over a certain period of time

Body Mass Index
A proportion of weight to height

Figure 9.6 Body Mass Index Table

To use the table, find the appropriate height in the left-hand column labeled Height. Move across to a given weight (in pounds). The number at the top of the column is the BMI at that height and weight.

	BMI																					
Height	19	20	21	22	23	24	25	26	27	28	29	30	31	32	33	34	35	36	37	38	39	40
58"	91	96	100	105	110	115	119	124	129	134	138	143	148	153	158	162	167	172	177	181	186	191
59"	94	99	104	109	114	119	124	128	133	138	143	148	153	158	163	168	173	178	183	188	193	198
60"	97	102	107	112	118	123	128	133	138	143	148	153	158	163	168	174	179	184	189	194	199	204
61"	100	106	111	116	122	127	132	137	143	148	153	158	164	169	174	180	185	190	195	201	206	211
62"	104	109	115	120	126	131	136	142	147	153	158	164	169	175	180	186	191	196	202	207	213	218
63"	107	113	118	124	130	135	141	146	152	158	163	169	175	180	186	191	197	203	208	214	220	225
64"	110	116	122	128	134	140	145	151	157	163	169	174	180	186	192	197	204	209	215	221	227	232
65"	114	120	126	132	138	144	150	156	162	168	174	180	186	192	198	204	210	216	222	228	234	240
66"	118	124	130	136	142	148	155	161	167	173	179	186	192	198	204	210	216	223	229	235	241	247
67"	121	127	134	140	146	153	159	166	172	178	185	191	198	204	211	217	223	230	236	242	249	255
68"	125	131	138	144	151	158	164	171	177	184	190	197	204	210	216	223	230	236	243	249	256	262
69"	128	135	142	149	155	162	169	176	182	189	196	203	210	216	223	230	236	243	250	257	263	270
70"	132	139	146	153	160	167	174	181	188	195	202	209	216	222	229	236	243	250	257	264	271	278
71"	136	143	150	157	165	172	179	186	193	200	208	215	222	229	236	243	250	257	265	272	279	286
72"	140	147	154	162	169	177	184	191	199	206	213	221	228	235	242	250	258	265	272	279	287	294
73"	144	151	159	166	174	182	189	197	204	212	219	227	235	242	250	257	265	272	280	288	295	302
74'	148	155	163	171	179	186	194	202	210	218	225	233	241	249	256	264	272	280	287	295	303	311
75"	152	160	168	176	184	192	200	208	216	224	232	240	248	256	264	272	279	287	295	303	311	319
76"	156	164	172	180	189	197	205	213	221	230	238	246	254	263	271	279	287	295	304	312	320	328

Source: National Institutes of Health

Figure 9.7 BMI Classifications and Desirable Body Fat Percentage

BMI Classification		Desirable Body Fat Percentage	
Risk Category	BMI Measurement	Men	Women
Underweight	BMI <18	13-25%	17-29%
Healthy Weight	BMI 20-25	12 grams	50 grams
Overweight	BMI 25-29.9		
Obese	BMI > 30		

To calculate percent weight change, it's important to find the most reliable weight information possible for past data. Sources may include a medical record, the report from the client, or a report from a family member. Unfortunately, it is not always possible to obtain highly reliable information about past weights. Also, there is no specific time frame for a percent weight loss calculation. As you learned in Chapter 8, the following percent weight changes indicate nutrition risk:

- ✓ a weight loss of 5 percent over the past one month,
- ✓ a weight loss of 7.5 percent over the past 90 days, or
- ✓ a weight loss of 10 percent over the past six months.

Another method for comparing weight with height to gauge overweight or underweight is the **body mass index (BMI)**. BMI is often used today as a measure of overweight and obesity. It is calculated from your height and weight. The National Heart, Lung, and Blood Institute describes BMI as "an estimate of body fat." The higher your BMI, the higher your risk for certain diseases such as heart disease, high blood pressure, Type 2 diabetes, gallstones, breathing problems, and certain cancers. Although BMI can be used for most men and women, it does have some limits:

- ✓ It may overestimate body fat in athletes and others who have a muscular build.
- ✓ It may underestimate body fat in older persons and others who have lost muscle.

Figure 9.6 shows a reference table for determining BMI. A final way to measure body mass is to examine the percentage of body weight that is fat. Obviously, as body fat percentage increases, so does the health risk. Figure 9.7 shows BMI classifications and desirable body fat percentage.

Body fat is most often measured by using special calipers to measure the skinfold thickness of the triceps and other parts of the body. Skinfold thickness is a measurement of the fleshy part of the body at a specified location. Because half of all body fat is under the skin, this method is quite accurate. Standards exist for comparing the measurements and using them to gauge not only percent body fat, but also overall nutritional status (protein and calorie nutrition). Other anthropometric measurements include mid-arm circumference and mid-arm muscle circumference.

Biochemical Tests. Biochemical tests, or laboratory tests, can be very helpful in assessing a client's nutritional status. Some typical standards for interpreting these test values appear in Figure 9.8. The normal values for each of these tests are determined by the facility. Following are some of the laboratory tests with nutritional significance:

Serum albumin. More than half of all the protein in the blood is albumin. Serum albumin is a good indicator of nutritional status, particularly protein status, but it takes time to change. Therefore, a client with a low serum albumin has been in poor nutritional status for some time. Serum albumin decreases in trauma, severe infection, or protein-calorie malnutrition. Serum albumin can also be affected by hydration.

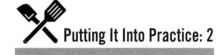

Putting It Into Practice: 2

Ava is 4'9" tall and has a small frame. What is her ideal body weight? Ava currently weighs 80 lbs. What is her percent of IBW?

(Check your answer at the end of the chapter)

Figure 9.8 Selected Laboratory Tests with Nutritional Significance

Serum Albumin (alb)

Normal Range*: 3.5-5.0 gm/dl (Centers for Medicaid Services uses 3.4 – 4.8 gm/dl for individuals over 60 years of age)

Significance: Can measure protein status; 3.0 – 3.4 may indicate mild protein depletion; 2.1 – 2.9 may indicate moderate protein depletion. May appear high due to dehydration, which concentrates the blood. Takes about 2-3 weeks to change in response to protein status.

Serum Prealbumin (PAB)

Normal Range*: 16-35 mg/dl

Significance: Can measure protein status; 11-15 mg/dl may indicate mild protein depletion; <10 mg/dl suggests significant protein depletion. PAB takes only a few days to change in response to protein status. With adequate nutrition support of a malnourished client, this value should rise approx. 2 mg/dl each day.

Serum Transferrin

Normal Range*: 180-380 gm/dl

Significance: Can measure protein status; takes about 10 days to change in response to protein status; may be elevated with iron-deficiency anemia.

Total Lymphocyte Count (TLC)

Normal Range*: 3,000-5,000 cells/mm

Significance: This is a count of lymphocyte cells in the immune system; can measure protein status; 1,500-1,800 may indicate mild protein depletion; 900-1,500 suggests moderate depletion. TLC may be high in infection.

Fasting Blood Sugar/Glucose (FBS or FBG)

Normal Range*: 80-120 mg/dl

Significance: Elevated FBS suggests diabetes or poor control of blood sugar for a person with diabetes. Slight elevations may occur with age. Note that random blood sugar (e.g. after a meal) may be higher (up to about 140 mg/dl). BS of approx. 300 mg/dl is dangerously high, leading to severe confusion and possible coma. Very low BS (< 60 mg/dl) is hypoglycemia and requires immediate treatment.

Glycosylated Hemoglobin (HbA1c)

Normal Range*: < 5%

Significance: This value indicates control of blood sugar over a recent period of several months. It is valuable in evaluating ongoing blood sugar control for a person with diabetes. A low figure indicates good control. A high figure (e.g. > 7%) suggests blood sugar may have been consistently or frequently high.

Hemoglobin (Hgb or Hb)

Normal Range*: 12-15 g/dl (adult female); 14 - 17 g/dl (adult male)

Significance: Low Hgb with low HCT together often indicate anemia due to inadequate iron, folate, vitamin B6, vitamin B12, or other nutrients in the body. It is also low following blood loss, e.g. from internal bleeding, trauma, or surgery, and during cancer. Slightly low levels may occur with aging.

Hematocrit (HCT)

Normal Range*: 36 - 46% (adult female); 41 - 53% (adult male)

Significance: Measures number and size of red blood cells; low Hgb with low HCT together often indicate iron-deficiency anemia; may be high (or appear normal) in dehydration.

Serum Cholesterol (chol)

Normal Range*: < 200 mg/dl

Significance: High levels represent risk of cardiovascular disease

High Density Lipoprotein (HDL) Cholesterol

Normal Range*: 40 – 60 mg/dl +

Significance: "Good" cholesterol; < 40 mg/dl represents risk of cardiovascular disease; high levels are desirable (see Chapter 6)

Low Density Lipoprotein (LDL) Cholesterol

Normal Range*: < 100 mg/dl optimal; 100 – 129 mg/dl near optimal

Significance: "Bad" cholesterol; elevated levels represent risk of cardiovascular disease (see Chapter 6)

Serum Triglyceride (TG)

Normal Range*: < 150 mg/dl

Significance: High levels may mildly increase risk for cardiovascular disease; very high levels may suggest a blood lipid disorder; can lead to fatty deposits in the body (e.g. in liver); can also suggest uncontrolled diabetes

Serum potassium (K)

Normal Range*: 3.5 – 5.0 mEq/l

Significance: Becomes elevated during renal failure and other conditions; may become low with medications (e.g. potassium-wasting diuretics) or diarrhea; elevated or very low levels can become life-threatening; important to monitor for a client placed on either a high or low potassium diet

Blood Urea Nitrogen (BUN)

Normal Range*: 8-20 mg/dl

Significance: An important measure of renal function; high levels may indicate renal failure, dehydration, or other medical conditions

* Note that standards for normal ranges are set by institution and may vary slightly. Also note that many clinical factors, such as fluid retention, dehydration, medication regimens, diseases of major organs, and many others can affect laboratory value readings. Thus, it is important to review the entire clinical picture, and consult with other members of the healthcare team in interpreting laboratory values.

Sources: National Institutes of Health, Centers for Medicare & Medicaid Services (CMS), American Family Physician

Figure 9.9   Nutrition-Related Clinical Information

Medical Factors

- Cancer
- Diabetes
- Heart and circulatory disease
- High blood pressure
- Kidney disease
- History of alcohol use and/or abuse

- GERD
- H/O Depression
- Liver disease
- Lung disease
- Illness with increased metabolic needs: burns, infection, trauma, protracted fever

- Malabsorption syndromes
- Surgery of gastro-intestinal tract
- Overweight
- Underweight
- Recent unplanned weight loss
- Certain medications

- Chemotherapy/radiation therapy
- Pressure ulcers
- Chewing/swallowing problems
- Inadequate fluid intake
- Declining cognition

Social Factors

- Living and eating alone
- Not enough money for food

- Inadequate facilities for storing and preparing food

- Problems shopping for food

- Declining mobility

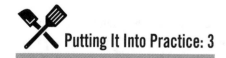

Putting It Into Practice: 3

Steven weighs 240 lbs. and is 6'2" tall. How would he be classified based on his BMI? He weighed 210 lbs. when he was admitted. What is his percent weight change?

(Check your answer at the end of the chapter)

Serum transferrin. Like albumin, transferrin is a protein found in the blood. Transferrin carries iron to where red blood cells are made. Serum transferrin levels are considered a more sensitive indicator of protein deficiency than albumin because transferrin levels change more quickly in response to changes in nutritional status.

Serum prealbumin. This is a protein made by the liver and is considered one of the most sensitive and reliable indicators of protein status. Unlike serum albumin, it is not affected by hydration. It is a good measure for effectiveness of nutrition support, because it will begin to change within approximately four days. Even though it is produced by the liver, prealbumin is not affected by most forms of liver disease.

Total lymphocyte count (TLC). Lymphocytes are white blood cells involved in fighting infection. In the case of protein deficiency, the total number of lymphocytes decreases. Certain drugs also decrease total lymphocyte count.

Hematocrit and hemoglobin. Hematocrit is the percent of red blood cells found in blood. Hemoglobin is the oxygen-carrying pigment of the red blood cells. A low hemoglobin level may indicate iron-deficiency anemia.

Clinical Information. Some of the clinical information that can have a bearing on nutrition screening and assessment is available in the medical record. Certain diagnoses or conditions, for example, may indicate a need for nutritional evaluation. We've already reviewed the idea that pressure ulcers are one of these conditions. A client whose symptoms include ongoing diarrhea and/or fever would be another. A client on a tube feeding would be yet another example. Figure 9.9 lists medical and social factors that may affect nutritional status.

Yet another type of clinical information that is important in understanding the nutritional picture for any client is medications. The effects foods and drugs have on each other can determine whether medications do their jobs and

Figure 9.10 Medications with Possible Nutrition-Related Effects

Drug	Possible Effects
Analgesic (Pain Killer)	
Aspirin	Gastric pain or bleeding, nausea and vomiting
Acetaminophen	Gastrointestinal disturbance, liver toxicity
Antibiotic	
Amoxicillin	Diarrhea, nausea and vomiting
Ampicillin	Diarrhea, glossitis (inflammation of the the tongue), stomatitis (mouth ulcers), nausea and vomiting
Cephalexin	Abdominal pain, diarrhea, nausea and vomiting
Erythromycin	Abdominal cramping, diarrhea, nausea and vomiting
Penicillin	Diarrhea, glossitis, stomatitis, nausea and vomiting
Tetracycline	Anorexia, diarrhea, dysphagia, glossitis, nausea and vomiting, decreases vitamin K synthesis
Antipsychotics/Antidepressants	
Nearly all affect appetite and/or weight change	
High Blood Pressure	
Atenolol	Diarrhea, nausea
Propranolol	Abdominal cramping, constipation, diarrhea, nausea and vomiting, decreased carbohydrate tolerance
Bronchodilator	
Theophylline	Anorexia, gastric irritation, nausea, vomiting
Diuretic	
Chlorthalidone	Anorexia, constipation, cramping, diarrhea, gastric irritation, electrolyte imbalance
Furosemide	Abdominal cramping; anorexia; constipation; diarrhea; dry mouth; thirst; fluid and electrolyte imbalance; nausea and vomiting; decreased blood potassium, magnesium, sodium; increased urinary potassium, magnesium, sodium
Hydrochlorothiazide	Anorexia, constipation, diarrhea, gastrointestinal irritation and ulceration, nausea and vomiting
Estrogen Replacement Therapy	
Estrogens	Abdominal cramping, bloating, edema, nausea and vomiting, carbohydrate intolerance
Ulcer	
Cimetidine	Bitter taste, constipation, decreased absorption of calcium and iron
Non-Steroidal Anti-inflammatory	
Ibuprofen	Abdominal cramping, constipation, diarrhea, edema, flatulence, gastrointestinal bleeding and ulceration, heartburn, nausea and vomiting
Naproxen	Abdominal pain, constipation, diarrhea, gastrointestinal bleeding and ulceration, heartburn, nausea and vomiting, stomatitis
Steroidal Anti-inflammatory	
Prednisone	Abdominal distention, fluid and electrolyte imbalance, fluid and sodium retention, indigestion, nausea and vomiting, negative nitrogen balance, peptic ulcer, decreased carbohydrate tolerance, less vitamin D activity, increased appetite, increased weight

Source: US Public Health Service

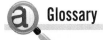 **Glossary**

Food Record
A diary of food and beverages consumed, usually for a given number of days

Food Frequency Questionnaire
A checklist or questionnaire that tracks how often a client eats each of a variety of foods

Calorie Count
Calculation of actual amount consumed from a food record a 24-hour time period

I/O (In and Out) Record
A document of all fluids consumed and excreted over a 24-hour time period

Meal Observation
A tool that helps to identify individuals who are having eating problems such as swallowing, chewing, or self-feeding

Nutrition Assessment
A comprehensive approach by a Registered Dietitian using multiple data sources to determine nutritional status

Basal Energy Expenditure (BEE)
The energy (calories) needed to maintain basic bodily functions such as breathing, brain function, and keeping the heart beating

Caloric Needs Estimate
An estimate of the total amount of calories needed (e.g. for one day) and includes the BEE plus the activity factory and, if needed, an injury factor (Activity Kcal: sedentary, moderate/strenuous)

Figure 9.11 Sample Food-Drug Interactions

Drug	Purpose of the Drug	System Affected	Possible Nutrient Drug Interaction	Nutrition Side Effects
Fosomax®	Antisteoporosis	Decreases Absorption	Absorption: 60% if taken with coffee or juice. No absorption **at all** if taken with food.	
Ciprofloxacin®	Antibiotic	Decreases Absorption	Decreases if taken with dairy products	Consumption of dairy products may be affected
Cefuroxime®	Antibiotic	Increases Absorption	Increases with food intake	
Diflucan®	Antifungal	Decreases Absorption	Decreases if taken with dairy	
Mthotrexate®	Cancer	Decreases Absorption	Reduces folate absorption	Causes folate deficiency
Progesterone®		Increases Absorption	Requires dairy products to work	Complications for those who are lactose intolerant
Tetracycline®	Antibiotic	Decreases Absorption	With the intake of dairy products and iron supplements	Complications occur if iron supplements are eliminated; can cause diarrhea, nausea, and vomiting
Altenolol®	Lowers Blood Pressure	Decreases Absorption	Orange juice decreases absorption	Can cause diarrhea and nausea; may require a low-salt diet
Coumadin®	Prevents Blood Clots	Decreases Metabolism	Keep intake of vitamin K from food consistant	
Nardil®, Parnate® (MAO Inhibitor)	Depression	Decreases Metabolism	Avoid foods high in tryamine	Can raise blood pressure to dangerous levels
Lasix®, Furosemide®	Diuretic	Increases Excretion	Increases excretion of potassium, sodium, chloride, calcium and magnesium	May cause an electrolyte deficiency
Digoxin®	Cardiovascular	Increases Appetite		May cause weight loss
Motrin®, Colchicine®, Dulcolax®, Metamucil®, Levothyroxine®	Pain reliever, Gout, Bowel, Medications, Thyroid	Decreases Appetite		May cause weight loss

Note: These are only a small number of the vast amount of medications. Use the Physician's Desk Reference to check other medications or Food and Medications Interactions by Pronsky.

whether the body gets the nutrients it needs. Medications can interfere with the way the body digests, absorbs, or uses a nutrient. A medication that causes taste changes or gastrointestinal discomfort may reduce a person's food intake over time. This may cause weight loss and/or loss of nutritional well-being. Conversely, dietary factors can affect how medicines function in the body. This interchange can be mild or life-threatening. It depends on the medication and many other factors. Figure 9.10 lists some commonly used drugs that may have nutrition-related effects. Figure 9.11 provides sample food/drug interactions.

Diet History. Diet history is the final part of nutrition screening. A diet history may include one or more tools designed to develop a snapshot of a client's eating habits. Chapter 8 described one tool; we'll review a few others in this chapter.

A Registered Dietitian may request a food record, which is a diary of food and beverages consumed. A common **food record** is kept for any number of days. A meaningful food record must include all condiments and additions to foods—such as mayonnaise used on a sandwich, or margarine and jelly spread on toast. Also, measurements of foods consumed are important. If a client has to tell how many ounces of roast beef he consumed, for example, this can be challenging. Sometimes, it helps to go over measurements and reporting with a client before the record begins. Food models (pieces of plastic molded to look like real foods) are useful for explaining portion sizes. The food record is then reviewed with the client to be sure all foods are listed and all portion sizes and preparation methods are accurate. Figure 9.12 shows a sample food record form.

Another tool is a **food frequency questionnaire**. This is a checklist that identifies how often a client eats each of a variety of foods. This provides information about eating habits and preferences that may not show up on a brief food record. Today there are many programs on the web to enter food frequency information such as myPyramid Tracker at myPyramid.gov.

In addition to diet histories, the Registered Dietitian/Certified Dietary Manager or nursing staff can record what the client eats and drinks for three days and then do a nutrient analysis to quantify intake of calories, protein, and/or other nutrients. This is called a **calorie count**, or *nutrient intake analysis*. Observing and/or recording actual intake as in a food record is extremely important for understanding a client's nutritional needs. Industry research shows that about 75 percent of nursing home residents eat less than three-quarters of their food, which can have a tremendous impact on health.

Now, remember that water is a nutrient and that dehydration is a major risk among older Americans. Thus, monitoring fluid intake is important, too. Nursing staff and other team members may monitor fluid intake for certain patients. From a clinical perspective, they may also want to know more about how kidneys or other body organs are functioning. Thus, a typical review of fluid becomes an I/O record. An **I/O (in and out) record** is a document of all fluids consumed and excreted over a 24-hour time period.

In a healthcare setting, nursing, foodservice, and other caregivers also review a resident's ability to eat and feed himself. **Meal observation** is a key assessment tool that helps to identify individuals who are having problems with appetite,

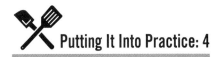

Putting It Into Practice: 4

You have just conducted a nutrition screening on Roberta. This is the information you have so far: She weighs 147 lbs, is 5'3" in height with a small frame; her BMI is 26; she is 85 years old; her serum albumin is 2.1; she has pancreatic cancer; she has no family in the area; she usually eats one main meal a day at the Senior Center, otherwise she just snacks. Can you identify each part of the nutrition screen?

(Check your answer at the end of the chapter)

chewing, swallowing, alertness, self-feeding, or many other factors that may influence nutritional well-being. Based on observations, members of the team may begin to form strategies for helping a client eat well and enjoy meals.

Finally, a nutrition assessment includes a broader background on lifestyle and social factors that may influence nutrition. Any of the factors described in Chapter 1—such as cultural influences, religious beliefs, attitudes, and more—may be relevant in a diet history. For example, a person's ability to shop for and prepare food at home is very important. Awareness of support systems and knowing who is responsible for meals sets groundwork for nutrition education that may be needed later in the nutrition care process. Developing a solid

Figure 9.12   Food/Beverage Intake Record

- Record all foods and beverages you consume. Include meals, snacks, juices, supplements, condiments, sugar, butter, and jelly.
- Describe the amount eaten (ml, oz, cup, etc.) and include careful measurements.

Your Name: _____   Date: _____

Meal	Food or Beverage	Amount (oz, tsp, cups)	Where Eaten
Breakfast			
Lunch			
Supper			
Snack			
Snack			

Figure 9.13 **Clinical Responsibility Assignments**   *Source: Carolina Nutrition Consultants, Inc. Revised August 2008*

Responsibility	Dietary Manager	Registered Dietitian
Food Preferences	X	
Nutrition Screen	X	
Estimation of Nutritional Needs		X
Enteral Initial Assessment		X
Enteral Follow-up, Changes		X
Family Request (refer to Registered Dietitian as appropriate)	X	
Wound Assessment		X
Wound Follow-up		X
Weight Change Progress Note	X	
Weight Change Assessment & Recommendations		X
Nutrition Recommendations for Interventions		X
Progress Note to Document Communication with Family or Resident	X	
*MDS Section K	X	
*Raps	X	
*Nutrition Care Plan	X	
Initial, Annual, Significant Change, Re-Admit, Quarterly Assessment		X
Diet Consult & Diet Instruction		X

* *High risk nutrition issues (TF new or changes, wounds, significant weight changes, dehydration; dx of malnutrition, FTT, anorexia, cachexia must be referred to the Registered Dietitian within 72 hours.*

diet history usually involves gathering information directly from the medical record, from other caregivers in a healthcare facility, from the client, and sometimes from family or significant others. The ability to gather accurate information depends on interpersonal rapport and solid communication skills. Talking with others to gather information requires interviewing skills. Upon completion of a nutrition assessment, a caregiver lists all nutrition problems identified, and then recommends a plan for addressing each problem.

Nutrition Assessment

Once the nutrition screening is completed, the next step is dependent upon the results of the screening. If the nutrition screening suggests a concern such as overweight, high blood sugar, cancer, etc., then an in-depth evaluation of a client's nutritional well-being will need to be done. This is called a **nutrition assessment**. The Registered Dietitian uses a comprehensive approach to determine nutritional status and will need the screening information you provide. The Registered Dietitian uses interviews, laboratory data, clinical information, body measurements, information gathered from healthcare team members, and other tools to develop an assessment. The Certified Dietary Manager and the Registered Dietitian work as a team and the determination of specific duties should be made as a team and stated in the facility policy and procedure manual. Figure 9.13 shows a sample of how clinical duties can be delineated. In some facilities, other members of the healthcare team may help to gather information for the nutrition assessment. It is typically the responsibility of

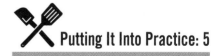 **Putting It Into Practice: 5**

You recently admitted a male client who is just recovering from surgery. His height is 67" and his weight is 135 lbs. What is his daily protein and fluid requirement?

(Check your answer at the end of the chapter)

the Registered Dietitian to make a final evaluation of the complete set of information. The nutrition assessment forms a basis for determining a nutrition diagnosis and developing a personalized nutrition care plan. Chapter 14 and 15 address nutrition care planning and explain some of the follow-up required to assure effectiveness of a nutrition care plan.

BEE and Nutrient Needs

Another aspect of nutritional assessment is an estimation of nutrient needs. Some assessments involve comparing these estimations with actual intake, in order to evaluate whether a client is able to nourish himself adequately. Estimating nutrient needs also forms a foundation for planning individual menus and meals, as well as for planning tube feedings and parenteral nutrition regimens. Most often, the estimation of nutrient needs will be the responsibility of a Registered Dietitian. However, here is some background that helps to demystify these seemingly magic numbers.

BEE. Basal metabolism is a term that describes how much energy the body needs when it is completely at rest. **Basal energy expenditure (BEE)** is the energy (calories) needed to maintain functions such as breathing, maintaining

Figure 9.14 Formulas for Calculating BEE for Clients Over the Age of 18

Men

Harris-Benedict Equation:
BEE = 66 + (13.7 x weight in kg) + (5 x height in cm) - (6.8 x age in years)
Alternate Formula: BEE = 1.0 x (weight in kg) x 24

Women

Harris-Benedict Equation:
BEE = 655 + (9.6 x weight in kg) + (1.8 x height in cm) - (4.7 x age in years)
Alternate Formula: BEE = 0.9 x (weight in kg) x 24

Notes: *To convert pounds to kilograms, divide by 2.2 (2.2ib = 1kg). To convert inches to centimeters, multiply by 2.54 (1in = 2.54cm).*

There are height-weight percentile tables for clients under age 18.

Figure 9.15 Caloric Needs Estimate for Clients Over the Age of 18

Activity Factors (Add These to the BEE)	Injury Factors (Also add these to the BEE)
0.2 x BEE for a paitent who is in bed most of the time	0.2 x BEE following surgery
0.3 x BEE for an individual who is ambulatory and/or moderately active	0.35 x BEE following skeletal trauma (bone fractures)
0.5 x BEE for an individual who is very active	0.1 - 0.4 x BEE following other trauma
	0.1 x BEE for each degree (F) of fever
	2.1 x BEE for severe burn

For Protein-calorie malnutrition

Add an amount for weight gain/growth. This might be 500-1,000 calories per day.

To achieve weight loss (for an overweight individual)

Subtract 500-1,000 calories per day to promote a loss of 1-2 lbs./week.

Figure 9.16 Estimating Daily Protein Needs

- For a healthy adult: 0.8 grams x body weight in kg

- For a malnourished client: 1.2-1.5 grams x body weight in kg

- Following surgery: 1.0-2.0 grams x body weight in kg

- Following trauma, severe burn, or multiple fractures: 2.0 grams x body weight in kg

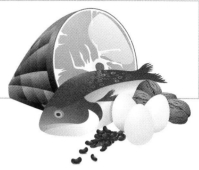

Figure 9.17 Estimating Daily Fluid Needs

Formula	What Disease Factors <u>Increase</u> Fluid Requirements	What Disease Factors <u>Decrease</u> Fluid Requirements
For Average Adults 30 mL/kg For Adults with Infection or Draining Wounds: 35 mL/kg For Adults with CHF or Renal Disease: 25 mL/kg	Fever Draining wounds Diarrhea Vomiting Hyperventilation Respirator Excessive perspiration Pressure ulcer (states II, III, IV)	Congestive Heart Failure (CHF) Cardiac disease Renal disease Edema or Ascites

Indicators of Dehydration

- Client consumes less than 1500 ml of fluids daily (review chart in Chapter 2 for food sources of water)

- Client has clinical signs of dehydration

- Client loses more fluids through vomiting, fever, diarrhea than he/she consumes

brain function, and keeping the heart beating or body functions at rest. It is usually expressed as calories per day. There are many formulas for calculating BEE, which differs between men and women and varies according to age. Figure 9.14 shows a sample set of formulas for adults. BEE calculations may also be automated through use of computer software. These calculations are based on weight in kilograms (kg). To convert pounds to kilograms, divide by 2.2. See Appendix H for a chart to convert pounds to kilograms. BEE accounts for only about two-thirds of calories in an average person's daily needs. Above and beyond the total resting state, the body needs more calories for digesting food, for moving and exercising, for growing or healing, and more. When a fever is present, the body uses a tremendous amount of energy to produce the fever. A fever is heat, and heat is energy. A **caloric needs estimate** is an estimate that accounts for the total amount of calories needed, e.g. for one day. It is built on the BEE, but includes additional factors to account for other energy needs. As with BEE, there are many models and formulas for calculating this. Figure 9.15 identifies some guidelines. Note that these guidelines are for adults only and are quite general. Furthermore, an estimate is only an estimate. In practice, any nutritional plan must be monitored. Follow-up assessment always includes weight monitoring, and adjustments to an initial plan are common.

Other common clinical nutrition calculations include an estimation of protein needs (Figure 9.16) and an estimation of fluid needs (Figure 9.17) For additional nutrient needs estimates, the RDIs described in Appendix B provide guidance for healthy people. Many medical conditions can alter the needs for calories, protein, fluids, and other nutrients. For fluids, it is particularly important to be aware of a physician's order. Fluid restrictions are common among healthcare clients.

Sources for Nutrition Screening Tools

As you have already noticed, many sources and standards exist for nutrition screening. Tools vary from one facility to another. If you join the staff of a healthcare facility, you will most likely find that there is a tool in place. Your job, then, will be to become familiar with the tool and to apply it. Often, a Registered Dietitian or Clinical Nutrition Manager will help to locate and/or develop a screening tool. Some facilities develop nutrition screening tools in-house, drawing on the expertise of Registered Dietitians and healthcare team members. On the other hand, a screening tool may come from professional organizations, such as The Academy of Nutrition and Dietetics (AND) [formerly known as The American Dietetic Association (ADA)]or other dietetics group. It may come from researchers or educational institutions. It may come from a provider of products to support medical nutrition therapy. Nutrition screening standards and forms are sometimes components of diet manuals. Finally, nutrition screening may be built into a clinical nutrition management software package. Software-based systems may have default screening criteria and scoring values built-in. Typically, however, a Registered Dietitian can select indicators and thresholds in the software in order to customize scoring to institutional policies and procedures. Another advantage of using software support in the screening process is that most programs can then generate a report or list for follow-up assessment. If a priority system is used (e.g. Level 1 Risk, Level 2 Risk, etc.), software may sort the list by priority level. Software also automates the calculations involved in nutrition screening.

Regardless of the choice of tools, an effective nutrition screening process:

✓ Uses meaningful screening criteria, as identified by a qualified individual (e.g. Registered Dietitian)

✓ Sets meaningful thresholds that correspond to known risks

✓ Is applied to every client

✓ Is implemented quickly upon admission

✓ Is implemented uniformly and consistently

The screening process is implemented uniformly and consistently through the use of standardized forms, such as the examples in Figure 9.1. Using a form ensures that as you screen, you review the same key indicators among all clients, without overlooking any piece of the screening standard. It's like a shopping list; it ensures you won't forget anything! A software program accomplishes the same objective, but through an electronic process. By following a methodical process for nutrition screening, you can be reasonably confident that you are finding the clients whose personal health may benefit from medical nutrition therapy. You can ensure that each of these clients receives a nutrition assessment.

Furthermore, nutrition screening is generally dictated by relevant healthcare regulations, both federal and state. Guidelines from the Joint Commission on Accreditation of Healthcare Organizations (JCAHO) also apply to most healthcare facilities. Standards may require that nutrition screening be conducted within a given timeframe after admission and again at prescribed intervals. Based on regulations, the role of a Certified Dietary Manager in screening may vary from one facility to another. Likewise, the method of documenting screening activities may also vary. Thus, it is imperative to become familiar with all relevant regulations and standards at any place of employment, and to follow them. Each healthcare facility needs to develop a policy and procedure for nutrition screening that achieves the objective of identifying clients at risk and stipulates a mechanism for assuring regulatory compliance and documentation.

END OF CHAPTER

 Putting It Into Practice Questions & Answers

1. Can you name the anthropometric measurements commonly used in nutrition screening?

    A. *Remember anthropometric measurements are measurements of the body. Typical anthropometric measurements are height, weight, wrist measurements, and body fat measurements using calipers.*

2. Ava is 4'9" tall and has a small frame. What is her ideal body weight? Ava currently weighs 80 lbs. What is her percent of IBW?

    A. *4'9" = 57" (4x12" in a foot + 9"); To determine IBW for heights less than 60" or 5', subtract 2.5 lbs for each inch below 60". 60"-57" = 3"; 2.5 x 3" = 7.5 lbs; IBW = 100-7.5 = 92 lbs*

    B. *IBW = actual weight ÷ IBW so 80 ÷ 92 = .869 or 87%*

3. Steven weighs 240 lbs and is 6'2" in height. What would be his risk category based on his BMI? He weighed 210 lbs when he was admitted. What is his percent weight change?

    A. *Use the chart to determine his BMI (Figure 9.6) and then compare to Figure 9.7. BMI = 31; risk category is Obese.*

    B. *To determine percent weight change, first subtract the actual weight from the usual weight and then divide by the usual weight. 210 – 240 = 30 lbs ÷ 210 = .1428 = 14.3% weight change*

4. You have just conducted a nutrition screening on Roberta. This is the information you have so far: She weighs 147 lbs, is 5'3" in height with a small frame; her BMI is 26; she is 85 years old; her serum albumin is 2.1; she has pancreatic cancer; she has no family in the area; she usually eats one main meal a day at the Senior Center, otherwise she just snacks. Can you identify each part of the nutrition screen?

    A. *Anthropometric = height, weight, BMI*

    B. *Biochemical - serum albumin*

    C. *Clinical = pancreatic cancer*

    D. *Diet History = eats one meal a day plus snacks*

5. You recently admitted a male client who is just recovering from surgery. His height is 67" and his weight is 135 lbs. What is his daily protein and fluid requirement?

    A. *Daily protein needs following surgery: 1.0-2.0 g x weight in kg. Weight in kg is divided by 2.2. 135 ÷ 2.2 = 61.36 x 1.0 = 61 gm of protein per day*

    B. *Fluid requirement: 30-35 ml x body weight in kg = 61.36 x 35 ml (due to surgery) = 2147.6 or 2148 ml per day.*

CHAPTER 10

Utilize Nutrient Intake, Such as Calories and Sodium

Overview and Objectives

Utilizing nutrient intake means translating nutrition needs into food choices. For a client receiving medical care, the focus is on consuming adequate nutrients in the form of food to maintain nutrition status.

After completing this chapter, you should be able to:

✓ Identify the food components and their contribution to calorie intake

✓ Calculate percent of calories from carbohydrate, protein, and fat

✓ Calculate fluid intake

✓ Identify sources of nutrition information for determining nutrient intake

✓ Explain the uses of nutritional analysis software

✓ Use a Nutrition Facts Label to identify nutrient intake

✓ Use the Exchange Lists to calculate intake of carbohydrate, protein, fat, and calories(s)

✓ Use a carbohydrate counting system to express carbohydrate intake

As the Certified Dietary Manager, you are the food expert. Once you and the Registered Dietitian have completed the nutrition screening and nutrition assessment, it is your job to translate the nutritional needs into food choices for the client. In Chapter 3 and 5, you learned that the percent of calories from nutrients (carbohydrate [CHO], protein, and fat) can make a difference in overall health. Recommendations for a healthy diet often use guidelines based on percentages of these nutrients. In addition, we use guidelines for percentages of CHO, protein, and fat in diets to treat high blood cholesterol, diabetes, and other conditions. Therefore, it is important for a Certified Dietary Manager to be able to determine how many calories are in food.

Three macronutrients provide calories. These are:

✓ Carbohydrate (CHO): 4 calories per gram

✓ Fat: 9 calories per gram

✓ Protein (PRO): 4 calories per gram

Also, alcohol provides calories at the rate of seven calories per gram. Knowing this, we can calculate calories and percent calories of any food or diet, as long as we know the grams of carbohydrate, fat, and protein—and alcohol, if applicable. Figure10.1 shows the formula for calculating total calories. Once we know total calories for any food, meal, or food record, we then can calculate the percent of calories contributed by each component. Percent of calories is simply a way to express the proportions, or how much each macronutrient (and alcohol, if applicable) is contributing to the total calories. This is also called caloric distribution. Figure 10.2 shows the math for calculating total calories. Figure 10.3 shows a sample calculation of calories and percent calories.

Figure 10.1 Calculating Total Calories

This formula works for a single food, a meal, or any food record.
To calculate a calorie distribution:

Step 1: **Find out how many grams of carbohydrate, fat, protein and alcohol are present.**

____ grams of carbohydrate

____ grams of fat

____ grams of protein

____ grams of alcohol (remember calories from alcohol are non-nutritious)

Step 2: **Multiply each by its calorie contribution**

____ grams of carbohydrate . . . . .x 4 cal/gm = ____ cal from carbohydrate

____ grams of fat . . . . .x 9 cal/gm = ____ cal from fat

____ grams of protein . . . . .x 4 cal/gm = ____ cal from protein

____ grams of alcohol . . . . .x 7 cal/gm = ____ cal from alcohol

Step 3: **Add the sub-totals you obtained in Step 2**

____ calories from carbohydrate

____ calories from fat

____ calories from protein

____ calories from alcohol

Total Calories . . . . =_____

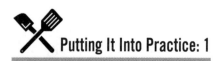

Putting It Into Practice: 1

A diet order says, 212 gm CHO, 48 gm protein, and 40 gm fat. How many total calories will the client consume? What will be the percentage of fat in this diet?

(Check your answer at the end of the chapter)

To calculate caloric distribution for a meal, a one-day menu, or a food record, you can use the same formulas shown in Figures 10.1 and 10.2. For the Figure 10.1 calculation, simply total grams of carbohydrate, fat, protein, and alcohol from all the foods in the diet for Step 1. Here are a few words of caution about interpreting the percent of calories information: We do not want to compare the caloric distribution of each individual food in a diet to the Dietary Guidelines for Americans or other standards. Let's say that we are aiming to achieve a caloric distribution of 50 percent of calories from carbohydrate, 20 percent of calories from protein, and 30 percent of calories from fat. Is it all right to eat the two graham crackers we examined in Figure 10.3? View the sample calculation

Figure 10.2 **Calculating Percent Calories**

Take another look at Step 2 in Figure 10.1. Use the sub-totals you obtained in Column 1 of this calculation. Now, take a look at the total calories you obtained in Step 3 in Figure 10.1. Enter this figure (total calories) in Column 2 below.

Column 1: Calorie Type

_____ Cal from carbohydrate

_____ Cal from fat

_____ Cal from protein

_____ Cal from alcohol

Column 2: Total Calories

_____

_____

_____

_____

Column 3: % Calories from this Component

Cal from carbohydrate ÷ Total calories = _____

Cal from fat ÷ Total Calories = _____

Cal from protein ÷ Total calories = _____

Cal from alcohol ÷ Total ca,ories = _____

Now, round each figure to two decimal places. Next, remove the decimal point (or multiply by 100) to change each figure to a percentage. To check your work, you can add the percentages together. Your total should come close to 100%. (Depending on rounding, you may obtain a total like 99% or 101%. This is OK.)

Figure 10.3 **Sample Calculation: Calories and Percent of Calories of a Specific Food**

We are determining calories for 2 full graham crackers. So far, we know that this serving contains 24 gm of carbohydrate, 3 gm of fat, and 2 gm of protein.

24 grams of carbohydrate   x 4 Cal/gm = 96 Cal from carbohydrate +

3 grams of fat   x 9 Cal/gm = 27 Cal from fat +

2 grams of protein   x 4 Cal/gm = 8 Cal from protein =

Total calories   = 131 Cal

Column 1:	Column 2: Total Calories	Column 3: % Calories from this Component
96 Cal from carbohydrate	131	96 ÷ 131 = 0.73 or 73%
27 Cal from fat	131	27 ÷ 131 = 0.21 or 21%
8 Cal from protein	131	8 ÷ 131 = 0.06 or 6%

To check the calculation, we can add the three percentages, and see if they total close to 100%:

73 + 21 + 6 = 100%

in Figure 10.2 to determine the answer. The answer is: they exceed the caloric distribution of 50 percent of the calories from carbohydrate. When applying caloric distribution guidelines, don't worry about individual foods. Simply review the total for the day.

However, if you find daily totals are not balanced, it can be helpful to look at the caloric distribution of individual foods. For example, if the daily total is too high in fat, we might look at which individual food(s) provided the highest percentage of fat, and reduce portion sizes of these foods to bring the diet into balance.

Calculating Fluid Intake

Water/fluid is also an essential nutrient. Managing fluids is a critical part of clinical care. It is important when there is a concern about dehydration—a common condition among those who are elderly, those who are eating poorly, and those who are undergoing various forms of medical stress. Certain conditions may require a diet order that includes an instruction to push fluids.

Conversely, there are times when the body cannot rid itself of water adequately. For example, a person experiencing end stage renal failure is not able to excrete water. As water builds up in the bloodstream, it dilutes the rest of the blood's contents. It often raises blood pressure and disrupts the sensitive balance of electrolytes (chemicals) in the blood. Fluid restriction may be required to avoid potentially life-threatening conditions. Other conditions that may require fluid restriction include advanced liver failure, congestive heart failure, and certain hormonal disorders.

When a fluid restriction is needed, a physician specifies the restriction along with the rest of the diet order. Fluid restrictions are expressed in milliliters (ml) or cubic centimeters (cc). Although these are equivalent, ml is the preferred term by the Joint Commission. They recommend that "ml" is less likely to be mis-read in a medical record. It is important to note that the Centers for Medicare and Medicaid Services (CMS) require the use of cc's. A number indicates how many ml's should be consumed per day. For example, a diet for an individual in renal failure may read:

60 gm protein, 2 gm Na, 2 gm K, 1000 ml.

This means the diet is limited to 60 grams of protein, 2 grams of sodium, 2 grams of potassium, and 1000 ml of fluid per day.

To honor an order such as this one, nursing and foodservice staff must communicate and work together. Some of the fluid may be served with meals. Other fluid may take the form of a drink offered by the nurse, e.g. with medications. Thus, the first step in implementing a fluid-restricted diet order is to find out which part you should provide through foodservice. Your facility may have a universal standard—80 percent from foodservice and 20 percent from nursing services, for instance. That would be 800 ml from foodservice and 200 ml from nursing services. If there is no standard, you and a nurse may need to specify and agree upon a split. You should document a distribution for the dietary allowance of fluid on your care plan or kardex card, and keep it consistent. For example, you may have a 1200 ml restriction, with 400 ml provided by nursing. You may distribute the remaining 800 ml as: 240 ml—breakfast; 240 ml—lunch; 240 ml—dinner; 80 ml—snack. You will need to manage menus and trays meticulously to stay in compliance.

As you plan a day's worth of menus, how do you count fluid? First, you need a conversion factor. One cup or 8 fluid ounces = 240 ml. Figure 10.4 lists some related conversions. Next, you need to decide what menu items count as fluids. This is specified in the diet manual, and you should use the manual as a reference. Also, refer again to Figure 3.20 in Chapter 3. Generally, anything that *looks* like a liquid at room temperature counts as fluid. Examples include: broth, juice, soft drinks, milk, shakes, coffee, tea, fruit ices, ice cream, sherbet, liquid nutritional supplements, gelatin, and popsicles. Pudding, custard, yogurt, hot cereal, and gravy do NOT count as fluid. Like calorie counting and carbohydrate counting, fluid counting is not 100 percent precise. We know, for example, that many fruits and vegetables contain water, but most systems do not count that as fluid.

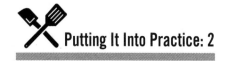

Putting It Into Practice: 2

You are counting fluid at a lunch meal. How will you count 6 oz. of cranberry juice?

(Check your answer at the end of the chapter)

If you are planning a fluid-restricted menu, consider menu needs. For example, most people want to have milk with cold cereal. Also, special portion sizes of fluid-containing items may be in order. The milk, for example, may be one-half cup instead of one cup. Fruits may come through as whole, fresh fruits or drained, canned fruits rather than juice. As a practical matter, most foodservice departments also provide a message on menus or tray tickets for fluid-restricted meals. One facility may use a red stamp to mark "Fluid Restriction." Another may generate a special message through a software program that prints tray tickets. Usually, nursing staff also post an alert near a patient's bed. To protect a resident's privacy, many facilities use only color-coding to signal special restrictions.

Figure 10.4 **Fluid Conversions**

Volume	Fluid Ounce	Milliliters
1 cup	8 fluid oz.	240 ml
3/4 cup	6 fluid oz.	180 ml
1/2 cup	4 fluid oz.	120 ml
1/3 cup	2.7 fluid oz.	80 ml
1/4 cup	2 fluid oz.	60 ml
2 Tbsp.	1 fluid oz.	30 ml

Sources of Nutrient Information

By now, you are prepared to calculate the amount of calories and fluid in the diet and, from Chapter 3, you can determine micronutrients as well. But where do you obtain figures for these calculations? Nutrient information is available from several sources. We will examine three: USDA Nutrient Database, nutrient analysis software, and Nutrition Facts Label.

USDA Nutrient Database

Historically, almost all nutrient data came from laboratory research conducted by the USDA. Over the years, the USDA has vastly augmented its information, adding nutrients such as dietary fiber and trace minerals—and now, caffeine, lycopene, isoflavones (a food component in soybeans), trans-fatty acids, and many others. For the most part, nutrient data in other books and software programs comes from the USDA database. Following are six points to keep in mind with USDA data.

1. Much of the USDA data is available per 100 gram portion. For a small serving of meat, this might be realistic (100 grams is just over 3 ounces). However, for some foods, it is not a "usual fit" with dietary habits. For instance, one cup of circular-shaped oat cereal is only 30 grams. When using USDA data, be sure to check units of measure carefully and select a unit that applies to your need. Also, you may have to convert weights to volume measurements. If the data is not available in the format you need, you can use a conversion table from another source, such as *Food for Fifty*, a quantity food production cookbook.

2. Using USDA nutrient data requires careful attention to edible portion and/ or product yield. Edible portion is the amount of a food you can actually eat after preparation is complete; product yield is the final volume of the cooked food. Consider that meat shrinks when it is cooked, and grain products like rice and pasta expand. If you want the nutrient values for a ground beef patty, you need to determine the final weight of the cooked patty, and match it to "cooked" ground beef in the database. Imagine you start with a six-ounce patty, and it cooks down to four ounces. If you calculate nutrients based on USDA data for six ounces of cooked ground beef, you will over-report nutrients. You would want to match "ounces" and "cooked" to the nutrient database. Now consider macaroni. Nutrients for a cup of uncooked macaroni may be about three times higher than nutrients for a cup of cooked macaroni. You need to match macaroni to a weight or volume and then carefully select "dry" or "cooked".

3. Your calorie total and the USDA calorie total may not match. If you conduct your own calculation of total calories based on grams of carbohydrate, fat, and protein (as in Figure 10.1), your calorie total and the one you see in USDA data may not match perfectly. This is OK. USDA uses more highly refined techniques for determining calorie information.

4. USDA data is primarily built on individual foods. Each time you have a recipe or combination dish, the most accurate way to determine nutrients is to calculate them based on individual ingredients. This is a cumbersome process. However, USDA data does include some combination dishes. You may need to decide how closely a USDA item matches your own recipes or sources for foods.

5. Historically, USDA nutrient data was all for generic foods. Today, the USDA maintains quite a bit of information by brand name. This is useful, as many people eat not only brand-name foods—but also packaged and convenience foods that would be difficult to calculate any other way.

6. Some data simply is not available. Despite the massive research conducted by the USDA, the task of determining nutrient values for thousands of foods is no small feat! As a result, certain nutrient values may be absent. This can lead to false zeroes. A false zero is a report that a nutrient is absent in food, when in fact we just don't have the data.

Nutrient Analysis Software

Because calculating nutrients in a recipe, meal, or menu can be a great deal of work, many dietary professionals use software for the job. Nutrient analysis software is readily available within a range of budgets. Some programs are built into foodservice management software packages. This can be convenient because they draw on lists of foods and recipes that are already in the system. Be aware, though, that any software does initially require you to enter data, such as an inventory list, individual recipes, and menus.

If you are selecting a program for nutrient analysis, look carefully at the sources of nutrient data. Generally, nutrient databases are built on USDA data, which is freely available. Some packages use the USDA database in its entirety. Others use a small proportion of USDA data. So, look at the number of foods contained in a program's database. Also check whether you can add foods to the database yourself, using Nutrition Facts Labels.

In addition, some software developers invest immense effort into expanding the database by adding nutrient data available from food manufacturers, restaurants and other sources. A database offering significantly more foods than USDA has most likely undergone development to list more brand-name and convenience foods. Some developers use sources beyond the USDA to eliminate false zeroes in the database through mathematical calculations and estimations. This eliminates the problem of under-reporting certain nutrients. Which nutrients and food components are included varies by software package.

Another consideration with software is portion sizes or units of measure. Some packages offer more choices for portion sizes and units of measure, as compared with the USDA database. This can improve accuracy and efficiency for a program user. If you are evaluating options, also take a look at how you find and enter foods. This should be a straightforward and convenient process. Finally, review the types of reports available. Most software will compare calculated totals with nutrient standards, such as myPyramid, RDAs, diabetic exchanges, and/or many others. Some reports are graphic and easy to read. Reports may be available for individual foods, recipes, menus, or averages for a series of days.

Let's look at how you might use the computer to get a nutrient analysis for one portion of a recipe.

✓ First, you may type the name of an ingredient (or part of the name), and the computer lists choices so that you can choose a match.

✓ Then you type in how much of that ingredient you want to be used in the analysis, such as one cup—or you select a measurement from a drop-down list.

✓ After entering all the ingredients, you can have the computer divide the results by the yield, such as 12 portions.

✓ Then the computer will tell you exactly how much of each nutrient (and the percent of the RDA) is contained in one portion.

Most computer analysis programs can also give you a percentage breakdown of calories from protein, fats, carbohydrate, and alcohol. Of course, these figures can be printed on a printer and/or stored in the computer. A sample nutrient analysis for a recipe appears in Figure 10.5.

Nutrition Fact Labels

The Nutrition Labeling and Education Act of 1990 requires labeling for most foods, except meat and poultry. The FDA notes that Nutrition Facts Labels are designed to offer consumers the following:

✓ Nutrition information about almost every food in the grocery store

✓ Distinctive, easy-to-read formats that enable consumers to find the information they need to make healthful food choices

✓ Information about the amount of nutrients per serving

 Utilize Nutrient Intake, Such as Calories and Sodium

Figure 10.5 **Sample Nutrient Analysis**

Recipe: French Toast (2 slices)
Serving size: 3.5 oz.

Calories	558.74 Kcal	20.7%
Protein	11.67 gr	20.8%
Fat	13.90 gr	15.4%
Carbohydrate	98.53 gr	26.5%
Calcium	179.71 mg	22.5%
Iron	3.66 mg	36.6%
Sodium	702.11 mg	26.0%
Potassium	257.63 mg	5.6%
Vitamin A	0.00 RE	0.0%
Ascorbic Acid	0.17 mg	0.3%
Folic Acid	47.67 mcg	11.9%
Cholesterol	57.50 mg	19.2%
Nutrient 13	0.00 mg	0.0%
Nutrient 14	0.00 mg	0.0%
Nutrient 15	0.00 mg	0.0%

Do you want a bar chart for this data (1=Yes, 2=No, 99=End)?

Recipe Number: 2002 French Toast (2sl)   Number of Servings 574

Code

No.	Item Name	Quantity Needed
47	Milk, Non-Fat Dry	2 Pounds + 2.44 Ounces (weight)
179	Water, Cold	2 Quarts + 1.74 Pints
96	Eggs, Fresh, Ex. Large	14 Pounds + 5.60 Ounces (weight)
68	Spices, Nutmeg	1.952 Ounces (weight)
48	Sugar, Cane-Gran Domino	5 Pounds
174	BK-FS Bread, White (weight)	140 Pounds + 10.08 Ounces
57	Syrup Pancake Maple	8 Gallons + 2.44 Quarts
104	Margarine One LB SPEC PRNT	14 Pounds + 5.60 Ounces (weight)

Dissolve Dry Milk in Water
Beat Eggs, Add to Milk
Mix Sugar and Nutmeg, Add to Mixture
Dip Bread in Mixture
Fry on 375 F° Grill Covered with Margarine
Cook Until Golden Brown
Serve with 2 oz. of Syrup

Nutritional Analysis

Name:	SAMPLE	Age: 23-50	
Date:	09-14-1984	Weight: 154 Pounds	Activity Level: Light
Prescribed Diet:	RDA, Safe & Adequate	Height: 70 inches	Lactating: No
Recipe:	French Toast (2 slices)	Sex: Male	Pregnant: No

Nutritional Category

		0	25	50	75	100	125
Calories	21%						
Protein	21%						
Fat	15%						
Carbohydrate	27%						
Calcium	22%						
Iron	37%						
Sodium	26%						
Potassium	6%						
Vitamin A	0%						
Ascorbic Acid	0%						
Folic Acid	12%						
Cholesterol	19%						
Nutrient 13	0%						
Nutrient 14	0%						
Nutrient 15	0%						

✓ Standardized serving sizes, which make nutritional comparisons of similar products easier

✓ Nutrient reference values, expressed as percent Daily Values, that help consumers see how a food fits into an overall daily diet

✓ Uniform definitions for terms that describe a food's nutrient content such as "light," "low-fat," and "high-fiber"—to ensure that such terms mean the same for any product on which they appear

✓ Claims about the relationship between a nutrient or food and a disease or health-related condition, such as calcium and osteoporosis, or fat and cancer. These are helpful for people who are concerned about eating foods that may help keep them healthy.

✓ Declaration of total percentage of actual juice in juice drinks

A Nutrition Facts Label (Figure 10.6) must include information about: total calories, calories from fat, total fat, saturated fat, trans fat, cholesterol, sodium, total carbohydrate, dietary fiber, sugars, protein, vitamin A, vitamin C, calcium, and iron. Optionally, a label may include: calories from saturated fat, polyunsaturated fat, monounsaturated fat, potassium, soluble fiber, insoluble fiber, sugar alcohols, other carbohydrate, percent of vitamin A present as beta-carotene, and other essential vitamins and minerals. If a label makes a claim regarding one of these optional items, then it must provide the nutrition facts

Figure 10.6 Sample Nutrition Facts Label for Macaroni & Cheese

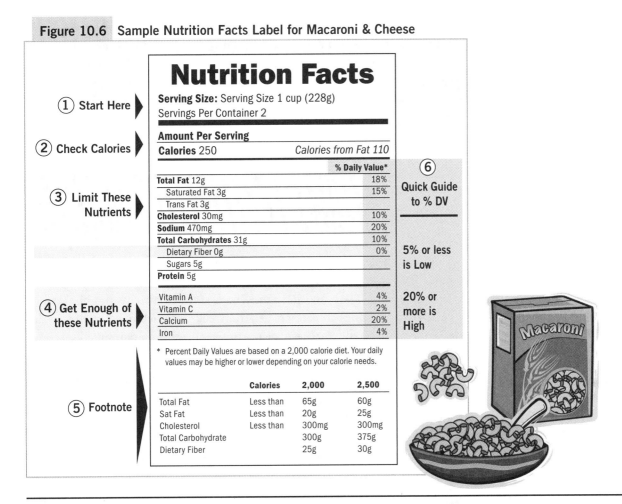

for the item. For instance, if the label claims "high fiber," it must list the fiber content and meet the definition for "high fiber" as described above.

Let's review each section of the Nutrition Facts Label. Figure 10.6 is labeled with the sections we will review.

1. Serving Size

This is the first place to look on a nutrition label and one that is extremely important because it can be very misleading for your clients. Serving sizes are standardized and are provided in standard units such as cups or pieces. The most important part of this section is the Servings Per Container line. Many people assume that the information on the label is the total for the package or container. For instance, they might assume that a 12 ounce bottle of juice is one serving where in reality, it is two servings. Since the serving size listed is what influences the data, including the calories, you could be consuming twice as many calories.

Another fact to watch is the number of items per serving on larger packages. A good example of this is different types of snack chips. Here are three snack chips with the serving size all different but all are a one-ounce serving:

✓ 1 ounce (33 chips)

✓ 1 ounce (12 chips)

✓ 1 ounce (9 chips)

2. Check Calories

If the Servings Per Container is two, you will need to double all of the calories and other nutrient numbers, including the % Daily Values. In this example of macaroni and cheese, how many calories would you consume if you ate the entire package? The FDA provides the following information to help consumers judge calories:

General Guide to Calories

✓ 40 calories is low

✓ 100 calories is moderate

✓ 400 calories or more is high

3. Limit These Nutrients

This section lists key nutrients macronutrients: Total Fat including Saturated Fat, Trans Fat, Cholesterol; Sodium; Total Carbohydrate including Dietary Fiber, Sugars; and Protein. The first four nutrients (highlighted in yellow) are the ones consumers generally eat too much of according to the new dietary guidelines. These are the nutrients we should limit. Please note these are not highlighted on the actual Nutrition Facts Label.

This section of the label expresses each nutrient as a percentage of the Daily Value. **Daily Values (DVs)** are reference intake levels devised specifically for nutrition facts labeling. They allow the food manufacturer to compare the amount of iron in a food to the amount that you, as a consumer, need. By using the % Daily Values column, you can determine if a food is high or low in a nutrient. These are generalized figures for nutrient that can be

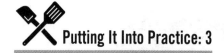

Putting It Into Practice: 3

Would wheat bread that contains one gram of fiber per serving be considered an adequate source of fiber? Why or why not?

(Check your answer at the end of the chapter)

applied to healthy people as a single group. Think of them as a generic set of "one-size-fits-all" nutrient recommendation for consumers. These differ from the Recommended Daily Allowances you learned about in Chapter 2 where the RDAs are broken down by age. For labeling purposes, when there is variation in actual RDAs, daily values reflect the higher values within ranges.

This section also contains Total Carbohydrates with sugars and dietary fiber broken out separately. Dietary fiber is highlighted in blue because according to the dietary guidelines we need to add more fiber in our diets. Use the dietary fiber information to help you increase your fiber intake by looking for foods with more grams of dietary fiber.

4. Get Enough of These Nutrients

These are micronutrients we should consume more of: vitamin A, vitamin C, calcium, and iron. They are expressed as a percentage of Reference Daily Intakes (RDIs) that you learned about in Chapter 2. Obviously, not all of the essential nutrients are listed on the nutrition facts label. For nutrition facts labeling, the FDA has selected only some key nutrients that relate to common health concerns.

5. Footnote

The footnote section highlights the fact that the label data is based on a 2,000 calorie diet. The remaining information will only be on the label if there is room on the package. The optional data represents general information for all Americans and is not specific to the food product. As you can see, it tells you what the recommended total fat grams should be for a 2,000 calorie diet as well as other nutrients. This information can be very useful when comparing the label data to this information. This food product has no dietary fiber, yet the % Daily Value indicates that we should consume 25 g each day. If you follow the dietary advice, you would want to increase your fiber intake throughout the remaining meals of the day.

As you can see, daily values used for nutrition facts labeling are less precise than RDAs. They are quite generalized. If you need to conduct detailed nutrient evaluation for an individual, your first choice of reference should be RDAs. However, nutrition facts labels do provide an excellent educational tool for consumers. They offer consistency and give consumers a way to compare nutritional values of foods.

Note that many labels also provide a set of nutrient information based on common serving or preparation practices. For cereal, you'll see values for the cereal alone, and for the cereal plus milk. For a bakery mix, you may see values for the mix alone (the contents of the package), and also for the mix prepared with added ingredients, according to preparation instructions on the package. Some labels vary based upon intended use. Infant formulas, for example, will not carry reference information about calories from fat or cholesterol. The reason is to prevent parents from mistakenly believing that they should restrict infants' fat intake.

Finally, labeling standards govern the use of special terminology to describe foods. Figure 10.7 (Food Label Dictionary) describes this terminology. Foods

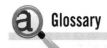

Glossary

Daily Values (DVs)
Reference intake levels for nutrition labeling for the general public

must meet specific criteria to make certain labeling claims. In addition, many terms have legal definitions when it comes to labeling statements. Just like the nutrition facts, these claims are based on per-serving information.

Now, let's consider the nutrition facts label as a source of nutrient information. Let's say you are planning a menu. You want to be sure it falls within certain dietary recommendations, and you want to be sure that the menu contains enough of key nutrients. You would like to include a frozen casserole—a convenience item. How can you identify the nutrients? If this product is not available in the USDA nutrient database (or in a nutrient analysis software system you use), you need to identify the nutrients from a label. Here are some pointers:

✓ First, compare the serving size. Determine whether it matches the serving size you will use. If not, use an adjustment factor. For example, imagine a product shows a serving size of 1⁄2 cup, but you plan to serve it as 3⁄4 cup. You will need to adjust all the nutrients by a factor of 1.5. You will multiply each nutrient value by 1.5 to get the nutrients for your serving size.

✓ Next, use the label to obtain calories and any of the following: fat, saturated fat, cholesterol, sodium, carbohydrate, fiber, sugars, and protein. (These are nutrients that have Daily Reference Values.)

Note: To determine the adjustment factor, divide the new amount (3/4 cup or .75) by the old amount (1/2 cup or .5). **.75 ÷ .50 = 1.5**

In addition, nutrient information is available from a book called *Bowes and Church's Food Values of Portions Commonly Used*, or the *USDA Nutrient Database for Standard Reference*. The USDA nutrient data is available in the form of free downloads from the Internet. You can also do an online search of any food to retrieve its nutrient information. Or, you can display lists of foods containing a selected nutrient. The Web address for searching USDA data appears in Appendix A—Chapter 10.

As you have seen, there is no actual amount of vitamin A, vitamin C, iron, and calcium, only the percent of RDIs. Generally, if the food provides a minimum of 20 percent of the Daily Value for these four nutrients, you can consider it an adequate source. If you want to know the exact amount of the four nutrients, you will have to do some math. Figure 10.8 is the FDA's Reference Values for Nutrition Facts Labeling. Let's say you want to know how many grams of calcium the food item in the label example in Figure 10.6 provides. You know from the label that this product contains 20 percent of calcium per serving. Now look at Figure 10.7; it shows you that the reference value for calcium is 1000 milligrams. You can calculate the exact milligrams of calcium by multiplying 1000 by 20 percent or 0.2 x 1000 = 200 milligrams of calcium.

Calculating Nutrients Based on Exchange Lists

In some situations, a full-blown nutrient analysis is more than you really need. For example, if you are performing a calorie count for a nursing home client, you may be interested in finding out how much protein and how many calories the client consumes in a day. Or, if you are trying to evaluate whether a particular diet provides fewer than 30 percent of calories from fat, you may not need to pull

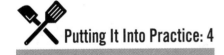

Putting It Into Practice: 4

You need to know how many milligrams of vitamin C are in a specific food product. The label says it contains 20%. How many milligrams does the product contain?

(Check your answer at the end of the chapter)

Figure 10.7 Food Label Dictionary

Nutrient Content Claim	Definition
Calories	
Calorie free	less than 5 calories
Low calorie	40 calories or less
Reduced or fewer calories	at least 25% fewer calories*
Light or lite	one-third fewer calories or 50% less fat*
Sugar	
Sugar free	less than 0.5 grams sugars
Reduced sugar or less sugar°	at least 25% less sugars*
No added sugar	no sugars added during processing or packing, including ingredients that contain sugars, such as juice or dry fruit
Fat	
Fat free	less than 0.5 grams of fat
Low fat	3 grams or less of fat
Reduced or less fat	at least 25% less fat*
Light	one-third fewer calories or 50% less fat*
Saturated Fat	
Saturated fat free	less than 0.5 grams of saturated fat and less than 0.5 grams of trans fat
Low fat free	1 gram or less of saturated fat and no more than 15% of calories from saturated fat
Cholesterol	
Cholesterol Free	less than 2 milligrams cholesterol and 2 grams or less of saturated fat
Reduced or less cholesterol	at least 25% cholesterol* and 2 grams or less of saturated fat
Sodium	
Sodium free	less than 5 milligrams of sodium
Very low sodium	35 milligrams or less of sodium
Low sodium	140 milligrams or less of sodium
Reduced or less sodium	at least 25% less sodium*
Light in sodium	50% less*
Fiber	
High fiber	5 grams or more
Good source of fiber	2.5 to 4.9 grams
More or added fiber	at least 2.5 grams more
Other Claims	
High, rich in, excellent source of	20% or more of Daily Value*
Good source, contains, provides	10% to 19% of Daily Value*
More, enriched, fortified, added	10% or more of Daily Value*
Lean**	less than 10 grams of fat, 4.5 grams or less of saturated fat, and 95 milligrams of cholesterol
Extra Lean**	less than 5 grams of fat, 2 grams of saturated fat, and 95 milligrams of cholesterol

* As compared with a standard serving size of the traditional food
** On meat, poultry, seafood, and game meats
Source: FDA

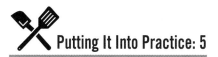

Putting It Into Practice: 5

How many calories would there be in a menu containing 75 gm CHO, 12 gm protein, and 10 gm fat?

(Check your answer at the end of the chapter)

Figure 10.8 **FDA Reference Values for Nutrition Facts Labeling**

Nutrient	Unit of Measure	Daily Values
Total Fat	grams (g)	65.0
Saturated fatty acids	grams (g)	20.0
Cholesterol	milligrams (mg)	300.0
Sodium	milligrams (mg)	2400.0
Potassium	milligrams (mg)	3500.0
Total carbohydrate	grams (g)	300.0
Fiber	grams (g)	25.0
Protein	grams (g)	50.0
Vitamin A	International Unit (IU)	5000.0
Vitamin C	milligrams (mg)	60.0
Calcium	milligrams (mg	1000.0
Iron	milligrams (mg)	18.0
Vitamin D	International Unit (IU)	400.0
Vitamin E	International Unit (IU)	30.0
Vitamin K	micrograms (µg)	80.0
Thiamin	milligrams (mg)	1.5
Riboflavin	milligrams (mg)	1.7
Niacin	milligrams (mg)	20.0
Vitamin B6	milligrams (mg)	2.0
Folate	micrograms (µg)	400.0
Vitamin B12	micrograms (µg)	6.0
Biotin	micrograms (µg)	300.0
Pantothenic Acid	milligrams (mg)	10.0
Phosphorus	milligrams (mg)	1000.0
Iodine	micrograms (µg)	150.0
Magnesium	milligrams (mg)	400.0
Zinc	milligrams (mg)	15.0
Selenium	micrograms (µg)	70.0
Copper	milligrams (mg)	2.0
Manganese	milligrams (mg)	2.0
Chromium	micrograms (µg)	120.0
Molybdeum	micrograms (µg)	75.0
Chloride	milligrams (mg)	3400.0

Source: FDA

out reference books or launch a software program. As you learned in Chapter 5, the exchange lists for meal planning group foods according to their content of carbohydrate, fat, protein, and calories. Any time you need a shortcut method of estimating these same four items, you can use the exchange lists.

Figure 10.9 shows the overall exchange groups with the grams of carbohydrate, protein, fat, and calories. Within the exchange lists are foods grouped together because they are alike. Each serving of a food has about the same amount of CHO, protein, fat, and calories. Foods within each list can be exchanged or traded for each other without affecting the CHO, protein, fat, or calories of a meal. The full list of exchanges appear in Appendix C. The steps below take you through a quick method of estimating the amount of CHO, protein, fat, and calories in a meal.

Step 1

Match the food(s) you wish to analyze to exchanges. Assign each food an exchange group and identify how many exchanges it represents. For mixed dishes you may be listing more than one exchange group. Do not count foods in the "free foods" exchange list at all.

Step 2

Total the exchanges for each group.

Step 3

For each exchange group, multiply the total number of exchanges by the standard carbohydrate, fat, protein, and calorie figures for that exchange group.

Figure 10.9 shows a worksheet for performing these steps, and Figure 10.10 shows an example of how you can apply it.

If you are obtaining a calorie count or calculating intake from a food record, your estimates will be only as good as the original records. Calorie counts in facilities can be challenging. To collect the best records possible:

✓ Inform everyone who may be involved in care that a calorie count is in progress. This includes the client, visitors, nurses, and other caregivers.

✓ Post a notice or make another visible reminder (as permitted by your policies and procedures).

✓ Keep printed menus or try a ticket from meal trays. Ask each person to record the percent consumed next to each menu item. Percents (rather than actual measurements) are useful. They do not require others to guesstimate portion sizes. However, you can refer to your actual menu and food production information to determine what the portion size is.

✓ If possible, review records frequently throughout the day. If a meal has not been recorded, check with the caregiver, or (if appropriate) with the client directly.

✓ Ask all caregivers to record any additional items the resident consumes, even if they are not printed on the menu. Example: A resident asks for a can of ginger ale. Or: A nurse offers a patient a cup of apple juice for taking medications. Or: A visitor brings in a cookie.

Obtaining a valid calorie count requires excellent communication, as well as vigilance and monitoring.

Figure 10.9 **Exchange Groups**

Group	Carbohydrate (grams)	Protein (grams)	Fat (grams)	Calories
Carbohydrate Group				
Starch	15	3	0-1	80
Fruit	15	—	—	60
Milk				
Fat-free	12	8	0-3	90
Reduced-fat	12	8	5	120
Whole	12	8	8	150
Other				
Other Carbohydrates	15	Varies	Varies	Varies
Nonstarchy Vegetables	5	2	—	25
Meat & Meat Substitutes Group				
Very lean	—	7	0-1	35
Lean	—	7	3	55
Medium-fat	—	7	5	75
High-fat	—	7	8	100
Fat				
Fat Group	—	—	5	45

Carbohydrate Counting

Carbohydrate counting may be used as a method of managing dietary concerns for an individual who has diabetes. This system revolves around one simple idea: Foods that contain carbohydrate become glucose in the body. Glucose is blood sugar. (Note that fiber does not become blood sugar because it is not digested.) In a diet for managing diabetes, the bottom line is often how much glucose enters the body and how often.

Carbohydrate counting is based on a prescribed level of carbohydrate intake. For example, one client may be aiming for 220 gm carbohydrate per day; another may be aiming for 185. Generally, this carbohydrate intake needs to be distributed throughout the day to prevent surges in blood glucose levels. How rigid this distribution needs to be is dictated by the diabetes itself and medication regimens. It varies tremendously among individuals. Carbohydrate counting is done in conjunction with blood glucose monitoring, and members of the healthcare team evaluate any necessary fine-tuning in carbohydrate totals and distribution.

To count carbohydrates, simply tally grams of carbohydrate in each food consumed. You need to count the carbohydrate in starches as well as sugars. Starchy foods include grain products, potatoes, dried beans, peas, and corn.

Foods with sugar include fruit, sweets, soft drinks, and milk. (Milk contains lactose, or milk sugar.) An easy way to track all of this is with exchange lists. You can use the same method shown in Figure 10.9 to count carbohydrates. Enter a food on the worksheet only if it contains carbohydrate. Omit foods that fall into the exchange lists for meats or fats. Do count foods that fall into these exchange groups: starch, fruit, milk, other carbohydrates, or vegetables. In Figure 10.10, total the grams of carbohydrate. You do not need to calculate grams of protein, fat, or calories.

Figure 10.10 Sample Calculation for a Calorie Count

John is a client in a nursing home. The healthcare team is not sure he is eating enough to maintain his nutritional health. You are conducting a calorie count. You have a food record of everything he has eaten over the course of the day, including breakfast, lunch, dinner, and snacks. Note the exchange values for chicken noodle soup come from the combination foods list. You enter each food into the worksheet, and calculate nutrients as shown below.

		Number of Exchanges						
Food	Serving Size	Starch	Fruit	Milk*	Other Carb.	Vegetable	Meat**	Fat
Orange Juice	1/2 cup		1					
Toast	1 slice	1						
Margarine	1 tsp.							1
Chicken Noodle Soup	1 cup				1			
Applesauce	3/4 cup		1.5					
Meatloaf	1 oz.						1	
TOTALS		1	2.5	0	1	0	1	1

				Number of Exchanges					
Exchange Group	No. of Exchanges	CHO GM	Your Total	PRO GM	Your Total	Fat GM	Your Total	Cal.	Your Total
Starch	1	x 15 =	15	x 3 =	3			x 80 =	80
Fruit	2.5	x 15 =	38					x 60 =	150
Milk	0	x 12 =		x 8 =				x 90 =	
Other Carb.	1	x 15 =	15					x 60 =	60
Vegetable	0	x 5 =	1.5	x 2 =				x 25 =	
Meat	1			x 7 =	7	x 5 =	5	x 75 =	75
Fat	1					x 5 =	5	x 45 =	45
TOTALS			68 gm CHO		10 gm PRO		10 gm fat		410 calories

Conclusion: John's intake for this day was 68 gm carbohydrate, 10 gm protein, 10 gm fat, and a daily total of 410 calories.

What if a food does not appear on the exchange lists? Nutrition facts labels can be useful. Check the product label for grams of carbohydrate. Count every 15 grams of carbohydrate shown as one exchange in the Other Carbohydrates group. Or, simply add the grams of carbohydrate from product labels to your tally.

END OF CHAPTER

 Putting It Into Practice Questions & Answers

1. A diet order says, 212 gm CHO, 48 gm protein, and 40 gm fat. How many total calories will the client consume? What will be the percentage of fat in this diet? Remember that a carbohydrate is 4 calories per gram, protein is 4 calories per gram, and fat is 9 calories per gram.

   A. *212 x 4 = 848*

   48 x 4 = 192

   40 x 9 = 360

   Total = 1400

   b. To calculate the percentage of calories from fat, divide the total calories from fat by the total calories. = 360/1400 = 26%

2. You are counting milliliters of fluid at a lunch meal. How will you count 6 oz. of cranberry juice?

   A. *There are approximately 30 ml per ounce so 6 x 30 = 180 ml.*

3. Would wheat bread that contains one gram of fiber per serving be considered an adequate source of fiber? Why or why not?

   A. *You have to remember that the recommended amount of fiber is about 25 grams per day. To determine the percentage of fiber in the bread, divide one (1) by 25 = 4%. For a food source to be considered a good source, it should be 20%, so no, wheat bread with only one gram of fiber per serving is not an adequate source of fiber.*

4. You need to know how many milligrams of vitamin C are in a specific food product. The label says it contains 20%. How many milligrams does the product contain?

   A. *Review the Figure 10.8 to determine the daily value for vitamin C. It is 60 mg. To determine the exact number of mg in the product, multiply 60 x 20% or .20 = 12 mg.*

5. How many caloires would there be in a menu containing 75 gm CHO, 12 gm protein, and 10 gm fat?

   A. *75 x 4 = 300*

   12 x 4 = 48

   10 x 9 = 90

   Total = 438 calories

Identify Nutrition Problems and Resident Rights

Overview and Objectives

As a prospective Certified Dietary Manager, you should see a pattern emerging with these chapters. You have interviewed clients, conducted screening, utilized the nutrient intake information and now you are going to identify clients who might need nutritional interventions and honor client rights in the process.

After completing this chapter, you should be able to:

✓ Explain the role of the Certified Dietary Manager in identifying nutrition problems

✓ Classify the types of information that are relevant to nutrition care

✓ Verify information to ensure accuracy

✓ Explain the rational for reviewing medications

✓ Compare nutrient intake to nutrient standards

✓ Review documentation for nutritional care follow up

✓ Honor client rights while providing nutritional care

✓ Identify significant nutrition related laboratory values

These past few chapters have focused on some of the clinical responsibilities of a Certified Dietary Manager. Clinical nutrition tasks that may appear on a Certified Dietary Manager's job description include: obtaining a diet history, nutrition screening, reviewing medical records for information relevant to nutrition, calculating nutrient intake, documenting nutrition care, planning individualized menus according to diet orders, counseling clients about basic dietary restrictions, and communicating with the client and the healthcare team. In many long-term care facilities, a Certified Dietary Manager attends to nutrition-related needs on a daily basis, while a part-time or consulting Registered Dietitian provides intermittent assessment and planning. The Certified Dietary Manager will be the first to identify nutrition problems and may be responsible for bringing it to the attention of others. Providing clinical nutrition care requires an understanding of what information to look for and using that information to identify potential problems.

Nutrition-Related Information

By now, you know that nutrition-related information may take the form of anthropometric measurements, biochemical tests, clinical information, and diet histories. Sources for this information include the medical record, direct observations and interviews, nutrition care documents, and communications with the healthcare team. Let's examine the process of gathering information from these sources in order to identify nutrition problems.

Medical Record

The medical record contains the formal documentation of all aspects of care for each individual client. Members of the healthcare team record their activities here. This includes the Certified Dietary Manager. It is the communication tool that allows the healthcare team to provide continuity of care. The record contains all orders written by the physician. Diet order is one of these. The medical record is the first document a Certified Dietary Manager will review in performing nutrition screening. Pertinent data here includes a report of laboratory tests performed, as well as history forms completed by the physician, the nurse, and other team members. Be alert to overlaps in these records with some of the pertinent questions for a diet history. For example, a nurse may note the patient's concerns with eating and previous diet patterns. Height and weight are usually in the medical history and/or the nursing intake notes, and weight must be obtained (not just estimated or copied) using standardized procedures. How the record is organized is somewhat unique to each facility. However, your job is to become familiar with it, and use it as a resource for information on an ongoing basis. However it is organized, remember it is a legal document. It must contain enough evidence to justify the progress and care of the client. Figure 11.1 summarizes information to check in the medical record.

Direct observation and interviews. The best way to understand your clients, including their nutrition-related needs and their progress, is to visit with them and observe them. As much as possible, it's a good idea to visit at meal times.

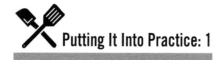

Putting It Into Practice: 1

As you begin your nutrition screening activities, what section of the medical record would most likely contain height/weight information?

(Check your answer at the end of the chapter)

Figure 11.1   Nutrition-Related Information in the Medical Record

• Diet order	• List of medications
• Diagnosis	• Care plan
• Medical history	• Progress notes
• Social history	• Nursing intake notes
• Laboratory tests	• Nursing notes
• Height and weight	• MDS Form
• Laboratory values	

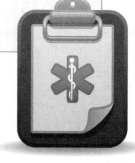

What should you be looking for?

✓ Focus on Food. What is the client eating; how much; what foods are they avoiding, enjoying; is the client chewing and swallowing without any problems?

✓ Focus on Fluid. How much is the client drinking; is there any coughing, drooling, or choking occurring?

✓ Focus on Feeding Issues. Is the client able to initiate eating; can the client position him/herself for a meal; can the client open/handle food packages; can the client use utensils?

If a client does not consume 75 percent or more of food for two out of three days, or does not consume all/almost all of the fluids for two out of three days, there is cause for concern. When a visual observation of intake suggests a problem, the next step is often a calorie count, and review with the healthcare team.

A visit with clients at meals or at other times, is a perfect opportunity to ask them if they have any questions or concerns regarding the diet. A client may not understand why bacon is not being offered on his low sodium diet, and you can explain this. Another important question to ask is if the client is consuming any other food (not provided by the facility). Family members can also be a valuable source of information.

Nutrition Care Documents

In most facilities, the foodservice department maintains its own detailed documents for managing day-to-day nutritional care. The system varies, but may include a nutrition care plan or kardex card. Here, the Registered Dietitian, Certified Dietary Manager, dietetic technician and other dietary personnel note information that will help with planning and meal management. A diet history may be recorded here. A Certified Dietary Manager or Registered Dietitian may copy pertinent facts from the medical record to this plan. A weight record is important. Each weight should be recorded with a date for ongoing monitoring. If you are monitoring certain laboratory values, you may also record these here. Having a policy and procedure for weight monitoring helps to assure consistency in weight records. See Figure 11.2 for a sample weight monitoring policy.

Meal planning details that appear in a nutrition care document include: the physician's diet order, a list of food likes and dislikes, a meal plan (if the client is following an exchange system diet or other meal pattern), and any special requests or needs. Foodservice staff use this information when planning individual menus for each meal. In some long-term care facilities, food preferences are recorded on a tray card, which accompanies a tray along a conveyor during tray assembly. In other facilities, nutrition care documents are maintained in a dietary computer system. The menu itself is also a critical nutrition care document. Whether by computer or by hands-on intervention, foodservice staff review menu offerings or nutritionally equivalent alternatives for clients and assure that each meal served meets the diet order and client preferences.

After reviewing weight records and diet histories, the next step is to identify clients who meet the criteria for at-risk weight loss or those who are having obvious problems eating. As you have learned from the chapter on nutrition screening, this is the information you share with the Registered Dietitian, take to care planning, and/or share with the interdisciplinary team members.

Communications with the Healthcare Team

Healthcare involves the cooperative efforts of many professionals. Each contributes expertise to address a broad range of needs for clients. Each team member has direct contact with the client, as well as with family and others. Each has observations to share. Nutrition-related information is always a piece of a bigger picture. Direct communication with team members helps a Certified Dietary Manager become aware of nutrition-related issues, gain perspective, and implement nutrition care effectively.

Figure 11.2   Policy on Weight Monitoring

Subject: Weight Monitoring Program

Policy:

Each resident or patient's weight will be monitored consistently and closely by the interdisciplinary team. All residents with patterned or significant weight change will be assessed by the facility's interdisciplinary team as indicated. Interventions to address nutritional issues will be initiated and incorporated into the resident's care plan and re-evaluated on a timely and periodic basis.

Procedure:

1 Upon admission to the facility, the nursing staff will weigh each resident, establish an accurate weight, and document the weight. The dietetics professional will determine ideal/desired body weight and document in the medical record.

2 Weights are to be taken (by nursing staff) at least monthly, weekly, as ordered by the physician, or as outlined in the nutrition risk protocol. If a patterned or significant weight loss or gain is noted, the resident is to be re-weighed using consistent scale.

3 Scales should be checked routinely for accuracy. Nursing or other designated staff is responsible for reviewing weekly weights, notifying appropriate disciplines of significant changes, initiating corrective actions, and completing documentation.

4 In the event of a patterned or significant, unplanned weight loss/gain of at least 5% in 30 days, or 10% in 180 days, the following interventions will be carried out:

   • Notification of attending physician and family member/responsible party by nursing staff.

   • Notification of dietetics professional by nursing staff. The dietetics professional will assess the resident, document the assessment, and make recommendations in the resident's medical record. Orders may be obtained for nutritional supplements or other interventions.

   • Nursing staff will initiate a new MDS if indicated, schedule an interdisciplinary conference, and revise the care plan.

   • The Director of Nursing is responsible for determining the need for initiation or discontinuation of weights other than weekly or ordered by physician.

   • Request lab work if necessary.

   • Nursing will initiate a 3-day calorie count.

5 If the resident's weight significant loss/gain is explainable (i.e., weight reduction program, dialysis, diuretic therapy), then the facility will not be required to complete a new MDS. If the facility does not complete a new MDS, documentation must be entered into the resident's medical record to support this determination, with appropriate revisions made to the resident's care plan.

http://www.RD411.com Used with permission.

Food-Drug Interactions

A Certified Dietary Manager needs to devote specific attention to the topic of food-drug interactions. The effects foods and drugs have on each other can determine whether medications do their jobs, and whether the body receives the nutrients it needs. The extent of interaction between foods and drugs depends on the drug dosage and on the individual's age, size, and specific medical condition. Adverse interactions occur more likely under the following circumstances:

✓ Drugs are taken over many years

✓ Several drugs are taken daily

✓ Nutrition status is poor

In general, the presence of food in the stomach and intestines can influence a drug's effectiveness by slowing down or speeding up the time it takes the medicine to go through the gastrointestinal tract to the site in the body where it is needed. Elderly people with chronic diseases are most vulnerable.

Food also contains natural and added chemicals that can react with certain drugs in ways that make the drugs virtually useless. Alternately, components in foods can enhance the action of certain drugs, sometimes triggering a medical crisis or, in rare instances, even death.

A major way food affects drugs is by impeding absorption of the drug into the bloodstream. A classic interaction is the one between tetracycline (an antibiotic) compounds and dairy products. The calcium in milk, cheese, and yogurt impairs absorption of tetracycline. The solution is to avoid dairy products close to the time of taking tetracycline. Another example is a drug called Fosamax®. It must be taken without food, especially coffee and orange juice. Otherwise, it may not be used by the body. In general, it is unwise to take drugs with soft drinks, acid fruit, or vegetable juices. These beverages can result in excess acidity that may cause some drugs to dissolve quickly in the stomach instead of in the intestines where they can be more readily absorbed into the bloodstream. For a summary of drug-nutrient interactions, see Figure 11.3.

Excessive consumption of foods high in vitamin K, such as liver and leafy green vegetables, may hinder the effectiveness of anticoagulants. Vitamin K, which promotes clotting of the blood, works in direct opposition to these drugs, which are intended to prevent blood clotting.

Some of the potassium-sparing diuretics (drugs that remove excess water from the body) can interact with large quantities of potassium in the diet. As potassium builds up in the bloodstream, heartbeat can become irregular. Even though high-potassium foods are ordinarily a great idea, a patient taking one of these medications must moderate potassium intake by avoiding excess orange juice, bananas, potatoes, tomatoes, and other high-potassium foods. However, other types of diuretic drugs remove potassium from the body. These are called potassium-wasting diuretics. Clients taking these drugs need to boost potassium intake to help maintain safe blood potassium levels.

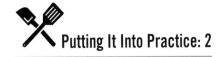 **Putting It Into Practice: 2**

An elderly client you are working with is taking the following medications:

Norvasc® for angina, Atenolol® for blood pressure, Levothyroxine® for thyroid, and Lasix®, a potassium-wasting diuretic.

What, if any, nutrient-drug interactions should you be concerned about and what should you do with the information?

(Check your answer at the end of the chapter)

Figure 11.3 **Summary of Drug-Nutrient Interactions**

DRUGS can alter food intake absorption, metabolism, or excretion by:	FOOD can alter absorption, metabolism or excretion by:
• Changing the acidity of the digestive track • Changing digestive juices • Altering the movement of the digestive tract • Damaging the lining of the digestive tract • Binding with nutrients • Interfering with the metabolism of vitamins	• Changing the acidity of the digestive track • Increasing the secretion of digestive juices • Changing the rate of absorption of the drug • Binding with drugs • Blocking absorption in the intestine

Specific Concerns:

• Grapefruit with Fosomax®, Statins

• Foods high in vitamin K (leafy greens, cauliflower, broccoli, brussel sprouts, kale) with Coumadin®

• Folate deficiency with cancer therapy (Methotrexate)

• MOA Inhibitors with foods containing tyramine (aged cheese, alcohol, liver, figs, bananas, avocados, soy sauce, fava beans, colas, coffee, chocolate, raisins)

• Alcohol and any medications

• Antacids and clients on low-sodium diets

What Can the Certified Dietary Manager Do?

• Look for long-term drug usage.

• Review drug and diet histories of clients

• Identify clients who are likely to develop drug-nutrient interactions (e.g. the elderly, those taking multiple medications)

• Re-assess nutrition status often for those clients who might be at risk

Perhaps the most hazardous food-drug interaction is the one between mono-amine oxidase (MAO) inhibitors, drugs prescribed for depression and high blood pressure, and tyramine in foods. The reaction can raise blood pressure to dangerous levels, sometimes causing severe headaches, brain hemorrhage, and, in extreme cases, death. To prevent a possible reaction, anyone taking MAO inhibitor drugs should avoid high tyramine foods. (Note: this diet is rarely prescribed today.)

Alcohol, which is a drug itself, does not mix well with a wide variety of medications, such as antibiotics; anticoagulants; hypoglycemic drugs, including insulin; antihistamines; high blood pressure drugs; MAO inhibitors; and sedatives. Alcohol combined with antihistamines, tranquilizers, or antidepressants causes excessive drowsiness that can be especially hazardous to someone driving a car, operating machinery, or performing some other task that requires mental alertness. Alcohol can also dissolve coatings on time-released medications. The result is that a medication surges into the bloodstream too quickly.

Just as some foods can affect the way drugs behave in the body, some drugs can affect the way the body uses food. Drugs may act in various ways to impair proper nutrition by hastening excretion of certain nutrients, by hindering absorption of nutrients, or by interfering with the body's ability to convert nutrients into usable forms. Nutrient depletion of the body occurs gradually, but for those taking drugs over long periods of time, these interactions can lead to deficiencies of certain vitamins and minerals, especially in children, the elderly, those with poor diets, and the chronically ill.

Some drugs inhibit nutrient absorption by their effect on the walls of the intestines. Among these are colchicines, drugs prescribed for gout, and mineral oil, an ingredient used in some over-the-counter laxatives. Mineral oil can interfere with absorption of vitamin D, vitamin K, and carotene.

A number of drugs affect specific vitamins and minerals. The antihypertensive drug hydralazine and the antituberculosis drug INH can deplete the body's supply of vitamin B6. They can do this by inhibiting production of the enzyme necessary to convert the vitamin into a form the body can use, or by combining with the vitamin to form a compound that is excreted. Similarly, anticonvulsant drugs that are used to control epilepsy can lead to deficiencies of vitamin D and folic acid because they increase the turnover rate of these vitamins in the body.

Quite a few drugs—such as the antibiotic neomycin and oral hypoglycemic agents—can impair absorption of vitamin B12. But because most Americans have good stores of vitamin B12 in their livers, it takes prolonged ingestion of these drugs to cause a deficiency. Anticonvulsant medications, such as dilantin, reduce the body's supplies of vitamin D and folacin. To prevent deficiency, clients may need to drink more milk, eat folacin-rich foods, and/or take vitamin supplements. Drugs readily available without prescription can also lead to nutrition problems. For example, chronic use of antacids can cause phosphate depletion, a condition that in its milder form produces muscle weakness and in more severe form leads to a vitamin D deficiency. Aspirin can cause vitamin C loss. Modifying the diet to include more foods rich in the vitamins and minerals that may be depleted by certain drugs is preferable to taking vitamin or mineral supplements. In fact, supplements of some vitamins can counter the effectiveness of certain drugs. For a summary, refer to Figure 9.10 in Chapter 9 (Medications with Possible Nutrition Related Effects).

Comparing Nutrient Intake to Standards

Often, a Certified Dietary Manager needs to use the results of nutrient calculations to identify nutrition problems. Let's say you have calculated the results of a one-day food record for a client. You need to make some comments about whether the intake would meet her nutritional needs. The first step is to select nutrients you need to report. Using the same nutrients ordinarily displayed on a Nutrition Facts Label is usually a good approach. For each nutrient, identify the Dietary Reference Intake—Recommended Dietary Allowances (DRI-RDA) for your client's age and sex. Then, calculate total intake as a percentage of the DRI-RDA. To calculate percentage, divide the actual intake of a nutrient by the recommended intake of the nutrient, then remove the decimal point. Following, is an example.

Case #1: Mary

Mary consumes 11 mg of iron in one day. Her DRI-RDA is 18 mg of iron. Percentage of DRI-RDA is 11 ÷ 18 = 0.61 or 61 percent. For calories, you can estimate energy needs, and then compare.

Is it necessary to have 100 percent of the DRI-RDAs for each nutrient? Not always. Consider Mary again, with the low iron intake for one day. Here are conclusions we cannot draw:

✓ Mary is deficient in iron.

✓ Mary never eats foods containing iron.

Here is a conclusion we can draw:

✓ Mary's intake of iron for one day was marginal.

What's next? Other information that would help in evaluating Mary's iron situation includes:

✓ Laboratory Data. Serum hemoglobin and hematocrit will help to determine whether Mary actually has iron-deficiency anemia.

✓ Physician's Diagnosis. Does the physician say Mary has iron-deficiency anemia?

✓ Diet History. More than a single day, we would like to know whether Mary frequently consumes less iron than the DRI-RDA. We may want to check food intakes for other days, or even calculate an average intake over many days.

✓ Food Frequency. We can examine how often Mary eats iron-rich foods.

In many situations, a comparison with Choose MyPlate standards is a convenient and meaningful tool for evaluation. You can tally the number of servings a client has consumed from each food group and compare these with recommended servings.

Nutritional Data and Dietary Management

By now, it's clear that a Certified Dietary Manager needs to consider many factors at once to provide effective dietary care. Let's consider another example.

Case #2: Connie

Connie has Type 2 diabetes, as well as hypertension. What information do we need to review to understand her nutritional care? Here are some pieces of data that will be especially important:

✓ Blood Sugar Levels. By noting blood sugar levels first thing in the morning (fasting blood sugar), following meals, and at bed time, we can find out whether Connie's diabetes is under control on a daily basis.

✓ Blood Pressure Readings. Usually part of the nurse's notes, blood pressure readings help us understand whether Connie's blood pressure is under control.

✓ Meal Time Observation. We need to know how well Connie is tolerating and following her therapeutic diet.

✓ Weight, Percent Body Weight, Weight Changes. If Connie happens to be overweight, weight reduction is likely to improve management of both the diabetes and the hypertension.

✓ Hgb Alc Lab Values Medications. Drugs that may affect blood sugar levels such as oral medications, insulin, or sliding scale insulin.

If blood sugar or blood pressure consistently run too high, team members may confer to decide on adjustments. Solutions may involve changes in medication and/or diet. It's important to recognize that these are closely intertwined. In addition, decisions are based on an understanding of the unique person receiving care. A physician makes a final decision based on input from team members. What can you offer as a Certified Dietary Manager? You can note how well Connie understands and complies with her diet, and give your judgment as to how effective a dietary change might be, based on the information you've collected. For example, if you find that she is not tolerating her diet well, you may recommend further restrictions. A physician may then decide to accomplish more with medications.

Let's imagine Connie is a resident in a long-term care facility. Since admission six months ago, she has paid careful attention to her diet and has lost 17 pounds. Now, you notice that her blood sugar levels and blood pressure levels are making a gradual decline. In the past few days, she has had two episodes of hypoglycemia (very low blood sugar), and the nurse has given her juice to bring her blood sugar back up to safe levels. This could be a signal that Connie's weight loss has improved her health, and it may be time for an adjustment to her care plan. Can you as a Certified Dietary Manager be absolutely certain? Can you make changes on your own? The answer to both questions is no. The reason is that the nutrition-related data you are reviewing is not quite the whole clinical picture. It's always possible that there are other medical factors at play. The physician is responsible for an actual diagnosis and medical assessment. What is your role as a Certified Dietary Manager in this situation? Because you have the background and expertise to focus on the nutrition-related information, you are the prime candidate to point out Connie's weight changes, to highlight a possible relationship between her weight and clinical changes, and alert other team members. Your information may signal a need for further evaluation and possible adjustments to the overall treatment plan.

Case 3: Ricky

Let's consider another situation. Ricky is a resident of a long-term care facility and has been bedridden for more than a year. He developed two pressure ulcers (Stage I) several months ago. At the time, you noted that he was underweight and his serum transferrin level was below normal. You and the Registered Dietitian agreed that Ricky was experiencing some protein-calorie malnutrition. He has been following a high-protein, high-calorie diet. What information is most pertinent to understand his nutritional needs today? Here are some ideas:

✓ Weight. You need to monitor his weight to see whether it is up, down, or remaining stable.

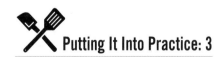

Putting It Into Practice: 3

As you read about Ricky, consider this information:

- June weight: 140 lbs.
- July weight: 135 lbs.

What would you do with this information?

(Check your answer at the end of the chapter)

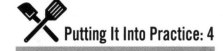

✓ Serum Transferrin (or other blood indicator of protein status preferred in your facility). You want to determine whether his protein status is improving in response to the diet.

✓ Pressure Ulcers. You want to know whether the pressure ulcers have improved, remained stable, or advanced to another stage. You want to know whether any new ulcers have developed.

✓ Diet Tolerance/Intake. To balance the above information with the overall nutrition care, you need to know whether Ricky is eating his food and tolerating it comfortably and consistently.

✓ Calorie Count. If your observations raise concern, you may perform a calorie count to quantify the situation. You can compare intake of calories and protein with estimated needs.

All of this information feeds into the ongoing monitoring of Ricky's nutritional status. It becomes critical to identify nutrition problems to assure that his nutritional status is raised and maintained at optimal levels. We already know that nutritional status is a major factor in the development and healing of pressure ulcers.

Case #4: Marilyn

Here is one more scenario. Marilyn is a client in a nursing home. She entered in excellent nutritional status, and was in the early stage of Alzheimer's disease. She was also following a diet to manage high blood cholesterol levels. Since her admission, she has experienced an advancement of Alzheimer's and has lost more than 6 percent of her body weight within the past month. As you monitor her ongoing nutritional care, you may be concerned with:

✓ Weight. You want to know how Marilyn's actual weight compares with her ideal body weight. You need to monitor weight and percent weight change as indicators of overall nutritional status.

✓ Serum Transferrin (or other blood indicator of protein status preferred in your facility). You want to evaluate protein status and find out whether she is maintaining or losing lean body mass.

✓ Clinical Information. You need to know what stage her Alzheimer's disease is in and whether any new symptoms have arisen.

✓ Diet Tolerance/Intake. Mealtime observation is essential to find out how Marilyn is eating and drinking—and whether the Alzheimer's disease is affecting her food intake. She may be inattentive to meals, or may be exhibiting behaviors that interfere with nutritional intake. You also may wish to evaluate whether dietary restrictions for high blood cholesterol are affecting her nutrient intake.

✓ Calorie Count. If your observations raise concern, you may perform a calorie count to quantify the situation. You can compare her intake of calories and protein with estimated needs.

Notice that Marilyn's blood cholesterol levels are not high on the priority list. This is a matter of clinical judgment. Because of her rapid weight loss, her nutritional status has advanced to the forefront as a nutritional concern. Her protein calorie status takes priority. With a decline or threatened decline in nutritional status, it's much more important to protect her overall and immediate health.

Putting It Into Practice: 4

In the hallway of your facility, a granddaughter stops a foodservice employee to ask about the condition of her grandmother. The foodservice employee comments that she must be doing better as she just ate all of her breakfast. Have the client's rights been violated? Why or why not?

(Check your answer at the end of the chapter)

Most likely, one of your suggestions for Marilyn will be to liberalize her diet. You may need more flexibility in offering high-fat foods to provide a diet that is dense in calories. You and the care planning team may contact the responsible person for Marilyn. That person may have historical data about the progression of the disease and the potential for further weight loss.

Each facility may have its own policies, regulatory concerns, and standards that influence a Certified Dietary Manager's actions in providing nutrition care. Some standards of practice or standards of quality management actually dictate what information will be reviewed in monitoring clinical conditions. Regulations addressing financial reimbursement to the facility may require specific monitoring and documentation. Concerns for clients' rights will affect how strong a role a client plays in making decisions about his or her own care. An institutional policy and/or regulatory requirement may identify the role of the Certified Dietary Manager differently in various locales.

Honor Client's Rights While Providing Nutrition Care

HIPAA is the federal law intended to protect the privacy of healthcare clients. Besides HIPAA regulations, nursing home clients have patient rights and certain protections under the law. The nursing home must list and give all new clients a copy of these rights. Examples of these rights are in Figure 11.4. As you are interviewing clients, recording information from the medical record, and calculating nutritional intake, it is important to consider both HIPAA and Residence Rights. Here are some ways to put those regulations into practice:

✓ Actively seek dietary information from the clients.

✓ When visiting during their meals, get down to eye level with the client, especially if they are hard of hearing.

✓ When observing during their meals, keep some distance away so the client doesn't feel like you are standing over them while they are eating.

✓ Try to eliminate trays in the dining room to provide a more home-like atmosphere.

✓ When and where you communicate information about the clients to interdisciplinary team members, make sure to do so in a way that protects the confidentiality of the information and the dignity of the client.

Figure 11.4 Nursing Home Residents Rights

Residents Rights Usually Include:

Respect: You have the right to be treated with dignity and respect.

Services and Fees: You must be informed in writing about services and fees before you enter the nursing home.

Money: You have the right to manage your own money or to choose someone else you trust to do this for you.

Privacy: You have the right to privacy, and to keep and use your personal belongings and property as long as it doesn't interfere with the rights, health, or safety of others. You have the right to privacy during your visits or meetings, in making telephone calls, and with your mail.

Medical Care: You have the right to be informed about your medical condition, medications, and to see your own doctor. You also have the right to refuse medications and treatment. You have the right to receive care in a manner which promotes and enhances your quality of life. This includes food of the quantity and quality to meet your needs and preferences.

Source:http://www.medicare.gov/Nursing/ResidentRights.asp, accessed September, 2010.

END OF CHAPTER

 Putting It Into Practice Questions & Answers

1. As you begin your nutrition screening activities, what section of the medical record would most likely contain height/weight information?

   A. *Medical records frequently contain a section titled height/weight. The information could also be in the nursing notes. Information about height and weight prior to admission should be in the medical history section. Flowsheets. Many electronic medical records rely on flowsheets.*

2. An elderly client you are working with is taking the following medications: Norvasc® for angina, Atenolol® for blood pressure, Levothyroxine® for thyroid, and Lasix®, a potassium wasting diuretic. What, if any, nutrient-drug interactions should you be concerned about and what should you do with the information?

   A. *Since Lasix® depletes potassium in the body, you will want to consult with the Registered Dietitian or take this information to the interdisciplinary team as a potential problem. There should be a plan to increase the intake of high potassium foods such as potatoes, bananas, fish, or honeydew melon.*

3. As you read about Ricky, consider this information: June weight: 140 lbs; July weight: 135 lbs. What would you do with this information?

   A. *You already know that he has Stage 1 pressure ulcers and is underweight. He is on a high-protein, high-calorie diet. As his weight is continuing to drop, you should alert the registered dietitian right away or the director of nursing.*

4. In the hallway of your facility, a granddaughter stops a foodservice employee to ask about the condition of her grandmother. The foodservice employee comments, "She must be doing better as she just ate all of her breakfast." Have the client's rights been violated? Why or why not?

   A. *The scenario above is a HIPAA violation. The foodservice employee doesn't know if the grandaughter is listed as one of the people who are allowed to receive status updates about the grandmother. The foodservice employee should have referred the granddaughter to the charge nurse who would have the information as to who is allowed to receive status updates about the grandmother.*

Implement Diet Plans or Menus Using Appropriate Modifications

Overview and Objectives

Food and meal services are one component of a Certified Dietary Manager's responsibilities in supporting nutritional care. Planning menus both for client groups and individuals requires a synthesis of much of what you have learned so far. In specialized cases, a unique set of procedures and service mechanisms is required for nutritional support. A Certified Dietary Manager needs to understand how these concepts interplay.

After completing this chapter, you should be able to:

✓ Implement nutrition plan into meals/foods to be served

✓ Identify menu planning needs for infants, children, and older adults

✓ Modify menus to suit fiber content, texture, or feeding needs

✓ Modify menus to control for calories, carbohydrates, proteins, fats, and minerals

✓ Modify menus to suit various racial, cultural and religious differences; and to suit medical or other personal condition(s) (nutritional supplements, enteral products, enteral tube feeding and parenteral nutrition)

In any facility, a menu drives every activity in the kitchen and is the fundamental tool for planning diets. The menu is the blueprint for what clients will be served. A menu must meet the nutritional needs of each client. It must supply adequate calories, protein, carbohydrate, fat, vitamins, minerals, and fluid. It is up to the Certified Dietary Manager to acknowledge and address the specialized nutrition needs of each client group.

Nutritional needs may be affected due to medical conditions. They are also affected by changes in metabolism throughout a person's life cycle. While the basic nutrients and their functions remain constant throughout a lifetime, the amounts change based on our developmental stage or medical condition. This chapter will address menu planning for both the nutritional needs throughout the life cycle and the nutritional needs for medical or other personal conditions.

Menu Planning for Pregnancy

Pregnancy is not really the time to "eat for two." As a matter of fact, a mother who eats for just one and one-half will gain too much weight! The current recommendation is for women of normal weight to gain between 25 and 35 pounds during pregnancy. Underweight women should gain 28 to 40 pounds, and overweight women should gain 15 to 25 pounds. These weights are the most appropriate to produce a baby of optimal size: between six and one-half to nine pounds. In addition, optimal weight gain supports a healthy outcome for both mother and infant. Inadequate weight gain during pregnancy is associated with premature birth. Overweight women run a higher risk for pregnancy-related complications, such as hypertension, gestational diabetes (a blood sugar disorder that occurs during pregnancy), and stillbirths.

Most women gain approximately three pounds during the first three months (also called the first trimester) and one pound a week thereafter. A woman's weight gain is distributed as follows for a total weight gain of 22 to 28 pounds:

Fetus . . . . .6½ to 9 pounds

Placenta . . . . .1½ pounds

Amniotic fluid. . . . . .2 pounds

Increase in size of uterus, breast, & blood volume. . . . . .9 pounds

Fat . . . . .2-8 pounds

The developing infant is called a fetus. The placenta is a new organ that develops in the first month of pregnancy and provides an exchange of nutrients and wastes between the fetus and the mother. The amniotic fluid is the fluid surrounding the fetus. This stage of development does require increased amounts of some nutrients.

Energy, Protein and Fat

Energy needs increase during pregnancy and lactation. During the second trimester, women should eat an additional 300 calories per day. During the third trimester, women should eat approximately 425 more calories per day. Those amounts are similar to the increase for lactating women with 330 calories more per day during the first six months and 400 calories per day for the second six months. Protein increases by 25 grams for a total of 71 grams per day. Since many women already exceed the Dietary Reference Intake—Recommended Dietary Allowances (DRI-RDA) of protein, it may not be necessary to add additional protein. A woman who follows a vegetarian diet or eats very little meat and dairy products may need to increase sources of protein in the diet. While fat sources should be monitored as much in pregnancy and lactation as in the normal diet, it is important to consume adequate amount of essential fatty acids such as omega-3. Eating foods such as high-fat fish (salmon, tuna, mackerel), nuts, seeds, and using polyunsaturated oils such as soybean oil is important for healthy growth in the fetus. See Figure 12.1 for a summary of the changes of key nutrient requirements during pregnancy and lactation.

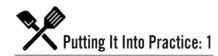

Putting It Into Practice: 1

Following the increase in calorie recommendation for pregnancy, what foods would you add to a general menu throughout the day and why?

(Check your answer at the end of the chapter)

Figure 12.1   Key Nutrient Changes for Pregnant and Lactating Women

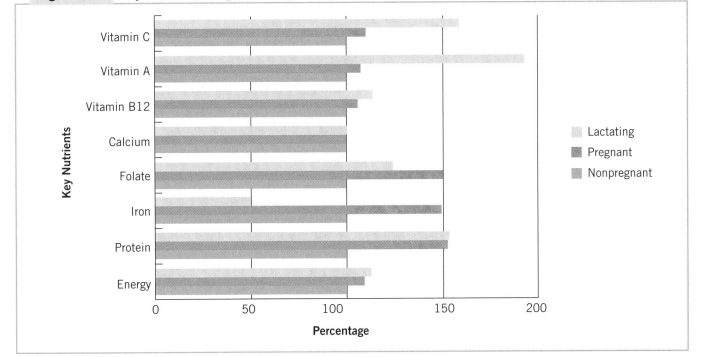

Minerals of Special Interest

The DRI-RDA for iron in pregnancy takes a big jump, from 18 mg to 27 mg per day. Iron is essential for producing the extra blood volume required to nourish a developing fetus. In addition, the fetus stores the extra iron during development, so that after birth, an infant has adequate iron stores to last about four to six months. Since many women do not have adequate iron stores when they become pregnant, an iron supplement is recommended during pregnancy.

Inadequate calcium intake by pregnant women can result in fetal bone development at the expense of the mother's bone health. A pregnant woman with inadequate calcium intake may actually lose calcium from her own bones to build the baby's bones. While the DRI-RDA for calcium does not change for pregnancy, maintaining adequate intake becomes particularly critical. A woman whose diet does not include adequate milk and other dairy products may need a calcium supplement.

Vitamins of Special Interest

The need for folate increases 50 percent during pregnancy. It is needed to sustain the growth of new cells and the increase in blood volume during pregnancy. Folate is critical in the first four to six weeks of pregnancy (when most women don't even know they are pregnant) because the neural tube, the tissue in the embryo that develops into the brain and spinal cord, forms at this time. Without enough folate, birth defects of the brain and spinal cord, such as spina bifida, can occur. In spina bifida, parts of the spinal cord are not fused together properly, so gaps are present. Because of the importance of folate during pregnancy and the difficulty most women encounter trying to get adequate folate through diet, the Food and Drug Administration has required manufacturers of certain foods to fortify them with folate, and folate supplementation is generally recommended, even prior to conception. Women eating folate-fortified foods should not assume that these foods will meet all their folate needs. They should still seek out folate-rich foods, such as leafy green vegetables (spinach, cabbage, romaine), oranges and orange juice, dry beans, peas, and lentils.

Vitamin B12 works with folate to create new cells. Women who are vegans and exclude animal products should consume foods fortified in Vitamin B12 or take a vitamin supplement containing Vitamin B12.

It is important to note that the DRI-RDA for both vitamin A and vitamin C increase during pregnancy and lactation. Women should consume extra servings of fruit and vegetables during pregnancy and lactation. Figure 12.2 provides a daily food guide for pregnant and lactating women. The increase demand for some nutrients can be met through a balanced diet of fruits, vegetables, whole grains, lean meats, and low-fat dairy products. A simple approach is to add one extra serving from each food group to account for added nutrient needs.

The following tips can help in planning menus for pregnant women:

✓ Offer a varied and balanced selection of nutrient-dense foods. When there is such an increased need for so many nutrients, empty calories are rarely an acceptable choice.

✓ In addition to traditional meat entrees, provide some entrees based on legumes and/or grains and dairy products.

✓ Avoid frying foods and using rich sauces.

✓ Use low-fat milk and milk products.

✓ Use assorted fruits and vegetables in all areas of the menu, including appetizers, salads, entrees, and desserts.

✓ Use iodized salt to provide adequate iodine.

✓ Offer some iron-rich foods such as meats, egg yolk, seafood, green leafy vegetables, legumes, dried fruits, and whole grain and enriched breads and cereals.

✓ Offer foods rich with fiber such as legumes, whole grains, fruits, and vegetables.

✓ Use folate-fortified breads and cereals.

✓ To avoid mercury in fish, choose shrimp, light tuna, salmon, pollock and catfish. Avoid shark, swordfish, mackeral, and tilefish.

✓ Increase fluid intake when increasing fiber intake.

Various medical experts, including the U.S. Surgeon General, advise pregnant women to avoid alcohol during pregnancy. Alcohol can cause fetal alcohol syndrome, which exhibits itself as facial malformations and impaired development in children.

Dieting, particularly low-carbohydrate dieting, is not appropriate during pregnancy and may result in deformities. It has not been shown that caffeine and sugar substitutes adversely affect the fetus, but it is recommended to use these

Figure 12.2 Daily Food Guide for Pregnancy and Lactation

Food Group	Servings	Serving Size
Meat or Meat Alternative	6 during pregnancy to include 1 serving legumes 6 during lactation	1 oz. cooked lean meat, poultry, or fish 1 egg 1 oz. cheese ¼ cup cottage cheese ½ cup dried beans or peas 2 Tbsp. Peanut butter
Milk	3 during pregnancy 4 during lactation	1 cup yogurt, pudding or custard 1 to 1½ oz. cheese 1 to 1½ cups cottage cheese
Vegetables	3⁺ during pregnancy and lactation	½ cup cooked or juice 1 cup raw
Fruits	2⁺ during pregnancy and lactation	Portion commonly served, such as a medium apple or banana
Grain	6⁺ during pregnancy and lactation	1 slice whole grain or enriched bread 1 cup ready-to-eat cereal ½ cup cooked cereal or pasta ½ bagel or hamburger roll 6 crackers 1 small roll ½ cup rice or grits
Fats and Sweets*		Includes butter, margarine, salad dressings, mayonnaise, oils, candy, sugar, jams, jellies, syrups, soft drinks, and any other fats or sweets

* In general, the amount of these foods to use depends on the number of calories you require. Get essential nutrients in the other food groups first before choosing foods from this group.

substances in moderation. Furthermore, use of herbal supplements can be especially hazardous during this critical time, as some may interfere with hormonal balance or affect the developing fetus. A pregnant woman considering use of herbal supplements should first seek advice from a qualified health professional. During pregnancy, several diet-related changes and complaints are common and may require changes in menu planning as shown in Figure 12.3.

Lactation

Lactation, also called breast feeding, substantially increases the mother's needs for many nutrients, such as protein, calcium, phosphorus, and magnesium, as these nutrients are secreted into the milk. Because a mother typically produces less milk during the second six months of an infant's life (about 20 ounces per day versus 25 ounces per day in earlier months), nutrition needs for that period

Figure 12.3 **Pregnancy Conditions That May Effect Menu Planning**

Condition	Menu Adjustment
Nausea and Vomiting May be due to hormonal changes during pregnancy	Dietary advice in the past has concentrated on frequent, small, carbohydrate-rich meals. Recent advice allows women to eat whatever food they think will stay down.
Taste Changes and Cravings May result from hormonal changes	Some women may develop an aversion to certain foods such as meats, strong smelling vegetables, or caffeinated drinks, or, they may request salty or sweet foods.
Constipation The GI tract slows down and begins relaxing during pregnancy	Some women may need to increase their fiber and fluid intake.
Heartburn Is caused by the growing fetus crowding the stomach; the muscle that controls the passage of food into the stomach also relaxes	Some women may need small, frequent meals, avoiding caffeine, or not lying down after eating. They may need to sleep with their head elevated.

may be somewhat lower. During lactation, mothers need 500 extra calories a day, and plenty of fluids (typically 8-10 cups per day). If the mother is not eating well, the quantity of milk may be adversely affected. Small amounts of caffeine are acceptable. Very little or no alcohol is advised.

Feeding and Menu Planning for Infants

The nutrient needs of a newborn are very high due to a rate of growth that will never again be duplicated. Babies actually triple their weight by the end of the first year; weight doubles in just the first four months. For the first four to six months, the only food necessary is mother's milk or infant formula. Figure 12.4 provides feeding guidelines for this period. Breast milk is the food of choice for infants. Besides these benefits, breast milk provides some protection from later development of food allergies, asthma, and possibly even cardiovascular disease. As compared with bottle-feeding, breast feeding promotes better tooth and jaw alignment.

Formula

Infant formula is made to resemble breast milk (except formula has added vitamin D and breast milk doesn't) and all formulas must meet nutrient standards set by the American Academy of Pediatrics. Formulas come in three different forms: ready-to-feed, liquid concentrate, and powdered. Infant feedings must be handled in a sanitary manner to prevent contamination and food-borne illness. If a baby is allergic to the protein in milk-based commercial formulas, there are other special formulas, such as soy-based formulas, that can be used. Supplemental fluoride drops are recommended for infants receiving breast milk or formulas prepared with non-fluoridated water. Fluoride is important to form healthy, strong teeth that are resistant to decay. Breast-fed babies also may need vitamin D supplementation, as breast milk is a poor source.

Semi-Solid Foods

A baby is ready to eat semisolid foods such as hot cereal when he can sit up and open his mouth for them. This usually occurs between four and six months of age. Some other signs that the baby is ready to begin spoon-feeding are when the baby:

✓ has doubled his/her birth weight, or

✓ drinks more than a quart of formula per day, or

✓ often seems hungry

The food guide for infants in Figure 12.4 shows the order in which foods should be introduced. The first solid food is iron-fortified baby cereal mixed with breast milk or formula. Rice cereal is usually offered first because it is the grain least likely to cause an allergic reaction. Cereals should not be put in the infant's bottle unless advised by a physician for a special-needs infant. Once the baby is accustomed to various cereals, strained vegetables and fruits may be introduced. New foods should be added to the infant's diet one at a time (and in small quantities) so that if there is an allergic reaction, you will know which food caused the reaction. Babies adjust differently to new tastes and new textures. If the baby does not like a certain food, offer it a week or two later. Always try new foods when the baby is hungry, such as at the beginning of the meal. While solid foods should not be introduced too early, it is important to introduce them when an infant is ready. A child who is not weaned appropriately may miss iron-rich foods in the diet and later develop iron-deficiency anemia.

Juices

Fruit juice that is fortified with vitamin C can be started about the fifth month. Although some babies get two or more bottles a day of apple juice (or other type of juice), it is a good idea to limit juice to one-half cup or four fluid ounces daily. Sometimes a baby who drinks too much juice starts drinking less mother's milk or formula. Another problem can occur when a baby goes to sleep with a bottle in her mouth. The natural sugars in the juice can cause devastating tooth decay, which is called nursing bottle syndrome. This can also result from sleeping with a bottle of formula in the mouth, as formula contains monosaccharides, which favor tooth decay. By ten months of age, an infant may be ready to begin drinking juice from a cup. Fruit-flavored beverages and soft drinks should not be given because the baby needs the vitamin C found in most juices. Unless the juice is labeled 100 percent juice, there may be added sugars and other ingredients in the juice drink. Remember that the label "contains 100 percent daily Vitamin C" does not mean it is 100 percent juice. Beverages labeled "juice drink, cocktail, punch, sparkler, blend, or beverage" are usually not 100 percent juice. Read the label to see the actual percent juice contained in the beverage. If during an illness such as vomiting and diarrhea, a physician recommends feeding the baby an electrolyte replacement beverage, the beverage is appropriate only during the illness. Once the illness is resolved, the extra nutrients in these products may make the baby sick.

Figure 12.4 **Food Guide for Infants**

Age	Food	Amount
0-4 Months	Breast milk or formula*	21-29 oz. formula, 5-8 feedings daily or 6-8 nursings
4-6 Months	Breast milk or formula	27-39 oz. formula, 4-6 feedings daily or 4-5 nursings
	Iron-fortified infant cereal (usually starts at 5 months)	Give 1 Tbsp. with mother's milk or formula to start. Start with rice cereal. Give once or twice daily. Can work up to 1½ Tbsp. twice daily.
	Strained vegetables and fruits (usually starts at 6 months; introduce vegetables first)	Give 1-2 tsp. once or twice daily. First fruits can be applesauce, pears, peaches, and bananas. First vegetables can be carrots, squash, and sweet potatoes. Slowly increase to 2 Tbsp. twice daily.
	Fruit juice fortified with non-acid Vitamin C (usually starts at 5 months)	Start with 2 oz. watered-down juice, usually apple juice. Limit fruit juice to ½ cup daily.
6-9 Months	Breast milk or formula	30-32 oz. formula, 3-5 feedings daily or 3-5 nursings
	Iron-fortified infant cereal	3 Tbsp. plus mother's milk or formula twice daily
	Strained fruits & vegetables	3 Tbsp. twice daily
	Strained plain meats	1 to 2 Tbsp. twice daily
	Crackers, plain toast	When baby has teeth, offer these foods or teething biscuit after other foods are eaten.
9-12 Months	Breast milk or formula	24-32 oz. formula, 3-4 feedings daily or 3-5 nursings
	Fruit juice (Vitamin C fortified)	½ cup daily
	Iron-fortified infant cereal	3-4 Tbsp. plus mother's milk or formula twice daily
	Vegetables, cut up	3-4 Tbsp. twice daily
	Fruits, cut up	3-4 Tbsp. twice daily
	Meats, cut up	2-3 Tbsp. twice daily
	Egg yolk (usually at 10 months)	Mix with a little milk or add to cereal
	Egg white (usually at 12 months)	1 egg=1 serving of meat
	Bread and bread products	½ slice four times daily

Avoid the following foods in the first year because of possible allergic reactions: chocolate, nuts, berries, tomatoes, shellfish.

* *Physician may request iron-fortified formula by third or fourth month.*

Finger Foods

Before a baby can move on to finger foods, he has to be able to eat lumpy foods, control the location of the food in his mouth, move his jaw up and down to mash it, and control swallowing. At seven to ten months, a baby learns to grasp objects and can try picking up pieces of finger foods to transfer to the mouth. About this time infants can also start eating protein foods. Poultry and fish must be very tender, and meat will have to be chopped or cut very fine. Between 10 and 12 months of age, many infants are eating table foods with the family.

Foods to Avoid

Several foods should be avoided during the first year. Honey may be contaminated with harmful bacteria and may cause food-borne illness. Infants represent one of the groups that is most highly susceptible to food-borne illness, so this is not an advisable risk. Certain foods cause choking because they are just the right size to lodge in the throat. Examples include nuts, raisins, hot dogs, popcorn, grapes, and chunks of apple. The American Academy of Pediatrics recommends no hot dogs, peanuts, or hard candy until age three. If hot dogs are offered later, they should be sliced like coins. Certain foods are apt to cause allergies: milk, eggs, wheat, nuts, chocolate, shellfish, and soy. Whole milk may be offered after twelve months of age, but not earlier, according to the American Academy of Pediatrics.

Infant Calorie Needs

Between the ages of one and three, a child needs approximately 1,300 calories a day. Between ages four and six, needs jump to 1,800 calories and then to 2,000 calories for children between the ages of seven and ten. Growth, of course, increases the demand for all nutrients. Protein, calcium, phosphorus, magnesium, and zinc are of particular importance. Some of the nutrients taken in during childhood will actually be stored and used for the upcoming growth spurt. Foods containing few nutrients, such as cookies, candy and soda should not be encouraged during childhood; they contribute to poor nutrition and possible obesity. Even though the first cow's milk for an infant (12+ months) should be whole milk, the USDA recommends gradually changing from whole milk to lower fat dairy products such as 2 percent, 1 percent, or fat-free milk by age five.

After the first birthday, as a child's physical capabilities and desire for independence increase, he or she will become more capable of feeding himself. By 18 months, many children can successfully use a spoon without too much spilling. However, exploring food with fingers is an important part of a child's development, so plenty of finger food that a child can handle without utensils is appropriate. By 24 months, most of the child's teeth are in and most children can drink well from a cup.

Menu Planning for Preschoolers

Preschoolers exhibit some food-related behaviors that may alarm parents. For example, many toddlers go through food jags, when they want to eat just one food continually. Preschoolers also often pick at foods or refuse to eat vegetables or drink milk. Lack of variety and erratic appetites are typical of this age group. These menu planning tips deal with preschoolers' food habits:

✓ Offer meals and snacks on a regular schedule.

✓ Offer food in child-friendly portions. For a preschooler, the USDA suggests a typical portion size is about 2/3 of the usual adult portion. An even smaller portion may encourage a child to try a new food.

✓ Let the child participate in food selection and preparation.

✓ Make sure the child has appropriately sized utensils and can reach the table comfortably.

✓ Offer foods in a variety of ways such as raw, cooked, individually or mixed.

There are several factors that make planning a menu for preschoolers challenging. A child's mouth is more sensitive to hot and cold than an adult's, so serve foods warm, not hot. Avoid strong-flavored and highly salted foods because children have more taste buds than adults, so these foods may taste too strong to them. Smooth textured foods such as pea soup or mashed potatoes should not have any lumps, because children often find this disturbing. Offer simply prepared foods and avoid mixed dishes if the child prefers separate foods on the plate. Try to make sure each meal includes:

✓ one soft or moist food that is easy to chew

✓ one crisp or chewy food (important for developing chewing skills)

✓ one colorful food, such as carrot sticks

✓ two finger foods

Vegetables are more likely to be accepted if served raw and cut up as a finger food. If serving celery, however, be sure to take off the strings. When serving cooked vegetables, it is better to serve them under-cooked. For children who won't eat vegetables, you can also hide vegetables in tomato sauce on spaghetti, on pizza, and in chili. Soups and casseroles are great places to add vegetables. Child development professionals have stated that children need to try a new food seven times and maybe in different preparation methods before they will accept new foods.

Most preschoolers love carbohydrate-rich foods, including cereals, breads, and crackers, as they are easy to hold and chew. Use them often as snack foods. Cut fruit and vegetables also make good snacks. Let the preschooler spread peanut butter on crackers or use a spoon to eat yogurt. Snacks are important to preschoolers because they need to eat more often than adults to get the nutrients they need. They may enjoy smoothies made with yogurt and fresh or frozen fruit. Cottage cheese with fruit may be another good snack.

Before the age of four, at which time the skills to cut up food start to develop, serve foods in bite-size pieces that are either eaten as finger foods or with a

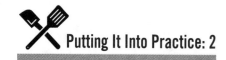

Putting It Into Practice: 2

Modify the following menu to meet the needs of preschoolers:

- Tator tot casserole
- Green beans
- Canned pears

(Check your answer at the end of the chapter)

spoon or fork. For example, cut meat into strips or use ground meat, cut fruit into wedges or slices, cut sandwiches into quarters, and serve pieces of raw vegetables instead of a mixed salad. Other good finger foods include cheese cut into sticks, wedges of hard-boiled eggs, dry ready-to-eat cereal, fish sticks, arrowroot biscuits, and graham crackers.

Menu Planning for School-Age Children

Among elementary school-age children, a few more nutritional considerations apply. Energy needs vary, depending on a child's age, size, activity, and pattern of growth. In general, it's important to understand that the entire growth process involves building new tissue at a rapid rate. This places many key nutrients in high demand, including protein, calcium, and iron. As a child grows, total protein requirements grow, too. The need for calcium remains stable at 800 mg per day from one year of age until 11 years of age, when it increases again. Consuming an adequate amount of calcium is very important at this time (and beyond), as it is essential for healthy bone growth. Adequate calcium in early years may also prevent osteoporosis in later years. Milk and milk products are an important source of calcium. Iron needs range from roughly 8 to 10 mg per day. According to current research, iron may be critical for brain development and functioning, as well as for red blood cell formation. Slight iron deficiency, before it reaches a stage that would be diagnosed as iron-deficiency anemia, may reduce attention span and intellectual performance. It may even have long-term effects on intellectual development.

Good snack choices are important for school-age children, as they do not always have the desire or the time to sit down and eat. Snacks can include fresh fruits and vegetables, juices, breads, unsweetened cereals, popcorn, tortillas, muffins, milk, yogurt, cheese, pudding, custard, sliced meats and poultry, eggs, or peanut butter.

According to the *Report of the DGAC on the Dietary Guidelines for Americans, 2010,* "The single most significant adverse health trend among U.S. children in the past 40 years has been the dramatic increase in overweight and obese children." There is strong research evidence to suggest that adolescents and school-age children should consume nutrient-dense, minimally processed foods and eat a healthy breakfast to combat this obesity trend. The following menu planning suggestions are from the DGAC:

✓ Greatly reduce intake of sugar-sweetened beverages

✓ Increase intake of vegetables and fruits

✓ Smaller amounts of fruit juice, especially for overweight children

✓ Smaller portions of foods and beverages

✓ Infrequent consumption of meals from quick service (fast food) restaurants

✓ Habitual consumption of breakfast

Another concern in childhood years is the prevalent concern of hyperactivity, or Attention Deficit Hyperactivity Disorder (ADHD). This is characterized by difficulty in paying attention and a certain amount of impulsive behavior. The condition is poorly understood, and both parents and educators find cause for

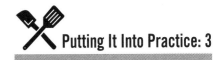

Putting It Into Practice: 3

Given the recommendation of the Report of the DGAC on the Dietary Guidelines for Americans, 2010, what would you recommend for breakfast for a school-age child?

(Check your answer at the end of the chapter)

concern when a child is diagnosed with ADHD. While pharmaceutical treatments are common, so is the belief that ADHD is a nutritional disorder—and that dietary restrictions can cure it. Dietary approaches include avoiding sugar and avoiding food colorings. Unfortunately, there is no dietary quick-fix for ADHD, and research has not confirmed the value of any dietary treatments for this condition.

Nutrition for Adolescents

The beginning of adolescence is marked by a growth spurt that results in physically mature adults. Most girls are in this rapid growth spurt by age 11. For boys, this spurt starts later, usually between 12 and 13 years of age. The growth spurt ends at about age 15 for girls and age 19 for boys. Both boys and girls get taller and heavier. Boys put on twice as much muscle as girls, while girls deposit more fat. During the adolescent growth spurt, approximately 20 percent of adult height and 50 percent of ideal body weight are gained.

Whereas parents are the main providers of food for young children, adolescents make many of their own food decisions. Of course, it helps to have healthy foods available to them to eat at home. Eating patterns of adolescents are influenced by peers, lifestyles, body image, popular media, and food preferences. Meal skipping (usually breakfast and/or lunch) and snacking are common. Although snack foods can be nutritious and make a contribution to the overall diet, popular teen snack foods may gravitate towards choices such as chips, cookies, candies, soft drinks, caffeinated energy drinks, and ice cream. Eating disorders often start during adolescence. **Anorexia nervosa**, self-induced starvation and highly distorted body image, is particularly common among adolescent girls. Another disorder called **bulimia** involves binge eating and forced vomiting. Both are unhealthy approaches to controlling weight and require intensive, long-term treatment.

Anorexia nervosa and bulimia are still nutritional concerns for adolescents. Another concern today is obesity. According to the *Report of the DGAC of the Dietary Guidelines for Americans Committee, 2010,* "among children and adolescents ages 2 through 19 years, 11.9 percent are at or above the 97th percentile of the body mass index (BMI) for age growth charts, 16.9 percent are at or above the 95th percentile, and 31.7 percent are at or above the 85th percentile. Again, minority children have a higher prevalence of both overweight and obesity."

Adolescents need four glasses of milk (or equivalent) daily and lots of high-iron foods such as meats, egg yolk, seafood, green leafy vegetables, legumes, dried fruits, whole grain and enriched breads and cereals. Teenagers often drink empty-calorie beverages, such as soft drinks and caffeinated energy drinks, instead of more nutritious choices such as milk or juice. Nutrients that may be lacking in an adolescent's diet include calcium, iron, vitamin A, vitamin C, and sometimes even calories and protein. Adolescent girls are at higher risk for nutritional deficiencies than boys because girls must get in more nutrients in fewer calories than boys. See Figure 12.5 for key nutrient changes from preteens to teens.

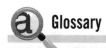

Glossary

Anorexia Nervosa
An eating disorder characterized by self-induced starvation and distorted body image

Bulimia
An eating disorder involving binging (eating large amounts of food) and then purging (forced vomiting or other methods of getting rid of the food)

Menu Planning for Adolescents

In planning menus for adolescents, it is a good idea to include nutritious snack choices that are portable and can be eaten on-the-run, such as:

✓ Small packages of nuts or sunflower seeds

✓ Fresh fruit

✓ Individually packaged, unsweetened cereals

✓ Mini muffins

✓ Mini bagels

✓ Yogurt

✓ Popcorn

✓ Fig bars

✓ Oatmeal raisin cookies

To meet the increased nutrient needs shown in Figure 12.5, consider the following:

✓ Fiber—whole grain pancakes or waffles with fruit, whole grain toast or muffins, cereals with fresh fruit, whole grain bagels with peanut butter

✓ Protein and iron—lean meats or fish

✓ Vitamin A and C—yellow vegetables, citrus fruits, tomatoes, and leafy greens combined in whole wheat tortillas with low-fat cheese

✓ Calories—Emphasize nutrient-dense foods such as nuts and seeds

Figure 12.5   Key Nutrient Changes for Pre-Adolescent to Teens

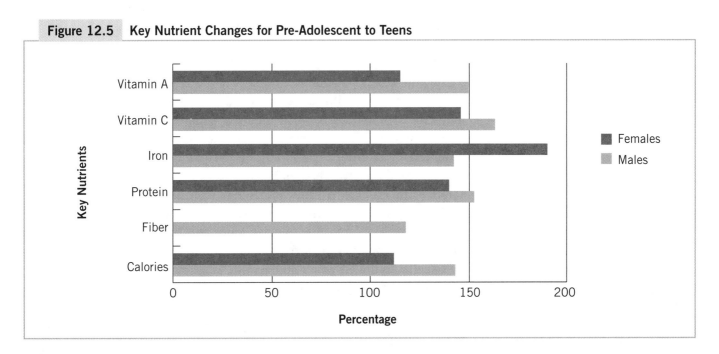

National School Lunch Program

Legislation that established the National School Lunch Program was signed by President Harry Truman in 1946. Through its National School Lunch Program, the USDA supports nutritious, low-cost or free breakfasts and lunches to more than 25 million children each school day. School districts and independent schools that choose to take part in the lunch program receive cash subsidies and donated commodities from the USDA for each meal they serve. In return, they must serve lunches that meet federal requirements, and they must offer free or reduced price lunches to eligible children. Schools can also be reimbursed for snacks served to children through age 18 in after-school educational or enrichment programs.

School lunches must meet the applicable recommendations of the Dietary Guidelines for Americans, with no more than 30 percent of calories from fat, and less than 10 percent from saturated fat. Regulations also establish a standard for school lunches to provide one-third of the DRI-RDA's for protein, vitamin A, vitamin C, iron, calcium, and calories. School lunches must meet federal nutrition requirements, but decisions about what specific foods to serve and how they are prepared are up to school foodservice administrators.

The last update for quality standards for school foodservice was 2000. With the epidemic of childhood obesity, Congress is currently reviewing the quality standards. In 2010, the USDA suggested changes that reflect the recommendations for school-age children: more fruits and vegetables, whole grain products, and less fat and sodium. Watch for changes in the reimbursement and commodity products along with the suggested menu changes.

Nutrition for the Elderly

Among the U.S. population, the number of older Americans is growing most quickly. As you have already read, the older population will escalate between the years 2010 and 2030, when the baby boom generation reaches age 65. With advances in medicine, average life spans are increasing. What does all this mean for a Certified Dietary Manager? Among other things, it means that a typical food service operation is likely to be serving more and more older adults. Numbers of elderly individuals in nursing homes are expected to triple within the next few decades. Correspondingly, the eldercare foodservice industry, which provides nutrition to older Americans through a variety of models (not just nursing homes), is growing quickly. To serve this client group well, it's essential to understand a number of changes that occur during the aging process—and the impact they have on nutrition.

Elderly is a loose term, and there is no defined age at which the body undergoes dramatic aging-related changes. What happens when we age? Metabolism changes and body systems and organs lose their peak efficiency. The rate of decline is typically very gradual, and shows great individual variation. Both genetic and environmental factors (such as nutrition) affect the rate of aging. Conversely, changes brought about by the aging process affect nutrition status. Of particular importance are those changes that affect digestion, absorption, and metabolism of nutrients.

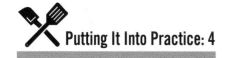

Putting It Into Practice: 4

Plan a portable snack for teenagers that would include calcium, iron, and fiber.

(Check your answer at the end of the chapter)

The basal metabolic rate (baseline energy requirement) declines about 5 percent each decade in adult life, and is accompanied by a 25 to 30 percent loss in muscle mass. Combined with a general decrease in activity level, these factors clearly indicate a need for decreased calorie intake, which generally does take place during aging. But the elderly don't have to lose all that muscle mass. Studies have shown that when the elderly do regular weight training exercises, they increase their muscular strength and basal metabolism, and improve appetite and blood flow to the brain. Overall, the functioning of the cardio-vascular system declines with age. The workload of the heart increases due to atherosclerotic deposits and less elasticity in the arteries. The heart does not pump as hard as before, and cardiac output is reduced in elderly people who do not remain physically active. Blood pressure increases normally with age. Lung capacity decreases by about 40 percent throughout life. This decrease does not restrict the normal activity of healthy, older persons but may limit vigorous exercise. Kidney function deteriorates over time, and the aging kidney is less able to excrete waste. Adequate fluid intake is very important, as is avoiding mega-doses of water-soluble vitamins because they put a strain on the kidneys to excrete them. Lastly, loss of bone occurs normally during aging, and osteoporosis is common.

Factors Affecting Nutrition Status

The nutrition status of an elderly person is greatly influenced by many variables, such as physiological, psychosocial, and socioeconomic factors, as outlined below.

Physiological Factors:

Illness. The presence of illness, both acute and chronic, and use of modified diets can affect nutrition status. The most prevalent nutrition-related problems of the elderly are chronic conditions that require therapeutic diets. Certain chronic diseases are associated with anorexia or loss of appetite. Examples include gastrointestinal disease, congestive heart failure, renal disease, neurological impairment, depression, and cancer. Other diseases, such as stroke, are not associated with anorexia but can affect ability to eat.

Caloric intake. An individual who adjusts caloric intake downwards to accompany decline in basal energy expenditure and muscle mass faces a new challenge: that of nutrient density. With even fewer calories, nutrient-dense food choices become increasingly crucial.

Dentition. Approximately 50 percent of Americans have lost their teeth by age 65. Despite widespread use of dentures, chewing still presents problems for many elderly people. According to the American Heart Association, poor oral health is linked to coronary heart disease.

Functional disabilities. Functional disabilities interfere with the ability of the elderly to perform daily tasks, such as the purchasing and preparation of food, and eating. These disabilities may be due to arthritis/rheumatism, stroke, visual impairment, heart trouble, or dementia (deterioration in mental functioning such as thinking and memory). One study reports that 39 percent of the elderly subjects need help food shopping and 26 percent need help making meals.

Taste and smell. Around age 60, there is a decline in the ability to taste and smell. Taste buds in the tongue are less sensitive, and the nerves in the nose that detect aromas need extra stimulation to detect smells. That's why seniors may find ordinarily seasoned foods too bland.

Changes in the gastrointestinal tract. The movement of food through the gastrointestinal tract slows down over the years, causing constipation, a frequent complaint of older people. Constipation may also be related to low fiber and fluid intake, medications, or lack of exercise. Other frequent complaints include nausea, indigestion, and heartburn. Intestinal changes typical of aging also reduce absorption of the vitamin B12 produced in the body.

Medications. More than half of seniors take at least one medication daily and many take six or more a day. Medications often alter appetite or the digestion, absorption, or metabolism of nutrients. More information about the effects of medications appears in Chapter 8.

Thirst. Many elderly people have a diminished perception of thirst that can cause problems, especially when they are not feeling well. Because the aging kidney is less able to concentrate the urine, more fluid is lost, setting the stage for dehydration.

Psychosocial Factors:

Ability to think. Poor thinking may affect nutrition—or perhaps poor nutritional status is contributing to poor thinking. If an elderly person is confused part of the time, this can affect meal patterns.

Social support. An individual's nutritional health results in part from a series of social acts. The purchasing, preparation, and eating of foods are social events for most people. For example, elderly people may rely upon each other for a ride to the supermarket, cooking, or sharing meals. The benefits of social networks or support are largely due to the companionship and emotional support they provide. This support can have a positive effect on appetite and dietary intake.

Socioeconomic Factors:

Education. Higher levels of education are positively associated with increased nutrient intakes.

Income. Money spent on food is a significant predictor of dietary quality.

Living arrangements. The elderly, particularly women, are more likely to be widowed. The trend has been for widows and widowers in the U.S. to live alone after the spouse dies. Research indicates that living alone is a risk factor for dietary inadequacy for older men, especially those over 75 years of age, and for women only in the youngest age group (55 to 64 years old).

Availability of federally funded meals. The availability of nutritious meals through federal programs such as Meals-on-Wheels, in which meals are delivered to the home, is crucial to the nutritional health of many elderly people. Many communities also have Senior Centers that provide meals, and educational and social programs.

Figure 12.6 Menu Planning Techniques for the Elderly

Technique	Special Considerations
Serve moderately sized meals	Healthy older adults have a slower metabolism and need to reduce calories. They also hate to see food wasted.
Add complex carbohydrate and high-fiber foods	Older people requiring softer diets will prefer high-fiber foods that are soft in texture such as cooked beans and peas, bran cereals soaked in milk, oatmeal, canned fruits, and cooked vegetables.
Use fat sparingly	Use lean meats and low-fat dairy products.
Offer adequate protein	To help balance the budget, offer lower-cost protein sources such as dried beans and peas, cottage cheese, macaroni and cheese, eggs, liver, Greek yogurt. Add nonfat dry milk to gravies.
Use herbs and spices to make foods flavorful	The sense of taste decreases with age so adding herbs and spices will make food more appealing.
Provide variety	Include traditional menu items as well as ethnic and regional cuisine.
Encourage fluid intake	Offer a variety of beverages such as flavored coffees and teas or liquid foods such as soup, ices, and gelatin desserts or fruit flavored water. Limit caffeine intake, which may be dehydrating.
Make sure foods are nutrient dense	Older people need fewer calories but the same or added nutrients such as vitamin D, calcium, and zinc. Make sure snacks and desserts are nutrient dense by reducing fat and sugar and adding complex carbohydrates.

Menu Planning for the Elderly

Basic guidelines for menu planning for older adults need to address a range of factors. They need to stimulate eating through aroma, taste, and visual appeal. They need to provide nutrient-dense choices, and adapt comfortably to any physical limitations. If chewing is a problem, menus must offer softer foods. Chapter 5 presents guidelines for offering a mechanical soft diet, which may be helpful. Figure 12.6 includes some other useful techniques and ideas for meal planning.

At Risk Populations

Individuals in various states of illness are at risk for developing nutritional problems. For example, a patient who has cancer may suffer loss of appetite along with increased nutrient needs due to the demands of a growing tumor. Experts estimate that in nursing homes, 17-65 percent of clients are affected with some degree of protein and calorie malnutrition. A client of a nursing home who is unable to move about may be at risk for developing pressure ulcers. Sound nutrition is crucial for protecting against this common problem. An individual who has difficulty swallowing, or one who is afflicted with Alzheimer's disease may not be able to consume adequate amounts of food. Some of your clients need to follow sodium restrictions. Others are following diets that are controlled for saturated fat and cholesterol. Others are following portion-controlled diets for management of diabetes. Yet others are eating pureed foods.

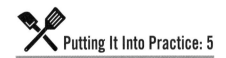 **Putting It Into Practice: 5**

How would you change the following menu to meet the menu planning suggestions in Figure 12.6?

- Pork chops and gravy
- Tossed salad with carrots, radishes, celery
- Mashed potatoes
- Lemon meringue pie

(Check your answer at the end of the chapter)

Interestingly, two extremes in age also present another type of food-related risk—that of food-borne illness. The FDA identifies certain populations as being more susceptible to contracting food-borne illness. These include pre-school age children and older adults. Within these groups, immune response may not be as strong as it is during other phases of the life cycle. Sound food safety and sanitation becomes even more crucial in serving these populations. How can you manage menu planning in a way that you will be able to serve it to all these clients and meet their unique needs?

Overall Menu Planning Guidelines

A menu must meet the nutritional needs of your clients, regardless of what growth stage or wellness stage they are in. It must supply adequate calories, protein, carbohydrate, fat, vitamins, minerals, and fluid. There may be specific nutritional standards for meal programs:

✓ USDA school lunch program

✓ senior congregate meal sites

✓ preschool childcare centers

✓ correctional facilities

In most of these settings, as well as in many healthcare facilities, a common standard for nutritional evaluation is the DRI-RDA. An analysis of the DRI-RDA is most effective when it spans a period of days. For example, if there is a seven-day cycle menu, we can analyze the percent of DRI-RDAs met for key nutrients, including vitamins and minerals, as averaged over seven days. This is a cumbersome task, and is best accomplished with the help of computer software designed for nutrient analysis. DRI-RDAs are designed for application to groups of people. However, DRI-RDA values vary based on age and sex. It is best to select the standards most representative of the group being served.

Another tool that will help you know if your menus comply with the Dietary Guidelines for Americans is the myPyramid model. There are models for ethnic groups, child care, and older Americans. To verify your menu compliance, simply total the number of servings in each group and compare it with the myPyramid recommendations. With certain therapeutic diets, it is not always possible to meet all nutritional needs. For example, you learned in Chapter 5 that a typical clear liquid diet is lacking in protein and calories as well as major vitamins and minerals. Unless liquid nutritional supplements are incorporated, a full liquid menu may be inadequate in key nutrients.

There are many other factors involved with the menu planning process. This textbook only addresses the nutritional factors. See the chapter in *Managing Foodservice and Food Safety* that addresses menu planning.

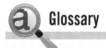

Glossary

Fixed Menu
A menu that doesn't change from day to day such as what is found in restaurants

Cycle Menu
A menu that repeats itself over a defined period of time)

Single Use Menu
Menus used for special meals that are not repeated

Selective Menu
An adaptation of a cycle menu where clients have the opportunity to make choices or selections in advance of meal service

Types of Menus

There are three common types of menus: Fixed, Cycle, and Single Use. The most common menu planning tool in the institutional setting is called a **cycle menu**. It is a menu that repeats itself over a defined period of time. You will have different menu cycles for different facilities. For instance, in a hospital, because the client doesn't stay as long, you might have a four, five, six, or seven-day cycle menu. In a long-term care setting or a school foodservice, you would want a much longer cycle menu such as four, five, or six week cycle. An odd-week cycle, such as five days or five weeks, often works better so the client doesn't notice that roast turkey is served every fourth day or week.

A **fixed menu** is often found in restaurants. The menu is the same every day. Some healthcare facilities have adopted the fixed menu. The **single use menu** is a menu planned for a special occasion or a specific day such as a Mother's Day Brunch or a Chinese New Year. These are often called monotony breakers to help break up the monotony of a cycle menu.

In order to meet the many needs of clients today, healthcare facilities are adopting a **selective menu**. This is an adaptation of the cycle menu where clients have the opportunity to make choices or selections in advance of meal service.

Diet Spreadsheets

In a facility serving clients who follow a variety of therapeutic diets, a menu must be versatile enough to provide nutritious, satisfying meals on every diet. This detail is mapped out on a diet spreadsheet. A diet spreadsheet displays the menu offerings and portion sizes for each diet, for each meal, and for each day of the cycle menu. Figure 12.7 shows a segment of a diet spreadsheet for a lunch meal. Note that with the trend in liberalization of therapeutic diets in healthcare, diet spreadsheets are developed to be as simple as possible, with no more restriction than is therapeutically necessary. At the same time, the strategy of making all menus "healthy" means that menu planners strive to limit total fat, saturated fat, cholesterol, and sodium in even a general (unrestricted) diet. Implementing healthful guidelines may also mean providing a variety of fruits and vegetables, including high-fiber foods in a menu, and more. Thus, a healthy "general" diet emerges that may be suitable for certain therapeutic needs as well.

In all, the goal is to keep a list of therapeutic diets reasonably short. This can lead to optimal health for all clients, while providing the best possible range of choices for each client. Management considerations apply, too. It is ideal to plan a menu in which many products are common to all diets. This minimizes the need to produce many different products at once, and also minimizes food waste, which is essential to controlling food costs. Sometimes, portion sizes vary among diets. Unique portion sizes are specified on the menus. A foodservice operation must be able to produce foods on a given menu in a manner that meets standards for quality and budget, while accommodating the unique therapeutic and nutritional needs of each client.

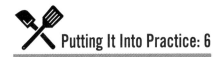

Putting It Into Practice: 6

At an assisted living facility, foodservice employees take orders in the dining room each day. Clients are offered two entreé choices for each meal. What type of menu is this?

(Check your answer at the end of the chapter)

Figure 12.7   Segment of a Diet Spreadsheet—Lunch For Cycle Day 3

General Diet	Sodium Controlled Diet	Diabetic Diet	Renal Diet	Pureed Diet	Full Liquid Diet
Tossed salad w/ low-fat dressing	Tossed salad w/ low-fat dressing	Tossed salad w/ low-fat dressing	Tossed salad w/ low-sodium dressing x 2	½ cup pureed vegetable medley	1 cup strained cream of chicken soup
Roast turkey sandwich: 3 oz. turkey on wheat bun with lettuce and tomato	Roast turkey sandwich: 3 oz. turkey on wheat bun with lettuce and tomato	Roast turkey sandwich: 3 oz. turkey on wheat bun with lettuce and tomato	Roast turkey sandwich: 3 oz. turkey on wheat bun with lettuce and low-sodium mayonnaise	Pureed turkey and noodle portion with parsley flakes	
Assorted fresh fruit	Assorted fresh fruit	Assorted fresh fruit	Fresh apple	½ cup pink applesauce	1 cup strained fruit juice
Cookie	Cookie	½ cup sugar-free gelatin	½ cup regular gelatin [count in fluid restriction]	½ cup regular gelatin	½ cup regular gelatin
Coffee, tea, or beverage of choice	Coffee, tea, or beverage of choice	Coffee, tea, or beverage of choice	½ cup fruit punch [Count in fluid restriction]	Coffee, tea, or beverage of choice	Coffee, tea, or beverage of choice
Skim or low-fat milk	Skim or low-fat milk	Skim or low-fat milk	Potassium and sodium free candy as desired, e.g. gum drops	Skim or low-fat milk	1 cup milkshake
Condiments as desired	Mayo, sugar, pepper, herb-based sodium-free seasoning as desired (No potassium-based salt substitute without a physician's order)	Sugar substitute, salt, pepper as desired	Low-sodium mayonnaise, herb-based sodium-free seasoning, sugar, pepper as desired (no potassium-based salt substitute without a physicians order)	Condiments as desired	Condiments as desired
Notes	Note that if a fresh roast turkey product low in sodium is used, the same meat is appropriate on sodium-controlled menus	Adjust portion sizes of bread, fruit, and milk if needed for specific meal pattern or carbohydrate count	Mayonnaise is not reduced for fat, as fat is an important source of calories in a renal diet. Omit tomato because it is high in potassium; add low-sodium mayonnaise for extra fat calories.	Adjust consistency of products as needed to meet individualized orders for national dysphagia diet.	

Another consideration in menu planning is providing thickened liquids for some therapeutic diets. For example, including chilled, thickened water at bedside may increase hydration. There are different degrees for thickened liquids, such as honey or nectar. You will also need to work with others in your facility to make sure that your clients are receiving appropriate thickened liquids throughout the day.

Aesthetic Concerns

As we know, nutrition is not just a matter of nutrients. Thus, engineering menus to meet diet orders alone is not enough. A Certified Dietary Manager also needs to ensure that menus as planned and served are enjoyable, appealing, and satisfying to clients. Ultimately, the appeal of a menu can have a great effect on nutritional well-being of clients. Many therapeutic diet restrictions make this a special challenge. One example is a pureed diet. Simply puréeing foods and spooning them into dishes does not make for an appealing meal.

Certified Dietary Managers can use a number of approaches to improve the aesthetic value of pureed foods. For example: puree whole entrees (rather than individual components) to provide appealing flavors; form pureed foods into molds; add a thickening agent to pureed foods to form a souffle, or layer pureed meats, sauces, and noodles to form lasagna. This can be sliced and presented on a plate, offering a more eye-appealing presentation. Add garnishes, gravies, and sauces to make them look pleasing and interesting.

A mechanical soft diet is another meal type in which modified consistency may require attention to look attractive. Some foods appropriate for this diet are easy to handle, such as a tuna noodle casserole or ground beef pie. However, a roast meat that is chopped for a mechanical soft diet may need a sauce, a gravy, and/or a garnish. Another diet that presents challenges is a sodium-controlled diet. Anyone who is accustomed to high-sodium foods and table salt may have difficulty adjusting to the blandness of this diet. Once again, it is not enough to simply prepare recipes without salt. For flavor, other seasonings need to take the place of salt. A Certified Dietary Manager can incorporate seasonings such as herbal blends, spices, lemon juice, low-sodium sauces, and other low sodium seasonings to improve enjoyment. Garnishes, such as the simple parsley sprig, lemon wedge, or carved vegetable can cast a very positive impression of food.

All menus should provide variety in color, shapes, and texture (as possible) to create a positive presentation on a tray. Theme meals, special events involving food, and the dining environment itself contribute greatly to enjoyment of meals. It is up to a Certified Dietary Manager to think creatively and apply culinary skills to assure that special diets do not look and feel like deprivation to clients. Instead, all meals should be able to hold their own with respect to aesthetic value.

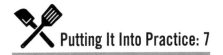

Putting It Into Practice: 7

What would you add to the following therapeutic diet to enhance the appearance and taste?

- Pureed scrambled eggs
- Pureed sausage
- Pureed biscuit
- Thickened orange juice

(Check your answer at the end of the chapter)

Regulatory Issues

In long-term care facilities subject to Centers for Medicare & Medicaid Services (CMS) regulations, some specific advice applies to menu planning. The menu planning considerations include the following:

✓ Each client receives, and facility provides, at least three meals daily, at regular times comparable to normal mealtimes in the community.

✓ There must be no more than 14 hours between a substantial evening meal and breakfast the following day (or 16 hours if a nourishing snack is provided at bedtime).

✓ An evening meal should provide at least 20 percent of the day's total nutritional requirements.

✓ The facility must offer snacks at bedtime daily.

✓ Food is attractive and palatable, incorporating needs as identified through observation, client and staff interviews, and review of client council minutes.

✓ If a food group is missing from the client's daily diet, the facility has an alternative means of satisfying the client's nutrient needs.

✓ Substitutes of similar nutritive value are offered to clients who refuse food served.

CMS regulations emphasize clients' rights—their options to exert control over their own care. This certainly extends to meals and menus. Both the menu as planned and the manner in which Certified Dietary Managers implement it must address these rights. If a client specifically refuses a food or requests a substitute, it is up to the Certified Dietary Manager to be of service in every way that is practical. If the facility uses a nonselective menu, it is especially important to make alternates available upon request. A client also has the right to refuse treatment, including a therapeutic diet. In making choices, a client should be well informed. It is up to the Certified Dietary Manager to work with other members of the healthcare team, as needed, to review any diet-related concerns and assure that clients' rights are being honored. In long-term care, a client council is a committee composed of clients who provide feedback and suggestions about care—including dietary services. In other institutional settings, there may be a similar body of clients. In a university, for example, there may be a council of students and/or other patrons who provide comments and suggestions for menu planning. A Certified Dietary Manager must solicit and respond to input from client groups such as these when planning menus and serving meals.

Menu Planning for Nutritional Support

The dual role of meeting nutritional needs and satisfying the personal menu requests of your clients is a challenge. Some degree of protein and calorie malnutrition is strikingly prevalent in today's healthcare facilities, so your job is essential. Supporting sound nutrition can reduce complications and improve outcomes for nearly every medical treatment imaginable—from surgery to cancer treatment to healing of fractures and more. **Nutrition support** is a general term describing providing foods and liquids to improve nutritional status and supporting good medicine.

Glossary

Nutrition Support
General term describing providing food and liquids to improve nutritional status and supporting good medicine

Enteral Nutrition
Feeding or formulas, by mouth or by tube, into the gastrointestinal tract

In the hospital or nursing facility, there are always some clients in poor nutritional status, or with high nutrient needs, whose diets simply do not meet their nutritional requirements. These clients are often in need of concentrated sources of nutrition. **Enteral nutrition** refers to the feeding, by mouth or by tube, of formulas that contain essential nutrients. It requires that the gastrointestinal tract be functioning. The most simple form of nutritional support is a high-protein, high-calorie diet. Generally, there are two approaches to providing added protein and calories. One is to use conventional foods, selecting those that are particularly nutrient-dense. Another is to add commercial nutritional supplements to menus.

Each has its pros and cons. Conventional foods have the advantage of familiarity, and are often readily accepted by clients. To make effective dietary recommendations, it is important to complete a diet history and discuss food tastes, preferences, and tolerances with a client. This helps to identify good candidates for menu enhancements. Figure 12.8 lists examples of simple menu planning techniques that can add calories to foods. When there is a nutritional problem, there may also be changes in appetite, taste sensation, or chewing ability. There may be mouth sores or other factors that affect nutrient intake. Consider these together to devise a workable solution. For example, a client undergoing cancer therapy may find the aromas of hot foods distressing. Here, it may be helpful to substitute chilled items for hot entrees. One client may enjoy a cottage cheese and fruit plate more than a hot meatloaf sandwich. Very large serving sizes and

---

Figure 12.8 Menu Planning Techniques for Nutrition Support

- Use margarine liberally on bread, toast, vegetables, rice, pasta, and in sandwiches.
- Add gravies or sauces to entrees and side dishes.
- Add sour cream to potatoes, casseroles, and fruits.
- Use whipped cream on top of desserts and fruits.
- Add 2 tablespoons dried milk powder to each cup of whole milk. Use for drinking and when making cream soups, hot cereal, pudding, custard, hot chocolate, mashed potatoes, casseroles, milkshakes, and creamed dishes.
- Add dried milk powder to scrambled eggs, gravies, casseroles, meatloaf, and meatballs.
- Spread peanut butter on toast or English muffins, on crackers and cookies, and on apple slices and celery sticks.
- Add cheese to sandwiches, scrambled eggs, casseroles, vegetables, and sauces.
- Add chopped eggs and diced or ground meat to salads, sauces, casseroles, and sandwiches.
- Use mayonnaise liberally on sandwiches.
- Choose desserts such as custard, bread pudding, rice pudding, and fruited yogurt. Serve with whipped cream or ice cream.
- Offer whole milk products or cream in place of skim milk or, offer milkshakes as beverages.
- Cook cream soups or hot cereal with whole milk; add margarine or butter.
- Serve six small meals rather than three large ones.
- Add ice cream to enteral products as a milkshake.
- Use enteral pudding supplements as a topping for cake desserts.
- Use olive oil or flavored oils to potatoes and vegetables.

packed meal trays can be overwhelming to a person whose appetite or ability to eat is limited. The visual impact of a tray should feel comfortable to a client.

Also consider lactose tolerance when using conventional foods to boost protein and calories. Many typical choices involve dairy products. If a client is not accustomed to these or has lactose intolerance, discomfort may ensue. Increase dairy products in the diet slowly, and monitor tolerance. If lactose creates concerns, consider lactose-free alternatives, or incorporate a commercial lactose-free supplement.

Specialized commercial products exist for providing nutrition support. A standard enteral formula provides one calorie per milliliter (ml); about 240 ml equals one cup. A complete enteral product contains a nutritional balance of protein, carbohydrates, fat, vitamins, and minerals. Some products are modified in carbohydrate content for routine use by individuals with diabetes. Highly specialized enteral formulas exist for patients in liver failure, renal failure, or pancreatic illness.

Many enteral formulas are flavored so they can be taken orally to supplement intake of ordinary food. This is helpful for an individual who needs a high-calorie, high-protein diet and is not able to eat enough food to provide these nutrients. Commercial nutritional supplements offer several advantages over conventional foods. Complete nutritional supplements provide controlled and measured amounts of nutrients. When a client is not able to consume a variety of foods, these products offer one means of assuring adequate nutrition. In addition, they are available with key dietary modifications, such as lactose-free formulations, high-fiber formulations, and so forth. Commercial products are available in calorically dense concentrations, in ranges from one to two calories per ml of liquid product. This means an eight-ounce glass of a supplement may provide about 240-480 calories—a significant nutritional addition to a diet.

Disadvantages to commercial supplements include acceptance and cost. Client acceptance may vary, as clients may perceive a flavor described as "medicinal" or tasting "like vitamin supplements." On the other hand, these products are available in a variety of flavors and textures that may help to overcome this drawback. When offering commercial supplements, it's helpful to allow a client to taste several products and choose what seems most enjoyable. A client may also need variety in supplement flavors and textures, just as with conventional foods. Many commercial supplements taste best when chilled, rather than served at room temperature. It is also possible to combine commercial products with conventional foods. For example, a client who does not enjoy a liquid supplement may enjoy a milkshake made from the supplement plus ice cream. For clients who prefer it—or for certain dysphagia diets—specialized nutritional pudding products represent another choice. Pudding supplements that are nutritionally similar to liquid products are available. A garnish of whipped cream, chocolate shavings, or fruit may also make these products more appealing.

Incomplete nutritional supplements offer another way to boost nutritional intake. For example, a product of carbohydrate powder with minimal flavor can

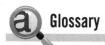

Glossary

Tube Feeding
Enteral feeding given through a tube

be stirred into beverages, soups, applesauce, and other foods to add almost invisible calories. This type of product does not provide protein. Therefore, it can be added to foods on a renal diet to boost calories without breaching a protein restriction. Yet another commercial product is a protein powder, which may be added to mashed potatoes, hot cereal, soup, or other products to boost protein content. If a client has developed an aversion or intolerance to meats and other high-protein foods, this can be a means of boosting protein content in the diet. As compared with a conventional dry milk powder, a commercial protein additive can be low in lactose.

A disadvantage of commercial nutritional supplements is that they tend to be more expensive than conventional foods. In many healthcare situations, third-party insurers reimburse for nutritional supplements if they are specified in physicians' diet orders. Another disadvantage may be how the commercial nutritional supplements are handled in your facility. In some facilities, the pharmacist or nursing orders them, and in others, they are ordered through dietary. Make sure your facility has a policy and procedure on who is responsible for these supplements from the ordering to serving. The Certified Dietary Manager should monitor that the supplements are actually presented to the client in a timely manner and are consumed. Some may need assistance to open them and encouragement to consume them. A list of formulas available should be maintained.

Tube Feeding

When drinking an enteral feeding is not possible or practical, enteral feedings may be given through a tube. This type of enteral feeding is called a **tube feeding**. Tube feedings are given through a pliable tube, most often inserted through the nose in a nonsurgical procedure. A common tube enters from the nasal cavity directly into the stomach. This is called a nasogastric (NG) tube. If the tube is passed to the intestine, it may be either a nasoduodenal (ND) tube (the tube ends at the duodenum) or a nasojejunal (NJ) tube (the tube ends at the jejunum). Feeding tubes can also be inserted, when necessary, through surgically created openings in the esophagus (esophagostomy), stomach (gastrostomy), or jejunum (jejunostomy). These types of tube feedings may be necessary for clients who will need to be fed enterally for long periods of time, such as three to six months. Figure 12.9 shows sites of feeding tubes and semi-permanent openings for tubes. Tube feedings may be used in clients:

✓ who are not able to swallow or take food by mouth, such as after head/neck surgery, stroke, trauma; or due to inflammation.

✓ whose caloric and protein needs are greater than can be ingested orally (such as with cancer or burns), and attempts to provide adequate nutrition through food and oral supplements have been unsuccessful.

✓ who have medical conditions that require modified diets the client can't tolerate orally (e.g. an elemental diet in which proteins are provided as amino acids, such as for treatment of Crohn's disease or pancreatitis).

✓ who will not eat (such as anorexia nervosa).

✓ who are in a coma (nasogastric route is not used).

In cases where the gastrointestinal tract is not functioning, enteral nutrition is not an appropriate choice.

Tube feedings can be administered continuously or intermittently. A pump is often used to administer continuous drip feedings over a 12-24 hour period. This type of feeding allows more formula to be given and decreases the chances of diarrhea. Once tube feeding tolerance is well established, a feeding may be changed to an intermittent schedule. Intermittent feedings or bolus feedings are usually given four to six times each day by gravity drip for a period of 30 to 60 minutes. One advantage of intermittent feedings is that they give the client freedom of movement between feedings. For jejunal feedings, which enter low in the gastrointestinal tract, intermittent feedings usually aren't practical, as they are quite likely to cause diarrhea. A typical jejunal feeding remains on a continuous drip regimen. A client receiving feedings by gastronomy tube may also be allowed to eat regular foods as desired.

Figure 12.9 Sites of Tube Feedings

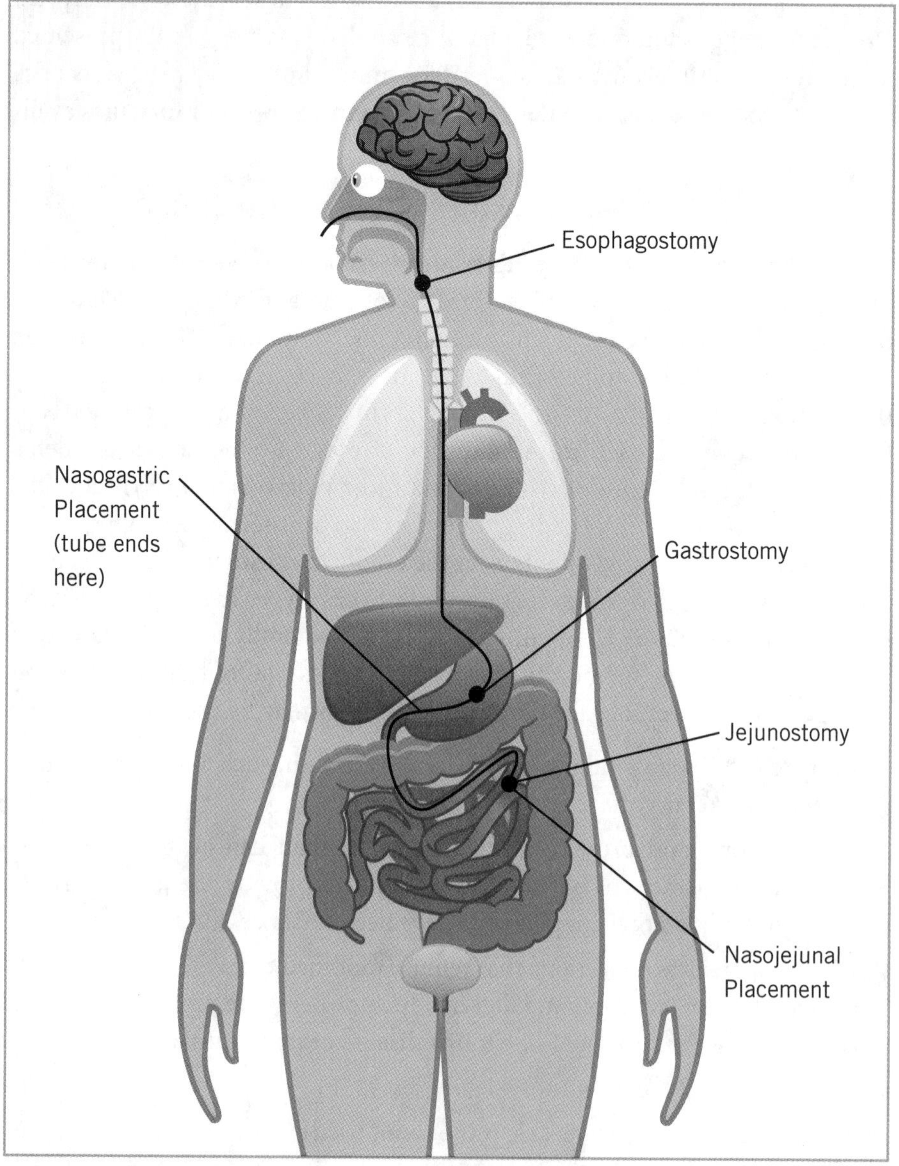

There are three types of complications that can occur in tube fed clients: gastrointestinal disturbances, metabolic complications, and mechanical complications. The most common gastrointestinal disturbance is diarrhea, due to the fact that enteral products are concentrated. Concentrated components tend to pull water into the intestines. Sometimes this is a function of how quickly the feeding is administered. Fiber content of formulas may also play a role. To prevent diarrhea, it is usually necessary to begin a tube feeding at low concentrations (i.e. diluted with water) and a slow rate of administration, building up gradually as the feeding is tolerated. If diarrhea occurs, it may respond to drug therapy or a change in formula. Sanitation is essential during the preparation, storage, and administration of the enteral formula. This will prevent bacterial contamination that could cause food-borne illness. Feeding containers must be changed daily.

Metabolic complications of tube feeding, such as electrolyte imbalance, frequently occur due to inadequate fluid intake, diarrhea, and/or vomiting. Tube feeding frequently serves as a client's sole source of fluid, so careful attention must be paid to fluid requirements. Fluid intake should be adequate to make up for normal losses. There is about a 500 ml difference between input and output over 24 hours. Fluid intake should accommodate unusual losses associated with increased body temperature, vomiting, and diarrhea.

Note that nursing personnel typically bear most of the responsibility for administering and managing tube feeding's. The Registered Dietitian is involved in recommending a product, concentration, and rate of administration that will provide adequate nutrients. Like a menu, a tube-feeding regimen is a type of diet that must be matched to estimated nutrient needs and specific therapeutic needs. As a feeding progresses, a Certified Dietary Manager often assists in monitoring tolerance and administration while coordinating with the Registered Dietitian.

One type of enteral formula that is used for tube feeding but rarely for oral supplementation is a chemically defined formula. Whereas usual formulas require some digestion, chemically defined formulas (also called elemental or hydrolyzed formulas) are almost completely digested so they require only minimal digestion. These formulas are absorbed quickly and are useful for clients with severe digestive problems, such as pancreatitis. Chemically defined formulas generally cost more than other types of formulas and are less palatable.

In selecting an enteral product for oral or tube feeding, a nutrition caregiver should consider the product concentration; the need for a nutritionally complete formulation; needs for modification in carbohydrate, fat, or protein composition; tolerance of lactose; location of the feeding tube; and whether or not to include fiber. A Certified Dietary Manager should be aware of taste, texture, and individual client acceptance as well.

Parenteral Nutrition

Parenteral nutrition is the administration of simple essential nutrients into a vein. Parenteral solutions may contain dextrose, lipids, amino acids, electrolytes, vitamins, and trace elements. They may be used in cases where the client's gastrointestinal tract is no longer able to digest and absorb food properly, or to maintain fluid and electrolyte balance both before and after surgery, or when a client is not receiving enough nourishment by other feeding methods. Other examples of situations that may require parenteral feedings include the following:

✓ severely malnourished clients with a nonfunctional gastrointestinal tract.

✓ clients with diseases of the small intestines who are not absorbing nutrients.

✓ clients with sepsis or burns who have very high nutrient needs.

When a client receives his or her total nutrient needs via parenteral nutrition, it is called total parenteral nutrition (TPN). Parenteral nutrition may use a central or peripheral vein. In central parenteral nutrition (CPN), a central vein near the heart is used because these veins are large in diameter. At other times, a peripheral vein (a vein in the arm or leg) is chosen, and this is called peripheral parenteral nutrition (PPN). PPN is used when only short-term support is needed and the client is not severely malnourished. PPN may be used to supplement ordinary eating. CPN is used in more severely malnourished clients who may also need more long-term nutrition support.

Although parenteral nutrition is very helpful to certain clients, it has its disadvantages. Inserting a catheter (tube) for parenteral nutrition is a surgical procedure, and once it is inserted, the catheter must be well cared for to prevent infection, a complication of parenteral nutrition. Also, when the gastrointestinal tract is not used for a long time, intestinal cells involved in absorption shrink in size, making a transition back to enteral feeding challenging. Furthermore, clients fed by vein have to forgo the usual satisfaction characteristic of eating, with all its social and emotional meanings. Lastly, parenteral solutions are very costly compared to enteral feedings.

In parenteral nutrition, an evaluation of nutritional status and an estimation of nutrient needs provide useful starting points for planning therapy, usually conducted by the Registered Dietitian. If a client is going to make a transition from parenteral feeding to conventional foods, the Certified Dietary Manager may be involved in the transition.

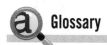 **Glossary**

Parenteral Nutrition
Administration of simple essential nutrients into a vein

END OF CHAPTER

Putting It Into Practice Questions & Answers

1. Following the increase in calorie recommendation for pregnancy, what foods would you add to a general menu throughout the day and why?

    A. *The extra 300 calories during the day can easily come from one extra serving of lean meat, vegetables, fruits, a slice of bread, and a cup of low-fat milk.*

2. Modify the following menu to meet the needs of preschoolers: tator tot casserole, green beans, canned pears.

    A. *The modified menu should have finger foods and individual foods (not mixed as in a casserole). You could adjust this menu by serving a mini hamburger with carrot and celery sticks and keep the canned pears but add a little maraschino cherry juice for color.*

3. Given the recommendation of the Report of the DGAC on the Dietary Guidelines for Americans, 2010, what would you recommend for breakfast for a school-age child?

    A. *A breakfast burrito (6 " whole grain tortilla or a breakfast pizza) containing scrambled eggs and low-fat sausage bits. Serve a piece of seasonal fruit such as strawberries, apple, or orange slices. This would be low-fat, low-calorie, higher in fiber, and provide a good protein source.*

4. Plan a portable snack for teenagers that would include calcium, iron, and fiber.

    A. *A crepe made with whole grain tortilla, 4 TBSP of Nutella (a chocolate hazelnut spread that is low in mono-unsaturated fat and provides both calcium and iron), or a cup of chili with shredded cheese and corn chips to dip.*

5. How would you change the following menu to meet the menu planning suggestions in Figure 12.6? (Pork chops and gravy; tossed salad with carrots, radishes, celery; mashed potatoes; and lemon meringue pie)

    A. *You will want to emphasize complex carbohydrate foods that are easy to chew, have a moderate fat intake, are nutrient dense. You could change the menu as shown below:*

    - *Pork chops with low-fat gravy*
    - *Mixed broccoli, cauliflower, and carrots (cooked)*
    - *Mashed potatoes (add non-fat dry milk for more protein)*
    - *Pumpkin pie or pumpkin custard (pumpkin pie filling without the high-fat crust)*

6. At an assisted living facility, foodservice employees take orders in the dining room each day. Clients are offered two entrée choices for each meal. What type of menu is this?

    A. *The facility will be using a cycle menu that provides choices for the entrées*

7. What would you add to the following therapeutic diet to enhance the appearance and taste? (puréed scrambled eggs, pureed sausage, pureed biscuit, and thickened orange juice)

    A. *Chop the scrambled eggs and add a small amount of cheese sauce; add the pureed sausage to a gravy and serve over a regular biscuit that is cut up. The biscuit will soak up the gravy and be tolerable for a pureed diet.*

CHAPTER 13

Implement Physician's Dietary Orders

Overview and Objectives

Like the menu in the kitchen, the physician's dietary orders drive the clinical activities in the foodservice department.

After completing this chapter, you should be able to:

✓ Recognize medical and nutrition terminology

✓ Demonstrate sensitivity to patient needs and food habits

✓ Provide needed diets from kitchen

✓ Determine availability of foods from the kitchen

✓ Exhibit competency in suggesting the correct diet orders for clients

✓ Include patient input on diet prescribed by physician

✓ Recognize appropriateness of diet order for diagnosis

The menu drives everything that is done in the kitchen, from the equipment that is needed, to the number of staff. But what drives the menu? In healthcare, one of the factors that drive the menu is the physician's diet order.

Physician Diet Order

How you receive the physician's diet order may vary depending upon the type of facility. For instance, in the hospital, you may receive a phone call from the floor nurse giving you diet order information for a new client. At this point, it is important to ask for written documentation of the diet order to assure accuracy. Your facility may have a policy and procedure as to how diet orders are communicated. There are standardized forms that many facilities use. See Figure 13.1 for a sample diet order.

Another method of obtaining the diet order is to review the medical record. There is often a section in the medical record called Physician's Orders. With the advent of electronic medical records, physicians may issue their orders electronically. No matter how the order is received, it is up to you to interpret it and implement it for your clients.

To interpret the Physician Diet Order, you will have to know standard medical terminology such as t.i.d, CHF, Dx, NPO, and others. Review the terminology chart in Chapter 7 and keep it handy as you read the physician's orders.

Figure 13.1   Sample Diet Order & Communication Form

DIET ORDER & COMMUNICATION

Resident Name: **Room #:**   **Date:**

COMMUNICATION: ○ Diet   ○ New Resident   ○ Discharge   ○ Room Change to Room:

CHANGE NOTICE: ○ Hospital   ○ Re-admit   ○ Hold Tray Until   ○ Change to Table:

○ Dining Room Change to:

○ Leave of Absence Until:

DIET ORDER:

○ NPO
○ Clear Liquids
○ Full Liquids
○ Regular
○ High Protein
○ Other: _____

RESTRICTIONS:

○ Low Salt
○ No Added Salt
○ Low Concentrated Sweets
○ CHO Controlled
○ Renal
○ Fluid Restrictions _____ mLs/24 hrs
○ Other: _____

TEXTURE:

○ Solids/Semi Solids
  ☐ Pureed   ☐ Advanced
  ☐ Mechanical Altered ☐ Regular
○ Thickened Liquids
  ☐ Thin   ☐ Honey-Like
  ☐ Nectar-Like ☐ Spoon-Thick

ALERGIES:

○ See Resident as soon possible
○ Registered Dietitian consult needed
○ Start/Change Snack:

_____

○ Start/Change Supplement:

_____

○ Weight Loss   ○ Abnormal Lab Values
○ Skin Breakdown   ○ Chewing/Swallowing Problems
○ Food Complaints   ○ Decline in Food/Fluid Intake

○ Known Food/Beverage Intolerances:

_____

○ Adaptive Equipment:

_____

BEVERAGE PREFERENCES:

Breakfast:_____

Lunch:_____

Supper:_____

Signature: **Title:**   **Date:**

Diet Manual

Once you have the physician's diet order, the next step is making sure you have an approved diet manual for your facility. The diet manual helps you and other healthcare professionals interpret the diet order. The purpose of the diet manual is to establish a common resource with practice guidelines for all healthcare professionals to use as a guide when providing nutritional care for clients. There are many diet manuals on the market and the choice to decide on the diet manual should be one made by your interdisciplinary team. Use these guidelines as you evaluate your options:

1. Make sure the manual includes the most current information on diets based on research findings.

2. Choose a manual that uses a standard such as the Dietary Reference Intakes (DRIs).

3. Look for manuals that include diets routinely ordered in your facility.

4. Use only as a guide.

When you have decided on a diet manual, customize it to your facility:

✓ Add standard diet terminology from your facility to assist in providing a common language.

✓ Have a sign off sheet so that each member of your interdisciplinary team and the physician has approved the diet manual.

✓ Place the manual on all floors, at each nursing station, or each unit, in the diet office, and in the kitchen.

✓ Make sure everyone knows where it is and how to use it.

Interpreting the Diet Order

As the Certified Dietary Manager, you help the client interpret their clinical treatment (physician diet order) through their food choices. This begins when you conduct your diet interview as part of nutrition screening. An important part of your job is to demonstrate sensitivity to patient needs and food habits. How do you respond to clients who don't want to follow their diet order? There is a paradigm shift occurring in institutional care: To involve clients in choices about their diet, their meal times and their dining locations. Centers for Medicare and Medicaid Services (CMS) guidelines have an increased focus on providing person-centered care, giving client/family/guardians more voice about desires and will of the client. The 2010 Position Paper of the The Academy of Nutrition and Dietetics (AND) [formerly known as The American Dietetic Association (ADA)]: *Individualized Nutrition Approaches for Older Adults in Health Communities* adds support for this evolving philosophy. (See *Nutrition in the News* at the end of this chapter for the full position paper.) The paper states, "**Health care communities** differ from **acute care facilities** in that long-term treatment and lifestyle goals take precedence over short-term clinical goals." Let's examine how to improve a client's quality of life through food in a long-term care facility.

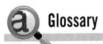

Glossary

Health Care Communities
The Position Paper of the The Academy of Nutrition and Dietetics (AND) [formerly known as The American Dietetic Association (ADA)]: *Individualized Nutrition Approaches for Older Adults in Health Communities* identifies the following as healthcare communities: "assisted living facilities, group homes, short-term rehabilitation facilities, skilled nursing facilities, and hospice facilities."

Acute Care Facilities
Hospitals or urgent care centers that provide emergency and surgical treatment or care for acute illnesses or injuries

Implementing the Diet Order

In long-term care facilities, preventing weight loss and malnutrition may override the need for clients to follow a strict therapeutic diet. Healthcare professionals are finding that general diets may improve outcomes because clients are more willing to eat foods that have not been modified for therapeutic diets. According to the The Academy of Nutrition and Dietetics (AND) [formerly known as The American Dietetic Association (ADA)] position paper referenced above, "...elderly nursing home residents with diabetes can receive a regular diet that is consistent in the amount and timing of carbohydrate, along with proper medication...." The American Diabetes Association no longer recommends the AND diet terminology (e.g. 1800 calorie AND diet), and suggests a "carbohydrate counting diabetes meal plan" as an alternative.

Let's use the example of an elderly client with diabetes and her physician's diet order of an 1800 calorie AND diet. How do you implement this diet order to comply with CMS guidelines and current recommendations for diabetic diets? The first step is to meet with the interdisciplinary team to discuss the idea of a change in the diet manual to a carbohydrate counting menu. It is important to note here that even if your current diet manual lists a carbohydrate counting diet, the physician's order may differ from what is in the current diet manual. You may receive a diet order that doesn't match the standard diets offered by the facility. Who is responsible to request the change should be determined by your facility policies. If no policy exists, confer with your Registered Dietitian.

The second step is to work on menu development. Look at the regular menu and decide if you need to make any changes to the regular menu to offer a carbohydrate counting diet. Look at foods containing carbohydrates such as dairy products, vegetables, fruits, and bread. It is helpful to keep in mind that about 15 grams of carbohydrate is equal to one exchange. You can count one carbohydrate exchange as one 'carb' on a carbohydrate counting diet. For a regular diet that also complies with a carbohydrate counting diet, you would want to offer about three to five 'carbs' at each meal to provide 1500 – 2000 calories per day. If you have desserts that are more than three 'carbs', you might consider eliminating them from the regular menu. The menu will be more in line with the Dietary Guidelines and myPyramid.

Remember in Chapter 12 where you learned about menu extensions? By making your general menu fit the carbohydrate counting diet, you will be able to eliminate a menu extension. Each time you can eliminate a diet extension, you will save food budget dollars and staff preparation time. By developing a regular menu that also meets a carbohydrate counting diet, you have eliminated a diet extension and are serving a healthier menu. Better yet, your clients with diabetes will be more satisfied with their diet.

The third step is education for clients, staff, and family members. They may not understand why the client/family member is being served a piece of pumpkin pie instead of a gelatin dessert. For staff, use your interdisciplinary team members to hold in-service training sessions. You and your Registered Dietitian may want to develop handouts for physicians, nurses and foodservice staff. See Figure 13.2 for an example of a training handout.

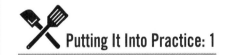

Putting It Into Practice: 1

According to your estimate, how many 'carbs' are in this regular menu?

- 3/4 cup minestrone soup
- 1 ea. soft taco (made with hamburger, cheese, lettuce, taco sauce)
- 1/2 cup pasta salad (made with pasta, peas, shredded carrots)
- 2 oz. carrot cake with frosting

(Check your answer at the end of the chapter)

The fourth step is to follow-up with clients. How do they like the diet? Do they understand the diet? The client may still prefer dietetic jellies and syrups. It will be important to monitor the amount of food consumed for clients with diabetes as well as their fasting blood glucose to make sure that the regular diet is appropriate.

In acute care/hospital facilities, some of the same steps to implementing the physician's diet orders apply. Using the same scenario as above, the first step would be meeting with the Registered Dietitian and other appropriate staff members to promote the idea of using a carbohydrate counting menu.

The second step, menu development, will be a little different than in long-term care, particularly if clients select their own food choices. If you have a room service menu, you may want to identify all the carbohydrate foods and label them either with the number of 'carbs' or the grams of carbohydrate for each food. Include directions at the top of the menu to explain that the client should select, for example, three to five 'carbs' or 45 to 75 grams of carbohydrate for each meal.

Again, the third step is the same as in long-term care—providing education to clients, staff, physicians, and families. How you provide that education may change for the clients. For instance, you might be preparing them for reading food labels because they will be going home in the near future. Because this is acute care, understanding counting carbohydrates will be critical for floor nurses that might be providing food substitutions for pediatric clients.

Figure 13.2 Training Handout

Sample Training Aid for Carbohydrate Counting Diet*

What is the Carbohydrate Counting Diet?
A diet where the client has more control over their food choices while trying to maintain a consistent amount of carbohydrate at every meal, every day. Instead of having a specific calorie level, the diet has a specific amount of carbohydrate for each day.

Where are carbohydrates found?
Starchy vegetables such as peas, corn, potatoes, squash; dairy products; breads/grains; fruits; sweet desserts.

Why is the facility adopting a Carbohydrate Counting Diet instead of the regular AND diet?
Both the American Diabetes Association and the The Academy of Nutrition and Dietetics (AND) [formerly known as The American Dietetic Association (ADA)] recommend using a carbohydrate counting approach to the diabetic diet because it is less restrictive and compliance is improved.

What are the advantages of using a Carbohydrate Counting Diet?
- Clients with diabetes can include a small amount of a sweet dessert or sweetened beverage as long as it is consumed with the meal.
- Medication can be adjusted based on the amount of carbohydrate consumed.
- Clients have more control over their diet because they can select from a list of food choices that each contain 15 grams of carbohydrate. If the client refuses to eat vegetables, he/she can select more fruits or low-fat dairy products to keep the carbohydrate content consistent.

How can I help implement a Carbohydrate Counting Diet?
- Help family members understand why and how it is OK for their loved one to have sweetened foods and beverages.
- Help clients select an appropriate substitute if they refuse a particular food. Use the term Carbohydrate Counting Diet instead of AND diet.

* This might be a handout provided during an in-service training of non-dietary staff.

Follow-up, or the fourth step, will also be a different process. Your clientele may not stay for more than a few days. Your follow-up may be part of a quality survey that is handled by the facility. If they return for a diabetic outpatient visit because they are having trouble balancing their carbohydrate choices and insulin doses, it may mean they need additional training.

Provide Needed Diets from the Kitchen

Part of implementing physician's dietary orders is providing the needed diets from the kitchen. You will have the opportunity to respond to client requests to have foods that may not be on their diet order. For example, a diabetic client may want potatoes for supper and it is not on the diet extension for a diabetic diet. This is another reason why moving to a carbohydrate counting diet will benefit your clients. With a carbohydrate counting diet, you can alter the diet to honor the client request.

You also have to comply with other diet orders such as a 2-gm sodium diet or a restricted fat diet. Your menu extensions will provide the information about meeting the diet order. For example, if your menu has glazed ham as an entrée, your menu extension would have a different entrée selection for a 2-gm sodium diet, such as roast pork. What if your client who is on the 2-gm sodium diet asks for glazed ham? How do you implement the physician's

Figure 13.3   When Clients Ask for a Food Not on their Prescribed Diet

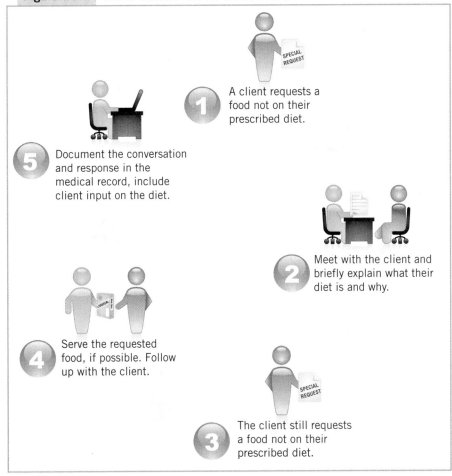

1. A client requests a food not on their prescribed diet.

2. Meet with the client and briefly explain what their diet is and why.

3. The client still requests a food not on their prescribed diet.

4. Serve the requested food, if possible. Follow up with the client.

5. Document the conversation and response in the medical record, include client input on the diet.

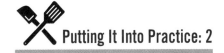 **Putting It Into Practice: 2**

Given the acute care selective breakfast menu below, how would you label it for your clients on a carbohydrate counting diet?

- Juice
- Bread
- Cereal
- Beverage
- Entree
- Condiment

(Check your answer at the end of the chapter)

dietary orders and meet the client's request? Remember, according to the CMS guidelines, there is an increased focus on providing person-centered care. Your response should be to explain to the client what their diet order is and why, and if they still insist on having glazed ham, provide them with the glazed ham. Then, it is very important to document your conversation with the client and his/her menu choice in the medical record. (see Figure 13.3)

Appropriateness of the Diet Order

Not only is it important to provide the needed diets from the kitchen, it is also essential to be able to recognize the appropriateness of the diet order for the diagnosis. To determine if the diet order is appropriate for the diagnosis, begin with the medical record. The medical record provides both the diet order and the diagnosis. This is where you apply the information you learned in previous chapters. For instance, when you conduct the nutrition screening, compare your results to the diagnosis and the diet order. The nutrition screening for a new client, Herbert, shows the following information:

✓ Age at admission: 80

✓ Height: 5'9"

✓ Weight: 117 lbs

✓ BUN: 97 g/sL

✓ Creatinine: 7.9 mg/dL

✓ Albumin: 2.9 mg/dL

✓ Potassium: elevated

✓ Blood Pressure: 150/92

✓ History: Herbert has had only had one kidney since he was a child. Last year, after prostrate surgery, he went into acute renal failure. Tests show his only kidney is declining in function. Herbert does not want dialysis or a transplant.

✓ Diet Order: 20 gms protein, 2 gm NA, and 2 gm K (potassium)

Is this diet order appropriate for Herbert? This may not be an appropriate diet order. This diet order is a strict renal diet. Herbert does not want dialysis or a transplant and putting him on a strict renal diet will not improve his kidney function. He is already very underweight. In keeping with the CMS and The Academy of Nutrition and Dietetics (AND) [formerly known as The American Dietetic Association (ADA)] new guidelines, Herbert might benefit from a general diet to encourage him to eat and enjoy the time he has left. You should refer your findings to the Registered Dietitian or contact the director of nursing with your concerns.

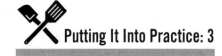

Putting It Into Practice: 3

List the steps you would take for a client who is insisting on having fried eggs for breakfast and she is on a low-fat, low-cholesterol diet.

(Check your answer at the end of the chapter)

Nutrition in the News

Position of the American Dietetic Association: Individualized Nutrition Approaches for Older Adults in Health Care Communities

Abstract

It is the position of the American Dietetic Association that the quality of life and nutritional status of older adults residing in health care communities can be enhanced by individualization to less-restrictive diets. The American Dietetic Association advocates for Registered Dietitians to assess and evaluate the need for nutrition interventions tailored to each person's medical condition, needs, desires, and rights. Dietetic technicians, registered, assist Registered Dietitians in the assessment and implementation of individualized nutrition care. Health care practitioners must assess risks vs. benefits of therapeutic diets, especially for older adults. Food is an essential component of quality of life; an unpalatable or unacceptable diet can lead to poor food and fluid intake, resulting in under-nutrition and related negative health effects. Including older individuals in decisions about food can increase the desire to eat and improve quality of life. The Practice Paper of the American Dietetic Association: Individualized Nutrition Approaches for Older Adults in Health Care Communities provides guidance to practitioners on implementation of individualized diets and nutrition care.

Position Statement

It is the position of the American Dietetic Association that the quality of life and nutritional status of older adults residing in health care communities can be enhanced by individualization to less-restrictive diets. The American Dietetic Association advocates for Registered Dietitians to assess and evaluate the need for nutrition interventions tailored to each person's medical condition, needs, desires, and rights. Dietetic technicians, registered, assist Registered Dietitians in the assessment and implementation of individualized nutrition care.

Health Care Communities

Health care communities are living environments for persons with chronic conditions, functional limitations, or need for supervision or assistance. Health care communities include assisted living facilities, group homes, short-term rehabilitation facilities, skilled nursing facilities, and hospice facilities. Health care communities differ from acute care facilities in that long-term treatment and lifestyle goals take precedence over short-term clinical goals. Care for individuals who reside in health care communities must meet two goals: maintain health and preserve quality of life. These goals can compete when it comes to delivery of nutrition care. Food must meet nutrition needs but also enhance quality of life.

Trends in Health Care Communities

America is aging rapidly. By 2030, predictions indicate that the older than age 65 years population will increase to approximately 72.1 million, or 19.3% of the population (1). This equates to a remarkable 52% increase since 2007. The number of people aged 85 years or older is projected to increase from 5.5 million in 2007 to 6.6 million in 2020, a 20% increase in the oldest old (2). These increases in the older population will have dramatic effects on the nation's health care system in years to come.

In 2008, approximately 1.6 million (4.1%) of Americans aged 65 years and older lived in institutional settings. This percentage increases with age, ranging from 1.3% for those aged 65 to 74 years, 3.8% for those aged 75 to 84 years, and 15.4% of those older than 85 years of age (1). Residents of nursing facilities are often frail older adults. In 2004, approximately 15% of nursing home residents were dependent on others for eating, and up to 39% were dependent on others for activities

(Continued)

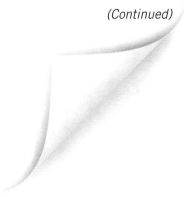

of daily living such as bathing and toileting (3). Older adults residing in any health care community are more likely to need assistance with activities of daily living and have cognitive impairment due to Alzheimer's disease or other dementias (1). As a result they are likely to experience physical and social problems that exacerbate poor health and alter food intake.

Health care communities have embraced new philosophies that reflect major paradigm shifts in culture from institutional care to more personalized living in a home-like environment. Improving quality of life and quality of care, allowing choices in daily living, and assisting individuals to make informed health care decisions are all major goals of culture change and person-centered care. Involving individuals in choices about food and dining such as food selections, dining locations, and meal times can help them maintain a sense of dignity, control, and autonomy.

Factors Affecting Nutritional Status

Physiological changes of aging can affect food intake, body composition, and weight. Food intake typically declines even in healthy older adults. This is often referred to as the "anorexia of aging" (4). Decreased appetite can be due to a decrease in olfaction, taste, and changes in levels of hormones that control satiety and food intake. As appetite diminishes, intake of energy and other nutrients decreases, which can result in weight loss and predispose an individual to increased risk of illness and infection. In addition, chronic disease, including cerebrovascular accidents, Parkinson's disease, cancer, diabetes, and dementia, can contribute to changes in appetite, metabolism, and weight. Older adults can be subject to sarcopenia, a loss of muscle mass associated with aging, and/or cachexia, a loss of weight and muscle mass associated with underlying illness. Depression, polypharmacy, drug nutrient interactions, or side effects such as anorexia,

nausea, vomiting; sensory loss that affects ability to see, smell, and taste food; and oral or dental changes that affect chewing or swallowing ability can all affect nutritional status. As a result of the physiological and psychological changes associated with aging, food can be less appealing, and food consumption may decline as a result. Restrictive diets may exacerbate poor food intake leading to unintended weight loss and under-nutrition.

The Risk for Under-Nutrition in Health Care Communities

Due to variations in definitions between under-nutrition and malnutrition, determining the scope of the problem in health care communities is difficult. According to a recent literature review that used the mini-nutrition assessment as a parameter, malnutrition was observed in 2% to 38% of institutionalized older adults, and 37% to 62% were considered at risk (5). Consequences of under-nutrition include increased mortality, loss of strength, depression, lethargy, immune dysfunction, pressure ulcers, delayed recovery from illness, increased chance of hospital admission, and poor wound healing (6). Older adults are at higher risk for pressure ulcer development due to age, skin frailty, unintended weight loss, and other factors. Although pressure ulcers have multiple causes, poor nutritional status is a contributing factor and is an important aspect of prevention (7). Since unintended weight loss can reflect poor intake or changes in metabolism of food and nutrients, it may be the best indicator of under-nutrition (4).

Risks vs. Benefits of Least-Restrictive Diets

A priority of nutrition care for most frail older adults in health care communities is to consume enough food to prevent unintended weight loss and under-nutrition. Although therapeutic diets are designed to improve health, they can negatively affect the variety and flavor of the food offered. Individuals may find restrictive diets unpalatable, resulting in reducing the pleasure of eating, decreased food intake, unintended weight loss, and under-nutrition—the very maladies health care practitioners are trying to prevent. In contrast, more liberal diets are associated with increased food and beverage intake (8). For many older adults residing in health care communities, the benefits of less-restrictive diets outweigh the risks. When considering a therapeutic diet prescription, a health care practitioner should ask: Is a restrictive therapeutic diet necessary? Will it offer enough benefits to justify its use?

(Continued)

Disease-Specific Conditions and Restricted Diets

Diabetes Mellitus

The risk of developing diabetes increases with age. By one 2002 estimate, 26.4% of all persons admitted to nursing homes had a diagnosis of type 2 diabetes (9). Although there are numerous evidence-based guidelines for treating diabetes, few of the data supporting interventions were obtained from research studies in older persons (10).

Blood glucose can be affected by factors other than diet, including infections, obesity, diseases of the pancreas, endocrine disease, genetic defects of beta cells or insulin action, and common medications (9). Since 2000, the American Diabetes Association has held the position that sucrose-containing foods can be substituted for other carbohydrates in the meal plan or covered with insulin lowering medications (11). There is no evidence to support prescribing diets such as no concentrated sweets or no sugar added for older adults living in health care communities, and these restricted diets are no longer considered appropriate (11). Most experts agree that using medication rather than dietary changes to control blood glucose, blood lipid levels, and blood pressure can enhance the joy of eating and reduce the risk of malnutrition for older adults in health care communities (11).

According to the American Diabetes Association position statement on nutrition recommendations and interventions for diabetes, elderly nursing home residents with diabetes can receive a regular diet that is consistent in the amount and timing of carbohydrates, along with proper medication to control blood glucose levels (11). The nutrition care plan should include education about appropriate food choices for managing diabetes.

Cardiovascular Disease

The use of low-fat, low-cholesterol diet prescriptions for older adults in health care communities is controversial. There are little data available to support the effects of lipid-lowering therapy on adults older than 75 years of age (12). However, the American Heart Association suggests that risks related to elevated blood lipid levels do not diminish with age and recommends treatment be considered for all older adults (12). Health care providers should be aware of cardiac problems while balancing an individual's condition, prognosis, and the threat of under-nutrition when making treatment decisions.

The relationship between congestive heart failure, blood pressure, and sodium intake in the elderly population has not been well studied. The American Heart Association recommends that older adults attempt to control blood pressure through diet and lifestyle changes (13) and recommends a sodium intake of 2 to 3 g/day for patients with congestive heart failure (14). However, a randomized trial of adults aged 55 to 83 years found that a normal-sodium diet improved congestive heart failure out-comes (15). A liberal approach to sodium in diets may be needed to maintain adequate nutritional status, especially in frail older adults (16). The Dietary Approaches to Stop Hypertension (DASH) eating pattern is known to reduce blood pressure and may also reduce rates of heart failure 1550 October 2010 Volume 110 Number 10(17). The DASH diet is low in sodium and saturated fat but also high in calcium, magnesium, and potassium.

The nutrition care plan for older adults with cardiac disease should focus on maintaining blood pressure and blood lipid levels while preserving eating pleasure and quality of life. Using menus that work toward the objectives of the Dietary Guidelines for Americans and/or the DASH diet can help achieve those goals. Physical activity that is based on each individual's abilities can also help facilitate cardiac health (14).

Chronic Kidney Disease

Older adults with chronic kidney disease often have increased protein catabolism and uremia (18). Anorexia, nausea, and vomiting are common side effects of uremia (19). Under-nutrition is especially difficult to define in this population because changes in body weight can be caused by shifts in fluid balance. Most experts agree that patients receiving dialysis lose protein with each treatment and, therefore, require an increase in dietary protein (20). Individualizing the diet prescription for

(Continued)

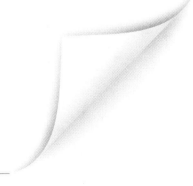

chronic kidney disease patients receiving dialysis may increase total energy and protein in-take and help prevent under-nutrition. Patients in earlier stages of chronic kidney disease may need an individualized diet if food intake is poor or weight loss is detected (20).

Obesity and Desired Weight Loss

In 2005-2006, 37% of individuals aged 65 to 74 years and 24% of those aged 75 years and older were classified as obese (3). Evidence suggests that weight loss in obese older adults improves physical functioning and quality of life and reduces medical complications (21). However, some experts suggest that adverse health outcomes of obesity and benefits of weight loss in older adults have not been proven (22). Weight loss in obese older adults results in both a loss of fat mass and lean body mass that could exacerbate sarcopenia (22,23), thus contributing to functional decline (24). If an individual desires weight loss, the care plan should provide adequate energy and protein along with regular physical activity to help preserve lean body mass (21). In most cases, a resident's usual body weight before decline or admission, rather than ideal body weight, is the most relevant basis for weight-related interventions. Caution should be applied in determining which older adults are appropriate for weight loss programs to avoid under-nutrition and complications such as pressure ulcers.

Alzheimer's Disease and Dementia

The prevalence of Alzheimer's disease in individuals aged 85 years is between 24% and 33% in developed countries (25). Unintended weight loss is common in people with Alzheimer's disease and is thought to be part of the disease process (26). Meal intake is often poor, usually due to cognitive decline. The goal of nutrition care for older adults with Alzheimer's disease or other forms of dementia is to develop an individualized diet that considers food preferences, utilizes nutrient-dense foods, and offers feeding assistance as needed to achieve the individual's goals.

Palliative Care

Supportive care is the most realistic goal for a dying patient. Decisions about care should be made with the patient and/or family. Accommodating individual food and fluid preferences is essential for acceptance and consumption (27). The nutrition care plan should allow provision of any food and beverage that the individual will safely consume, regardless of medical diagnosis. If texture modifications are recommended, education may be needed on the risks vs benefits of consuming certain foods. More information on this topic is available in the Position of The American Dietetic Association: Ethical and legal issues in nutrition, hydration, and feeding (28).

Compliance With Federal Long-Term Care Regulations

The State Operations Manual of the Centers for Medicare and Medicaid Services—Appendix PP-Guidance to Surveyors for Long Term Care Facilities—states, "A facility must care for its residents in a manner and in an environment that promotes maintenance or enhancement of each resident's quality of life" (29). Facilities must respect ethnic, cultural, religious, and other food and dining preferences, and protect and promote the rights of each resident (28). Providing a therapeutic diet against a resident's wishes is a violation of resident rights. (Note: proper counseling should be provided to ensure the resident understands the risks vs benefits of not following a therapeutic diet.) In an effort to enhance quality of life, respect resident rights, and promote person-centered care, many facilities are enhancing their dining programs to include creative ideas that demonstrate improvements in dining, food intake, and/or quality of life (8). The State Operations Manual (27) also addresses nutrition and recognizes the potential benefits of liberalized diets. According to the manual, "it is often beneficial to minimize restrictions consistent with a resident's condition, prognosis, and choices." Providing a more liberal diet may help prevent an F-325 citation (nutrition and unintended weight loss) because the intent is to ensure that residents maintain acceptable parameters of nutritional status (28).

The Role of Registered Dietitians and Dietetic Technicians, Registered

Registered Dietitians should utilize the Nutrition Care Process and develop an individualized care plan that is consistent with needs based on nutritional status, medical condition and personal preferences.

(Continued)

Position of the American Dietetic Association *(Continued)*

Registered Dietitians should assess nutritional status, determine a nutrition diagnosis, plan appropriate nutrition interventions, and monitor and evaluate outcomes. Dietetic technicians, registered, support Registered Dietitians in the Nutrition Care Process and may complete parts of the process as assigned by an Registered Dietitian (2). Collaboration between the patient, family, and members of the health care team will help achieve these goals. Registered Dietitians and dietetic technicians, registered, should be actively involved in developing facility policies and procedures and educating staff, residents, and family members on the benefits of a less-restrictive diet based on each individual's needs.

Conclusions

Under-nutrition, weight loss, poor food intake, satisfaction, and acceptance are serious issues in health care communities. Despite the growing body of evidence discouraging the use of therapeutic diets in older adults, these diets are still regularly prescribed. Research has not demonstrated benefits of restricting sodium, cholesterol, fat, and/or carbohydrate in older adults (9). Additional research is needed to help practitioners make evidence-based decisions about nutrition care of older adults in health care communities.

Registered Dietitians should evaluate each individual and assess the risks vs the benefits of a therapeutic diet. Maximizing meal intake can help prevent under-nutrition and unintended weight loss, which can lead to additional health complications. Individualizing to the least-restrictive diet can enhance nutritional status and improve quality of life, particularly for an older adult with poor food/fluid intake or unintended weight loss.

References

1. Profile of older Americans. US Department of Health and Human Services, Administration on Aging Web site. http://www.aoa.gov/aoaroot/aging_statistics/Profile/index.aspx. Accessed May 5, 2010.

2. American Dietetic Association Quality Management Committee. American Dietetic Association revised 2008 Standards of Practice for Registered Dietitians in nutrition care; Standards of Professional Performance for Registered Dietitians; Standards of Practice for dietetic technicians, registered, in nutri-tion care; and Standards of Professional Performance for dietetic technicians, registered. J Am Diet Assoc. 2008;108:1538-1542.

3. Older Americans 2008: Key indicators of well-being. Published March 2008. Federal Interagency F orum on Aging Related Statistics Web site. http://www.agingstats.gov/agingstatsdotnet/Main_Site/Data/2008_Documents/Health_Care.aspx. Accessed October 1, 2009.

4. Morley JI, Thomas DR, Kamel HK. Nutri- tional deficiencies in long-term care. Ann Long Term Care. 2004;2(suppl):S1-S5.

5. Pauly L, Stehle P, Volkert D. Nutritional situation of elderly nursing home residents. Z Gerontol Geriatr. 2007;40:3-12.

6. Challa S, Sharkey JR, Chen M, Phillips CD. Association of resident, facility, and geographic characteristics with chronic under- nutrition in a nationally represented sample of older residents in U.S. nursing homes. J Nutr Health Aging. 2007;11:179-184.

7. Dorner B, Posthauer ME, Thomas D. The role of nutrition in pressure ulcer prevention and treatment: National Pressure Ulcer Advisory Panel white paper. Advance Skin Wound Care. 2009;22:212-221.

8. Unintended weight loss (UWL) in older adults: Evidence-based nutrition practice guideline. American Dietetic Association Evidence Analysis Library. http://www.adaevidencelibrary.com/topic.cfm?cat 3651& library EBG. Accessed November 2, 2009.

9. Diabetes Management in the Long-Term Care Setting Clinical Practice Guideline. Columbia, MD: American Medical Directors Association; 2008.

10. American Geriatrics Society Panel on Improving Care for Elders with Diabetes. Guidelines for improving the care of the older person with diabetes mellitus. J Am Geriatr Soc. 2003;51(suppl):S265-S280.

(Continued)

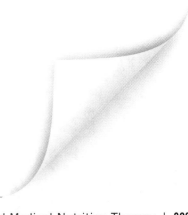

Position of the American Dietetic Association *(Continued)*

11. Nutrition recommendations and interventions for diabetes: A position statement of the American Diabetes Association. Diabetes Care. 2008;31(suppl):S61-S78.

12. Williams MA, Fleg JL, Ades PA, Chaitman BR, Miller NH, Mohiuddin SM, Ockene IS, Taylor CB, Wenger NK. Secondary prevention of coronary heart disease in the elderly (with emphasis on patients 75 years of age). Circulation. 2002;105:1735-1743.

13. Appel LJ, Brands MW, Daniels SR, Karanja N, Elmer PJ, Sacks FM. Dietary approaches to prevent and treat hypertension: A scien-tific statement from the American Heart Association. Hypertension. 2006;47:296-308. American Heart Association Web site. http:// hyper.ahajournals.org/cgi/content/full/47/2/296. Accessed November 3, 2009.

14. Riegel B, Moser DK, Anker SD, Appel LJ, Dunbar SB, Grady KL, Gurvitz MZ, Havranek EP, Lee CS, Lindenfeld J, Peter-son PN, Pressler SJ, Schocken DD, Whellan DJ. State of the science: Promoting self-care in persons with heart failure: A scientific statement from the American Heart Association. Circulation. 2009;120:1141-1163.

15. Paterna S, Gaspare P, Fasullo S, Sarullo FM, Di Pasquale P. Normal-sodium diet compared with low-sodium diet in compensated congestive heart failure: Is sodium an old enemy or a new friend? Clin Sci (Lond). 2008;114:221-230.

16. Niedert KC, Dorner B. Nutrition Care of the Older Adult. 2nd ed. Chicago, IL: American Dietetic Association; 2004:36.

17. Levitan EB, Walk A, Mittleman MA. Consistency with the DASH diet and incidence of heart failure. Arch Intern Med. 2009;160: 851-857.

18. Chronic kidney disease: Disease process. American Dietetic Association Nutrition Care Manual Web site. http://www. nutritioncaremanual.org/content.cfm?ncm content_ id 78551. Accessed October 30, 2009.

19. Lindemann RD. The aging renal system. In: Chernoff R, ed. Geriatric Nutrition: The Health Professional's Handbook. 3rd ed. Sudberry, MD: Jones and Bartless Publishers; 2006:295-306.

20. Niedert KC, Dorner B. Nutrition Care of the Older Adult. 2nd ed. Chicago, IL: American Dietetic Association: 2004:62.

21. Villareal DT, Shah K. Obesity in older adults-a growing problem. In: Bales CW, Ritchie CS. Handbook of Clinical Nutrition and Aging. 2nd ed. New York, NY: Humana Press; 2009:263-277.

22. Miller SL, Wolfe RR. The danger of weight loss in the elderly. J Nutr Health Aging. 2008;12:487-491.

23. Kennedy RI, Chokkalingham K, Srinivasan R. Obesity in the elderly: Who should we be treating, and why, and how? Curr Opin Clin Nutr Metab Care. 2004;7:3-9.

24. Janssen I. Sarcopenia. In: Bales CW, Ritchie CS. Handbook of Clinical Nutrition and Ag- ing. 2nd ed. New York, NY: Humana Press; 2009:183-205.

American Dietetic Association. Position of the American Dietetic Association: Individualized nutrition approaches for older adults in health care communities. J Am Diet Assoc. 2010; 110:1549-1553.

END OF CHAPTER

 Putting It Into Practice Questions & Answers

1. According to your estimate, how many 'carbs' are in this regular menu? (3/4 cup minestrone soup, 1 soft taco (made with hamburger, cheese, lettuce, taco sauce), 1/2 cup pasta salad (made with pasta, peas, shredded carrots), 2 oz. carrot cake with frosting.

   A. *Using the exchange list at the back of this text, look up the carbohydrate content for the foods that you know contain mostly carbohydrate.*

   Taco shell, pasta salad, carrot cake:

   - *Taco shell = 1 carb or 15 gm*
   - *Pasta 1/3 cup = 1 carb or 15 gm*
   - *Peas (starchy vegetable) 1/8 cup = 3.75 gm*
   - *Carrot cake: 2" frosted cake = 2 carb or 30 gm*

   That is a total of 63.75 gm of carbohydrate or 4.25 carbs (63.75 ÷ 15).

2. Given the acute care selective breakfast menu below, how would you label it for your clients on a carbohydrate counting diet?

   A. *For this breakfast menu, select a minimum of three carb sources and a maximum of five carb sources.*

Juice (1 carb each)	Orange Juice, Cranberry Juice, Apple Juice, Prune Juice
Cereal (1 carb each)	Oatmeal, Cream of Wheat®, Cold Cereal—Raisin Bran®, Corn Flakes®
Entree	Scrambled Eggs, Bacon, Pancakes (1 carb), Yogurt (1 carb)
Bread (1 carb each)	Whole Wheat Toast, Cinnamon Biscuit, Toaster Pastry
Beverage	Coffee, Tea, 2% Milk (1 carb), Water
Condiment	Margarine, Salt, Pepper

3. List the steps you would take for a client who is insisting on having fried eggs for breakfast. She is on a low-fat, low-cholesterol diet.

   A. *1. Cheerfully explain to the client that they may have a scrambled egg substitute for breakfast and why this is important for her diet. (e.g. Eggs are high in cholesterol and fried foods add unnecessary fat)*

   2. If she still insists on having fried eggs for breakfast, offer her one fried egg.

   3. Follow-up with the client to determine acceptance.

   4. Document your conversations in the medical record, including what was served and why.

Apply Standard Nutrition Care Procedures

Overview and Objectives

Regulations and standards governing the healthcare industry require that planning, documentation, and ongoing clinical care follow prescribed models. A Certified Dietary Manager plays a role in compliance to provide optimal care.

After completing this chapter, you should be able to:

✓ Explain the purpose of a care plan

✓ Review client's nutrition needs based on guidelines provided

✓ List the steps involved in developing a nutrition care plan

✓ Identify sources to consult to assist in implementing nutrition care plans

Clinical care revolves around a care plan. Every good outcome hinges on some advance planning. Imagine a simple everyday task, such as going to the grocery store. If you make a plan for what you will do there, you can be more effective. Let's say you want to buy food to prepare dinner this evening. If you go unprepared, you won't know what you need. When you get home, you might not be able to complete dinner preparation. Meanwhile, grocery aisles may tempt you with things you don't need. You may spend money on impulse items, yet not accomplish your original objective of being able to cook this evening.

If planning what you will do is useful for a mundane task like grocery shopping, imagine how critical it can be to providing medical care, where the stakes are high and the outcomes affect the quality of clients' lives profoundly. This is why a cornerstone of medical care is a care plan. A **care plan** is a written plan for medical care. It involves identifying the client's interests, preferences and abilities. It identifies objectives for helping a client reach the best possible physical, mental, social, and/or spiritual well-being. It describes steps members of the healthcare team will take to accomplish this and the disciplines that will carry out the approaches.

Each client has his/her own unique set of needs; thus they need a unique care plan written just for him/her. A care plan essentially charts the course for actions that members of the healthcare team will take to support and improve an individual's well-being. All members of the team use it as a focal point and driving force in their routine of care for clients. The care plan assures that team members' actions contribute toward established clinical needs and objectives that are entirely customized to each unique client. A care plan actually makes the work that each team member performs more effective. We will examine the idea of a comprehensive care plan, and then examine the steps involved in developing a plan of care that specifically addresses nutrition.

Comprehensive Care Plans

One of the ways to measure the quality of your comprehensive care plan is by looking at the quality of each client's life. The American Association of Homes and Services for Aging (AAHSA) has a perspective on defining quality of life. The following is an excerpt from that perspective.

> *Quality is also difficult to define because it is a concept that evolves with respect to the status of each person. Like most of us, recipients of long-term care services don't feel the same way about life from one period to the next. But unlike most of us, their source of quality may well depend on what people around them are willing and/or able to do, and how well they know the individual and what is meaningful to that person. In the world of long-term care, what is "quality" often reflects a judgment made by others for individuals who may not be able to communicate and whose condition is very fragile. This becomes particularly true as people approach the end of life.*

The focus of Centers for Medicare and Medicaid Services (CMS) guidelines is client centered. CMS expects each facility to interview their clients so interdisciplinary team (IDT) members can "know the individual and what is meaningful to that person." In the past, "quality often reflected a judgment made by others" in developing a comprehensive care plan. By striving to include the client, CMS hopes to have less judgment by others and more input from the client. In today's healthcare environment, emphasis on teamwork is primary. That team begins with the client and includes interdisciplinary contributions to the care planning process. There has to be coordination among members of the team and ongoing communication among team members, including the client, in order to improve a client's quality of life.

Care planning is part of the RAI (Resident Assessment Instrument) process as shown below:

As team members develop a care plan together, this becomes essentially a master plan that drives some of the details carried out by individual professionals. A care plan developed by members of a coordinated healthcare team and that addresses the multi-faceted needs of a client is called a **comprehensive care plan**.

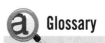 **Glossary**

Care Plan
A written plan for medical care

Comprehensive Care Plan
Developed by interdisciplinary team that addresses the multifaceted needs of the client

---

Figure 14.1   Overview of the Resident Assessment Instrument (RAI) and Care Area Assessments (CAAs)

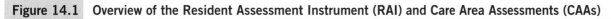

Assessment (MDS)	Decision-Making (CAA)	Care Plan Development	Care Plan Implementation	Evaluation

---

The facility must develop a comprehensive care plan for each client that includes measurable objectives and timetables to meet a client's medical, nursing, and mental and psychosocial needs, which are identified in the comprehensive assessment. The plan of care must deal with both the relationship of services ordered to be provided (or withheld), and the facility's responsibility for fulfilling other requirements in these regulations. According to CMS, a comprehensive care plan must be:

✓ developed *within seven days after the completion of the CAA (Care Area Assessment)*

✓ prepared by an interdisciplinary team that includes the attending physician, a registered nurse with responsibility for the client, and other appropriate staff disciplines as determined by the client's needs, and to the extent practicable, the participation of the client, the client's family, or the client's legal representative

✓ reviewed periodically and revised by a team of qualified persons after each assessment

CMS regulations further stipulate that an interdisciplinary team, in conjunction with the client, client's family, surrogate, or representative, as appropriate, should develop quantifiable objectives for the highest level of functioning the client may be expected to attain, based on the comprehensive assessment.

According to the CMS interpretative guidelines, "the interdisciplinary team should show evidence in the CAA summary or clinical record of the following:

✓ the client's status in triggered CAA areas (called CATs);

✓ the facility's rationale for deciding whether to proceed with care planning; and,

✓ evidence that the facility considered the development of care planning interventions for all CAAs triggered by the MDS."

The care plan must reflect intermediate steps for each outcome objective if identification of those steps will enhance the client's ability to meet his/her objectives. Facility staff will use these objectives to monitor client progress. Facilities may, for some clients, need to prioritize their care plan interventions. This should be noted in the clinical record or on the plan of care.

The requirements reflect the facility's responsibility to provide necessary care and services to attain or maintain the highest practicable physical, mental, and psychosocial well-being, in accordance with the comprehensive assessment and plan of care. However, in some cases, a client may refuse certain services or treatments that professional staff believe may be indicated. Desires of the client should be documented in the comprehensive assessment and reflected in the plan of care.

Following are some questions to consider when care planning:

✓ Does the care plan address the needs, strengths, and preferences identified in the client assessment, including the RAPs?

✓ Is the care plan oriented toward preventing avoidable declines in functioning or functioning levels?

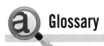
Glossary

RAI
Resident Assessment Instrument consists of three components and is utilized to assess each nursing home or swing bed client's functional capacity and needs

MDS
Minimum Data Set is the starting point of the RAI and is a standardized tool collecting information that is the core of the RAI

CAA
Care Area Assessment is the second component of the RAI and is used to make decisions about areas suggested by the MDS

CAT
Care Area Triggers are related to one or more items in the MDS and are the flags for the interdisciplinary team member

IDT
Interdisciplinary team of health professionals that collaborate in the completion of the RAI

✓ How does the care plan try to manage risk factors?

✓ Does the care plan build on the client's strengths?

✓ Does the care plan reflect standards of current dietetic practice?

✓ If the client refuses treatment, does the care plan explain alternatives to address the problem?

✓ Is the care plan evaluated and revised as the client's status changes?

✓ Does the care plan identify the healthcare professional that will carry out the approaches?

✓ Do treatment objectives have measurable outcomes?

✓ Does the care plan corroborate information regarding the client's goals and wishes for treatment?

To summarize, the comprehensive care plan is completed seven days after completion of the RAI. Developing a comprehensive care plan is the responsibility of the interdisciplinary team. Although the physician must participate as part of the interdisciplinary team, he or she may arrange with the facility for alternative methods, other than attending care planning conferences, such as one-on-one discussions and conference calls.

Although the MDS and supplemental assessments give much information about the client's problems, they won't always identify or trigger them all. One purpose of the care plan conference is to help identify additional problems or needs. The Registered Dietitian and/or Certified Dietary Manager needs to identify a client's nutrition-related problems, set measurable goals with time limits, and determine appropriate interventions.

In long-term care, the care plan, which is part of the client's medical record, is updated at least quarterly and as the client's condition changes. The date of the quarterly review is entered on the care plan. When a problem is no longer a problem, this needs to be noted on the care plan by highlighting it (with a yellow highlighter pen) and writing, "Resolved" with the date of resolution next to it, or noting resolution in a computerized system.

Steps in Developing a Nutrition Care Plan

The nutrition care process involves screening clients for nutrition risk, assessing each client identified by the screening process as being at risk, and then developing a nutrition care plan for each client.

All care planning relates to a list of specified problems. These problems are pinpointed by various members of the healthcare team as they complete their respective assessments. As described above, members of the team tackle this list together. Aspects of the care plan are tightly interwoven among disciplines, and many plans require the efforts of multiple disciplines to succeed. Completing the detail of a plan is often up to the individual professionals involved. Once a plan is developed, the specifics of how it will be implemented follow. Afterwards, it is important to evaluate the effectiveness of care.

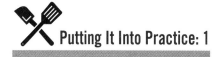

Putting It Into Practice: 1

Mrs. S. hasn't been feeling well. She had the flu two weeks ago and still isn't eating more than 25% of her meals. Normally, a cheerful person, she cries easily and frequently seems confused. She has lost 5% of her total body weight since the beginning of the month. Should Mrs. S. be reassessed? Why or why not? If yes, what should the time frame be for her reassessment and care planning?

(Check your answer at the end of this chapter)

For clients who are not new admissions, you should be alert for significant changes in the client's health. Those changes can be either a decline or an improvement. Not all changes in a client's health status require a new care plan. If a client has the flu for a week and then recovers, a care plan isn't required. If the decline or improvement is consistent over two weeks and it covers two or more areas of decline or improvement, you should begin a comprehensive reassessment. Refer to Figure 14.2 for characteristics of decline or improvement according to MDS 3.0. For clients with no significant changes, a comprehensive reassessment including care planning is required every quarter or every 90 days.

For new clients, care planning must be completed within seven days after the CAAs are completed. Whether for a new client or a current client, the overall care plan should focus on the following:

- ✓ preventing avoidable declines in functioning or functional levels or clarifying why another goal takes precedence
- ✓ managing risk factors to the extent possible or indicating the limits of the interventions
- ✓ addressing ways to try to preserve and build upon client strengths
- ✓ applying current standards of practice in the care planning process
- ✓ evaluating treatment of measurable objectives, timetables and outcomes of care
- ✓ respecting the client's right to decline treatment such as refusing to eat
- ✓ offering alternative treatments as applicable
- ✓ using an appropriate interdisciplinary approach to care plan development to improve the client's functional abilities
- ✓ involving client, client's family and other client respresentatives as appropriate
- ✓ assessing and planning for care to meet the client's medical, nursing, mental and psychosocial needs
- ✓ addressing additional care planning areas that are relevant to meeting the client's needs in the long-term care setting

Figure 14.2 Characteristics of Decline or Improvement

Characteristics of Decline	Characteristics of Improvement
• Client's ability to make decisions for themselves declines	• Any improvement in an ADL physical functioning area such as a change from Limited Assistance to Independent
• Change in client's mood or an increase in the symptom frequency	• Decrease in the number of areas where behavioral symptoms are coded as being present and/or the frequency of a symptom decreases
• Any decline in an ADL physical functioning area such as from Limited assistance to Extensive assistance	• Client's ability to make decisions for themselves improves
• Client's incontinence pattern changes or there is placement of a catheter	• Client's incontinence pattern improves
• Unplanned weight loss (5% change in 30 days or 10% change in 180 days)	• Overall improvement of client's condition
• Client begins to use trunk restraint or a chair that prevents rising when it was not used before	
• Overall deterioration of resident's condition	

Source: CMS's RAI Version 3.0, Chapter 3

Here are some basic steps for the nutrition care planning process summarized from the CMS RAI Version 3.0 Manual.

Step 1. Identify Nutrition Problems

To determine the need for care planning, CAAs are developed from items coded on the MDS. The MDS is a preliminary assessment to identify potential client problems, strengths, and preferences. Care areas are triggered by MDS item responses that indicate the need for additional assessment based on problem identification. There are 20 CAAs in Version 3.0 of the RAI (refer to Figure 7.10 in Chapter 7). Ideally, the RAI is completed by the IDT that will develop the client's care plan. The following guidelines can help you develop a meaningful statement of the problem:

✓ be as specific as possible

✓ state the problem as it relates to the client

✓ identify possible reasons for the problem, including the client's perspective

✓ identify any strength the client has that will help in overcoming the problem.

IDT role. Uses clinical problem solving and decision making steps (see Figure 14.3) to make decisions. The team may find several problems/issues/conditions that have a related cause or they might be unrelated. Goals and approaches for each issue/condition may overlap and the IDT may decide to address those areas collectively in the care plan. The care planning issue should be documented as part of the CAA review documentation.

Certified Dietary Manager/Registered Dietitian role. Collect or verify data needed to determine nutrition problems. Care Area Triggers (CATs) of greatest interest to the Certified Dietary Manager and Registered Dietitian include falls, nutritional status, feeding tube, dehydration/fluid maintenance, and pressure ulcers. Care planning should include provisions for monitoring the client during mealtimes and during activities that include the consumption of food. You will want to consider the following:

✓ What risk factors for decline of eating skills did you identify?

- decrease in the ability to chew and swallow food
- deficit in the ability to move food onto a utensil and into the mouth
- oral health status affecting eating/chewing ability
- depression or confused mental state

✓ What care is the client receiving to address risk factors to maintain eating abilities?

- assistive devices to improve client's ability to grasp or coordination
- seating arrangement to improve sociability
- seating in a calm, quiet setting for clients with dementia

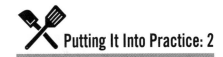

Putting It Into Practice: 2

What might a goal statement be for a client who has lost 6% of their total body weight in the past 30 days?

(Check your answer at the end of this chapter)

Interview the client to determine if the triggered condition affects the client's functioning or well-being. If it isn't a concern for the client, it should not be addressed on the care plan. Make sure you address issues such as the timing of the meals with the client. For instance, the client may request a late breakfast. In this case, the client's wishes should be honored and documented in the clinical record and alternatives should be offered before the care plan is finalized.

Step 3. Gather Data

IDT role. Gather data for their respective areas. The IDT will want to document how identified conditions are a problem for the client or how the condition affects the client's well-being.

Figure 14.3 Clinical Problem Solving and Decision Making Process Steps and Objectives

Process Step/Objectives	Key Tasks
Recognition/Assessment *Gather essential information about the individual*	• Identify and collect information that is needed to identify an individual's condition that enables proper definition of their conditions, strengths, needs, risks, problems, and prognosis • Obtain a personal and medical history • Perform a physical assessment
Problem Definition *Define the individual's problems, risks, and issues*	• Identify any current consequences and complications of the individual's situation underlying condition and illnesses, etc. • Clearly state the individual's issues and physical functions, psychosocial strengths, problems, needs, and deficits and concerns
Diagnosis/Cause-and-Effect Analysis *Identify physical, functional, and psychosocial causes of risks, problems, and other issues, and relate to one another and to their consequences*	• Identify causes of, and factors contributing to, the individual's current dysfunctions, disabilities, impairments, and risks • Identify pertinent evaluations and diagnostic tests • Identify how existing symptoms, signs, diagnoses, test results, dysfunctions, impairments, disabilities, and other findings relate to one another • Identify how addressing those causes is likely to affect consequences
Identifying Goals and Objectives of Care *Clarify purpose of providing care and of specific interventions and the criteria that will be used to determine whether the objectives are being met*	• Clarify prognosis • Define overall goals for the individual • Identify criteria for meeting goals
Selecting Interventions/Planning Care *Identify and implement interventions and treatments to address the individual's physical, functional, and psychosocial needs, concerns, problems, and risks*	• Identify specific symptomatic and cause-specific interventions (physical, functional, and psychosocial) • Identify how current and proposed treatment and services are expected to address causes, consequences, and risk factors, and help attain overall goals for the individual • Define anticipated benefits and risks of various interventions • Clarify how specific treatments and services will be evaluated for their effectiveness and possible adverse consequences.

Source: CMS's RAI Version 3.0, Chapter 4, pg. 4-9

Certified Dietary Manager role. As the Certified Dietary Manager, you may need to determine how many calories, how much protein, and how much fluid is needed by the client. Refer to Chapter 9 for methods of estimating needs for these nutrients. Also, be aware that your own facility or the Registered Dietitian may provide alternate methodologies. Calculation schemes may also be part of policies and procedures, nutrition care protocols, standards of practice, and/or regulations with which you must comply. **Standards of practice** are documents that define what constitutes quality in practice. They are standards addressing what you do. For example, a standard of practice will outline how a Certified Dietary Manager documents in the medical record. In standardized terminology developed by The Academy of Nutrition and Dietetics (AND) [formerly known as The American Dietetic Association (ADA)], there are 62 specific phrases to describe nutrition diagnoses. **Care protocols** are documents that outline a care process related to a specific medical condition. For example, a facility may have a care protocol for pressure ulcers that lists some standard steps that must be taken and describes how each member of the healthcare team will contribute. AND has developed a systematic process to describe care for clients. This process is called the Nutrition Care Process. You will need to become familiar with the standards that apply in your place of employment, and work with your Registered Dietitian to apply them consistently.

Keep in mind that disease states can affect needs for calories, protein and fluid. For example, a client experiencing renal failure or congestive heart failure may need to curtail fluid intake. In these scenarios, the physician should stipulate a fluid restriction in the diet order. This fluid order overrides the standard fluid calculations of 30 cc per kg of body weight; you will honor the diet order. A client experiencing pressure ulcers may need more protein and calories. As you apply standards and formulas, be sure to consider the client's unique disease factors, and consult with your Registered Dietitian as needed to clarify nutrient needs.

Step 4. Agree on Intermediate Goal(s)

IDT role. Agrees upon goal(s) that will lead to outcome objectives. The goal(s) and objectives must be pertinent to the client's condition and situation, be measurable, and have a time frame for completion or evaluation. Parts of the goal statement should include: The subject [first or third person, the verb, the modifiers, the time frame, and the goals(s)]. (See Figure 14.4 for example) Types of goals may include improvement, prevention, treatment to alleviate disease symptoms, or maintenance of current status. Goals should be prioritized based on client preferences if possible.

Figure 14.4 **Example Care Planning Goal Statement**

Subject	Verb	Modifiers	Time Frame	Goal
Mr. Jones	Will consume	24 oz. liquid daily	The next 30 days	In order to maintain hydration and prevent UTIs

Certified Dietary Manager role. If the Registered Dietitian is not present, the Certified Dietary Manager is responsible for understanding and relaying any nutrition diagnoses and care standards that the Registered Dietitian has identified. You must confirm that the nutrition goal is feasible and can be served/produced/monitored.

Step 5. Identify Specific Steps or Approaches

IDT role. Using input from the client, family, and/or client representative, the IDT identifies specific steps, approaches, or tasks that will be taken to help the client achieve his or her goals(s). These approaches serve as instructions for client care and provide for continuity of care by all staff. They should include precise and concise instructions to help staff understand and implement interventions.

The client has the right to participate in the care planning and the right to refuse treatment. The final care plan should be agreed to and discussed with the client or the representative.

Certified Dietary Manager role. Writing the goal(s) and specific steps/approaches may be an electronic process in your facility. You will need to become familiar with the documentation process for care planning in your facility and apply this information to that process. The Registered Dietitian may be responsible for writing the care plan. The nutrition care documentation should comply with the regulations and document the steps taken to meet the client's requests/needs/strengths.

Some examples of approaches for a goal to increase food intake might be: enhancing the taste and presentation of food; assisting the client to eat; addressing food preferences; and increasing finger foods and snacks for individuals with dementia.

Step 6. Communicate the Goal(s) and Objectives

IDT role. The goals and objectives/approaches should be communicated to other direct care staff who were not directly involved in developing the care plan. Changes to the care plan should occur as needed in accordance with professional standards of practice and documentation (e.g. signing and dating entries to the care plan). IDT members should communicate as needed about care plan changes.

Certified Dietary Manager role. You should communicate the goal(s) and objectives/approaches to your staff. You are responsible for alerting the Registered Dietitian to any changes in the client's condition, especially significant changes that may require a reassessment. Follow your facility policy and procedures for communicating with the Registered Dietitian and the IDT. You may need to schedule staff training, depending upon the goal(s) and objectives/approaches.

Step 7. Evaluate the Effectiveness of the Care Plan
This final step will be addressed in Chapter 15.

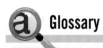

Glossary

Standard of Practice
Standards for what you normally do that constitute quality in practice

Care Protocols
Documents that outline a care process related to a specific medical condition

END OF CHAPTER

 Putting It Into Practice Questions & Answers

1. Mrs. S. hasn't been feeling well. She had the flu two weeks ago and still isn't eating more than 25% of her meals. Normally, a cheerful person, she cries easily and frequently seems confused. She has lost 5% of her total body weight since the beginning of the month. Should Mrs. S. be reassessed? Why or why not? If yes, what should the time frame be for her reassessment and care planning?

   A. *Mrs. S. has two areas of decline: weight loss and behavioral/mood change. Complete the MDS and review what was triggered before. Complete a CAA for the MDS item responses that indicate the need for additional assessment based on problem identification within 14 days. Interview the client or her family for their input and collaborate with the Registered Dietitian and the IDT to decide whether or not to develop a care plan for triggered care areas. If a care plan is warranted, it must be completed within 7 days after the CAAs.*

2. Write a goal statement for Mr. J. who has lost 6% of his total body weight in the past 30 days.

   A. *Mr. J will consume 50% of all meals during the next 30 days in order to maintain weight and gain strength.*

CHAPTER 15

Review Effectiveness of Nutrition Care Plan

Overview and Objectives

To be effective, nutritional care must be dynamic. A Certified Dietary Manager and the Interdisciplinary Team must routinely assess new information and apply findings to ongoing plans for quality care.

After completing this chapter, you should be able to:

✓ Describe interdisciplinary relationships

✓ Identify effectiveness of the nutrition care plan

✓ Suggest cooperative ways to solve problems

✓ Identify methods of communicating with other departments

✓ Evaluate care plans for individuality and specific needs

The Interdisciplinary Team

You've seen the words, interdisciplinary team (IDT), but who are they? The IDT is a group of professionals, each with unique training and expertise, who contribute to the overall care of a client. Thus, a Certified Dietary Manager works closely with others. Let's take a look at some typical roles and a partial list of responsibilities, particularly as they relate to nutrition care.

Administrator (in a Nursing Home)

✓ Ensure that a nutritional screening/assessment system exists

✓ Ensure adequacy of staffing to implement and maintain the system

✓ Support all staff members in performing their duties

Registered Dietitian

✓ Assume primary responsibility and accountability for nutrition screening and assessment and client nutrition care planning

✓ Select and sets up a nutrition screening/assessment system (in cooperation with the nursing service and facility administration); train facility staff as needed

✓ Monitor the screening system

✓ Perform nutritional assessments; may complete the Resident Assessment Instrument (RAI) and care plan

✓ Develop nutrition care plan

✓ Record assessment findings, recommendations, and follow-up plans in medical record and client care plan

✓ Alert other team members to any part of the nutritional care plan needing their cooperation

✓ Define the role of a Certified Dietary Manager and provide training

✓ Provide nutrition counseling

✓ Monitor the accuracy of diet service

✓ Participate in quality management

Certified Dietary Manager (Clinical Duties)

✓ Interview clients for diet history

✓ Conduct routine nutrition screening/collects data for assessment

✓ Calculate nutrient intake

✓ Implement diet plans

✓ Document nutrition information on clients' medical records

✓ Counsel clients on basic diet restrictions; specify standards and procedures for food preparation to comply with diet restrictions

✓ Review effectiveness of nutrition care plans

✓ Assist in nutrition care process according to established policies and procedures

Nurse

✓ Assess client needs; develop, implement, and monitor care plan

✓ Deliver direct nursing care

✓ Ensure that client consumes food: organize the client feeding responsibilities, distribute the workload, determine need for adaptive eating devices with input from occupational therapist

✓ Assist with mealtimes and feeding

✓ Record accurate and meaningful information about client's food and fluid intake

✓ Provide education to clients

✓ Completes RAI

Occupational Therapist

✓ Evaluate needs related to fine motor skills

✓ Recommend assistive eating devices and other techniques to help clients feed themselves

✓ Provide therapy to develop fine motor skills

Physician

✓ Evaluate medical conditions and develop medical diagnoses

✓ Plan, oversee, and monitor treatment

✓ Possess major responsibility for the nutritional status of the client (in conformance to acceptable standards of practice)

✓ Write diet orders and/or approve protocol for standard orders

✓ Order other treatments which affect nutritional status

✓ Utilize information provided by other members of the healthcare team

Social Worker

✓ Evaluate social and support needs

✓ Assist clients and families with decision-making

✓ Help clients and families plan care upon discharge from a healthcare facility

✓ Assist with applying for other healthcare services, such as home-delivered meals or home care

✓ Identify resources

✓ Provide counseling

Speech Pathologist

✓ Evaluate the chewing and swallowing function of clients

✓ Recommend appropriate therapy for dysphagia

✓ Provide evaluation and therapy for speech-related needs

Policies and procedures must be developed and followed for optimal nutrition care. Whether dealing with clients in a hospital, long-term care facility, or other healthcare setting, the nutrition care process uses the same methods and principles. However, depending on your facility's policies and procedures and state regulations, the Certified Dietary Manager's exact role in the nutrition care process will vary.

Note that in current Centers for Medicare and Medicaid Services (CMS) guidelines for client care, the client and family members or significant others also play crucial roles. The client, for example, has a great deal of information and insight to offer in developing an understanding of his condition and needs. The client also has the right to contribute to care planning, and to play a well-informed role in deciding upon care. Ultimately, the client must participate in care for it to be effective.

Gathering and Sharing Information

As each member of the team contributes specialized training, knowledge, and experience to the care of clients, all members participate in such basic tasks as:

✓ Assessing client needs

✓ Developing a plan of care

✓ Evaluating a plan of care

✓ Providing education to clients

While the details of a nutrition care plan may differ from the details of a nursing care plan or a speech therapy care plan, the overall objectives are in unison. For example, team members may work together to improve a client's nutritional status as follows:

✓ A physician orders a diet.

✓ A Certified Dietary Manager conducts a diet history to find out how the client usually eats and to determine food preferences and intolerances.

✓ A speech therapist recommends an appropriate diet for dysphagia and specifies techniques to manage a swallowing disorder.

✓ An occupational therapist helps a client develop the strength and skills to feed himself effectively.

✓ A nurse or nursing assistant provides hands-on set-up and assistance at mealtime and encourages a client to eat—or feeds a client.

✓ Both a nurse and a Certified Dietary Manager may help monitor diet tolerance and food intake.

✓ A Certified Dietary Manager develops a menu and manages food production to ensure that the client receives appropriate foods, and that they are appetizing and wholesome.

This chapter is about how the effectiveness of IDT participates in monitoring the plan of care.

To attain the best outcomes, team members have to share information. As each views the client's needs from a unique perspective, each has observations and ideas to offer. Thus, sharing information and communicating effectively are critical to clinical care. How do team members share information? One means is through the medical record itself. A good starting point is the list of problems (if a problem-oriented medical record system is used). Each team member documents assessments, plans, and progress in the record. Each time any team member works with a client, the first step is to open the medical record and review the documentation provided by other members of the team.

Now you have completed your comprehensive care plan. During the care planning meeting, each member of the IDT listens to others to understand the comprehensive clinical picture. Each member contributes ideas to help meet a client's needs.

However, care does not end with a plan. The plan is only the beginning. This is particularly true in long-term care environments, in which a client may be receiving care for weeks, months, or years. After documenting and implementing the plan, the final two steps in providing nutrition care are to: re-assess the client at defined intervals, and (as appropriate), revise the plan. In re-assessing a client, we are answering the questions: Is the nutrition care plan working? How do we know?

As you begin to evaluate the effectiveness of nutrition care, let's look at some of the questions that surveyors will be asking to assess the effectiveness of your care:

✓ Has the client's ability to eat or eating skills improved, declined, or stayed the same?

✓ Was any deterioration or lack of improvement avoidable or unavoidable?

✓ If the client's eating abilities have declined, is there any evidence that the decline was unavoidable?

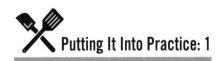

Putting It Into Practice: 1

As you are observing a client in the dining room, you notice that Mr. H is having trouble grasping his utensils. His coordination seems to be declining. To what member of the IDT would you refer Mr. H?

(Check your answer at the end of this chapter)

✓ What risk factors for decline of eating skills did the facility identify in the care plan?

✓ Is there sufficient staff time and assistance provided to maintain eating abilities (e.g., allowing clients enough time to eat independently or with limited assistance)?

✓ Were Care Area Triggers (CATs) and the Care Area Assessment (CAA) process used to assess reasons for decline, potential for decline, or lack of improvement?

✓ Were individual objectives of the plan of care periodically evaluated, and if the objectives were not met, were alternative approaches developed to encourage maintaining eating abilities?

✓ Was the care plan driven by client's strengths identified in the comprehensive assessment?

✓ Was the care plan consistently implemented? What changes were made to treatment if the client failed to progress or when initial rehabilitation goals were achieved?

As you can see from these questions, you are expected to closely monitor the implementation of the care plan. Whenever you monitor the care plan objectives, it needs to be documented in the medical record to show the other IDT members what progress is being made. Even in this follow-up period for the care plan, it will be important to communicate with the client to assess how well he/she feels the plan is working. It is also critical to communicate with the Registered Dietitian if you see any decline or improvement as the result of the care plan approaches.

Let's look at some specific data that will assist you in monitoring the effectiveness of your care plan.

Hydration and Dehydration

The regulation requires that the facility must provide each client with sufficient fluid intake to maintain proper hydration and health. Among the most common clinical concerns in a long-term care setting is dehydration, or a lack of sufficient water in the body. As you have learned in earlier chapters, water is a nutrient. Inadequate water in the body can lead to a drop in blood volume, with serious consequences. In addition, older individuals may lose some of the sense of thirst, which normally protects us from become dehydrated. Some restrict their own fluid intake to avoid bathroom issues. Figure 15.1 lists possible signs of dehydration. Remember that thirst itself is not a reliable sign of dehydration. It is possible to become dehydrated without experiencing thirst. This situation can also occur under severe heat stress. Other factors that can lead to dehydration include fever, bleeding, severe burns, vomiting, diarrhea, or certain metabolic disorders.

Consider these risk factors for the client becoming dehydrated:

✓ Coma/decreased sensory ability

✓ Fluid loss and increased fluid needs (e.g. diarrhea, fever, uncontrolled diabetes)

✓ Fluid restriction secondary to renal dialysis

Figure 15.1 Possible Signs of Dehydration

- Decrease in urinary output or dark urine
- Sudden weight loss (e.g. 5% or more of body weight)
- Sunken eyes
- Hollow cheekbones
- Dry mucous membranes
- Cracked lips
- Skin turgor (resilience) is poor
- Change in state of alertness (in extreme dehydration)
- Deep, gasping breathing

✓ Functional impairments that make it difficult to drink, reach fluids, or communicate fluid needs

✓ Dementia in which the client forgets to drink or forgets how to drink

✓ Refusal of fluids

As you are assessing the effectiveness of your hydration care plan, consider asking/answering these questions:

✓ Have you and other staff members provided clients with adequate fluid intake to maintain proper hydration and health? How do you know?

✓ What approaches were taken to ensure adequate fluid intake? (e.g. fluids were kept next to the client at all times with staff assisting or cuing the client to drink)

✓ Are staff members aware of the need for maintaining adequate fluid intake?

✓ If adequate fluid intake is difficult to maintain or the client is refusing fluids, have alternative treatment approaches been offered such as popsicles, gelatin and other similar non-liquid foods?

Remember, too, that for clients with renal or cardiac distress, an excess of fluids can be detrimental.

Certain clinical conditions create a different kind of problem—water retention. Unhealthy water retention is called edema. This may occur, for example, when the heart is not functioning properly and/or kidneys are not removing excess water. Signs of edema appear in Figure 15.2. Edema is not a disease; it is a symptom. Fluid retention can make the heart and lungs work harder, and can eventually lead to a medical crisis. To manage diseases in which edema occurs, a physician may order restriction of dietary fluids. For any client following a fluid restriction, part of the follow-up evaluation will be to check on how the edema has changed.

Figure 15.2 Possible Signs of Edema

- Visible swelling in legs, ankles, feet, and/or abdomen
- Elevated blood pressure
- Sudden weight gain (e.g. more than 5% of body weight)

Monitoring Diabetes

If one of the problems you are monitoring is diabetes mellitus, there are several indicators that help you understand how well the client is doing. A goal of diabetes management is to maintain blood glucose levels at defined levels to prevent complications. What pieces of information will tell you this?

✓ Blood glucose measurements such as fasting blood glucose. Taken in the morning over a period of days

✓ Measurements of glucose and ketones in the urine. Normally, both should be zero. Presence of glucose in the urine generally indicates recent high blood glucose values. Ketones can indicate that the body has gone into an abnormal type of metabolism in an attempt to nourish cells.

Ongoing management of blood glucose levels is also measured in glycosylated hemoglobin. This laboratory measurement gives a snapshot of management over time. Depending upon a client's needs and goals, blood lipid levels and total body weight may also be important.

In monitoring diabetes, it is important to talk to the client regularly and find out what concerns exist. Check for any symptoms that indicate high glucose levels—such as thirst, excessive hunger, and excessive urination. Also check nursing notes for any reports that the client has experienced hypoglycemia (low blood sugar). In addition, you will want to observe meal intake and menu management. Consider how the client is doing with managing the form of dietary control being used, such as carbohydrate counting, exchange lists, or other system. Is this system proving a good match for the client? Is the client able to apply it? Is the client enjoying meals? Is the client eating any additional foods not on the menu (e.g. gifts from family or visitors)? Is the diet providing an adequate level of control for blood glucose? You would want to review the medication regimen, and note whether medicines and/or dosages have changed as well. As you gather this information and check with other members of the healthcare team, you can develop a solid picture of how the diabetes management plan is working, and make dietary suggestions and/or a referral to the Registered Dietitian as appropriate. For example, a client who is having frequent episodes of hypoglycemia may need liberalization of medications (determined by the physician) and/or of diet. A client whose blood glucose levels run consistently higher than a clinical goal may need a boost or change in medication, a boost in exercise, and/or a more tightly controlled meal plan.

Monitoring Nutritional Status/Weight Loss

A variety of clinical conditions relate to nutritional status, such as protein-calorie malnutrition. There are many reasons a client may experience weight loss (see Figure 15.3). About one-third of these reasons are easy to correct, e.g., toileting before meals or assisting clients with dental hygiene. Any time improvement of nutritional status is one of the clinical goals, a Certified Dietary Manager needs to take an active role in monitoring progress. Here is some objective information to review (as available): weight changes, percent ideal body weight (IBW), skinfold thickness, serum transferrin or albumin, prealbumin, and total lymphocyte count. In monitoring weight, remember to weigh a client the same way, in the same amount of clothing, on the same scale, and at the same time of day each time for a good comparison. If you have performed a calorie/protein count, review this carefully, and compare it with estimated nutrient needs.

Nursing notes can be a helpful source of information about food intake and meal tolerance from day to day. Review them for trends and any notations of concerns or problems related to eating. You can also check intake and output records to find out whether the client is consuming adequate fluids.

Examine the current medication list and identify any changes. Many medications affect sense of taste. Some cause dry mouth, nausea, or other symptoms that can profoundly affect food intake.

Remember that your care plan is individualized to each client and your assessment of the effectiveness needs to be individualized as well. The following are questions you may want to ask a client to help you assess an objective to gain weight, eat more, or eat less:

✓ How is your appetite?

✓ Are you having any problems or concerns with eating?

✓ Are you having any problems in chewing?

✓ Are you have any problems in swallowing?

✓ Are you experiencing any digestive concerns, such as nausea, vomiting, diarrhea, or constipation?

Check carefully for tolerance of the current diet. Update food preferences, because they can change. A new medication or other condition may alter how a client tolerates a particular food. In a long-term care environment, repetition of foods may also reduce intake. A client may simply become bored with the same foods. Look for changes in dental health, and any other conditions that may affect a client's ability to feed him/herself, swallow, and maintain interest and alertness at mealtimes.

If the client is not able to communicate, look for this same information through observation, asking family members, or through consultation with others who are involved in their care.

If you have implemented special dietary plans to improve nutritional status, review the success of these. You may be including nutritional supplements and/ or high-calorie, high-protein foods in the daily menu. Who is responsible for ordering the supplements? Consider how well the client is tolerating these. Is the client enjoying these foods? How much is the client consuming? Is there enough variety to keep meals appetizing? The bottom line, of course, is improvement in nutritional status.

Monitoring Pressure Ulcers

For a client with pressure ulcers, nutritional monitoring is also essential. Maintaining or improving nutritional status can contribute greatly to resolving this clinical problem. Thus, you would want to evaluate changes in nutritional

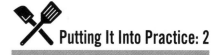

Putting It Into Practice: 2

If your care plan goal was to have the client maintain their weight and, after one month, the client is continuing to lose weight, what steps should you take. What questions would you ask?

(Check your answer at the end of this chapter)

Figure 15.3 **101 Reasons for Weight Loss in Long-Term Care**

1 Uncontrolled diabetes
2 Severe COPD
3 Shortness of breath
4 Fear of aspiration
5 Dehydration
6 Poor vision
7 Inadequate staff to feed
8 Poor plate presentation
9 Dry mouth
10 Drugs
11 Therapeutic diets
12 Inability to open food packages
13 Unable to cut meat
14 Unable to feed self
15 Food does not taste good
16 Overmedicated
17 Unacceptable food texture
18 Unable to chew food
19 Many food dislikes
20 Unable to communicate needs
21 Recent change in physical condition
22 Mental confusion
23 Pacing; inability to keep still
24 Food preferences not honored
25 Unable to get food to mouth
26 Inappropriate portion size
27 Improper positioning

28 Not enough time to eat
29 Adaptive equipment not used
30 Depression
31 Recent loss of a significant person
32 Renal disease
33 Liver disease
34 Cancer
35 Ill-fitting dentures
36 Too weak to eat
37 Poor dental hygiene
38 Sore mouth
39 Pain
40 Unhappiness with table mates
41 Failure to get snacks/nourishments
42 Unfamiliar foods
43 Hungry between meals
44 Repetition in meals—especially special diets
45 Menus not changed in years
46 No substitutes given
47 Frequent infections
48 Body image distortions
49 Psychological problems
50 Dining room unattractive
51 Care plan does not adequately address needs
52 Inappropriate snacks between meals
53 Inappropriate remarks about food

54 Boredom
55 Not toileted before meals
56 Recent surgery
57 Family does not visit
58 Food allergies/food intolerances
59 Contractures in hand
60 Wanders
61 Anorexia
62 Too tired to eat
63 Fear of eating
64 Facial paralysis
65 Cold food
66 Too long a wait for meal
67 Refusal to swallow
68 Diarrhea
69 Vomiting
70 Increased calorie needs
71 New on diuretic
72 Mood disorders
73 Agitated at meals
74 Decline in eating abilities
75 Dementia
76 Slow eaters
77 Chronic bowel disease
78 Refusal to eat
79 Refusal to take liquids
80 Fever
81 Nurse aides not trained to feed
82 Using food to get attention
83 Amputation

84 Expectation of weight loss as normal
85 Lack of encouragement
86 Elderly failure to thrive
87 Anxious
88 Treatment for malignancy
89 Hyperthyroidism
90 Taste alterations
91 Spitting or throwing of food
92 Constipation
93 Food intakes not accurate
94 Weight control
95 Dining room too distracting
96 Client does not understand nutrition needs
97 Failure to follow care plan
98 Decreased ability to smell
99 Attitude regarding placement
100 Need for control
101 Desire to die

AND MORE...

- Food activities too close to meal time
- Foodborne illness
- Boredom with nourishments
- Loss of preferred caretaker
- Inaccurate weight

status, weight changes, percent IBW, skinfold thickness, serum transferrin or albumin, prealbumin, and total lymphocyte count. It is also imperative to consider protein, calorie, and fluid intake, and review whether the overall diet provides a reasonable balance of other essential nutrients. Furthermore, check on the staging of a pressure ulcer and ask whether it has advanced, stayed the same, or improved. Note whether new pressure ulcers have occurred.

Documenting Progress

As with all professional activity, an evaluation of the effectiveness of care should be documented in the medical record. The purpose of the progress note is to summarize how the client is responding to treatment as well as to document the degree of success in achieving goals identified in the care plan.

Progress notes are written in a specific, accurate, objective, concise and thorough manner. Whatever documentation method your facility uses, your progress note may address questions such as the following:

✓ How has the client responded to treatment?

✓ Has there been progress in achieving the nutrition goals in the care plan?

✓ Are there any new nutrition-related problems?

✓ What has changed since the care plan and previous progress notes were written, such as medications, laboratory values, ability to feed self, etc.?

The timing of progress notes you write will depend on the type of facility you work in, as well as the facility's own policies and procedures. Normally, progress notes in long-term care facilities are written quarterly for all clients, monthly for those at risk, and more frequently for those with special circumstances.

END OF CHAPTER

 Putting It Into Practice Questions & Answers

1. As you are observing a client in the dining room, you notice that Mr. H is having trouble grasping his utensils. His coordination seems to be declining. To what member of the IDT would you refer Mr. H?

   A. *You should refer Mr. H. to the occupational therapist. The OT can recommend an assistive eating device or other techniques to help Mr. H. feed himself.*

2. If your care plan goal was to have the client maintain weight and, after one month, the client is continuing to lose weight, what steps should you take? What questions would you ask?

   A. *First, you should notify the Registered Dietitian and make a note of the client's weight loss in the medical record. You should look at the food intake records to see what percentage of the diet the client is consuming. Has something new such as a fever, UTI, or pressure ulcer changed the need for calories? Has there been a change in meds such as adding a diuretic that would explain the weight loss? Have you asked the client for his perspective?*

CHAPTER 16

Help Clients Choose Foods from Selective Menus

Overview and Objectives

Today's clients are more independent and want more choices, and the federal regulations Centers for Medicare and Medicaid Services (CMS) are also mandating more focus on the client. Providing exceptional nutritional care goes hand-in-hand with a culture change in meal service systems.

After completing this chapter, you should be able to:

✓ Determine dietary requirements of client

✓ Ascertain client's present knowledge and needs

✓ Choose appropriate resource materials

✓ Evaluate client's food preferences

✓ Suggest acceptable food substitutes

✓ Verify substitutes in terms of availability and facility practices

✓ Match food items identified with patient preferences

In an article in the Dietary Manager's Magazine, June, 2010, on Culture Change in Dining and Regulatory Compliance, Linda Handy, MS, RD, explains that "never before has the Certified Dietary Manager been needed more as a manager to use your skills to implement a more person-centered, client-driven dining program." The choices for healthcare communities for older Americans are expanding and the type of food and nutrition care will need to expand as well. With 2010 CMS regulations, F242, "your facility has to demonstrate that it's allowing clients' choice and self-determination in dining." At the same time, it is important to tailor a menu to the dietary requirements of the client. How do we accomplish this? This chapter will describe the culture change movement and menu options to support culture change.

Culture Change in Language

Culture change in dining begins with changing some of the language we use. Karen Schoeneman wrote about this in an "editorial" for the Pioneer Network Culture Change project. She asked people to come up with alternative words for 'bibs,' 'feeder,' 'elderly.' Figure 16.1 lists samples of dining terms that were suggested to help older adults maintain their dignity and healthcare facilities to become more person-centered.

Figure 16.1 Terminologies in Culture Change

Old Terminology	Suggested Terminology
Elderly	Elder, older adult, individual
Wing, unit	Household, neighborhood, street
Institutional care	Individual care
Feeder table	Dining table
Feeder	Person who needs help eating
Facility, institution, nursing home	Home life center, living center
Foodservice worker, Hey You	The person's name
Dietary service, foodservice	Dining services
Tray line	Fine dining
Nourishment	Snack
Bib	Napkin, clothing protector
Diabetic	Person who has diabetes
Mechanical soft food	Chopped food
Trays are here	It's dinner time; dinner is served

Source: http://www.pioneernetwork.net Used with permission.

Culture Change in Dining

The culture change movement in dining is driven in part by the large numbers of Americans who are aging and who will be entering the various healthcare communities as they age. It is also being driven by the change in regulations to implement more person-centered, client-driven dining programs. This is indeed an opportune time to showcase dining services and your ability to enhance the quality of life through food and dining choices.

As with any change, there is resistance based on concerns about cost, staffing, and coordinating the changes with regulations. The California Culture Change Coalition piloted a project in 2007 in 11 participating facilities. The purpose of the project was to identify and implement a new food-related practice in their facilities. They have provided information about their projects, lessons learned, and resources at this URL: http://www.calculturechange.org/services-dining. html. One of these resources is a decision-making tool with questions they needed to answer to move forward with restaurant style dining. (see Figure 16.2)

As you begin to adopt this culture change, there are many questions that need to be answered. Start with questioning your clients to help you decide what they want for dining services. You might ask questions such as:

✓ What time of day do you like to eat your meals?

✓ Do you snack regularly?

✓ How frequently during the day do you want coffee, tea, or water?

✓ Where do you prefer to eat your meals?

Figure 16.2 Decision-Making Tool for Culture Change to Restaurant Style Dining

Decision Making Tool: Critical Element—Restaurant Style Dining

- What equipment is needed for restaurant or waiter dining?
- Where will the mobile equipment be stored when not in use? Does it need to be locked?
- Is there adequate electrical and plumbing access for your plan?
- What existing equipment can be re-purposed for restaurant or waiter dining?
- Are there any physical plant changes that will be needed?
- Who will approve the expenditure?
- Can restaurant or waiter dining be operated on an interim basis with existing equipment while waiting for the capital budget?
- How many different food items can be offered?
- Will these menu food items be available to clients who do not dine in restaurant or waiter dining?
- Are there any client safety concerns such as pouring hot beverages?
- How will menu be communicated to clients?
- Will waiters take orders at the dining table or will menus be pre-selected the day or meal before?
- Can physician ordered diet restrictions be liberalized?
- How will items be labeled or designated for various dietary restrictions?
- Does the current facility budget cover the anticipated costs?
- How will costs be monitored or reported?
- What serving utensils or equipment will be needed?
- What glasses, dishes or utensils will be used by the clients?
- How will condiments such as salt, pepper, sugar packets be handled for clients on "No Added Salt" and diabetic diets?
- What disposable or re-usable items, including napkins, staff uniforms, table linens and clothing protectors will be needed?
- How will cross-contamination be avoided when serving clients?
- How many clients will participate in restaurant or waiter dining and how long will it take to serve them?
- How will staff be assigned to restaurant or waiter dining?
- What is the cost of staffing restaurant or waiter dining?
- How will dietary restrictions be communicated and provided?
- Who will monitor and document the client choice/consumption of food?
- Will this be documented in the medical record?
- Will staff track the waste, over-production or shortage of food?
- Do the facility policy and procedures need to be updated and approved for restaurant or waiter dining?
- Are there any forms needed for restaurants or waiter dining?
- Will you do client satisfaction surveys?
- How will you communicate about the new restaurant or waiter dining? To whom?
- Will you do a pilot test of restaurant or waiter dining?

Source: http://www.pioneernetwork.net Used with permission.

✓ What foods do you usually eat at breakfast, lunch, and dinner?

✓ Where should you begin with the culture change? (expanded snack program, restaurant services, selective menu)

Next, you will want to choose appropriate resources for changing your dining and/or menu options. The California Culture Change Coalition materials are a good start. You could survey other facilities in your area to determine how/if they have begun to implement a culture change. The Academy of Nutrition and Dietetics (AND) [formerly known as The American Dietetic Association (ADA)] published a practice paper in 2010: *Individualized Nutrition Approaches for Older Adults in Health Care Communities*. This practice paper is located in *Nutrition in the News* at the end of this chapter. Remember, the changes you make need to reflect your client's food and dining preferences.

Once you have data for what you want to do and why, the next step is to work with all of your facility departments. This will be a change for them as well and you want them to support your changes. Specifically, other departments that might be affected are maintenance, fiscal, and nursing. You will want to develop a policy and procedure that outlines every department's responsibility for each type of change you initiate. Communication and training will be key steps as you begin to implement a culture change in your facility. It is important to note that the a culture change is a process that takes some time to implement.

Menu Options

A selective menu is the way to implement current federal regulations and more importantly, enhance the quality of life and quality of care for your clients. A selective menu is one in which clients have the opportunity to make choices or selections in advance of meal service. For example, a selective menu usually offers at least two choices for an entrée, and multiple choices for most items on the menu. Typically, a selective menu is distributed to clients in advance of the meal (about a day or half a day before service, depending on the system). Clients note their selections, which are retrieved and used in the kitchen as trays or meals are prepared. Computer-based selective menu systems may use handheld computers and/or telephone systems for entry of choices into an automated system. Figure 16.3 shows an actual selective menu with options for general, carbohydrate counting, clear liquid, and full liquid diets. Notice that the modifications for the carbohydrate counting diet are the numbers of 'carbs' found in specific menu items. That way, the client who knows how many 'carbs' they can have, still has many choices. Menu options on a selective menu in a hospital should rotate daily for variety.

In healthcare facilities, or in any environment where the foodservice department is responsible for honoring therapeutic diets, it was standard practice to review menu choices before they are served. If clients make choices on a selective menu, a member of the foodservice staff then reviews these choices against a nutrition kardex card or computerized tray ticket. Common adjustments on selective menus that may need to be made are:

✓ Portion sizes of products that count as fluid, for a fluid-restricted diet

✓ Portion sizes of high-carbohydrate foods, for a carbohydrate counting diet

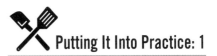

Putting It Into Practice: 1

List three steps you would need to take to implement a culture change in your facility.

(Check your answer at the end of this chapter)

Figure 16.3 Sample Selective Menu with Carbohydrate Count

Room Number: _____ Pt. Name: _____ Diet Order: _____

DOB: _____ Meal: **B L D** Time if advance: _____ Total Carb Choices: _____

Breakfast	Cereals	Fruits/Yogurt	Bakery/Breads
Scrambled eggs	Oatmeal: 1/2 cup = **1**	Apple = **1**	English Muffin: 1/2 = **1**
Egg beaters	Malt O Meal: 1/2 cup = **1**	Banana = **2**	Muffin: small = **2**; large = **4**
Pancake = **1**	Cream of Wheat: 1/2 cup = **1**	Orange Slices = **1**	White Toast: 1 slice = **1**
Waffle = **4**	Bran Flakes: 1 box = **1**	Fresh Fruit: 1/2 cup = **1**	Bagel: 1/2 = **2**
Bacon	Cherrios: 1 box = **1**	Applesauce: 1/2 cup = **1**	Coffeecake: 1 piece = **6**
Sausage link	Cornflakes: 1 box = **1**	Stewed Prunes: 4 = **1**	Dinner Roll: 1 = **1**
	Frosted Flakes: 1 box = **1**	Flavored Yogurt: 6 oz. = **2**	White Bread: 1 slice = **1**
	Fruit Loops: 1 box = **2**		
	Raisin Bran: 1 box = **2**		
	Rice Krispies: 1 box = **1**		

Entrees	Soups	Sides	Salads
Roast Turkey	Chicken Noodle: 1 cup = **1**	Mashed Potatoes: 1/2 cup = **1**	Tossed
Baked Chicken	Tomato: 1 cup = **1**	Baked Potato: 1/2 = **1**	Dressing
Roast Beef	Cream of Broccoli: 1 cup = **1**	Rice: 1/3 cup = **1**	Coleslaw
Chef Salad = **1**	Chili: 1 cup = **1**	Carrots or Peas:	Cottage Cheese
Taco Salad: 1 pkg. = **1**	Crackers: 3 = **1**	1/2 cup = **1**	Potato Salad: 1/2 cup = **1**
Cafe Special (Noon M-F)	LS Tomato: 1 cup = **1**	Corn: 1/2 cup = **1**	Pasta Salad: 1/2 cup = **1**
Ham	LS Chicken Noodle: 1 cup = **1**	Green Beans: 1/2 cup = **0**	
	LS Vegetable: 1 cup = **1**	Broccoli/Cauliflower:	
	LS Crackers: 3 = **1**	1/2 cup = **0**	
		Gravy: regular or large	
		Baked Beans: 1/2 cup = **1.5**	

Sandwiches	Desserts	Beverages	Milk/Juices
White, Whole Wheat, Bun*	Angel Food cake: 1 piece = **1**	Coffee	2%: 1 cup = **1**
Hamburger	Pie: 1 piece = **3**	Decaf Coffee	Skim 1 cup = **1**
Cheeseburger	Ice cream: 1/2 cup = **1**	Black Tea	Chocolate: 1 cup = **2**
Sliced Meat	Sherbet: 1/2 cup = **2**	Green Tea	Apple Juice: 1/2 cup = **1**
Turkey, Ham,	Cake: 1 piece = **2**	Decaf Tea	Cranberry Juice:
Chicken: 1/3 cup = **1**	Cookies: 1 = **1**	Iced Tea	1/3 cup = **1**
Grilled Cheese	Vanilla Wafers: 5 = **1**	Lemon Juice	Diet Cranberry Juice:
Grilled Chicken	Pudding: 1 = **2**	Crystal LIght	1 cup = **1**
Ham and Cheese		- Lemonade	Grape Juice: 1/3 cup = **1**
Ham (hot, cold)		- Raspberry	Orange Juice: 1/2 cup = **1**
Grilled Ham & Cheese			Tomato Juice: 6 oz. = **1/2**
Tuna salad, Egg salad			V8 Juice: 6 oz. = **1/2**
Ham salad			Prune Juice: 1/3 cup = **1**
			Pineapple Juice: 1/3 cup = **1**
*Each bread = **1**, Bun = **2**			Hot Chocolate = **1**
			SF Hot Chocolate = **1/2**

(Continued)

Figure 16.3 **Sample Selective Menu with Carbohydrate Count** *(Continued)*

Condiments*	Clear Liquids	Full Liquids
Butter	Apple Juice: 1/2 cup = **1**	Any clear liquid items
Margarine	Cranberry Juice: 1/3 cup = **1**	Orange Juice: 1/2 cup = **1**
Cream Cheese	Grape Juice: 1/3 cup = **1**	Milk, White: 1 cup = **1**
Light Cream Cheese	Diet Cranberry Juice: 1 cup = **1**	Milk, Chocolate: 1 cup = **2**
Sour Cream	Beef Broth	Hot Cereal: 1/2 cup = **1**
Creamer	Chicken Broth	Cream Soup (strained)
Non Dairy Creamer	Plain Gelatin: 1 = **1**	Pudding: 1/2 cup = **2**
Salt	Pop Treat: 1 = **2**	Ice Cream: 1/2 cup = **1**
Salt Substitute	Crystal Light	Sherbet: 1/2 cup = **2**
Sugar: 3 = **1**	Coffee/Tea	Creamer
Splenda, Equal, Sweet-N-Low	Creamer Breeze: 8 oz - 54g = **3.5**	V8 Juice: 6 oz = **1/2**
Syrup: 1 = **1**		Tomato Juice: 6 oz = **1/2**
Diet Syrup		Prune Juice: 1/3 cup = **1**
Jelly: 1 = **1**		Pineapple Juice: 1/3 cup = **1**
Pepper		Boost: 8 oz - 41g = ~ **3**
Mrs. Dash		
Catsup		
Mustard		
Mayonnaise		
Peanut butter		
* Condiments are okay: salt, sugar, Equal, Spenda, Sweet-N-Low, syrup, diet syrup. NOT PEPPER		

Source: Southwest Health Center, Platteville WI, 2010. Used with permission.

✓ Consistency of foods and liquids for specific dysphagia diets

✓ Special adjustments for diets with multiple restrictions

✓ Adjustments to incorporate a standing order such as the addition of a liquid nutritional supplement to meals

What happens if the client does not request enough food on a selective menu? What if the client selects food that is not on his/her diet? Foodservice staff should be trained to address a client's diet when they drop off the menu. (e.g. "Good morning Mrs. Smith; I know that you are on a sodium restricted diet and here are your menu selections for today"). This helps remind the client of their diet and sets the stage for their menu choices. If they see that the client has not selected very much food, the foodservice staff might say, "Oh, Mrs. Smith, our roast chicken is very tender and moist today; can I add that to your selection?" If the client insists on selecting something that is not on their menu such as bacon on a salt restricted diet, gently remind the client that their diet does not allow them to have bacon. Always treat the clients with respect and respond in such a way that they don't become defensive.

On a selective menu, there may also be items a client writes in as a special request. How this is handled depends on the facility policy. In general, health

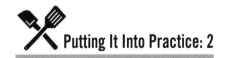

Putting It Into Practice: 2

What would be an appropriate substitute if a client does not like broccoli?

(Check your answer at the end of this chapter)

facilities attempt to honor write-in requests as practical. Many facilities develop a standardized list of write-in options to provide greater choice for clients.

A nonselective menu is one in which clients do not have the opportunity to make choices for main dishes. Instead, they receive a standard, predefined menu. This is more common in a group dining experience such as a nursing home or assisted living. Even with a nonselective menu, you can focus on the clients by following their individualized food preferences with appropriate substitutions. You may be able to work with the medical staff to implement more liberalized diets so that all clients receive the general diet except for texture modifications.

In a nonselective menu system, it is also important to review and modify standard menu choices to accommodate specific diet orders. If your facility has implemented a liberalized diet, there may be very few diet orders, other than texture modifications. You will still want to follow individual food preferences, which may mean substituting a food item. Menu substitutions must be

Figure 16.4 Food Substitutions*

Food Item	Substitute Choices	Vitamin A Content (per 1/2 cup serving)	Vitamin C Content (per 1/2 cup serving)
Dark Green Vegetables	Broccoli, frozen, boiled	50 ug	50 ug
	Asparagus, boiled	50 ug	7 mg
	Peas, frozen and boiled	84 ug	8 mg
	Green beans, canned	129 ug	4 mg
	Brussels sprouts, frozen, boiled	36 ug	35 mg
	Kale (use in soups)	260 ug	16 mg
	Romaine lettuce, 1 cup	163 ug	14 mg
	Mixed vegetables, frozen	195 ug	3 mg
	Green peppers, boiled	13 ug	60 mg
	Pea pods, boiled	43 ug	38 mg
Bright Orange Vegetables	Carrots, sliced, boiled	671 ug	2.8 mg
	Winter squash, baked	268 ug	10 mg
	Sweet potatoes, boiled and mashed	1000 ug	21 mg
White Vegetables	Cabbage, boiled	11 ug	30 mg
	Turnips	0	9 mg
	Parsnips	0	10 mg
	Rutabaga	0	16
	Celery	13 ug	2 mg
	Wax Beans	7 ug	3 mg
Red Vegetables	Tomatoes, fresh, diced	38 ug	11 mg
	Beets	1 ug	3 mg

* Note: Vegetables are often the foods that clients will have an aversion to. Remember that substitutions have to be equivalent in nutritional value so choose another vegetable (s) that is roughly equivalent to the content of the leader nutrients, vitamin A and vitamin C

of equal nutritional value. For instance, if someone doesn't like cabbage, the substitute should be a food that replaces the vitamin C, such as tomatoes. Since menus are planned to incorporate color, try to replace a food with a similar or additional color. Your facility should have a list of approved substitutes for your menu cycle. See Figure 16.4 for food substitution choices.

Service Options

Restaurant style service is another way of implementing a culture change in a nursing home, even with a nonselective menu. Your regular cycle menu entrée can be the daily special with an option of sandwiches, grilled items, vegetables, and salads. Restaurant style dining might include the following:

✓ Foodservice staff waiting on tables

✓ Food ordered and delivered in courses

✓ Food plated in the dining room

✓ Specials such as sandwiches, salads, or desserts offered tableside from a cart

Buffet Style Service

Buffet style service is offered in some long-term care facilities as a way to implement Culture Change. Be prepared to offer extra help for those clients who cannot serve themselves. Facilities offer the same number of choices as with restaurant style service, only clients cannot serve themselves.

Whatever menu or service style you use in your culture change, make sure there are adequate policies, staff training, and oversight to be able to justify when clients choose foods that are contrary to the therapeutic diet that was ordered for them. In addition, a facility needs to establish procedures and provide adequate staffing to assist with person-centered dining.

Case Study for Culture Change

Southwest Health Center, a small, rural 25-bed hospital in Platteville, WI, and their 84-bed nursing home in Cuba City, was one of the first healthcare centers in the state of Wisconsin to implement a culture change in 2005. They began the culture change in the nursing home with the implementation of a liberalized diet for all clients. The Southwest Health Center Manager of Food and Nutrition Services, Joan Bahr, MS, RD, met with the medical staff and gained their support to liberalize the diets in the nursing home. Now, the majority of their nursing home clients are on a general diet with the exception of texture modifications.

Then, in 2007, in the nursing home, they went from the traditional tray line in the kitchen to restaurant service in the dining room. Two staff members take orders from each client and then the food is dished up right in the dining room from a portable steam table. Think about how the sight and smell of this food might entice small eaters to consume more food. Another advantage is the foodservice staff has the opportunity to interact with the clients for whom they prepare the food. In order to bring in the concept of "home" as much as possible to the dining experience, Southwest Health Center has eliminated trays in the dining room. They purchased china dishes and cloth napkins for their

Figure 16.5 Plate Waste Study

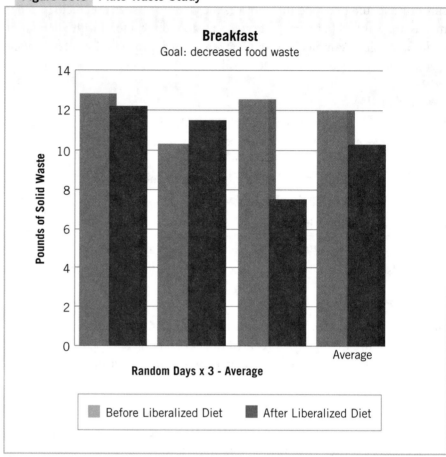

Source: Southwest Health Center, Platteville WI, Joan Bahr, MS, RD. Used with permission.

dining services. Foodservice staff also maintains the records of how much food is consumed by their clients.

Overall, they had four goals, all of which have been met, as they implemented this culture change:

✓ Improve resident satisfaction

✓ Decrease food waste

✓ Accomplish this without increasing blood glucose or A1C

✓ Decrease weight loss

Figure 16.5 shows how the results of a plate waste study and how food waste has declined since the implementation of this culture change.

In the hospital, they implemented the culture change through a selective menu and room service. Hospital clients are also served on china dishes with cloth napkins and a flower on each tray. The selective menu, seen in Figure 16.3, contains many regional preference choices as well as the number of carbohydrates for each menu Item. Also included in Figure 16.3 are the selective menus for both the clear liquid and full liquid diets. The room service menu is located in each room and the client is free to order anything from the menu at any time from 6:30 am to 7:00 pm. Foodservice staff delivers the meals, picks up the trays, and records the amount consumed for each client.

Southwest Health Center uses Press Ganey data as one of their quality measures. (Press Ganey is an outside company that helps healthcare facilities improve clinical and business outcomes, including customer satisfaction surveys.) Joan Bahr, MS, RD, tracked their satisfaction scores as compared to other Press Ganey facilities. They are consistently exceeding other benchmarked facilities for client satisfaction since they implemented the culture change. Figure 16.6 shows how the Press Ganey scores for overall meals (includes quality, temperature, friendliness of staff) has improved since the full implementation of the culture change in 2007.

Figure 16.6 Improvement in Press Ganey Meal Satisfaction Scores

Overall Meals
2004, 2007, 2008

[Line graph showing Mean Score (y-axis, 0–100) by month (Jan–Dec, x-axis) for SHC 2004, SHC 2007, and SHC 2008]

Source: Southwest Health Center, Platteville WI, Joan Bahr, MS, RD. Used with permission.

Nutrition in the News

Practice Paper of the American Dietetic Association: Individualized Nutrition Approaches for Older Adults in Health Care Communities

Abstract

It is the position of the American Dietetic Association that the quality of life and nutritional status of older adults residing in health care communities can be enhanced by individualization to less-restrictive diets. The Association advocates the use of qualified Registered Dietitians (RDs) to assess and evaluate the need for nutrition care according to each person's individual medical condition, needs, desires, and rights. Dietetic technicians, registered, provide support to RDs in the assessment and implementation of individualized nutrition care. Individual rights and freedom of choice are important components of the assessment process. An RD must assess each older adult's risks vs benefits for therapeutic diets. Older adults select housing options that provide a range of services from minimal assistance to 24-hour skilled nursing care. Food is an important part of any living arrangement and an essential component for quality of life. A therapeutic diet that limits seasoning options and food choices can lead to poor food and fluid intake, resulting in undernutrition and negative health effects. Including older individuals in decisions about food can increase the desire to eat and improve quality of life. The expansion of health care communities creates a multitude of options for RDs and dietetic technicians, registered, to promote the role of good food and nutrition in the overall quality of life for the older adults they serve. J Am Diet Assoc. 2010;110: 1554-1563.

Description of the Population

The number of older adults is expected to increase to 55 million in 2020 and the older than age 85 years population will reach 6.6 million, a 15% increase (1). The projected growth of this population challenges the health care system, as well as workforce demand for Registered Dietitians (RDs) and dietetic technicians, registered (DTRs), who provide nutrition care for an aging population residing in a variety of settings. Collaboration between RDs and DTRs will be important as they strive to implement the Nutrition Care Process (2).

In 2008, 4.1% of Americans aged 65 years or older (1.44 million) lived in an institutional setting such as a nursing facility where Medicaid is the primary payer for the care they receive (2). It is estimated that 83% of the Medicare beneficiaries residing in nursing facilities require assistance with one or more activities of daily living, and 67% have difficulty with three or more activities of daily living, including assistance with eating (2). Sensory impairments, including dentition, are prevalent in 32% of people older than age 85 years and 23% of people older than age 65 years, potentially leading to limited food selection (3).

The most common and costly chronic diseases diagnosed in older adults (older than age 65 years) are heart disease, stroke, cancer, and diabetes mellitus (4). These conditions contribute to decline in function and quality of life, and ultimately affect ability to continue to live independently.

Health Care Communities

As a result of the growth of the older adult population in the United States, the range of housing accommodations and community services has expanded. The type of food and nutrition care offered may depend on the living environment. RDs and DTRs must be flexible and willing to adapt their clinical skills to meet the needs of individuals in a variety of settings ranging from custodial care to skilled nursing care.

(Continued)

Position of the American Dietetic Association *(Continued)*

Long-Term Care and Short-Term Rehabilitation

The typical long-term care skilled facility changed dramatically when Medicare policy shifts created an influx of short-stay, post-hospitalization admissions with more medically complex conditions. In addition, state Medicaid policy modifications avoided or delayed admission for lower acuity long-term residents. These changes created two different patient populations: short-stay residents requiring intense rehabilitation and/or medically complex care; and older, more disabled long-term residents with medically complex conditions. The average length of stay for short-term rehabilitation residents is 33 days compared to 835 days for the longer-term stays (3).

A short-term stay resident is typically a younger person recovering from knee or hip replacement or a brief illness. An individual recovering from surgery requires additional energy and protein for healing vs a strict therapeutic diet. An RD has the opportunity to discuss the benefits of healthy eating before discharge or may assign this education component to a competent DTR. Offering specific recommendations focused on an individual's nutritional requirements, such as a consistent carbohydrate diet for a person with diabetes, is a proactive approach to improve chances for a positive recovery and improved future health. The educational process could include referral to an appropriate agency or program, such as home-delivered meals, or a postdischarge follow-up by an RD or competent DTR, as assigned by the RD.

The Centers for Medicare and Medicaid Services (CMS) and state agencies are the regulatory bodies for long-term care facilities. Licensed health care facilities, programs, and agencies must meet the conditions of participation to participate in Medicare and Medicaid programs and receive payment for beneficiary care. The conditions of participation are minimum health and safety legal requirements that are the foundation for improving quality and protecting the health and safety of beneficiaries and are published in the Code of Federal Regulations. The rules are available in Appendix PP—Guidance to Surveyors for Long Term Care Facilities of the CMS's State Operations Manual (5). Accreditation by The Joint Commission is voluntary and supplements the conditions of participation mandated by the CMS. In 2009 there were 1,100 long-term care facilities

accredited by The Joint Commission, which conducts performance improvement surveys every 3 years (6).

Long-term care facilities are surveyed by state or federal agencies at a minimum of every 9 to 15 months, with additional complaint surveys conducted in between if needed. Most state regulations mirror the federal survey and certification standards. Federal regulations require that "The facility must employ a qualified dietitian either full time, part time, or on a consultant basis." The CMS requires each facility to be licensed by the state to be certified for CMS payment. State facility licensure laws therefore meet or exceed CMS regulations. In the case of nursing facilities, all but two states expand on the CMS's definition of *qualified dietitian*. For example, some states require that the qualified dietitian be only an RD. Other states, particularly those with dietitian licensing or certification, may require a licensed/certified RD or an RD or licensed/certified dietitian. Other states require just education and training equivalent to RD training. All of these options technically meet CMS requirements.

State regulations may or may not define required RD hours each month. However, based on the current medically complex population in long-term care facilities, an RD's required time often exceeds any minimum state requirements. Because each facility is unique, an RD should negotiate hours based on the time required to achieve the goals of nutrition services for the facility and its residents.

In the State Operations Manual, each federal tag number is associated with a regulation that provides interpretive guidance to assist surveyors in determining if a facility is compliant with the regulation. F 325 Nutrition loosely follows the American Dietetic Association's (ADA's) Nutrition Care Process to assist in the management of an individual's nutrition care.

(Continued)

The Nutrition Care Process is designed to improve the consistency and quality of individualized care. There are four steps in the process: nutrition assessment, nutrition diagnosis, nutrition intervention, and nutrition monitoring and evaluation (7).

Interventions highlighted in F 325 interpretative guidance include resident choice, diet liberalization, weight related interventions, and meeting nutrition needs (8). Following the Nutrition Care Process, an RD or DTR as assigned, must individualize interventions, maintain or improve quality of life, and adhere to residents' rights. CMS tag F 150 Resident's Rights, which is linked to F 325 Nutrition, notes that facilities need to "determine if the resident's preference related to nutrition and food intake were considered" in making decisions related to his or her care (8). A resident has the right to refuse treatment, which may include a therapeutic diet.

Home- and Community-Based Services (HCBS)

HCBS, operated under the CMS Medicaid programs, include adult day care services, home care, home health/hospice programs, and the Program for All-inclusive Care for the Elderly. HCBS provide some overlapping but distinct services that differ from the 24-hour round-the-clock nursing care in a nursing facility (9). The HCBS waiver program established by the federal government under Section 1915 (c) of the Social Security Act may include home-delivered meals and nutrition counseling (10). Only 29 states have chosen this option as part of the Medicaid waiver program. Programs for All-inclusive Care for the Elderly vary by state and include day programs with supportive services such as rehabilitation aides, speech, and occupational therapists and perhaps a medical director and/or nutrition services. In 2009, 2.8 million senior citizens in the United States received Medicaid HCBS services and 300,000 individuals were on waiting lists.

States providing HCBS have evidence indicating that offering community-based services is less expensive than institutionalized care (11). Currently the role of RDs and DTRs is limited in HCBS. However, as the population ages, additional HCBS programs will open, providing potential opportunities for RD/DTR services. Availability of RD/DTR services may depend on reimbursement, making it imperative that RDs and DTRs work at the grassroots level to support public policy for these important services (12).

Assisted Living Facilities

The Department of Health and Human Services defines assisted living facilities as residential settings that provide either routine general protective oversight or assistance with activities necessary for independent living to mentally or physically limited persons. Assisted living is a philosophy of service that focuses on maximizing each individual's independence and dignity. It emphasizes flexibility, individualized supportive services and provision of health care. Involvement of the community, as well as the individual's family, neighbors, and friends, is encouraged (13).

In 2009, there were approximately 5,000 assisted living facilities in the United States that were either standalone buildings or part of a Continuing Care Retirement Community (CCRC). During 2006, 882 RDs were employed in assisted living facilities. In 2009, the majority of those residing in assisted living facilities were women (74%) requiring assistance with two or more activities of daily living, including eating (12%) and meal preparation (87%). According to the Assisted Living Resident Profile conducted by the National Center for Assisted Living, the average age of older adults in assisted living facilities in 2009 was 86.9 years. Due to higher acuity levels, about one third of individuals who live in this setting spend the last month of their lives in the facility (14). There are no federal regulations governing assisted living facilities; however, every state has its own regulatory oversight. Private pay is the primary funding source, but 41 states have some type of Medicaid Waiver or Medicaid State Plan, which supplemented care for 131,208 beneficiaries in 2009 (13).

One hundred fifty-three national aging and health experts were surveyed (15) on their perception of the state regulations for assisted living facilities' food and

(Continued)

Position of the American Dietetic Association *(Continued)*

Culture Change/Person-Centered Suggested Terminology for Dining	
Old Terminology	Suggested Terminology
Allow	Encourage, welcome
Elderly	Elder, older adult, individual
Wing, unit	Household, neighborhood, street
Institutional care	Individual care
Feeder table	Dining table
Feeder	Person who needs help eating
Facility, institution, nursing home	Home life center, living center
Dietary service, foodservice	Dining services
Tray line	Fine dining
Nourishment	Snack
Bib	Napkin, clothing protector
Diabetic	Person who has diabetes

Adapted with permission from reference 20: "The Language of Culture Change" by Karen Schoeneman. Pioneer Network http://www.pioneernetwork.net/Culturechange/Language.

nutrition services. The 18 indicators on the survey included questions on dining room environment, food safety and sanitation, number of employees, meal quality, menu standards, and therapeutic nutrition service. The indicator, "menus have nutrition standards," was included in 40 states' regulations; 32 states include "therapeutic diet order must be provided and ordered by a medical director" and only 28 states' regulations noted "if the resident needs a therapeutic diet, the facility policy is to contract with an RD to plan menus and supervise meal preparations." The authors concluded that voluntary standards and best-practice models for food and nutrition services for assisted living facilities may improve the quality of food and nutrition services. Individuals residing in assisted living facilities, as well as the staff, benefit from inclusion of an RD on the interdisciplinary team.

CCRCs

CCRCs promote independent living through long-term contracts that provide for housing, services, and nursing care, usually in one location. Housing choices may include independent living apartments, assisted living, and nursing facility care. The goal of CCRCs is to provide a seamless transfer between levels of care as

deemed appropriate for each individual. The number and type of CCRCs vary by state.

There are three basic financial contracts offered for residents of CCRCs: extensive contracts, with unlimited long-term nursing care at little or no increase in the monthly fee; modified contracts that include a specified amount of long-term nursing care with additional care being the responsibility of the individual; or a fee-for-service contract that includes a daily rate for long-term-care services (16). Some CCRCs are accredited by the Commission on Accreditation of Rehabilitative Services, a non-profit accrediting organization (17). The accrediting process includes voluntary evaluation of the facilities. The role of RDs and DTRs can vary

(Continued)

depending on the setting and how the CCRCs are licensed or regulated. Older adults residing in CCRCs may benefit from nutrition and fitness education for healthy aging.

Culture Change and Person-Centered Care

Following the 1987 Omnibus Budget Reconciliation Act, The CMS issued the Medicare and Medicaid programs survey, certification, and enforcement of skilled nursing facilities final rule. The focus of the 1987 Omnibus Budget Reconciliation Act was to improve the quality of life for individuals and increase their role in making informed decisions about their own care. In 1998 the Prospective Payment System legislated how skilled nursing facilities received payment for specific services (18). The Prospective Payment System emphasizes the medical vs the social model of providing care and services. In recent years, the model for long-term care settings has gone through a major paradigm shift from the traditional institutional, medical environment to more interactive communities that focus on quality of life, individual choice, and a more person-centered, home-like culture.

Culture change and person-centered care are national movements designed to transform services for older adults, regardless of their living arrangement. These movements are based on person centered values. The core values are dignity, respect, self-determination, and purposeful living (19).

Culture change challenges health care providers to adapt terminology that embraces the four core values. Schoeneman's article (20) on the language of culture change offers expressions that communicate the changing philosophy. The Figure indicates the old terminology vs the suggested new terminology related to dining (20). Although culture change or person-centered care is encouraged in all senior housing settings, the CMS has included the concept in many of the revised

interpretive guidelines for nursing home survey and certification. A CMS document published in 2008 acknowledged support of the culture change movement stating, "the principles behind culture change echo [the 1987 Omnibus Budget Reconciliation Act's] principles of knowing and respecting each nursing home resident and providing individualized care that best enhances each resident's quality of life" (21). A CMS Interpretive Guidelines memo dated April 10, 2009, outlines specific principles that embrace resident choice (22). Federal nursing home regulations, specifically 42 CRF §483.15(a) Dignity, addresses promoting resident independence and dignity in dining. For example, "Avoid using 'bibs' at meal time which are not age appropriate for an older adult, and instead offer napkins or clothing protectors." The interpretive guideline for PP/483. 15(b), F242 Self-Determination and Participation states: "Resident should choose activities/schedules, including dining times." PP/483.35(i), F371 Sanitary Conditions F Tag 371 Sanitation states, "The food procurement requirements for facilities are not intended to restrict resident choice. All residents have the right to accept food brought to the facility by any visitor(s) for any resident."

Freedom of choice encourages residents to determine when and where they will dine, what type and how much food they will select. Individualization of the diet provides RDs and DTRs a window of opportunity to promote healthy menus and choices that include foods abundant in nutrients, flavor, color, and variety.

Does Food Choice Improve Consumers' Perception of Dining in Health Care Communities?

Most people look forward to mealtime and the chance to enjoy good food and socialize with others. Eye-appealing, familiar menu options that meet nutritional needs may decrease the risk of undernutrition and unintended weight loss in older adults. Undernutrition has been defined as "protein and energy deficiency which is reversed solely by the administration of nutrients" (23). A strict, unappealing therapeutic diet is not beneficial unless it is actually consumed and can actually be detrimental to an older adult at risk of undernutrition or unintended weight loss (24).

The culture change movement expands dining options available in many heath care communities. Surveys

(Continued)

Position of the American Dietetic Association *(Continued)*

indicate a higher level of satisfaction when dining programs are individualized to meet a wide range of consumer expectations. Relaxing dietary restrictions and expanding choices includes consideration of several key areas. RDs and DTRs should collaborate with a facility's dining services director or chef to determine menu and food options and initiate an appropriate action plan. Staff training modules incorporated in the plan should include:

- dining options such as select menus, buffet dining, restaurant style service, and family-style dining;

- methods for seasoning food to enhance flavors such as using herbs and spices rather than high-sodium alternatives;

- menu options that offer consistent levels of carbohydrate;

- suggestions for increasing fiber and offering seasonal fresh fruits and vegetables;

- adhering to food safety and sanitation guidelines; and

- implementing budgetary and cost control measures while maintaining quality.

Regardless of the setting, older adults should be involved in decisions regarding menus and creative dining programs. Two studies on creative dining in nursing homes, such as buffet dining or meal portioning on the resident floors, resulted in both increased food consumption and meal satisfaction (25,26). Menus should reflect the cultural, ethnic, and individual choices of the client population and should be approved by an RD before implementation.

Menu Options and Suggestions

Selective Menus. Some facilities choose to offer a selective menu rather than a traditional nonselective menu with multiple therapeutic diets. To allow for individualized diets, consider several menu options in addition to the regular diet, such as a consistent carbohydrate diet for those with diabetes and altered texture diets for individuals with chewing or swallowing problems. Rotate the options on the selective menu to allow more variety in choices. Adding a meaningful icon next to the foods on the menus that are moderate in fat, sugar, or sodium can allow for a subtle form of education, which may help individuals choose appropriate foods to help manage hyperlipidemia, diabetes, or hypertension.

Nonselective Menus. Although allowing for choice is the ideal option, if a facility offers only nonselective menus, there are still ways to enhance variety and choice. Keep individual food preferences up to date to allow for appropriate substitution and to ensure that individuals receive foods they enjoy. Consider establishing a dining committee to incorporate favorite menu items or recipes into the menu plan. Expand the menu cycle beyond the traditional 4- or 5-week cycle to increase variety.

Restaurant-Style Menus. Restaurant-style menus provide the most popular foods from the community. Many facilities offer traditional daily cycle menus as the "special of the day" and add additional menu options such as vegetables, salads, sandwiches, or grilled items that can be prepared in advance or on demand. Waiter/waitress service allows for a more catered dining experience.

Dining Programs

Buffet-Style Dining. It is well known that the aroma of food stimulates the appetite. Consider relocating the steam table to the dining room for service or offering buffet-style service. Encourage individuals to participate in choosing foods from the buffet and provide assistance to those who need it. Individuals should be allowed to see and smell the food and select the type and quantity they desire. A choice of entrées, side dishes, desserts, soup, salad bars, and dessert bars allows for a variety of choices. Include a variety of soft foods for individuals on mechanical soft diets. Careful planning, flexible dining hours, and open seating allow for relaxed dining and reduce the need to rush meals. Several studies note increased meal consumption and weight gain with buffet-style vs tray service (27,28).

Green House and Neighborhood Living. Assisted living facilities, CCRCs, and some nursing homes are developing "neighborhoods" where accommodations

(Continued)

for up to 20 individuals are located around a central area that includes a kitchen, dining room, and living space. The Green House concept developed by William Thomas, MD, is generally a home with 10 bedrooms clustered around an open kitchen, dining, and living area with access to a courtyard. The staff who prepare and serve the food are often the same staff who assist residents with activities of daily living. Consistency in staffing assignments helps to create a family-like atmosphere. Individuals living in the facility may assume an active role in food selection and even food preparation as desired. Relaxed individualized diet plans are appropriate since family-style dining is common practice in these living situations.

Five Meals vs Traditional Three. The five-meal-a-day plan offers a continental breakfast, usually served in a person's bedroom, a brunch at midday in the dining room, a moderate lunch at midday, dinner in the dining room about 4:00 or 5:00 PM, followed by a nourishing snack in the evening. Individual selection is the cornerstone of this menu style. Communities using this plan have reported increased satisfaction and reduced food waste. One small study to determine whether five meals vs three meals would improve energy intake among older adults with dysphagia resulted in similar energy intake but improved fluid intake (29).

Family-Style Dining. Family-style dining is similar to how most people eat at home: serving food in bowls or platters that are passed around the table. Staff and residents dine together, which helps increase socialization at meal time. This works particularly well for individuals who are able to eat independently and/or those who have dementia. According to several studies, family-style dining had a positive effect on the food intake of older adults primarily because of the interaction between staff and residents, which created a positive social atmosphere (30).

Social Functions. Social functions offer the opportunity to collaborate with older adults, families, and staff to incorporate popular food selections at social functions that are tasty and healthy. Beverage stations offering a variety of selections such as juices, coffee, or tea encourage consumption of fluids and nutrients. The aroma created by bread machines, soup kettles, or popcorn machines located in common areas can result in increased energy consumption. For individuals who participate in cooking activities, recipes that are moderate in energy can be enjoyed by most individuals. These in-between-meals foods can have a positive benefit, especially for individuals struggling to consume an adequate diet at meal time. A recent study on the benefits of snacking reported that snacking made a significant contribution in terms of total energy consumed. Snacking contributed 14% of daily protein and approximately 25% of energy intake (31). A study conducted by Meals-on-Wheels Association of America examined community residing adults aged 60 to 90 years who had experienced weight loss, and compared a test group that received three meals and two snacks daily with a group that received the traditional three meals a day. The study concluded that weight loss was reversed in the test group (32).

Do all Older Adults in Health Care Communities Require Individualized Nutrition Interventions to Promote the Least-Restrictive Diet?

Regardless of the living environment chosen by an older person, the aging process results in physiological, psychological, and social changes that may have an effect on appetite and food consumption. A number of studies indicate that there is an association between aging and declining energy intake (33,34). Comparisons between 25- and 70-year-olds estimated that men's intake declines by 1,000 to 1,200 kcal daily and women's by 600 to 800 kcal daily (35). The Third National Health and Nutrition Examination Survey demonstrated a decrease in total energy intake leading to decreased protein intake. Adults older than age 60 years scored only 68 out of 100 points on the 2005 Healthy Eating Index. Data from the 2000-2001 Healthy Eating Index indicated more than 80% of older adults consumed diets that needed improvement. Recommended dietary improvements included consuming more whole grains, dark-green and orange vegetables, and low-fat dairy products (36). The 2005

(Continued)

Position of the American Dietetic Association *(Continued)*

Dietary Guidelines for Americans emphasize the need to consume a variety of foods within and among the basic food groups while staying within energy needs, to be physically active daily, and to choose fats and carbohydrates wisely for good health (36). Considering the impaired physical functioning and poor or declining dietary intake that occurs with aging, individualized nutrition care and education is appropriate for the majority of older adults in health care communities. For frail older adults, referral to an RD and/or DTR for individualized nutrition interventions to promote the least restrictive diet is appropriate.

Physical and Medical Factors Affecting Nutritional Status

Unintended Weight Loss

Unintended weight loss is defined as a gradual, unplanned weight loss that may occur slowly over time or have a rapid onset. In older adults, a 5% or more unplanned weight loss in 30 days often results in protein-energy undernutrition as critical lean body mass is lost (37). Skeletal muscle loss can occur from starvation, cachexia, or sarcopenia. Starvation is the inadequate consumption of protein and energy, which is reversed by intake of nutrients (37). Cachexia is severe wasting accompanying diseases such as cancer (37). Sarcopenia is the loss of skeletal muscle associated with aging, which leads to reduced strength and exercise ability (38). Thomas (39) noted that unintended weight loss in older adults is a significant risk factor for mortality, and Murden and Anslie (40) indicated a loss of 10% in 6 months was a strong predictor of mortality in older adults. Anorexia of aging factors that may lead to undernutrition includes weight loss, reduced appetite, and declining metabolic rate (39).

In October 2009, ADA's unintended weight loss task force completed guidelines for the ADA Evidence Analysis Library. The target population for these evidence-based guidelines is adults aged 65 years and older with unintended weight loss. The overall objective of the recommendations is to provide medical nutrition therapy guidelines for unintended weight loss that will increase energy, protein, and nutrient intake, improve nutritional status, and improve quality of life. Nutrition recommendations within the guideline include these topics: medical nutrition therapy, instruments for

nutrition screening, assessment of food, fluid and nutrient intake, collaboration for modified diet texture, eating assistance, and monitoring and evaluating nutritional status (41). The unintended weight loss guideline debuts the first nutrition diagnosis. Nutrition interventions associated with individualized diet plans include feeding assistance, dining environment, collaboration of texture-modified diets, evaluation and treatment of depression, and appetite stimulants. Access the guidelines on www.adaevidencelibrary.com.

Research supports a positive association between poor nutritional status, weight loss, and eating dependency, in particular for older adults requiring modified-texture diets (42, 43). Simple interventions may include opening packets, removing container lids, cutting meat at the point of service, buttering bread, and ensuring eye glasses or dentures are available as applicable. The key areas for individualized diet plans for older adults receiving texture-modified diets include increasing food choice, including snacks, attention to presentation, correct preparation, and enhanced taste (44-47). Based on studies reporting dissatisfaction and decreased enjoyment of texture-modified diets, RDs should collaborate with speech-language pathologists to ensure care plans are individualized (44-46).

As previously mentioned, creative dining programs can improve quality of life and meal intake. After reviewing 238 studies, Stroebele and De Castro (48) concluded that eating with others in a comfortable environment improved nutritional status. Playing music during meals had a positive effect on appetite and decreased feelings of anxiety and depression.

The relationship between weight loss, poor nutritional status, and depression is supported by research (48-50). When individualized interventions fail to improve or stabilize weight or meal intake, an RD should *(Continued)* recommend that a patient's physician consider a depression evaluation and antidepressant therapies as appropriate.

Unintended Weight Loss Case Study. An 80-year-old woman moved from her home of 40 years to an assisted living facility. Upon admission, the health care practitioner interviewing her and her son discovered the woman had gradually lost weight during the past year. Admission anthropometric values included height 63 in, weight 115 lb, and usual body weight 130 lb. When she lived at home, her advancing Parkinson's disease hindered her from preparing meals, so she usually ate soup or cereal. Since her husband's death several months ago, she was lonely and depressed. The physician ordered a 1,500-kcal diet, based on her diagnosis of type 2 diabetes. Two weeks after admission, her blood glucose levels were normal, but her weight was down to 110 lb and she rarely came to the dining room for meals. The assisted living facility staff contacted the staff RD and requested a nutrition assessment. During the initial interview, the RD discovered that the resident didn't come to the dining room due to difficulty chewing and the embarrassment it caused in front of others. She enjoyed desserts that were not offered on her current diet plan and rarely ate meat. The RD requested a regular diet, based on the 2008 position of the American Diabetes Association that food containing sucrose can be substituted for other carbohydrates in a meal plan (51). Evidence guidelines contain little research to support restrictive nutrition interventions for diabetes in older adults (52).

Problem. Inadequate intake of protein and/or energy based on recommended needs.

Etiology. Difficulty chewing, restrictive diet plan, and symptoms of depression.

Signs and symptoms. Gradual weight loss, rarely comes to the dining room, avoids difficult-to-chew protein foods, limited food choices, symptoms of depression.

Nutrition diagnosis. Unintended weight loss related to intake inconsistent with estimated energy and nutrient requirements as evidenced by continued weight loss of 5 lb in 2 weeks, limited diet prescription, and difficulty chewing; symptoms of depression evidenced by remaining in room at meal time.

Nutrition Interventions

- Collaborate with speech-language pathologist to determine appropriate diet texture;
- Recommend the physician change the diet order to a regular diet with ground meat based on nutrition diagnosis;
- Recommend a high-energy/high-protein supplement for evening snack;
- Collaborate with DTR/dining services director to identify food preferences and honor them;
- Collaborate with staff to encourage and accompany the resident to dine in the dining room;
- Collaborate with staff to offer assistance and monitoring at meal time to ensure adequate intake;
- Collaborate with social services to complete a Geriatric Depression Scale;
- Collaborate with physician to evaluate Geriatric Depression Scale and appropriate anti-depressive therapy;
- Collaborate with staff to evaluate weekly weights until stable as determined by the RD; and
- Collaborate with DTR/dining services director to complete a nutrient intake study.

Obesity

There is some evidence to support a planned weight loss program for obese older adults to improve their physical functioning and reduce medical complications (53). However, weight reduction in adults with obesity results in loss of both fat mass and lean body mass that may trigger sarcopenia (54,55) and functional decline (56). Individualized diet plans should be implemented with caution, using professional judgment based on the nutrition assessment and an individual's overall health goals and should include physical activity to assist with retention of lean body mass and increased losses of fat mass.

Position of the American Dietetic Association *(Continued)*

Obesity Case Study. After surgery for a total knee replacement, a 75-year-old man was admitted to a rehabilitation facility for physical therapy. Admission statistics included height 68 in, weight 285 lb, body mass index 43.3, and a physician's order for an 1,800-kcal diet. He expressed multiple food complaints, including hunger.

Problem. Inadequate oral food intake.

Etiology. Energy-restricted diet plan.

Signs and symptoms. Reported food complaints.

Nutrition diagnosis. Inadequate protein-energy intake compared to recommendation based on physiological needs.

Nutritional Interventions

- Recommend the physician order a regular diet based on nutrition diagnosis;
- RD and individual will agree on an education plan that includes diet and physical activity goals before discharge; and
- RD will negotiate post discharge follow-up for the individual to receive a nutrition evaluation.

Cardiac Disease/Hypertension

The risk of imposing a cholesterol controlled diet on an older person with poor nutritional intake outweighs the positive effect of a lipid lowering diet (57). Although the American Heart Association advocates a 2 to 3 g/day sodium diet as treatment for congestive heart failure, a randomized control trial of adults aged 55 to 83 years reported that a normal sodium diet improved congestive heart failure (58).

Nutrition interventions for older adults with cardiac disease who are at nutrition risk should focus on stabilizing blood lipid levels and blood pressure while preserving eating pleasure. RDs should collaborate with the dining services department and implement menus that work toward meeting the goals of the Dietary Guidelines for Americans and/or the Dietary Approaches to Stop Hypertension diet, which is rich in potassium, magnesium, calcium, protein, and fiber (59). Menus including whole-grain breads and cereals, juice packed fruits, low-fat foods such as low-fat dairy, low-fat salad dressings, brown rice, seasonal fruits, and fresh or frozen vegetables can help to meet these guidelines. Season foods with salt-free seasonings such as fresh or dried bay leaves, basil, celery seed,

thyme, garlic powder, onions, lemon juice, or parsley. Additional recommendations are included on the ADA Evidence Analysis Library's Hypertension Evidenced-Based Nutrition Practice Guidelines available at www.adaevidencelibrary.com.

Alzheimer's Disease

Alzheimer's disease is the fifth leading cause of death for individuals older than 65 years of age. Fifty percent of those suffering from Alzheimer's disease are older than the age of 85 years (60,61). Walking, pacing, and wandering are common in earlier stages of the disease, and it is sometimes difficult for these individuals to sit long enough to finish eating a meal. Nutrition concerns for individuals with Alzheimer's disease include unintended weight loss, fatigue, and poor nutritional intake. As Alzheimer's disease advances, cognitive and functional declines require increased assistance with eating and texture modified diets (62).

Alzheimer's Disease Case Study. A 70-year-old man with stage 4 (moderate cognitive decline) Alzheimer's disease was admitted to a secure unit in a skilled nursing facility. Assessment parameters included height 72 in, weight 150 lb, weight loss of 30 lb during the previous 6 months, a tendency to sleep in late and wander during the night. This individual would rarely sit down to eat and if redirected to go back and sit down, he became combative. He had a tendency to eat with his fingers, liked sweet foods, received antihyperlipidemic medication, and was receiving a low cholesterol diet, but he was only eating about 40% of his meals.

Problem. Increased energy expenditure and inadequate energy intake.

Etiology. Wandering during the night, inability to sit down at meal time, becomes combative due to Alzheimer's disease.

(Continued)

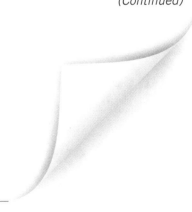

Signs and symptoms. Twelve percent weight loss in 6 months, 40% meal intake.

Nutrition diagnosis. Increased energy expenditure related to excessive wandering and 12% weight loss in 6 months.

Nutrition Interventions

- Recommend the physician modify the diet to a regular diet with finger foods;

- Collaborate with the DTR/dining services director to provide sandwiches, whole milk, ice cream sandwiches, and other high-energy snacks;

- Collaborate with the staff to evaluate weekly weights until stable as determined by the RD;

- Collaborate with staff to notify RD if unintended weight loss occurs;

- Collaborate with staff to provide a finger food diet, monitor intake, and offer substitutes when oral intake <50% of needs; and

- Collaborate with staff to provide assistance at meal time.

Palliative Care

The Position of the American Dietetic Association: Ethical and Legal Issues in Nutrition, Hydration, and Feeding supports an individual's right to request or refuse nutrition and hydration as medical treatment. When implementing nutrition care at the end of life, an RD should promote the rights of an individual in collaboration with the health care team (63). Terminally ill individuals experience loss of appetite and should be offered food and fluid as desired or requested. Contrary to popular belief, several reports indicate that absence of food at the end of life does not produce suffering or diminish quality of life (64,65).

Palliative Care Case Study. A frail, cachetic 90-year-old man with chronic obstructive pulmonary disease and failure to thrive was admitted to hospice. He was on continuous oxygen, drinking only 8 to 10 oz fluids daily, receiving routine pain medication, and according to his caregiver had lost 30 lb in 6 months. The caregiver expressed concern that he would die of starvation and requested an RD visit.

Problem. Inadequate intake of energy over prolonged period of time.

Etiology. Prolonged catabolic illness.

Signs and symptoms. Thirty pound weight loss in 6 months; underweight with muscle wasting; thin, wasted appearance; and terminal illness.

Nutrition diagnosis. Inadequate intake of energy and fluids over a prolonged period of time resulting in loss of fat stores and muscle wasting.

Nutritional Interventions

- Collaborate with the physician to coordinate medication and medication schedules, with a goal of maximizing the individual's food intake;

- Collaborate with caregiver and hospice staff and develop a routine for offering sips of liquid to lessen thirst sensations or small amounts of favorite foods and energy-dense foods, such as milkshake or commercial supplement, when alert and/or willing to accept nourishment;

- Educate the family/caregiver about the metabolic changes and sedative effect of dehydration at end of life (64); and

- Support caregiver's concern for client and suggest alternate ways to provide comfort, such as playing soft music or reading to him.

Education and Research

As health care communities expand, RDs and DTRs have a responsibility to inform administrators, surveyors, policymakers, legislators, families, and members of health care teams on the value of individualized nutrition intervention, including nutrition care for older adults.

Declining food intake can lead to loss of weight and/or muscle mass, frailty, and functional disability, which can all decrease quality of life and increase the cost of care. As an older adult's health declines, health care

(Continued)

Position of the American Dietetic Association *(Continued)*

costs can spiral due to increased need for assistance with activities of daily living, treatments, medications, and physician and hospital visits. Implementing the Nutrition Care Process, a standardized care process that incorporates the critical thinking and decision-making skills of RDs when providing care, can increase the reliability of outcomes measurement. RDs should document outcomes, including cost savings, associated with individualized diets for older adults and share these results with key administrative staff, policymakers, and other health care practitioners.

Important areas for research include evaluation of outcomes associated with RDs providing nutrition care and the cost benefits of applying the Nutrition Care Process in health care communities, including the positive effects of individualized nutrition interventions to promote the least-restrictive diet and culture change on quality of life. Research is needed to define appropriate energy and protein requirements for older adults, especially those older than age 85 years. As the minority population expands, research focusing on preserving ethnic values related to food and foodservice practices while maintaining nutritional status is also important.

Conclusions

Most people eat 1,000 meals annually, which is equivalent to 75,000 meals over a lifetime for a 75-year old. Food selections are influenced by preference, habit, religious beliefs, ethnic values, traditions, and emotional comfort. Food nourishes the spirit as well as the body. When older adults move into health care communities, meal satisfaction may help to prevent weight loss and additional health problems. Relaxing diet restrictions can make it easier to implement enhanced dining programs and provide older adults opportunities to interact with others in an atmosphere that encourages both increased food consumption and meal satisfaction.

RDs should use the Nutrition Care Process to evaluate each individual and determine appropriate nutrition interventions while assessing the risks vs the benefits of individualized nutrition interventions to promote the least-restrictive diet. The emphasis on resident rights and freedom of choice are components of the assessment process. The shift toward person-centered care affords RDs and DTRs the opportunity to strengthen relationships with residents, families, and staff with the ultimate goal of enhancing the quality of life for older adults in their care.

References

1. Profile of Older Americans. Agency on Aging Web site. http://www.aoa.gov/AoARoot/Aging_ Statistics/Profile/index. aspx. Accessed May 11, 2010.

2. American Dietetic Association Quality Management Committee. American Dietetic Association Revised 2008 Standards of Practice for Registered Dietitians in nutrition care; Standards of Professional Performance for Registered Dietitians; Standards of Practice for dietetic technicians, registered, in nutrition care; and Standards of Professional Performance for dietetic technicians, registered. *J Am Diet Assoc.*2008;108:1538-1542.

3. Use of health care services. Older Americans 2008: Key indicators of well-being. Federal Interagency Forum on Aging Related Statistics Web site. http://www.agingstats. gov/agingstatsdotnet/Main_Site/Data/2008_ Documents/ Health_Care.aspx. Accessed October 1, 2009.

4. Chronic diseases and health promotion. Updated October 7, 2009. Centers for Disease Control and Prevention Web site. http://www. cdc.gov/nccdphp/overview.htm. Accessed October 25, 2009.

5. State Operations Manual: Appendix PP— Guidance to surveyors for long term care facilities. Revised August 17, 2007. Center for Medicare and Medicaid Services Web site. http://www.cms.hhs.gov/CFCsAndCoPs/ Downloads/ som107ap_pp_guidelines_ltcf. pdf. Accessed October 30, 2009.

6. 2010 Long term care accreditation manual. The Joint Commission Web site. http://www. jointcommission.org/ AccreditationPrograms/ LongTermCare. Accessed October 30, 2009.

(Continued)

Position of the American Dietetic Association *(Continued)*

7. *International Dietetics and Nutrition Terminology (IDNT) Reference Manual: Standardized Language for the Nutrition Care Process.* 2nd ed. Chicago, IL: American Dietetic Association; 2009.

8. Survey and certification—Guidance to laws and regulations: Nursing homes. Revision 26, September 1, 2008. Centers for Medicare and Medicaid Services Web site. http://www.cms. hhs.gov/ GuidanceforLawsAndRegulations/12_ NHs.asp. Accessed October 30, 2009.

9. American Health Care Association, Alliance for Quality Nursing Home Care. 2009 Annual Quality Report. The Alliance for Quality Nursing Home Care Web site. http:// www.ahcancal.org/research_data/quality/ Documents/2009 AnnualQualityReport.pdf. Accessed October 1, 2009.

10. Deficit Reduction Act of 2005, Pub L No. 109-171, §6071, 6086, and 6087. http://frwebgate. access. gpo.gov/cgi-bin/getdoc.cgi?dbname 109_cong_ billsanddocid=f.s1932enr.txt.pdf. Accessed September 15, 2009.

11. Struglinski S. HCBS needs boost, report says. *Provider.* 2009;35:14-15.

12. Position of the American Dietetic Association, American Society for Nutrition, and Society for Nutrition Education: Food and nutrition programs for community-residing older adults. *J Am Diet Assoc.* 2010;110:463- 472.

13. Definition of assisted living. Long Term Care Education Web site. http://www. longtermcareeducation.com/ learn_about_ the_field/definition_of_assisted_living.asp. Accessed October 25, 2009.

14. Resident profile. National Center for Assisted Living Web site. http://www.ahcancal.org/ncal/resources/Pages/ ResidentProfile. aspx. Accessed October 30, 2009.

15. Chao S, Dwyer J, Houser R, Tennstedt S, Jacques P. What food and nutrition services should be regulated in assisted-living facilities for older adults? *J Am Diet Assoc.* 2009; 109:1022-1030.

16. Continuing care retirement communities— Definition and history. Medicine Encyclopedia Web site. http://medicine. jrank.org/ pages/368/Continuing-Care-Retirement-Communities-Definition-history.html. Accessed October 25, 2009.

17. Providers earn recognition for accredited services. Commission on Accreditation of Rehabilitation Facilities Web site. http://www.carf.org/Providers. aspx?content=content/ Accreditation/Opportunities/AS/ CCAC.htm. Accessed October 30, 2009.

18. Prospective payment system-general information: Overview. Centers for Medicare and Medicaid Services Web site. http://www.cms.hhs.gov/prospmedicarefeesvcpmtgen. Accessed November 1, 2009.

19. What is culture change? Pioneer Network Web site. http:// www.pioneernetwork.net/CultureChange/. Accessed October 30, 2009.

20. Schoeneman K. The language of culture change. The Pioneer Network Web site. http://www.pioneernetwork.net/ CultureChange/Language. Accessed July 31, 2010.

21. Centers for Medicaid and Medicare Services. The 2008 CMS action plan for (further improvement of) nursing home quality. The Pioneer Network Web site. http://www. pioneernetwork.net/Data/Documents/2008NHActionPlan. pdf. Accessed October, 30, 2009.

22. Nursing homes—Issuance of revisions to interpretive guidance at several tags, as part of Appendix PP, State Operations Manual (SOM), and training materials. Published April 10, 2009. Centers for Medicaid and Medicare Services Web site. http://www.cms.hhs.gov/ SurveyCertificationGenInfo/downloads/SCLetter09_31.pdf. Accessed October 30, 2009.

23. ASPEN Board of Directors and the Clinical Guidelines Task Force. Guidelines for the use of parenteral and enteral nutrition in adult and pediatric patients. *J Parenter Enteral Nutr.* 2002;26:22SA-24SA.

24. Splett PL, Roth-Yousey LL, Vogelzang JL, Medical nutrition therapy for the prevention and treatment of unintentional weight loss in residential healthcare facilities. *J Am Diet Assoc.*2003;103:352-362.

25. Bernstein MA, Tucker KL, Ryan ND, O'Neill EF, Clements, KN, Nelson ME, Evans WJ, Fiatarone Singh MA. Higher dietary variety is associated with better nutritional status in frail elderly people. *J Am Diet Assoc.* 2002;102:1096-1104.

26. Hetherington MM. Cues to overeating. Psychological factors influencing over consumption. *Proc Nutr Soc.* 2007;66:113-123.

27. Shatenstein B, Ferland G. Absence of nutritional or clinical consequences of decentralized bulk food portioning in elderly nursing home residents with dementia in Montreal. *J Am Diet Assoc.* 2000;100:1354–1260.

28. Remsburg RE, Luking A, Baran P, Radu C, Pineda D, Bennett RG, Tayback M. Impact of a buffet-style dining program on weight and biochemical indicators of nutritional status in nursing home residents: A pilot study. *J Am Diet Assoc.* 2001;101:1460–1364.

29. Taylor KA, Barr SL. Provision of small, frequent meals does not improve energy intake of elderly Alzheimer's disease. *J Gerontol A Biol Sci Med Sci.* 2006;106:1115-1118.

(Continued)

Position of the American Dietetic Association *(Continued)*

30. Nijs K, Graaf C, Kok FJ, van Staveren WA. Effect of family-style meal time on quality of life, physical performance and body weight of nursing home residents; a cluster RTC. *BMJ.* 2006;332:1180-1183.

31. Zizza C, Tayie F, Lino M. Benefits of snacking in older Americans. *J Am Diet Assoc.* 2007;107:800-806.

32. Kretser AJ, Voss T, Kerr WW, Cavadini C, Friedmann J. Effects of two models of nutritional interventions on homebound older adults at nutritional risk. *J Am Diet Assoc.* 2003;103:320-336.

33. Position of the American Dietetic Association: Nutrition across the spectrum of aging. *J Am Diet Assoc.* 2005;105:616-663.

34. Drewnowski A, Evans WJ. Nutrition, physical activity and quality of life in older adults: Summary. J *Gerontol A Bio Sci.* 2001;56:89-94.

35. Wakimoto P, Block G. Dietary intake, dietary patterns, and changes with age: An epidemiological perspective. *J Gerontol A Bio Sci Med Sci.* 2001;56:65-80.

36. Dietary Guidelines for Americans 2005: Executive summary. Health.gov Web site. http://www.health.gov/dietaryguidelines/dga2005/document/html/executivesummary.htm. Accessed October 30, 2009.

37. Sullivan DH, Johnson LE, Bopp MM, Roberson PK. Prognostic significance of monthly weight fluctuations among older nursing home residents. *J Gerontol A Biol Sci Med Sci.* 2004;59:M633-M639.

38. Thomas DR. Loss of skeletal muscle mass in aging: Examining the relationship of starvation, sarcopenia and cachexia. *Clin Nutr.* 2007;26:389-399.

39. Thomas DR. Unintended weight loss in older adults. *Aging Health.* 2008;4:191-200.

40. Murden RA, Ainslie NK. Recent weight loss is related to short-term mortality in nursing homes. *J Gen Intern Med.* 1994;9:648-650.

41. Unintended weight loss in older adults evidence-based nutrition practice guideline. American Dietetic Association Evidence Analysis Library. http://www.adaevidencelibrary.com/topic=cfm?cat3651&libraryEBG. Accessed November 4, 2009.

42. Ekberg O, Harndy S, Wolsard V, Wuttge-Hannig A, Ortega P. Social and psychological burden of dysphagia: Its impact on diagnosis and treatment. *Dysphagia.* 2002;17: 139-146.

43. Lorefait B, Granerus AK, Unosson M. Avoidance of solid food in weight-losing older patients with Parkinson's disease. *J Clin Nurs.* 2006;15:1404-1412.

44. Rypkema G, Adang E, Dicke H, Naber T, De Swart B, Disselhorst L, Goluke-Willernse G, Olde Rikkert M. Cost-effectiveness of an interdisciplinary intervention in geriatric inpatients to prevent malnutrition. *J Nutr Health Aging.* 2004;8:122-127.

45. Wright L, Cotter D, Hickson M, Frost G. Comparison of energy and protein intakes of older people consuming a texture modified diet with a normal hospital diet. *J Hum Nurt Diet.* 2005;18:213-219.

46. Colodny N. Dysphagic independent feeders' justification for noncompliance with recommendations by a speech-language pathologist. *Am J Speech Lang Pathol.* 2005;14: 61-70.

47. Stroebele N, De Castro JM. Effect of ambience in food intake and food choices. *Nutrition.* 2004;20:821-838.

48. Foley N, Finestone H, Woodbury MG, Teasell R, Greens-Finestone L. Energy and protein intake of acute stroke patients. *J Nutr Health Aging.* 2006;10:171-175.

49. Shum NC, Hui WW, Chu FC, Chai J, Chow TW. Prevalence of malnutrition and risk factors in geriatric patients of a convalescent and rehabilitation hospital. *Hon Kong Med J.* 2005;11:234-242.

50. Woods NF, LaCroix AZ, Gray SL, Aragaki AA, Cochrane BB, Brunner RL, Masaki K, Murray A, Newman AB. Frailty: Emergence and consequences in women aged 65 and older in the Women's Health Initiative Observational Study. *J Am Geriatr Soc.* 2005; 53:1321-1330.

51. American Diabetes Association. Nutrition recommendations and interventions for diabetes: A position statement of the American Diabetes Association. *Diabetes Care.* 2008; 31(suppl):S61-S78.

52. American Geriatrics Society Panel on Improving Care for Elders with Diabetes. Guidelines for improving the care of the older person with diabetes mellitus. *J Am Geriatr Soc.* 2003;51(suppl):S265-S280.

53. Villareal DT, Shah K. Obesity in older adults—A growing problem. In: Bales CW, Ritchie CS. *Handbook of Clinical Nutrition and Aging.* 2nd ed. New York, NY: Humana Press; 2009:263-277.

54. Miller SL, Wolfe RR. The danger of weight loss in the elderly. *J Nutr Health Aging.* 2008;12:487-491.

55. Kennedy RI, Chokkalingham K, Srinivasan R. Obesity in the elderly: Who should we be treating, and why, and how? *Curr Opin Clin Nutr Metab Care.* 2004;7:3-9.

56. Janssen I. Sarcopenia. In: Bales CW, Ritchie CS. *Handbook of Clinical Nutrition and Aging.* 2nd ed. New York, NY: Humana Press; 2009:183-205.

57. Schatz IJ, Masaki K, Yano K, Chen R, Rodriquez BL, Curb JD. Cholesterol and all-cause mortality in elderly people from the Honolulu Heart Program. *Lancet.* 2001;358: 351-355.

(Continued)

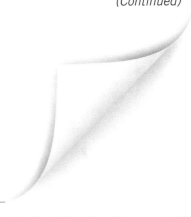

Position of the American Dietetic Association *(Continued)*

58. Paterna S, Gaspare P, Fasullo S, Sarullo FM, Di Pasquale P. Normal-sodium diet compared with low-sodium diet in compensated congestive heart failure: Is sodium an old enemy or a new friend? *Clin Sci (Lond).* 2008;114:221-230.

59. Your guide to lowering your blood pressure with DASH. National Heart, Lung, and Blood Institute Web site. http://www.nhlbi.nih.gov/health/public/heart/hbp/dash/new_dash.pdf. Accessed November 5, 2009.

60. Heron MP, Hoyert DL, XU J, Scott C, Tejada-Vera B. Death-preliminary data for 2006. *National Vital Statistics Reports.* Vol 56, No 16. Hayattsville, MD: National Center for Health Statics; 2009.

61. Wachterman M, Kiely DK, Mitchell SL. Reporting dementia on the death certificates of nursing home residents dying with endstage dementia. *JAMA.* 2008;300:2608-2610.

62. Stages of Alzheimer's. Alzheimer's Association Web site. http://www.alz.org/alzheimers_disease_stages_of_alzheimers.asp. Accessed May 12, 2010.

63. Position of The American Dietetic Association: Ethical and legal issues in nutrition, hydration, and feeding. *J Am Diet Assoc.* 2008;208:387-882.

64. McCann R, Hall W, Groth-Juncter A. Comfort care for terminally ill patients: The appropriate use of nutrition and hydration. *JAMA.* 1994;272:1263-1266.

65. Winter SM. Terminal nutrition: Framing the debate for the withdrawal of nutritional support in terminally ill patients. *Am J Med.* 200;109:723-741.

The authors thank the following people for their contributions in developing this Practice Paper. *Authors:* Becky Dorner, RD, LD, Nutrition Consulting Services & Becky Dorner & Associates, Inc, Akron, OH; Elizabeth K. Friedrich, MPH, RD, LDN, Nutrition and Health Promotion Consultant, Salisbury, NC; Mary Ellen Posthauer, RD, LD, M.E.P. Healthcare Dietary Services, Inc, Evansville, IN.

Reviewers: Jo Jo Dantone-Debarbieris, MS, RD, LDN (Nutrition Education Resources, Inc, LaPlace, LA); Sharon Denny, MS, RD (ADA Knowledge Center, Chicago, IL); Kristin A.R. Gustashaw, MS, RD, CSG (Rush University Medical Center, Chicago, IL); Mary H. Hager, PhD, RD, FADA (ADA Policy Initiative & Advocacy, Washington, DC); Sharon McCauley, MS, MBA, RD, LDN, FADA (ADA Quality Management, Chicago, IL); Management in Food and Nutrition Systems dietetics practice group (Susan M. McGinley, Sodexho Senior Services, Haddon Heights, NJ); Lynn Carpenter Moore, RD, LD, Nutrition Systems, INC, Jackson, MS; Esther Myers, PhD, RD, FADA (ADA Research & Strategic Business Development, Chicago, IL); Lisa Spence, PhD, RD (ADA Research & Strategic Business Development, Chicago, IL); Dietitians in Health Care Communities dietetics practice group (Lisa A. Weigand, RD, LD/N, Perferred Clinical Services, Ocala, FL).

Association Positions Committee Workgroup: Alana Cline, PhD, RD (chair); Dian O. Weddle, PhD, RD, FADA; Linda Roberts, MS, RD, LDN (content advisor).

END OF CHAPTER

Putting It Into Practice Questions & Answers

1. List three steps you would need to take to implement a culture change in your facility.

   A. *1. Interview your clients*

   2. Review/research resources

   3. Decide what your facility can/will offer for a culture change in dining

   4. Meet with other departments

   5. Refine ideas

   6. Communicate, communicate, communicate, train

2. What would be an appropriate substitute if a client does not like broccoli?

   A. *Green beans, asparagus, mixed vegetables with peas, beans, corn*

17

Conduct Nutrition Education

Overview and Objectives

Nutrition education enables clients to participate in caring for themselves. By developing basic skills in this area and adapting those skills to the educational needs of the client, a Certified Dietary Manager can be a valuable resource to clients.

After completing this chapter, you should be able to:

✓ Develop a plan for nutrition education

✓ Select educational materials and resources

✓ Utilize resource materials

✓ Evaluate client readiness and ability to learn

✓ Ascertain background and knowledge of clients

✓ Implement a teaching plan

✓ Suggest appropriate/available social resources

✓ Evaluate effectiveness of the teaching

A client takes part in the fine details of managing a diet. The client may choose particular foods for a selective menu. With knowledge, the client can choose foods that make meals enjoyable and support their own care by self-managing their own diet. Providing appropriate nutrition education will enable the client to make better choices for themselves. Using nutrition education materials begins with developing a plan for nutrition education.

The Academy of Nutrition and Dietetics (AND) [formerly known as The American Dietetic Association (ADA)], nutrition education is "a process that assists the public in applying knowledge from nutrition science and the relationship between diet and health to their food practices. It is a deliberate effort to improve the nutritional well-being of people by assessing the multiple factors that affect food choices, tailoring educational methodologies and messages to the public being reached, and evaluating results. It can help individuals develop a knowledge base, make a commitment to good nutrition, select nutritionally adequate diets, and develop decision-making skills." According to this definition, nutrition educators can enhance knowledge, encourage skills to make decisions and select nutritious diets, and help clients develop a positive attitude toward nutrition. It can also help clients utilize the knowledge toward positive lifestyle behavioral changes. Nutrition education is one form of nutrition intervention, as defined by the AND.

Developing Objectives

Before beginning any type of nutrition education, we first need to answer a simple, direct question: What do I want the client to learn? What do you want the outcome to be? Our answer to this is developing one or more learning objectives. A **learning objective** is a specific, measurable statement of the outcome of education. To develop a learning objective, think about what the client will be able to do when you have successfully competed nutrition education. An effective learning objective includes key elements, described in the acronym **RUMBAS**.

RUMBAS stands for:

R- Relevant

U- Understandable

M- Measurable

B- Behavioral

A- Attainable

S- Specific

Each learning objective should be relevant to the overall purpose of the instruction. For example, if you want to educate a client about managing hypertension, there is no need to toss in nutrition information about diverticulitis. You want to focus on what the client needs and address this in an objective. Next, you want the objective to make sense. In addition, you want the outcome you specify to be measurable. Why? So that you will be able to assess whether the education has been successful. Figure 17.1 lists examples of objectives that are and are not measurable. An effective objective is also behavioral. This means it describes what a client will do. Needless to say, an objective must be attainable and realistic. It should also be specific.

Figure 17.1   Measurable Objectives

Not Measurable:

Client will do better with choosing foods on the daily menu.

Measurable:

Client will choose foods on the daily menu that meet his 200-gram carbohydrate diet, within 10%.

Not Measurable:

Client will eat more calories.

Measurable:

Client will select foods that bring intake up to at least 1600 cal/day.

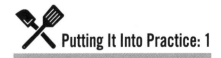 Putting It Into Practice: 1

Change the following objective so it meets the "rumbas" criteria: Client will explain why he should choose nutritious foods.

(Check your answer at the end of this chapter)

Group Instruction

Formal education of clients is most often accomplished through group instruction. An advantage of group instruction is that it allows clients to share experiences and develop a sense of group motivation. If the clients will continue to have contact after an educational session, they can encourage and support each other. A group may include clients, as well as family members and others involved in care. In any facility where a group of clients has common educational needs, this can be an excellent option. A Certified Dietary Manager may also combine group instruction with individual nutrition counseling (discussed later in this chapter).

After developing learning objectives, a Certified Dietary Manager planning group instruction needs to develop a class outline that includes motivation to the topic, organized detail for comprehension, some form of practice, and how to apply the material or application. Here are some tips for developing these sections of an outline.

Motivation

The motivation helps to pull the learner/client into the topic. It orients learners to the subject. It gives the Registered Dietitian/Certified Dietary Manager an opportunity to learn more about the clients. It can also be used to create client involvement and interest, by, for example, tasting a new low-fat food. When choosing a motivation, pick an opening that will quickly engage participants' attention. It may be a question, such as: *What do you find most confusing (or annoying) about your current diet?* Sometimes, a statistic can capture attention. An example is: *Ninety percent of people who go on weight loss diets end up heavier than when they started. Why is that?* The motivation needs to feel non-threatening. For example, you can ask each participant to state a favorite food. Make the opening relevant to the group, and design it to put people at ease. As clients share information about themselves, avoid making judgments. You want to encourage open communication, which requires absolute acceptance of each person in the group. If the client is doing something undesirable, your approach should be to present information and help the client draw personal conclusions. During this section, you also want to briefly describe the learning objectives. You may or may not include every detail you have used in planning. You may say something like: *When we are finished with this class, you will be able to determine the total amount of carbohydrates in your daily diet.*

Organized Detail/Comprehension

This part of the class outline describes the content, or what you teach; and the teaching methods, or how you teach it. For each learning objective, you must sketch out what you will say, and choose an appropriate teaching method. When choosing your current teaching material, pick information that is relevant and significant to the group. Be specific, and use examples.

Practice

When choosing your teaching methods, choose some that allow for participation. Research demonstrates that people remember only 20 percent of what they hear, 30 percent of what they see, but 50 percent of what they

Glossary

Learning Objective
A specific, measurable statement of the outcome of a lesson, inservice, or nutrition education session

RUMBAS Objective
A learning objective that is **R**elevant, **U**nderstandable, **M**easurable, **B**ehavioral, **A**ttainable, **S**pecific

hear and see (Metcalf 1997). By having clients actively participate in training, you can expect them to remember 90 percent of what they say and do. Activities may include checking sample food labels and deciding how they fit into a diet, or marking a selective menu according to a meal plan. They may include practice in modifying recipes to fit special dietary needs, or even simple food preparation.

Application

Application is where you ask the client to apply the information to his/her own diet or situation. They make their own choices, work on their own, and correct their own work when possible. For some clients, the application may occur after they've left the facility and you will follow up with them at another meeting.

Figure 17.2 shows a sample outline for group instruction. Figure 17.3 lists some ideas for achieving effective communication.

Here are some additional ideas to enhance your success in teaching groups:

✓ Start on time.

✓ Use a seating arrangement such as a circle that enhances communication and vision.

✓ Make eye contact. Smile and nod to show positive reinforcement.

✓ Pay attention to the pace, volume, and tone of your voice. Don't talk too fast, and be sure everyone can hear you.

Figure 17.2   Sample Education Session Outline: Carbohydrate Counting

Topic	Action
Motivation	Ask clients if they have any family members with diabetes. Ask them what type of diet they followed and what foods were restricted (It may be the exchange diet). Explain that the outcome today is for each client to be able to use a new diabetic eating plan where they have more choices and fewer restrictions. It is called carbohydrate counting.
Organized Detail/ Comprehension	Begin with an explanation of what a carbohydrate is and why it is important for diabetics to know where carbohydrates are found. Keep it simple for now...only talk about starch, sugar, and fiber. Hand out nutrition labels and help them not only find the grams of carbohydrate but also identify the sources of carbohydrate on the nutrition label. Explain how carbohydrates can be counted and demonstrate that with a handout they can keep and refer to.
Practice	Divide the group into smaller groups or a sharing pair where they pair up with someone nearby to work on the activity. Give each group or pair some empty food packages and ask them to determine how many 'carbs' each food would provide and what type of carbohydrate it is. Ask one person from each group to report back to the full group.
Application	Each client should know how many 'carbs' they have in one day and how it should be distributed. Ask them to select from the bin of food labels the foods they could have for one meal that would be equivalent to the number of 'carbs' they are allowed. Ask a few of the group to share their 'meals.'
Closing	Thank participants for their cooperation. Ask for questions and reactions. Summarize key points: What is a carbohydrate, why it is important and where to find them. Briefly review how to count carbohydrates. Give session evaluation if you use a formal evaluation or ask them to write one sentence about what they learned.

Figure 17.3 Keys to Effective Communication

 Respect Personal Space

When you first sit down to speak with clients, ask them to sit where they feel the most comfortable or let them tell you where to sit. This will allow people to choose the distance that feels right to them. Comfortable distance varies by culture and individual.

 Learn the Cultural Rules About Touching

Find out the cultural rules regarding touch for the ethnic groups with whom you work, including differences based on gender. In some Asian cultures, the head should not be touched because it is the seat of wisdom. In many Hispanic cultures, the head of a child should be touched when you admire the child. A vigorous handshake may be considered a sign of aggression by Native Americans.

 Establish Rapport

Take time to establish common ground through sharing experiences and exchanging information.

 Ask Questions

Do not be afraid to ask someone about something with which you are unfamiliar or uncomfortable. Nutrition educators suggest open-ended, honest questions that show an interest in the person, a respect for his culture, and a willingness to learn.

 Listen to the Answers

Really listen. Do not interrupt your client or try to put words in their mouth. Let them tell their own story. Appreciate and **use silence**. Observe your client to get a feel for how he or she uses silence. Do not feel that silence has to be filled in with small talk. Give people a chance to formulate their thoughts, especially if they are trying to speak in a language that is not their native tongue. Cultures that value silence learn to distinguish varying qualities of silence, which may be hard for others to discern. "Pause time" is different for different cultures.

 Notice Eye Contact

Notice the kind of eye contact your client is making with family members or your coworkers. Many cultures consider it impolite to look directly at the person speaking.

 Pay Attention to Body Movements

Movements such as upturned palms of the hands, waving one's hand, and pointing with fingers or feet convey varying messages. Observe your clients for clues.

Note Client Responses

Note that a "yes" response does not necessarily indicate that a client has understood or is willing to do what is being discussed. It may simply be an offering of respect for the health professional's status. Some clients may not ask questions because this would indicate a lack of clear communication by the provider. In some cultures, smiling and laughing may mask other emotions or prevent conflict.

✓ Ask clients what they already know about the topic to be discussed.

✓ Actively listen.

✓ Encourage and facilitate client participation.

✓ Ask open-ended questions.

✓ Praise and give encouragement.

✓ Use visual aids effectively.

Visual Aids

You can reinforce your points with visual aids, such as simple handouts, posters, models, slides, or transparencies (see Figure 17.4). Visual aids keep clients' attention, reinforce main ideas, save time, and increase understanding and retention. Visual aids are also useful in making comparisons. DVDs may also be useful, but do not use this to replace your teaching. Make sure you use terms that your audience will know and understand, avoiding medical jargon. Make key points simple, and design handouts to be readable, especially for anyone with a vision impairment. The most effective visual aid is limited to one idea that can be communicated within three to five seconds. If you have more ideas, use more aids! Special visual aids for nutrition education include food models, which are synthetic replicas of food; measuring cups and spoons; food packages; and nutrition facts labels from foods. Compare your visual aids to the checklist in Figure 17.5 before you use them.

Serving Sizes

It is important that your clients understand what an appropriate amount of food is in a standard serving size. Many clients have no idea that a serving of bread or starch is one ounce nor can they tell you how much one ounce is. For instance, one ounce of crackers or snack chips varies by the type of cracker or chip (e.g. 1 ounce of thin wheat crackers is 15 crackers; 1 ounce of soda crackers is 7 crackers.)

In Chapter 2, you reviewed the servings sizes listed on myPyramid. The serving sizes found on the Exchange System for Meal Planning differs from myPyramid. For instance, myPyramid lists one-half cup of vegetables or fruit as a serving. The Exchange System for Meal Planning lists half cup of most vegetables and fruits as a serving. If you use synthetic replicas of food as a visual aid, those are usually the serving size found on the Exchange System for Meal Planning. Serving sizes for the Exchange System can be found in Appendix C. Your clients may be eating considerably more or less amounts of food than a standard serving size, depending on the food group. Visual aids are an appropriate way to help your clients see what a standard serving is. It is also helpful for the clients to communicate to you how much they normally eat.

Adapting Teaching to Client Education Needs

Providing nutrition education in groups is easier if everyone attending is there for the same reason and on the same level in terms of their readiness and ability to learn. However, that rarely happens in groups. There will be some clients who are not as ready to learn or able to learn in the same way. What if

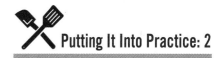

Putting It Into Practice: 2

What would be an effective visual aid when conducting a nutrition education session for a client following a low-fat diet?

(Check your answer at the end of this chapter)

Figure 17.4 Carbohydrate Counting

Your doctor wants you to count carbohydrates as part of a healthy eating plan. Carbohydrate counting can help you balance your carbohydrates to keep blood glucose levels within a target range. This can help prevent complications of diabetes. Carbohydrate counting can be used in place of other meal planning methods to help you choose what and how much to eat, and if you take insulin, to decide how much insulin to use.

Foods that are mostly carbohydrate affect blood glucose levels more than foods that are not high in carbohydrate. Foods that are mostly carbohydrate include breads/grains (chips, crackers, etc.), starchy vegetables (corn, peas, potatoes, etc.), sweets, fruits, milk and milk products. Foods that are not high in carbohydrate include meat/meat alternates, non-starchy vegetables (green beans, carrots, broccoli, etc.) and fats.

One carbohydrate serving equals 15 grams of carbohydrate.

Amount of Carbohydrate for Each Meal and Snack

The recommended number of servings of carbohydrate for each meal and snack is based on your weight, activity level, diabetes medications/insulin, and goals for target blood glucose levels. As a general guide, many people do well on 3 or 4 servings of carbohydrate foods at each meal, and 1 or 2 servings per snack.

In order to maintain a healthy, well balanced diet, meals and snacks need to include a variety of foods from all the food groups. Use the Food Choices lists for counting carbohydrates. Each Food Choice list notes the amount of carbohydrate for each food in the list. Again, one carbohydrate serving equals 15 grams of carbohydrate. For example:

* **Fruit**—Each serving contains 15 grams of carbohydrate
* **Bread/Grain**—Each serving contains 15 grams of carbohydrate
* **Milk**—Each serving contains 12 grams so it is rounded up to 15 grams and counted as 1 serving of carbohydrate
* **Starchy Vegetable**—Each serving contains 15 grams of carbohydrate

Using the Nutrition Facts on Food Labels

Check the label for the number of carbohydrate grams to determine serving size. One carbohydrate serving equals 15 grams of carbohydrate.

If one serving provides...	...then one serving of food is equivalent to:
A total of 15 grams of carbohydrate	1 carbohydrate serving
More than 15 grams of carbohydrate	Divide the total by 15 to determine the number of carbohydrate servings
Less than 15 grams of carbohydrate	Multiply the serving size to determine a serving size that will have 15 grams of carbohydrate to equal one carbohydrate serving

Your Pattern for Carbohydrate Counting

Total Calories per Day:_____

Carbohydrate Servings

Breakfast: _____

Lunch: _____

Snack:_____

Dinner: _____

Sample Menu Pattern

Carb. Servings	Veg.	Fruit	Milk	Bread/ Grain	TOTAL per Meal/Snack
Breakfast		1	1	2	4
Lunch	1			2	3
Snack	1				1
Dinner	1	1	1	1	4
Snack			1	1	2
TOTAL per Day	3	2	3	6	14

Source: Diet Instructions. Becky Dorner & Associates, Inc. Used with permission.

they don't speak English or are unable to read English? What if everyone in the group has a different ethnic background? Regardless of whether you have one person or six people, you need to adapt your teaching to what each client needs. The diet history for each person is the foundation of personalized diet planning and education. For example, if you learn in a diet history that a client frequently chooses fast foods, then you want to help the client learn to choose foods from a fast food menu as part of the education process. If you discover that a client is a vegetarian, you will need to be sure your recommendations are consistent with this dietary choice.

Figure 17.5 Checklist for Evaluating Printed Nutrition Education Materials

- The cover is attractive and clearly identifies the topic.
- The writing style is conversational and in an active voice.
- Technical jargon is not used. In cases when a technical term must be used, it is defined.
- The text is at the appropriate reading level, interesting, and lively.
- The emphasis is on "what to do," or specific behavioral changes.
- The illustrations are simple and relevant to the content.
- The print size is large enough and the font is plain enough to be easily read.
- There is contrast between the color of the print and the color of the paper so the words are easily read.
- The pages are not cluttered with too much information.
- The material is appropriate for the intended audience (gender, culture, age, level of education).
- The publication invites reader thought and/or participation, e.g. through a questionnaire, a recipe, a worksheet, or other techniques.

Figure 17.6 Communication Techniques for Effective Instruction

Topic	Action
Verbal Communication	• Describe behavior rather than judge it • Treat clients with respect and trust • Involve them in the problem solving • Empathize with the client • Be receptive to other ideas
Listening	• Be willing to hear a person out • Maintain good eye contact with the client • Restate, paraphrase or clarify statements as a way to allow the client to elaborate on their feelings
Promote Effective Communication	• Use understandable language with few medical terms • Allow for adequate time for the instruction • Become aware of the client's concerns and limitations before they can interfere with communication • Be genuine

It is important to be non-judgmental when teaching clients. Demonstrate respect for clients by making the time before you meet with them to learn as much as possible about their background and ability to learn. Then, make sure you have visual aids that reflect their backgrounds and ability to learn. If you have an older client, choose materials with larger print. If your client doesn't speak English, try to locate materials in their language or use food models or pictures without words. To adapt teaching to client educational needs, use the communication tips in Figure 17.6.

While some facilities develop their own teaching materials, this is a time-consuming proposition. Many high-quality materials are available either free or at low cost from government agencies, industry groups, health

Figure 17.7 Sources for Credible Educational Nutrition Resources

Source Name	URL
Health Associations	
Association of Nutrition & Foodservice Professionals	www.anfponline.org
The Academy of Nutrition and Dietetics (formerly known as The American Dietetic Association)	www.eatright.org
American Heart Association	www.heart.org/HEARTORG
American Cancer Society	www.cancer.org
American Dairy Association/Dairy Council	www.adadc.com
American Diabetes Association	www.diabetes.org
Federal Agencies	
Food & Drug Administration	www.fda.gov
National Digestive Diseases Information Clearinghouse	www.digestive.niddk.nih.gov
Food & Nutrition Information Center	http://fnic.nal.usda.gov/nal_display/index.php?info_center_48tax_level=1
Centers for Disease Control	www.cdc.gov
FDA Center for Food Safety and Applied Nutrition	www.fda.gov/food/foodsafety/default.htm
Others	
Harvard Medical School Consumer Information	www.intelihealth.com
Tufts University	Nutrition.tufts.edu
Mayo Clinic Health Information	www.mayoclinic.com
RD411	RD411.org
Meals for You	Mealsforyou.com
Institute of Food Science & Technology	www.ifst.org
SNAP Newsletters (for senior consumers)	http://recipefinder.nal.usda.gov/
Food & Health Communications	http://foodandhealth.com/

Note: This is a sample of highly rated sources; your instructor may have others

Figure 17.8 Sample Class Evaluation Form

Class Evaluation

Instructions: Please circle your answers to the following questions. Add any comments you'd like. Your feedback is very important to us. Thank you!

1. How well did this session match your interests about nutrition?

   Excellent Match   Fair Match   Poor Match

2. Was this material:

   Too Complex   Too Simple   Just Right

3. Please rate the activities (name them specifically on your form)?

   Excellent   Good   Fair

4. Please rate the handouts:

   Excellent   Good   Fair

5. Please rate the group leader's skills:

   Excellent   Good   Fair

6. What did you like most about this session?

7. What did you like least about this session?

8. Is there anything you will do differently after attending this session?

   No   Yes   If yes, what?

9. What other topics would you like to see in future classes?

Comments:

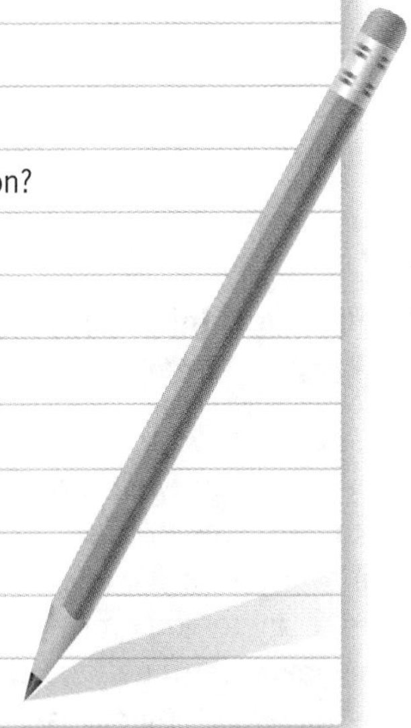

organizations, food manufacturers, cooperative extension services, and education institutions. Of course the World Wide Web has a multitude of resources; just make sure you abide by copyright laws if you use information from the Web.

If you are teaching someone who will be preparing meals at home, help develop a plan for meal preparation. You may want to develop a sample grocery list together, emphasizing choices that meet dietary needs. If you are working with the group, use the share/pair technique so the two can focus on what is practical for the client's abilities and lifestyle. You may recommend additional resources as relevant, such as a local Meals-on-Wheels program. See Figure 17.7 for a list of resources for credible education nutrition resources.

Whether you are teaching in a group or one-on-one, effective communication is the foundation. Dietary instruction generally involves some sort of recommended change on the part of the client. This may cause them to become defensive, which interferes with good communication.

Evaluate the Effectiveness of Your Education Session

The final, but very important component of any nutrition education program is evaluation. The key purpose of evaluation is to determine whether you have met the learning objectives. This is, in fact, one of the reasons we insist that learning objectives be measurable. A description of how to measure behavior, as written in an objective, gives us a solid gauge for evaluating the results of education. For instance, if the objective says, *Client will consume at least 80 percent of the nutritional supplements provided*, the evaluation will include determining what percentage of nutritional supplements were consumed.

A second reason for evaluating nutrition education is to obtain feedback about the educational approach itself. Particularly for group education, good practice dictates that we gather feedback from participants at the end. This information helps us refine educational techniques and related materials. Sometimes, it provides feedback to us as professionals to help us focus on how to work with a particular group or tackle a particular topic.

Following an educational session, three levels of evaluation may apply—client reaction, actual learning, and behavioral change. Here is more information about each:

Client reaction. Evaluation focused on client reaction answers the question: *How did the client(s) respond to the education sessions?* To evaluate client reaction for a group class, use a rating sheet such as a class evaluation, shown in Figure 17.8. Client reaction often provides feedback to group leaders, too. For example, we may find out which techniques worked best, or what questions may not have been addressed. We can use this information to revise outlines for future classes. Following a one-on-one nutrition counseling session, we also solicit the client's reaction. Usually, this is done informally, by asking questions such as:

✓ Was this session helpful to you?

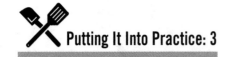

Putting It Into Practice: 3

You have a client with whom you have delivered two nutrition education sessions in the hospital over the past week. They are ready to go home. How can you determine if your sessions met your objectives?

(Check your answer at the end of this chapter)

✓ What questions have we left unanswered?

✓ Would you like to meet again to discuss your diet? If so, what would you like to talk about?

Actual learning. The second level of evaluation answers the question: *How much did clients learn?* To evaluate learning, you can use written and verbal questions, often given as a post-test. This is a test about facts and information presented. Some educational strategies require a pre-test before a session begins, and the same test at the end given as the post-test. This allows you to measure how much participants have learned. A drawback, however, is that many people feel intimidated by a formal test. Many people associate a test with uncomfortable situations in school and feel anxious. Two tests in one session can be even worse. Often, it helps to make a test a "quiz" and transform it into a fun, light-hearted activity. Written tests also require language competency and reading and writing skills of your clients. Sometimes this is not practical. An alternative to written tests is a friendly question-and-answer session.

Here are some examples of statements/questions that could be used to evaluate how much a client learned:

✓ Divide the list of foods into two groups, those with (e.g. high calories, the most vitamins, fat, sodium, etc) or (least vitamin C, low calories, low-fat, low-sodium)

✓ Write down one fact you learned that you will use

✓ What is the difference between (e.g. sugar content, fat content, sodium content) these food products?

✓ Choose, from this group of foods, the best source of (e.g. fiber, unsaturated fat, carbohydrate, calories, etc)

✓ What would be a better way to increase (e.g. calories, fiber, iron, vitamin A, etc.)

✓ Create a menu you would eat that meets your fluid restrictions

Behavioral change. The third level of evaluation answers the question: *Have dietary habits changed?* Refer to the learning objectives, and observe how behavior corresponds to the objectives themselves. In some cases, a food diary is useful. If clients are using a selective menu in a hospital or nursing facility, you can monitor how they make choices on menus. Likewise, if a client is choosing foods in a dining room, you can evaluate change by visiting the client at mealtime and making observations.

Refining Plans

If you find that education has not been as effective as you'd like, you need to try to identify reasons. A feedback tool such as the evaluation may help with this process. If you have already developed rapport with clients, you can discover many reasons simply by asking in a friendly, low-key manner. For example, three days after counseling a client about how to implement a high-calorie diet, you may say: *We are aiming to keep your daily calories up to 1500. Your calorie count for yesterday shows 900 calories. What do you think might be holding you back?* Keeping your responses non-judgmental makes it easier for clients to trust you. In turn, this helps you help them more effectively.

Consider all possible barriers to communication. These may include differences in language, ability to read (if you rely on printed materials), use of terminology a client does not understand, state of alertness, and many others. If any of these barriers exists, you may need to re-evaluate how best to communicate with a client. Also keep in mind that individual learning styles vary. One person may learn best by reading words. Another may learn best by glancing at images and graphics. One needs to hear information. Another needs to do things. Each of these styles is valid, and each requires different educational techniques. If you discover that a client has not understood information, try using a different educational approach.

As you evaluate progress, it's important to be flexible. Do not expect perfection from clients, especially if they are striving to change longstanding dietary habits. Try to notice every positive step towards achieving objectives. Encouragement reassures a client about putting information into practice, and tends to bring about more of the same behaviors.

In addition, it's critical to recognize the distinction between knowledge and behavior. This distinction crops up continually when we examine any type of health education. The client might know the information that will make them healthy. However, that doesn't mean they will automatically put it all into practice! Often, the challenge is not limited to explaining diets or relating information. The real challenge is to help motivate and support an individual in making subtle improvements in habits. This may hinge on much more than nutrition knowledge. In fact, dietary habits have many cultural and psychological undertones. Values, emotional needs, and other life priorities may easily affect the final outcomes of nutrition counseling. As possible, try to understand these factors, and help clients address them. As needed, mold your suggestions to the client's preferences, customs, and concerns. You may need to weave nutrition ideas into specialized plans creatively in order to match a client's needs.

Also consider the big picture. Nutrition education is only one component of a health plan. Consider the other components, and ask yourself how these fit together for the client. Is the client overwhelmed? Is nutrition high or low on a priority list? If there are many health-related objectives and regimens, it may help to show the client how nutrition can support other needs. For example, a client who has hypertension and is also obese may appreciate discovering how weight loss will likely help reduce hypertension, too. The bottom line is to articulate a payoff. Explain to the client how he will benefit, how he will feel, or what other desirable health effects he may expect from implementing dietary advice.

Furthermore, it is easy for a client to believe that sound nutrition is an all-or-nothing endeavor. This is key to the culture of dieting, and tends to affect our thinking as a culture when it comes to nutrition. Effective education depends on our ability to transform dietary advice into a series of small steps and to praise all positive changes. Any time a client experiences difficulty following a restrictive diet, we can provide reassurance and encouragement.

Sometimes, implementing dietary advice simply isn't practical for a client, due to one of various obstacles. As part of any re-assessment, be alert to problems that may interfere with meeting nutrition-related objectives. Factors such as medications, dental changes, or changes in swallowing ability can easily affect how a person eats. If obstacles exist, try to help remove them. If that is not possible, refine the plan and the education to make them realistic for the client.

Documenting Evaluation

Like any aspect of a nutrition care plan, nutrition education requires evaluation and documentation. If you provide nutrition counseling, include this information in a progress note. You want to tell who was involved (e.g. client and/or family members), what you covered together, and what objectives you have set. You should also name any handout(s) you have provided. You should assess a client's understanding of the educational content. As possible, state what you have seen that shows how the client can meet behavioral objectives. For example, you may write: *Client accurately selected foods to total 160 grams of carbohydrates on tomorrow's menu.* You should state your recommended follow-up. As you re-assess educational objectives, gather new information and provide your assessment. If you revise the plan for education, indicate this in the progress note.

Reinforcing Education

Typically, one nutrition education session does not change a person's dietary habits. The most effective education is delivered in manageable chunks, over a period of time. Education of any type requires reinforcement. If you have ongoing contact with clients, as in a school, retirement community, or long-term care facility, you have an excellent opportunity to provide intermittent education and reinforcement. Reinforcement can be as simple as:

✓ Providing a nutrition tip on a menu

✓ Preparing a bulletin board in your facility to highlight a nutrition topic

✓ Labeling foods in a group dining area with nutrition facts

✓ Chatting with a client about daily food choices

✓ Noticing when a client implements a dietary change at any meal, and providing praise

✓ Giving a client an opportunity to ask a follow-up question a day or two after an educational session

✓ Highlighting a special item on a menu and noting how it meets particular needs

Clearly, nutrition education is more than a one-shot endeavor. Quite often, Certified Dietary Managers are in roles where they can have a tremendous impact on clients' individual dietary choices.

END OF CHAPTER

 Putting It Into Practice Questions & Answers

1. Change the following objective so it meets the "rumbas" criteria: Client will explain why he should choose nutritious foods.

   A. *Client will select foods high in vitamin A and C at 75% of his meals; or, Client will consume at least 80% of nutritional supplements provided.*

2. What would be an effective visual aid when conducting a nutrition education session for a client following a low-fat diet?

   A. *Some examples are: labels from butter, oil, margarine products to see the difference in the types of fat; test tubes full of shortening or an amount of butter pats that are equivalent to the grams of fat in some foods that are high in fat such as fast food items; colorful handouts that show menu options that are low in fat and cholesterol.*

3. You have a client with whom you have delivered two nutrition education sessions in the hospital over the past week. They are now ready to go home. How can you determine if your sessions met your objectives? There are several ways to evaluate a nutrition education session.

   A. *To begin with, look at your objectives to see what you said was the outcome. If you used action verbs such as **will consume**…, you can measure plate waste to see if they are implementing your objectives. If your action verb was…**to gain or lose weight**…you might want to schedule a follow-up appointment to look at his/her weight over time. If your action verb was…**to select**…you can review their selective menus to determine if they are implementing your objectives.*

Participate in Regulatory Agency Surveys

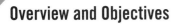

Overview and Objectives

The last few chapters have addressed how critical it is to focus on clients and their quality of care. State and federal regulations also focus on clients and their quality of care. You will learn what the regulations are, how to locate them, and some tips for following them.

After completing this chapter, you should be able to:

✓ Identify regulatory standards and recent revisions

✓ Develop an appropriate plan of correction

✓ Demonstrate professional interaction with surveyors

✓ Utilize regulatory agencies as professional resources

✓ Explain how regulations influence the quality management process

It is fitting that the last chapter in this textbook is about regulations. In many ways, regulations address everything that has been covered in this textbook. Let's look first at the regulatory agencies and the regulations that most impact the foodservice department.

Regulatory/Accrediting Agencies

The **Centers for Medicare and Medicaid Services (CMS)** is a branch of the U.S. Department of Health and Human Services. CMS is the federal agency that administers the Medicare program and monitors the Medicaid programs offered by each state. All healthcare facilities have mandatory state licensing requirements according to their state law. The facility is held to the strictest regulatory requirements, either state or federal. It is important to know and follow the local state regulations. Once a facility has a state license to operate, it can voluntarily seek a federal CMS survey to determine if it is compliant with all the federal 'certification' requirements for federal funding. The long-term care initial and annual federal survey, required by the Omnibus Budget Reconciliation ACT (OBRA) 1987, is usually provided by state agency surveyors who wear the federal hat. Acute care hospital surveys may have a CMS deem status and a survey process annually or every three years. Since a CMS validation survey can be conducted at any time, it is important to be "survey ready" at all times. Any healthcare facility that offers services to clients who are funded by

Medicare or Medicaid must follow the CMS regulations. CMS also oversees HIPPA, which was covered in Chapter 7, and is the act that assures privacy for all healthcare client information.

Regulations appear in a document called the CMS State Operations Manual (SOM). Information for accessing this manual and other information on CMS can be found in Figure 18.1. The operations manual contains a great deal of helpful information besides the regulations. Regulations cover all areas of a healthcare facility including the following that are specific to nutrition in dietary:

483.25 Quality of Care

✓ 483.25 (c) Pressure Sores

✓ 483.25 (g) NG Tubes

✓ 483.25 (i) Nutrition

✓ 483.25 (j) Hydration

483.35 Dietary Services

✓ 483.35 (a) Staffing

✓ 483.35 (d) Food

✓ 483.35 (e) Therapeutic diets

There are other dietary areas that will be covered in the *Managing Foodservice and Food Safety* textbook. There are many other regulatory tags throughout the SOM that overlap. Two key examples are:

✓ F 501 Medical Director and the requirements for effective nutrition policies and oversight.

✓ F 520 Quality Assessment and Assurance and the requirements for developing and monitoring effective client nutrition maintenance systems.

The following is an overview of CMS Federal regulatory requirements for Nutrition in Long Term Care and related tags for hospitals. It is challenging to keep up with regulatory revisions, survey expectations, and changing evidenced-based expectations in the industry. As interdisciplinary team members, in a very demanding area of care, it is imperative to keep current and knowledgeable. For additional information, study archived articles at www. anfponline.org under Publications > ANFP Magazine > Index and Archive > Section on Regulations/Compliance. Earn continuing education credits with timely webinar topics archived under The ANFP Marketplace. On the ANFP website, look up and join the state and national ANFP organizations to receive the ANFP magazine, network with colleagues, and learn of conferences with outstanding speakers and topics. CMS provides investigative protocols that provide guidance for the surveyors. The Investigative Protocol for Nutrition Status is found in Figure 18.2. CMS guidelines use "**F-Tag**" numbers to identify specific guidance for long-term care; they use "**A-Tag**" numbers for hospitals. On September 1, 2008, changes were implemented to improve quality of care. These changes make long-term care facilities more accountable for maintaining clients' nutrition status. An example of an F-Tag regulation for

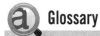

Glossary

CMS
Centers for Medicare and Medicaid Services

TJC
The Joint Commission

F-Tags
An identification number of a CMS guideline for long-term care

A-Tags
An identification number of a CMS guideline for general acute care hospitals

C-Tags
An identification number of a CMS guideline for small rural or critical access hospitals

Nutrition Status (F-Tag 325) is shown in Figure 18.3. Figure 18.4 shows the process for noncompliance for F-Tag 325. CMS uses quality measures to assess the quality of care in healthcare facilities such as: Percent of Low-Risk Residents Who Have Pressure Sores (looks back seven days).

Small rural hospitals or critical access hospitals use "**C-Tag**" numbers. Some hospitals have a subacute or rehab unit on their license and must meet the regulatory requirements of both the acute and the long-term care regulations. Nutrition departments staff, including Certified Dietary Managers, in collaboration with Registered Dietitians, should study and know all the regulatory requirements for all levels of care that they provide.

(Continued on page 397)

Figure 18.1 **How to Access Regulations & Surveyor Guidance for CMS**

www.cms.hhs.gov > Regulations/Guidance>Manuals> (right hand) "Internet Only"> Publications: 100-07 State Operations Manual (SOM)> scroll down to "Appendices"

Skilled Nursing:

SOM Appendix PP (revised 10/1/2010) are the OBRA Regulations (tags) & Guidance, Scroll down to the newly revised sections with Surveyor Investigative Protocols:

- **F 325** Nutritional Status, Last revised 9/1/08

- **F 371** Sanitation, Last revised 6/12/09

- **F 240-252** Quality of Life and Residents Rights of Choice Self Determination, and Reasonable Accommodation. Revised 6/12/09

- **F 441** Infection Control, Last revised 9/25/09

NOTE: At end of Appendix PP: Surveyor Resident Review Forms 8025 and 805 are excellent to use for your own QAA

SOM Appendix P are the NH survey protocols for surveyors, includes Traditional Survey and QIS Survey Protocols

Acute Care:
- SOM Appendix A , scroll down to 482.28 (a)
- A-0618-631, Condition of Participation: Food and Dietetic Services, starts on pg. 248
- Critical Care Hospitals: (Small, rural)
- SOM Appendix W, C-279

Federal QIS Surveyor Task Forms for New Survey Process for Skilled Nursing Homes

Even if the traditional, standard survey process is still being used in your area, the surveyor task worksheets are invaluable to use for your own QAA (F 520). in developing your own QAA, those who work in hospitals may gain tremendous insight into the recently revised regulatory requirements of Long Term Care. Surveyors are cross trained. CMS expert panel workgroups who revise the "Interpretive Guidance to Surveyors" and "Investigative Protocols" for each tag requirement, search the evidenced-based best practices and standards in updating these.

Example: Nutrition, Hydration, and Tube Feeding:
- 22 pages of what a surveyor should review while conducting a survey in a subacute or nursing home.
- Others include: Kitchen, Dining, QAA, Pressure Ulcers, etc.

Forms only: http://www.uchsc.edu/hcpr/qis_forms.php

Training and QIS : http://www.aging.state.ks.us/Manuals/QIS/TabIndex.html

Self Study Materials for Compliance, view and order: www.linda@handydietaryconsulting.com

Source: Handy, Linda, President Handy Dietary Consulting, W San Marcos Blvd #38, San Marcos, CA 92078, linda@handydietaryconsulting.com, 2010

Figure 18.2   Investigative Protocol—Dining and Food Service

Objectives:

- To determine if each resident is provided with nourishing, palatable, attractive meals that meet the resident's daily nutritional and special dietary needs;

- To determine if each resident is provided services to maintain or improve eating skills; and

- To determine if the dining experience enhances the resident's quality of life and is supportive of the resident's needs, including food service and staff support during dining.

Task 5C: Use

This protocol will be used for:

- All sampled residents identified with malnutrition, unintended weight loss, mechanically altered diet, pressure sores/ulcers, and hydration concerns; and

- Food complaints received from residents, families and others.

General Considerations:

- Use this protocol at two meals during the survey, preferably the noon and evening meals.

- Record information on the Form CMS-805 if it pertains to a specific sampled resident, or on the Form CMS-807 if it relates to the general observations of the dining service/dining room.

- Discretely observe all residents, including sampled residents, during meals, keeping questions to a minimum to prevent disruption in the meal service.

- For each sampled resident being observed, identify any special needs and the interventions planned to meet their needs. Using the facility's menu, record in writing what is planned in writing to be served to the resident at the meal observed.

- Conduct observations of food preparation and quality of meals.

Procedures:

1. During the meal service, observe the dining room and/or resident's room for the following:
   > Comfortable sound levels;
   > Adequate illumination, furnishings, ventilation; absence of odors; and sufficient space;
   > Tables adjusted to accommodate wheelchairs, etc.; and
   > Appropriate hygiene provided prior to meals.

2. Observe whether each resident is properly prepared for meals. For example:
   > Resident's eyeglasses, dentures, and/or hearing aids are in place;
   > Proper positioning in chair, wheelchair, gerichair, etc., at an appropriate distance from the table (tray table and bed at appropriate height and position); and
   > Assistive devices/utensils identified in care plans provided and used as planned.

3. Observe the food service for:
   > Appropriateness of dishes and flatware for each resident. Single use disposable dining ware is not used except in an emergency and other appropriate dining activities. Except those with fluid restriction, each resident has an appropriate place setting with water and napkin;
   > Whether meals are attractive, palatable, served at appropriate temperatures and are delivered to residents in a timely fashion.
   > Did the meals arrive 30 minutes or more past the scheduled mealtime?
   > If a substitute was needed, did it arrive more than 15 minutes after the request for a substitute?
   > Are diet cards, portion sizes, preferences, and condiment requests being honored?

4. Determine whether residents are being promptly assisted to eat or provided necessary assistance/cueing in a timely manner after their meal is served.

   Note whether residents at the same table or in resident rooms are being served and assisted concurrently. If you observe a resident who is being assisted by a staff member to eat or drink, and the resident is having problems with eating or drinking, inquire if the staff member who is assisting them is a paid feeding assistant. If so, follow the procedures at tag F 373.

5. Determine if the meals served were palatable, attractive, nutritious and met the needs of the resident. Note the following:
   > Whether the resident voiced concerns regarding the taste, temperature, quality, quantity and appearance of the meal served;
   > Whether mechanically altered diets, such as pureed, were prepared and served as separate entree items (except when combined with food, e.g., stews, casseroles, etc.);
   > Whether attempts to determine the reason(s) for the refusal and a substitute of equal nutritive value was provided, if the resident refused/rejected food served; and
   > Whether food placement, colors, and textures were in keeping with the resident's needs or deficits, e.g., residents with vision or swallowing deficits.

(Continued)

Figure 18.2   Investigative Protocol—Dining and Food Service *(Continued)*

Sample Tray Procedure

If residents complain about the palatability/temperature of food served, the survey team coordinator may request a test meal to obtain quantitative data to assess the complaints. Send the meal to the unit that is the greatest distance from the kitchen or to the affected unit or dining room. Check food temperature and palatability of the test meal at about the time the last resident on the unit is served and begins eating.

6. Observe for institutional medication pass practices that interfere with the quality of the residents' dining experience. This does not prohibit the administration of medications during meal service for medications that are necessary to be given at a meal, nor does this prohibit a medication to be given during a meal upon request of a resident who is accustomed to taking the medication with the meal, as long as it has been determined that this practice does not interfere with the effectiveness of the medication.

> Has the facility attempted to provide medications at times and in a manner to support the dining experience of the resident, such as:

> Pain medications being given prior to meals so that meals could be eaten in comfort;

> Foods served are not routinely or unnecessarily used as a vehicle to administer medications (mixing the medications with potatoes or other entrees).

7. Determine if the sampled resident consumed adequate amounts of food as planned.

> Determine if the facility is monitoring the foods/fluids consumed. Procedures used by the facility may be used to determine percentage of food consumed, if available; otherwise, determine the percentage of food consumed using the following point system:

> Each food item served except for water, coffee, tea, or condiments equals one point. Example: Breakfast: juice, cereal, milk, bread and butter, coffee (no points) equals four points. If the resident consumes all four items in the amount served, the resident consumes 100% of breakfast. If the resident consumes two of the four food items served, then 50% of the breakfast would have been consumed. If three-quarters of a food item is consumed, give one point; for one-half consumed, give .5 points; for one-fourth or less, give no points. Total the points consumed x 100 and divide by the number of points given for that meal to give the percentage of meal consumed. Use these measurements when determining the amount of liquids consumed: Liquid measurements: 8 oz. cup = 240 cc, 6 oz. cup = 180 cc, 4 oz. cup = 120 cc, 1 oz. cup = 30 cc.

> Compare these findings with the facility's documentation to determine if the facility has accurately recorded the intake. Ask the staff if these findings are consistent with the resident's usual intake; and

> Note whether plates are being returned to the kitchen with 75% or more of food not eaten.

8. If concerns are noted with meal service, preparation, quality of meals, etc., interview the person(s) responsible for dietary services to determine how the staff are assigned and monitored to assure meals are prepared according to the menu, that the meals are delivered to residents in a timely fashion, and at proper temperature, both in the dining rooms/areas and in resident rooms.

NOTE: If concerns are identified in providing monitoring by supervisory staff during dining or concerns with assistance for residents to eat, evaluate nursing staffing in accord with 42 CFR 483.30(a), F 353, and quality of care at 42 CFR 483.25(a)(2) and (3).

Task 6: Determination of Compliance:

Compliance with 42 CFR 483.35(d)(1)(2), F 364, Food

• The facility is compliant with this requirement when each resident receives food prepared by methods that conserve nutritive value, palatable, attractive and at the proper temperatures. If not, cite F 364.

Compliance with 42 CFR 483.35(b), F 362, Dietary services, sufficient staff

• The facility is compliant with this requirement if they have sufficient staff to prepare and serve palatable and attractive, nutritionally adequate meals at proper temperatures. If not, cite F 362.

NOTE: If serving food is a function of the nursing service rather than dietary, refer to 42 CFR 483.30(a), F 353.

Compliance with 42 CFR 483.15(h)(1), F 252, Environment

• The facility is compliant with this requirement if they provide a homelike environment during the dining services that enhances the resident's quality of life. If not, cite F 252.

Compliance with 42 CFR 483.70(g)(1)(2)(3)(4), F 464, Dining and Resident Activities

• The facility is compliant with this requirement if they provide adequate lighting, ventilation, furnishings and space during the dining services. If not, cite F 464.

Figure 18.3 **F325 Nutrition Status**

- **F 325** (Rev. 36; Issued: 08-01-08; Effective/Implementation Date: 09-01-08)
- **§483.25(i) Nutrition** Based on a resident's comprehensive assessment, the facility must ensure that a resident--
- **§483.25(i)(1)** Maintains acceptable parameters of nutritional status, such as body weight and protein levels, unless the resident's clinical condition demonstrates that this is not possible; and
- **§483.25(i)(2)** Receives a therapeutic diet when there is a nutritional problem.

Intent: §483.25(i) Nutritional Status

The intent of this requirement is that the resident maintains, to the extent possible, acceptable parameters of nutritional status and that the facility:

- Provides nutritional care and services to each resident, consistent with the resident's comprehensive assessment;
- Recognizes, evaluates, and addresses the needs of every resident, including but not limited to, the resident at risk or already experiencing impaired nutrition; and
- Provides a therapeutic diet that takes into account the resident's clinical condition, and preferences, when there is a nutritional indication.

Definitions

Definitions are provided to clarify clinical terms related to nutritional status.

- **"Acceptable parameters of nutritional status"** refers to factors that reflect that an individual's nutritional status is adequate, relative to his/her overall condition and prognosis.
- **"Albumin"** is the body's major plasma protein, essential for maintaining osmotic pressure and also serving as a transport protein.
- **"Anemia"** refers to a condition of low hemoglobin concentration caused by decreased production, increased loss, or destruction of red blood cells.
- **"Anorexia"** refers to loss of appetite, including loss of interest in seeking and consuming food.
- **"Artificial nutrition"** refers to nutrition that is provided through routes other than the usual oral route, typically by placing a tube directly into the stomach, the intestine or a vein.
- **"Avoidable/Unavoidable"** refers to a failure to maintain acceptable parameters of nutritional status:
- **"Avoidable"** means that the resident did not maintain acceptable parameters of nutritional status and that the facility did not do one or more of the following: evaluate the resident's clinical condition and nutritional risk factors; define and implement interventions that are consistent with resident needs, resident goals and recognized standards of practice; monitor and evaluate the impact of the interventions; or revise the interventions as appropriate.

- **"Unavoidable"** means that the resident did not maintain acceptable parameters of nutritional status even though the facility had evaluated the resident's clinical condition and nutritional risk factors; defined and implemented interventions that are consistent with resident needs, goals and recognized standards of practice; monitored and evaluated the impact of the interventions; and revised the approaches as appropriate.
- **"Clinically significant"** refers to effects, results, or consequences that materially affect or are likely to affect an individual's physical, mental, or psychosocial well-being either positively by preventing, stabilizing, or improving a condition or reducing a risk, or negatively by exacerbating, causing, or contributing to a symptom, illness, or decline in status.
- **"Current standards of practice"** refers to approaches to care, procedures, techniques, treatments, etc., that are based on research or expert consensus and that are contained in current manuals, textbooks, or publications, or that are accepted, adopted or promulgated by recognized professional organizations or national accrediting bodies.
- **"Dietary supplements"** refers to nutrients (e.g., vitamins, minerals, amino acids, and herbs) that are added to a person's diet when they are missing or not consumed in enough quantity.
- **"Insidious weight loss"** refers to a gradual, unintended, progressive weight loss over time.
- **"Nutritional Supplements"** refers to products that are used to complement a resident's dietary needs (e.g., total parenteral products, enteral products, and meal replacement products).
- **"Parameters of nutritional status"** refers to factors (e.g., weight, food/fluid intake, and pertinent laboratory values) that reflect the resident's nutritional status.
- **"Qualified registered dietitan"** refers to one who is qualified based upon either registration by the Commission on Dietetic Registration of the American Dietetic Association or as permitted by state law; on the basis of education, training, or experience in identification of dietary needs, planning, and implementation of dietary programs.

(Continued)

Figure 18.3 F325 Nutrition Status *(Continued)*

- "**Therapeutic diet**" refers to a diet ordered by a health care practitioner as part of the treatment for a disease or clinical condition, to eliminate, decrease, or increase certain substances in the diet (e.g., sodium or potassium), or to provide mechanically altered food when indicated.
- "**Usual body weight**" refers to the resident's usual weight through adult life or a stable weight over time.

Overview

Nutrients are essential for many critical metabolic processes, the maintenance and repair of cells and organs, and energy to support daily functioning. Therefore, it is important to maintain adequate nutritional status, to the extent possible.

Other key factors in addition to intake can influence weight and nutritional status. For example, the body may not absorb or use nutrients effectively.

Low weight may also pertain to: age-related loss of muscle mass, strength, and function (sarcopenia), wasting (cachexia) that occurs as a consequence of illness and inflammatory processes, or disease causing changes in mental status.

Changes in the ability to taste food may accompany later life. Impaired nutritional status is not an expected part of normal aging. It may be associated with an increased risk of mortality and other negative outcomes such as impairment of anticipated wound healing, decline in function, fluid and electrolyte imbalance/dehydration, and unplanned weight change. The early identification of residents with, or at risk for, impaired nutrition, may allow the interdisciplinary team to develop and implement interventions to stabilize or improve nutritional status before additional complications arise. However, since intake is not the only factor that affects nutritional status, nutrition-related interventions only sometimes improve markers of nutritional status such as body weight and laboratory results. While they can often be stabilized or improved, nutritional deficits and imbalances may take time to improve or they may not be fully correctable in some individuals.

A systematic approach can help staff's efforts to optimize a resident's nutritional status. This process includes identifying and assessing each resident's nutritional status and risk factors, evaluating/analyzing the assessment information, developing and consistently implementing pertinent approaches, and monitoring the effectiveness of interventions and revising them as necessary.

Assessment

According to the American Dietetic Association, "Nutritional assessment is a systematic process of obtaining, verifying and interpreting data in order to make decisions about the nature and cause of nutrition-related problems."

The assessment also provides information that helps to define meaningful interventions to address any nutrition-related problems.

The interdisciplinary team clarifies nutritional issues, needs, and goals in the context of the resident's overall condition, by using observation and gathering and considering information relevant to each resident's eating and nutritional status. Pertinent sources of such information may include interview of the resident or resident representative, and review of information (e.g., past history of eating patterns and weight and a summary of any recent hospitalizations) from other sources.

The facility identifies key individuals who should participate in the assessment of nutritional status and related causes and consequences. For example:

- Nursing staff provide details about the resident's nutritional intake.
- Health care practitioners (e.g., physicians and nurse practitioners) help define the nature of the problem (e.g., whether the resident has anorexia or sarcopenia), identify causes of anorexia and weight loss, tailor interventions to the resident's specific causes and situation, and monitor the continued relevance of those interventions.
- Qualified registered dietitians help identify nutritional risk factors and recommend nutritional interventions, based on each resident's medical condition, needs, desires, and goals.
- Consultant pharmacists can help the staff and practitioners identify medications that affect nutrition by altering taste or causing dry mouth, lethargy, nausea, or confusion.

Although the Resident Assessment Instrument (RAI) is the only assessment tool specifically required, a more in-depth nutritional assessment may be needed to identify the nature and causes of impaired nutrition and nutrition-related risks. Completion of the RAI does not remove the facility's responsibility to document a more detailed resident assessment, where applicable. The in-depth nutritional assessment may utilize existing information from sources, such as the RAI, assessments from other disciplines, observation, and resident and family interviews. The assessment will identify usual body weight, a history of reduced appetite or progressive weight loss or gain prior to admission, medical conditions such as a cerebrovascular accident, and events such as recent surgery, which may have affected a resident's nutritional status and risks. The in-depth nutritional assessment may also include the following information:

- **General Appearance**—General appearance includes a description of the resident's overall appearance (e.g., robust, thin, obese, or cachectic) and other findings (e.g., level of consciousness, responsiveness, affect, oral health and dentition, ability to use the hands and arms, and the condition of hair, nails, and skin) that may affect or reflect nutritional status.

(Continued)

Figure 18.3 F325 Nutrition Status *(Continued)*

- **Height**—Measuring a resident's height provides information that is relevant (in conjunction with his or her weight) to his/her nutritional status. There are various ways to estimate height if standing height cannot be readily measured. A protocol for determining height helps to ensure that it will be measured as consistently as possible.

- **Weight**—Weight can be a useful indicator of nutritional status, when evaluated within the context of the individual's personal history and overall condition. When weighing a resident, adjustment for amputations or prostheses may be indicated. Significant unintended changes in weight (loss or gain) or insidious weight loss may indicate a nutritional problem.

Current standards of practice recommend weighing the resident on admission or readmission (to establish a baseline weight), weekly for the first 4 weeks after admission and at least monthly thereafter to help identify and document trends such as insidious weight loss. Weighing may also be pertinent if there is a significant change in condition, food intake has declined and persisted (e.g., for more than a week), or there is other evidence of altered nutritional status or fluid and electrolyte imbalance. In some cases, weight monitoring is not indicated (e.g., the individual is terminally ill and requests only comfort care).

Obtaining accurate weights for each resident may be aided by having staff follow a consistent approach to weighing and by using an appropriately calibrated and functioning scale (e.g., wheelchair scale or bed scale). Since weight varies throughout the day, a consistent process and technique (e.g., weighing the resident wearing a similar type of clothing, at approximately the same time of the day, using the same scale, either consistently wearing or not wearing orthotics or prostheses, and verifying scale accuracy) can help make weight comparisons more reliable.

A system to verify weights can help to ensure accuracy. Weights obtained in different settings may differ substantially. For example, the last weight obtained in the hospital may differ markedly from the initial weight upon admission to the facility, and is not to be used in lieu of actually weighing the resident. Approaches to improving the accuracy of weights may include reweighing the resident and recording the current weight, reviewing approaches to obtaining and verifying weight, and modifying those approaches as needed.

Examples of other factors that may impact weight and the significance of apparent weight changes include:

- The resident's usual weight through adult life;
- Current medical conditions;
- Calorie restricted diet;
- Recent changes in dietary intake; and
- Edema

Food and fluid intake—The nutritional assessment includes an estimate of calorie, nutrient and fluid needs, and whether intake is adequate to meet those needs. It also includes information such as the route (oral, enteral or parenteral) of intake, any special food formulation, meal and snack patterns (including the time of supplement or medication consumption in relation to the meals), dislikes, and preferences (including ethnic foods and form of foods such as finger foods); meal/snack patterns, and preferred portion sizes.

Fluid loss or retention can cause short term weight change. Much of a resident's daily fluid intake comes from meals; therefore, when a resident has decreased appetite, it can result in fluid/electrolyte imbalance. Abrupt weight changes, change in food intake, or altered level of consciousness are some of the clinical manifestations of fluid and electrolyte imbalance. Laboratory tests (e.g., electrolytes, BUN, creatinine and serum osmolality) can help greatly to identify, manage, and monitor fluid and electrolyte status.

Altered Nutrient intake, absorption, and utilization. Poor intake, continuing or unabated hunger, or a change in the resident's usual intake that persists for multiple meals, may indicate an underlying problem or illness. Examples of causes include:

- The inability to consume meals provided (e.g., as a result of the form or consistency of food/fluid, cognitive or functional decline, arthritis-related impaired movement, neuropathic pain, or insufficient assistance)

- Insufficient availability of food and fluid (e.g., inadequate amount of food or fluid or inadequate tube feedings);

- Environmental factors affecting food intake or appetite (e.g., comfort and level of disruption in the dining environment);

- Adverse consequences related to medications; and

- Diseases and conditions such as cancer, diabetes mellitus, advanced or uncontrolled heart or lung disease, infection and fever, liver disease, hyperthyroidism, mood disorders, and repetitive movement disorders (e.g., wandering, pacing, or rocking).

The use of diuretics and other medications may cause weight loss that is not associated with nutritional issues, but can also cause fluid and electrolyte imbalance/dehydration that causes a loss of appetite and weight. Various gastrointestinal disorders such as pancreatitis, gastritis, motility disorders, small bowel dysfunction, gall bladder disease, and liver dysfunction may affect digestion or absorption of food. Prolonged diarrhea or vomiting may increase nutritional requirements due to nutrient and fluid losses. Constipation or fecal impaction may affect appetite and excretion. Pressure ulcers and some other wounds and other health impairments may also affect nutritional requirements. A hypermetabolic state results from an increased demand for

(Continued)

Figure 18.3 **F325 Nutrition Status** *(Continued)*

energy and protein and may increase the risk of weight loss or under-nutrition. Examples of causes include advanced chronic obstructive pulmonary disease (COPD), pneumonia and other infections, cancer, hyperthyroidism, and fever.

Early identification of these factors, regardless of the presence of any associated weight changes, can help the facility choose appropriate interventions to minimize any subsequent complications.

Often, several of these factors affecting nutrition coexist:

Chewing abnormalities—Many conditions of the mouth, teeth, and gums can affect the resident's ability to chew foods. For example, oral pain, dry mouth, gingivitis, periodontal disease, ill-fitting dentures, and broken, decayed or missing teeth can impair oral intake.

Swallowing abnormalities—Various direct and indirect causes can affect the resident's ability to swallow. These include but are not limited to stroke, pain, lethargy, confusion, dry mouth, and diseases of the oropharynx and esophagus. Swallowing ability may fluctuate from day to day or over time. In some individuals, aspiration pneumonia can complicate swallowing abnormalities.

> *NOTE: Swallowing studies are not always required in order to assess eating and swallowing; however, when they are indicated, it is essential to interpret any such tests in the proper context. A clinical evaluation of swallowing may be used to evaluate average daily oral function.*

Functional ability—The ability to eat independently may be helped by addressing factors that impair function or by providing appropriate individual assistance, supervision, or assistive devices. Conditions affecting functional ability to eat and drink include impaired upper extremity motor coordination and strength or reduced range of motion (any of which may be hampered by stroke, Parkinson's disease, multiple sclerosis, tardive dyskinesia, or other neuromuscular disorders or by sensory limitations (e.g., blindness). Cognitive impairment may also affect a resident's ability to use a fork, or to eat, chew, and swallow effectively.

Medications—Medications and nutritional supplements may affect, or be affected by, the intake or utilization of nutrients (e.g., liquid phenytoin taken with tube feedings or grapefruit juice taken with some antihyperlipidemics). Medications from almost every pharmaceutical class can affect nutritional status, directly or indirectly; for example, by causing or exacerbating anorexia, lethargy, confusion, nausea, constipation, impairing taste, or altering gastrointestinal function. Inhaled or ingested medications can affect food intake by causing pharyngitis, dry mouth, esophagitis, or gastritis. To the extent possible, consid-

eration of medication/nutrient interactions and adverse consequences should be individualized.

Goals and prognosis—Goals and prognosis refer to a resident's projected personal and clinical outcomes. These are influenced by the resident's preferences (e.g., willingness to participate in weight management interventions or desire for nutritional support at end-of-life), anticipated course of a resident's overall condition and progression of a disease (e.g., end-stage, terminal, or other irreversible conditions affecting food intake, nutritional status, and weight goals), and by the resident's willingness and capacity to permit additional diagnostic testing, monitoring and treatment.

Laboratory/Diagnostic Evaluation

Laboratory tests are sometimes useful to help identify underlying causes of impaired nutrition or when the clinical assessment alone is not enough to define someone's nutritional status.

Abnormal laboratory values may, but do not necessarily, imply that treatable clinical problems exist or that interventions are needed. Confirmation is generally desirable through additional clinical evaluation and evidence such as food intake, underlying medical condition, etc. For example, serum albumin may help establish prognosis but is only sometimes helpful in identifying impaired nutrition or guiding interventions. Serum albumin may drop significantly during an acute illness for reasons unrelated to nutrition; therefore, albumin may not improve, or may fall further, despite consumption of adequate amounts of calories and protein.

The decision to order laboratory tests, and the interpretation of subsequent results, is best done in light of a resident's overall condition and prognosis.14 Before ordering laboratory tests it is appropriate for the health care practitioner to determine and indicate whether the tests would potentially change the resident's diagnosis, management, outcome or quality of life or otherwise add to what is already known. Although laboratory tests such as albumin and pre-albumin may help in some cases in deciding to initiate nutritional interventions, there is no evidence that they are useful for the serial follow-up of undernourished individuals.

> *NOTE: If laboratory tests were done prior to or after admission to the facility and the test results are abnormal, the physician or other licensed health care practitioner, in collaboration with the interdisciplinary team, reviews the information and determines whether to intervene or order additional diagnostic testing.*

(Continued)

Figure 18.3 **F325 Nutrition Status** *(Continued)*

Analysis

Analysis refers to using the information from multiple sources to include, but not limited to, the Resident Assessment Instrument (RAI), and additional nutritional assessments as indicated to determine a resident's nutritional status and develop an individualized care plan.

Resultant conclusions may include, but are not limited to: a target range for weight based on the individual's overall condition, goals, prognosis, usual body weight, etc; approximate calorie, protein, and other nutrient needs; whether and to what extent weight stabilization or improvement can be anticipated; and whether altered weight or nutritional status could be related

to an underlying medical condition (e.g., fluid and electrolyte imbalance, medication-related anorexia, or an infection). Suggested parameters for evaluating significance of unplanned and undesired weight loss are:

Interval	Significant Loss	Severe Loss
1 month	5%	Greater than 5%
3 months	7.5%	Greater than 7.5%
6 months	10%	Greater than 10%

Figure 18.4 **Noncompliance with Tag F325**

After completing the investigative protocol, the survey team must analyze the data to determine whether noncompliance with the regulation exists. Noncompliance must be established before determining severity. A clear understanding of the facility's noncompliance with requirements (i.e., deficient practices) is essential to determine how the deficient practice(s) relates to any actual harm or potential for harm to the resident.

Noncompliance with Tag F325 may include (but is not limited to) one or more of the following, including failure to:

- Accurately and consistently assess a resident's nutritional status on admission and as needed thereafter;

- Identify a resident at nutritional risk and address risk factors for impaired nutritional status, to the extent possible;

- Identify, implement, monitor, and modify interventions (as appropriate), consistent with the resident's assessed needs, choices, goals, and current standards of practice, to maintain acceptable parameters of nutritional status;

- Notify the physician as appropriate in evaluating and managing causes of the resident's nutritional risks and impaired nutritional status;

- Identify and apply relevant approaches to maintain acceptable parameters of residents' nutritional status; and

- Provide a therapeutic diet when indicated.

Potential Tags for Additional Investigation

If noncompliance with 42 CFR 483.25(i) has been identified, the survey team may have determined during the investigation of Tag F325 that concerns may also be present with related process and/or structure requirements. Examples of related process and/or structure requirements related to noncompliance with Tag F325 may include the following:

- 42 CFR 483.10, Tag F150, Resident Rights
  > Determine if the resident's preferences related to nutrition and food intake were considered.

- 42 CFR §483.20(b)(1), Tag F272, Comprehensive Assessments
  > Determine if the facility assessed the resident's nutritional status and the factors that put the resident at risk for failure to maintain acceptable parameters of nutritional status.

- 42 CFR §483.20(k), Tag F279, Comprehensive Care Plans
  > Determine if the facility developed a comprehensive care plan for each resident that includes measurable objectives, interventions/services, and time frames to meet the resident's needs as identified in the resident's assessment and provided a therapeutic diet when indicated.

- 42 CFR §483.20(k)(2)(iii), Tag F280, Comprehensive Care Plan Revision
  > Determine if the care plan was periodically reviewed and revised as necessary by qualified persons after each assessment to maintain acceptable parameters of nutritional status and provided a therapeutic diet when indicated.

- 42 CFR 483.20(k)(3)(ii), Tag F282, Provision of Care in Accordance with the Care Plan
  - Determine if the services provided or arranged by the facility were provided by qualified persons in accordance with the resident's written plan of care.

- 42 CFR 483.25(j), Tag F327, Hydration Accordance with the Care Plan
  - Determine if the facility took measures to maintain proper hydration.

- 42 CFR 483.25(k)(2), F328, Special Needs
  - Determine if the facility took measures to provide proper treatment and care for Parenteral and Enteral Fluids.

(Continued)

Figure 18.4 Noncompliance with Tag F325 *(Continued)*

- 42 CFR 483.25, Tag F329, Unnecessary Medicines
  - > Determine if food and medication interactions are impacting the residents' dietary intake.
- 42 CFR 483.30(a), Tag F353, Sufficient Staff
  - > Determine if the facility had qualified staff in sufficient numbers to provide necessary care and services, including supervision, based upon the comprehensive assessment and care plan.
- 42 CFR 483.35(a)(1)(2), F361, Dietary Services—Staffing
  - > Determine if the facility employs or consults with a qualified registered dietitan. If not employed full-time, determine if the director of food service receives scheduled consultation from the registered dietitan concerning storage, preparation, distribution and service of food under sanitary conditions.
- 42 CFR 483.35(b), F362, Standard Sufficient Staff
  - > Determine if the facility employs sufficient support personnel competent to carry out the functions of the dietary service.
- 42 CFR 483.40(a)(1)(2), Tag F385, Physician Services–Physician Supervision
  - > Determine if a physician supervised the medical aspects of care of each resident, as indicated, as they relate to medical conditions that affect appetite and nutritional status.

- 42 CFR 483.75(h)(2)(ii), Tag F500, Use of Outsider Resources
  - > If the facility does not employ a qualified Registered Dietitian, determine if the professional services of a registered dietitan are furnished by an outside resource, meet professional standards and principles, and are timely.
- 42 CFR 483.75(i)(2)(i)(ii), Tag F501, Medical Director
  - > Determine if the medical director helped develop and implement resident care policies as they relate to maintaining acceptable parameters of nutritional status and the provision of therapeutic diets when indicated.
- 42 CFR 483.75(o), Tag F520, Quality Assessment and Assurance
  - > Related concerns may have been identified that would suggest the need for a review of facility practices. Such activities may involve a review of policies, staffing and staff training, contracts, etc. and interviews with management, for example. If there is a pattern of residents who have not maintained acceptable parameters of nutritional status without adequate clinical justification, determine if quality assurance activities address the facility's approaches to nutrition and weight issues.

Note: These regulations change continually. Your facility will have the updated regulations. These are printed to give you an idea of what to expect.

There are several for-profit agencies that offer voluntary accreditation according to their established standards of care. They are not to be confused with the requirements of a state license or for the requirement to certify for federal funds. The most well known is **The Joint Commissions (TJC)**, formerly the Joint Commission on Accreditation of Healthcare Organizations (JCAHO). Originally, the Joint Commission only accredited hospitals but it has moved into other healthcare facilities such as long-term care. In the past, CMS approved the authority for the Joint Commission accreditation programs. As of July 2010, The Joint Commission's hospital accreditation program will be subject to Centers for Medicare & Medicaid (CMS) requirements for accrediting organizations. According to the Joint Commission, their mission is: To *continuously improve healthcare for the public, in collaboration with other stakeholders, by evaluating healthcare organizations and inspiring them to excel in providing safe and effective care of the highest quality and value."* The Joint Commission has established standards that each facility is measured against.

(Continued on page 403)

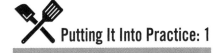

Putting It Into Practice: 1

What would be the outcome and quality indicator of an improvement plan for a client to gain one pound a week for the next month?

(Check your answer at the end of this chapter)

Figure 18.5 **Difference Between the QIS and Traditional Survey Process**

Traditional Survey Process	QIS Process
AUTOMATION	
• Survey team collects data and records the findings on paper • The computer is only used to prepare the deficiencies recorded on the CMS-2567	• Each survey team member uses a tablet PC throughout the survey process to record findings that are synthesized and organized by the QIS software
OFFSITE	
• Review OSCAR 3 AND 4 REPORT • Survey team uses QM/QIs report offsite to identify preliminary sample of residents (about 20% of facility census) and areas of concern	• Review the OSCAR 3 Report and current complaints • Download the MDS data to tablet PCs • The production-grade software (ASE-Q) selects a random sample of residents for Stage I
TOUR	
• Gather information about pre-selected residents and new concerns • Determine whether pre-selected residents are still appropriate	• No sample selection • Initial overview of facility
SAMPLE SELECTION	

• Sample size is determined by facility census.
• Residents selected based on QM/QI precentiles, and issues identified offsite and on tour
	• The production-grade software (ASE-Q) provides a randomly selected sample of residents for the following:
	  - Admission sample is a review of 30 current or discharged resident records
	  - Census sample includes 40 current residents for observation, interview, and record review.

SURVEY STRUCTURE	

• Resident sample is about 20% of facility census for resident observations, interviews, and record reviews.
  > Phase I: Focused and comprehensive reviews based on QM/QI report and issues identified from offsite information and facility tour
  > Phase II: focused record reviews
  > Facility and environmental tasks completed during the survey
	• Stage I: Preliminary investigation of regulatory areas in the admission and census samples and mandatory facility-level tasks started.
	• Stage II: Completion of in-depth investigation of triggered care areas and/or facility-level tasks based on Stage I findings.

GROUP INTERVIEW	
• Meet with Resident Group/Council • Includes resident Council minutes review to identify concerns	• Interview with Resident Council President or Representative

Source: CMS Quality Indicator Survey Demonstration Project, 2008

Figure 18.6 **Dining Observation**

DEPARTMENT OF HEALTH AND HUMAN SERVICES
CENTER FOR MEDICARE & MEDICAID SERVICES

Facility Name: _____   Facility ID: _____   Date: _____

Surveyor Name: _____

This review should concentrate primarily on determining whether necessary staff is available to assist residents and if the facility promotes a positive dining experience. Meal times and dining room locations should be identified during the entrance conference. If the facility has more than one dining area or residents are eating in their rooms, observations should occur in all of these areas. While the bulk of the information is obtained through observation, the surveyor should ask residents questions to confirm or validate observations and to assess food palatability and temperature. Surveyors should include a discussion of these observations at their team meetings. Team members not specifically assigned the responsibility of completing Dining Observation task should surveyor initiate Dining in the QIS DCT and answer only questions pertaining to observations made.

☐ Conduct a dining observation at the first full meal that occurs after the team enters the facility. The first full meal will be a meal that allows observations to occur from the start of meal service until residents have finished eating. Mark all areas of concern and follow up as needed with subsequent meal observations.

☐ Meal observations will also be conducted for Stage II sample residents who trigger because of related Quality of Care Indicators (e.g., weight loss, ADL decline, dehydration, etc.). Document these observations on the applicable resident's Critical Element Summary or Surveyor Notes Worksheet.

☐ Use this worksheet for each meal observation conducted throughout the survey. Findings on this worksheet should be entered into the QIS DCT on the Stage II—Critical Elements screen under the facility-level task, Dining.

Dining Experience	Dining Area/Room #: _____ Date: _____ Time: _____	Dining Area/Room #: _____ Date: _____ Time: _____
Frequency of Meals		
1. Are staff preparing, serving, and assisting with dining in the scheduled time frames? ☐ Yes ☐ No F353, F362		
2. Does the facility provide meals that are no greater than 14 hours between the evening meal and breakfast (or 16 hours with approval of a resident group and provision of a substantial evening snack)? ☐ Yes ☐ No F368		
If Question 1 or 2 is marked "No": Interview residents and/or staff to determine how often meals are served beyond the posted serving times.		
Assistance at Mealtime		
☐ Conduct staff interview to determine how the dining rooms and/or other locations where residents eat are monitored to assure the residents' needs are accommodated.		
3. **Do residents receive timely and appropriate assistance with meals?** ☐ Yes ☐ No F311, F312		*(Continued)*

FORM CMS-20053 (09/09)

Figure 18.6 **Dining Observation** *(Continued)*

DEPARTMENT OF HEALTH AND HUMAN SERVICES
CENTER FOR MEDICARE & MEDICAID SERVICES

Dining Experience	Dining Area/Room #: _____ Date: _____ Time: _____	Dining Area/Room #: _____ Date: _____ Time: _____
Meal Services		
Observe for proper handling techniques, such as:		
☐ Preventing the eating surfaces of plates from coming in contact with staff clothing;		
☐ Handling cups/glasses on the outside of the container; and		
☐ Handling knives, forks, and spoons by the handles.		
4. Does staff follow proper tableware handling techniques? ☐ Yes ☐ No F371		
☐ Observe whether staff used proper hygienic practices such as keeping their hands away from their hair and face when handling food.		
5. Does staff utilize hygienic practices? ☐ Yes ☐ No F371, F441		
☐ Observe whether staff had any open areas on their skin, signs of infection or other indications of illness.		
6. Are the staff who handle food products free of signs of infection? ☐ Yes ☐ No F441		
NOTE: The F tag offered in the QIS DCT is not consistent with this worksheet. If the facility is not in compliance with this question, mark the CE in the QIS DCT as "No," mark the offered Ftag (F443) as "N/A", and initiate F441.		
Dignity and Independence		
Observe whether staff:		
☐ Waited for residents at a table to finish their meal before scraping food off of plates at that table;		
☐ Talked with residents for whom they are providing assistance rather than conducting social conversations with other staff who are assisting other residents;		
☐ Are allowing residents the time needed to complete eating their meal; and		
☐ Are speaking with residents politely and respectfully.		

(Continued)

FORM CMS-20053 (09/09)

DEPARTMENT OF HEALTH AND HUMAN SERVICES
CENTER FOR MEDICARE & MEDICAID SERVICES

Figure 18.6 **Dining Observation** *(Continued)*

Dining Experience	Dining Area/Room #: _____ Date: _____ Time: _____	Dining Area/Room #: _____ Date: _____ Time: _____
7. Does staff act, or interact, with residents during meals in a manner to promote dignity? ☐ Yes ☐ No F241		
8. Are non-disposable cutlery and plates used and napkins available (e.g., plastic cutlery and paper/plastic plates are not used)? ☐ Yes ☐ No F241		
9. Are resident's desires considered when using clothing protectors? ☐ Yes ☐ No F241		
10. Are assistive devices provided as needed to promote independence? ☐ Yes ☐ No F369		
Positioning		
11. Are residents positioned to maximize eating ability (i.e., wheel chairs fit under tables so residents can access food without difficulty and resident is positioned in correct alignment)? ☐ Yes ☐ No F310		
Dining Room Atmosphere		
12. Is the lighting adequate? ☐ Yes ☐ No F464		
13. Is the ventilation adequate? ☐ Yes ☐ No F464		
14. Do noise levels promote socialization? Free of offensive odors? ☐ Yes ☐ No F253 If any one of Questions 1-15 is marked "No": ☐ Are there concerns with lighting, noise, ventilation, or furnishings that are negatively affecting the residents?		
Meal Substitutes		
16. Are meal substitutes offered when foods are refused? ☐ Yes ☐ No F366		

FORM CMS-20053 (09/09)

(Continued)

	Dining Area/Room #: _____ Date: _____ Time: _____	Dining Area/Room #: _____ Date: _____ Time: _____
Figure 18.6 Dining Observation *(Continued)*	DEPARTMENT OF HEALTH AND HUMAN SERVICES	CENTER FOR MEDICARE & MEDICAID SERVICES

Dining Experience

Furnishings and Space

Observe table height to determine if it provides the residents with easy visibility and access to food.

17. Are the dining areas adequately furnished to meet residents' physical and social needs?

☐ Yes ☐ No F464

18. Do the dining areas have sufficient space to accommodate all activities?

☐ Yes ☐ No F464

If Question 17 or 18 is marked "No":

☐ Can mobile residents enter and exit the dining room independently without staff needing to move other residents out of the way;

☐ Could residents be moved from the dining room swiftly in the event of an emergency; and

☐ Would staff be able to access and assist a resident who is experiencing an emergency, such as choking?

Food Quality

19. Does the facility serve the meals in an attractive manner (foods not combined together, variety of textures/colors)?

☐ Yes ☐ No F364

Liquids at Mealtimes

20. Does the facility provide the residents with sufficient liquids and provide assistance when needed?

☐ Yes ☐ No F327

If Question 20 is marked "No," conduct staff interview(s) for additional information to determine staff awareness of the need for maintaining adequate fluid intake:

☐ Were liquids provided?

☐ Were liquids within the resident's reach?

☐ Were the residents encouraged (or reminded) to consume liquids?

☐ When residents refuse liquids offered, does staff offer different beverages and/or foods with high fluid content (e.g., soup or broth, ice cream)?

☐ Are residents assisted with their liquids as needed (e.g., cued to drink, handed glasses, offered a variety of fluids)?

FORM CMS-20053 (09/09)

The Survey Process

Both TJC and CMS use surveys as part of their accreditation or enforcement effort. CMS and its contracted state agencies conduct on-site surveys of healthcare facilities.

As part of its enforcement effort, CMS and its contracted state agencies conduct on-site surveys of healthcare facilities. Each time a team of surveyors arrives to evaluate compliance of a healthcare facility with CMS regulations, all managers become involved. A survey is typically unannounced, and may occur on any day of the week. A standard LTC survey is designed to review compliance with CMS regulations, including all the detail of the various F-Tags.

A new survey process for long-term care was beta-tested in six states. It is called the CMS Quality Indicator Survey or QIS. National implementation of the QIS is progressing state by state as resources are available to conduct training of state and federal surveyors. The QIS process provides for the review of larger samples of clients based on the MDS, observations, interviews, and clinical record reviews. Figure 18.5 shows the differences between the QIS and the traditional survey process. This figure will help you follow the survey process whether it is traditional or the QIS.

To futher your understanding of the survey process, please review Figures 18.6 and 18.7. These are the electronic forms, including the corresponding F-Tag numbers that a surveyor who is using the QIS survey would use.

At the time of a survey, a Certified Dietary Manager may be asked to provide documentation and pertinent information. Surveyors will focus on quality indicators. They will review medical records and interview clients. Part of the survey may include a detailed tour of dietary areas. A Certified Dietary Manager should accompany a surveyor and cooperate fully. When the survey concludes, the survey team will state any deficiencies noted and reference F-Tag numbers (see Figure 18.4). A deficiency is a finding that the facility is not in compliance with CMS Guidelines. The facility is cited and instructed to correct the deficiency. Deficiencies are categorized by the level of risk/harm that may occur. If a problem is identified, the Certified Dietary Manager and other members of the interdisciplinary team need to follow up promptly and effectively to correct them. In all, a Certified Dietary Manager plays a critical role in assuring that the quality of dietary services meets the needs of clients, and that the end results of care are excellent.

Assuring Quality or Quality Assessment (QA)

Because a survey could occur at any time, a Certified Dietary Manager should always be prepared. In other words, a Certified Dietary Manager needs to manage the entire quality process from day-to-day, and assure that standards are being met. Having a quality assurance program is a critical approach to quality management. Quality assurance is a process of evaluating and verifying whether your services meet or exceed your client's expectations.

(Continued on page 417)

Figure 18.7 Stage II—Critical Elements for Nutrition, Hydration, and Tube Feeding Status

Facility Name: _____ Facility ID: _____ Date: _____

Surveyor Name: _____

Resident Name: _____ Resident ID: _____

Initial Admission Date: _____ Interviewable: ☐ Yes ☐ No Resident Room: _____

Care Area(s): _____

Use

Use this protocol for a sampled resident with the potential for, or identified with:

☐ Significant weight loss or gain;

☐ A naso-gastric/gastrostomy tube; or

☐ Hydration issues, such as not being able to reach, pour, and drink without assistance.

Procedure

☐ Briefly review the assessment, care plan, and orders to identify facility interventions and to guide observations to be made.

☐ Corroborate observations by interview and record review.

Observations

If the resident is still in the facility:

Observe whether staff consistently implement the care plan over time and across various shifts. Staff are expected to assess and provide appropriate care for residents from the day of admission. During observations of the interventions, note and/or follow up on deviations from the care plan as well as potential negative outcomes, including but not limited to the following:

☐ Observe to determine whether staff provide care in accord with the care plan. Note and follow up on negative outcomes and deviations from the care plan or accepted standards of practice. Note any signs that might indicate an altered nutritional or hydration status, such as:

- Decreased or absent urine output;

- Decreased tears, complaint of dry eyes;

- Poor oral health (including obvious dental problems);

- Dry chapped lips, tongue dryness, longitudinal tongue furrows, dryness of the mucous membranes of the mouth (resident may be mouth-breather that may mimic or contribute to dehydration);

- Gastrointestinal (GI) complications (e.g., diarrhea, vomiting, abdominal distention, constipation);

- Sunken eyes;

- Substantial muscle wasting; and

- Edema.

Notes:

FORM CMS–20075 (06/07)

DEPARTMENT OF HEALTH AND HUMAN SERVICES
CENTER FOR MEDICARE & MEDICAID SERVICES

(Continued)

Figure 18.7 Stage II—Critical Elements for Nutrition, Hydration, and Tube Feeding Status *(Continued)*

☐ In addition, note whether the resident's level of alertness and functioning permits oral intake, whether assistive devices and call bells are available for the resident who is able to use them, and whether staff provide assistance for the resident who is dependent upon staff for care. Note, for example, whether:

- The resident is resistant to assistance, refuses food or liquids, or is experiencing GI complications and how staff respond;

- The resident is receiving therapy or restorative care to improve swallowing or feeding skills, if the comprehensive assessment indicates the resident has deficits and restorative potential;

- The extent and type of assistance during and in-between meals:

    > Promotes resident dignity and maintains resident's rights (resident's appearance, staff approach to the resident); and

    > Meets the resident's needs and follows rehabilitation and restorative care schedules and instructions including the use of adaptive equipment; positioning to avoid aspiration of food (including positioning of the resident's head); fluids or tube feeding; positioning at the table; cueing or totally feeding; placement of food in the mouth; etc.

- Staff are alert to reduced food or fluid intake and the nature of the staff response, including the types of alternative approaches utilized or substitutes offered.

Notes:

For the resident with hydration concerns:

Observe to determine:

☐ Whether containers have fresh water (with or without ice according to resident preference), and a drinking glass/cup, or straw are available in the room and accessible to the resident, unless the resident is on fluid restriction or has swallowing precautions that would contradict the use of a straw (or for the dependent resident, staff offer assistance and encourage the resident to take fluids at each encounter, or on a routine basis);

☐ Whether fluids are provided at meal times and the resident is encouraged to drink them;

☐ If the resident is on fluid restrictions, how the restriction is monitored;

☐ If the resident has dysphagia, what approaches are being used to ensure adequate fluid intake; and

☐ Whether environmental issues such as exxessive heat may be contributing factors.

Notes:

DEPARTMENT OF HEALTH AND HUMAN SERVICES
CENTER FOR MEDICARE & MEDICAID SERVICES

(Continued)

Figure 18.7 **Stage II—Critical Elements for Nutrition, Hydration, and Tube Feeding Status** *(Continued)*

Observations

For the resident with issues related to maintenance of nutritional parameters:

☐ Review diet orders in the medical record on the care plan.

☐ Observe to determine whether:

- The resident receives nourishments and/or supplements, whether and to what extent the resident consumes what is offered, and whether the supplements are offered at times that minimize interference with intake at meals; and

- During the meal service, the food served was in accord with the diet and menu plan (compare what was served with the tray card and if no tray card is available, record what was served and compare with menu and recorded type of diet, beverage preference, likes, dislikes and allergies).

Notes:

For the resident who has a naso-gastric or gastrostomy tube:

☐ Review the orders for the type and amount of feeding.

☐ Observe the provision of care and services to determine whether:

- The resident displays behaviors or psychosocial consequences of tube use such as agitation, depression, self-extubation and staff approaches to address these consequences;

- Tube feeding is being administered as defined in the care plan and as ordered for flow rate, type of formula, free water, flushing, etc. (If unable to observe feeding, follow up with interview and record review);

- The insertion site is free of complications and staff provide care of the tube insertion site, in accord with standards of practice, to avoid dislodging the tube and to prevent infections and breakdown of the site;

- Staff practices for handling, hang-time and changing tube feeding bags are consistent with accepted standards of practice for infection control and manufacturer instructions;

- Staff check placement of tube, monitor and check for feeding residuals, and monitor resident's response to tube feeding;

- If medications are administered via the tube, liquids are used to flush the tubing before and after the medications (the type of liquid used to irrigate depends upon a combination of the following: physicians orders, condition of resident, facility policy/standard of practice and manufacturer's guidelines); the administration follows physician's orders and standards of practice, the medications are compatible with the tube feeding formula and the medication formulation is appropriate for administration through the tube, in accord with manufacturer's instructions (e.g., extended release tablets should not be crushed unless the goal is immediate release of the medication); and

Notes:

FORM CMS–20075 (06/07)

DEPARTMENT OF HEALTH AND HUMAN SERVICES
CENTER FOR MEDICARE & MEDICAID SERVICES

Figure 18.7 **Stage II—Critical Elements for Nutrition, Hydration, and Tube Feeding Status** *(Continued)*

• Staff verify the amount of fluid and feeding administered independent of the flow rate established on a feeding pump (if used), e.g., labeling the formula with the date and time the formula was hung and flow rate.	**Notes:**

Resident / Representative Interview

Interview the resident and/or family or responsible party (as appropriate) to determine: ☐ The level of involvement in the development of the care plan and goals, and whether the interventions reflect resident choices, preferences, portion sizes, meal or nourishment frequency, condiment requests, fluid/food restrictions, allergies and intolerances; ☐ Whether care and services are provided as written, including the type of assistance/encouragement provided at meal times (e.g., cues, hand-over-hand or extensive assistance), and at intervals to provide assistance/encouragement for fluid intake, and whether it is sufficient to meet needs; ☐ Whether necessary adaptive equipment is available for use; ☐ If the resident is on a special program for rehabilitation and restorative care, whether schedules and instructions were provided and are followed by staff; and whether supplements are offered at times that minimize interference with intake at meals; ☐ Whether the resident has demonstrated or complained of persistent fatigue, lethargy, muscle weakness or cramps, headaches, dizziness, recent nausea, vomiting, diarrhea, constipation and/or impactions, or acute illness; ☐ Whether there has been a condition change, a change in cognition (e.g., increasing and/or sudden confusion), an improvement or decline in condition, recent acute illness, weight loss or gain (including large recent weight changes or slow, insidious changes) and whether the resident is on a planned weight change program, or is in a hospice program, or is imminently at the end of life; ☐ If foods or fluids are refused, whether other interventions or substitutions were offered and whether staff provided counseling on alternatives and potential consequences of refusing food and fluid; ☐ Whether there is poor food or fluid intake because the resident "can't keep anything down," lacks an appetite or a sense of thirst, has difficulty getting to or using the bathroom, or there is a lack of staff assistance, etc.; ☐ Whether there are any concerns regarding how the food and fluids taste, the portions, variety, temperature, frequency of meals and fluids offered, etc. and if the current meal plan meets the needs of the resident; ☐ Whether the resident takes medications that may affect taste or appetite, such as chemotherapy, digoxin, or antibiotics and whether there have been changes in medications recently;	**Notes:**

DEPARTMENT OF HEALTH AND HUMAN SERVICES
CENTER FOR MEDICARE & MEDICAID SERVICES

(Continued)

Figure 18.7 **Stage II—Critical Elements for Nutrition, Hydration, and Tube Feeding Status** *(Continued)*

☐ Whether the resident is experiencing oral or other pain that might interfere with nutrient or fluid consumption and how it is managed; and

☐ Whether the resident is receiving a naso-gastric or gastrostomy tube feeding, and:
- What the facility did to maintain oral feeding prior to inserting a feeding tube (e.g., provided the appropriate level of assistance to eat and consume fluids, used assistive devices, honored preferences, etc.);
- What the facility is doing to assist the resident to regain normal eating skills, if possible, after admission with or insertion of a naso-gastric or gastrostomy tube;
- Whether the tube has been accidentally dislodged; and
- Whether the possibility of a gastrostomy tube has been discussed, if the resident has a naso-gastric tube.

Notes:

Staff Interviews

Interview staff on various shifts when concerns about hydration, nutrition, or naso-gastric or gastrostomy tube use have been identified. Interview staff to determine:

☐ How staff are monitoring the resident's food and fluid intake, including enteral feeding;

☐ Whether staff are aware of any evidence of potential nutrition or hydration deficits, e.g.,
- The resident's skin lacks its normal elasticity and sags back into position slowly when pinched up into a fold (slow retraction may also be due to loss of elasticity associated with aging);
- The resident has recent upper body muscle weakness, confusion, speech difficulty;
- The resident has a reduced sense of thirst (may be common among older adults);
- The presence of episodes of vomiting, frequent urination, hard or impacted stools and/or episodes of diarrhea, indications of acute illness such as sweating and/or fever, deep rapid breathing, or an increased heart rate; and
- Resident complaints of poor appetite or resident has poor intake of fluids.

☐ Whether staff are aware of any limitations or other factors affecting the resident's hydration or nutrition. For example:
- Difficulty getting to or using the bathroom (especially if requires staff assistance);
- Medications (e.g., diuretics);
- Limited intake of fluids due to a physician ordered restriction (ESRD); or
- Resident is imminently at the end of life.

☐ Whether staff are aware of facility-specific guidelines/protocols about what, when, and to whom to report changes in food intake.

Notes:

FORM CMS–20075 (06/07)

DEPARTMENT OF HEALTH AND HUMAN SERVICES
CENTER FOR MEDICARE & MEDICAID SERVICES

(Continued)

Figure 18.7 **Stage II—Critical Elements for Nutrition, Hydration, and Tube Feeding Status** *(Continued)*

For the resident who is being fed by a naso-gastric or gastrostomy tube:

Determine whether the nursing assistants know:	**Notes:**

☐ What, when, and to whom to report concerns with tube feedings or potential complications from tube feeding;

☐ What precautions are utilized for residents who are tube fed (e.g., positioning, protecting tube);

☐ The resident's ability to eat independently;

☐ How much assistance the resident needs with meal service;

☐ The resident's nutritional problems and risks, care plan interventions and how the resident is responding to interventions, etc.

Assessment

	Notes:

☐ Review the RAI and other documents such as history and physical; height and weight history; nutritional assessment; physician orders; progress notes; therapy notes if applicable, records of meal and fluid consumption, if available; enteral feeding consumption and/or nutritional supplements; and other progress notes or records that may have information regarding the assessment of the resident's nutrition and hydration status, underlying factors affecting the status, and whether those factors can and should be modified to improve the status. In addition, review to determine whether the rationale for the naso-gastric or gastrostomy tube was identified. Determine whether the assessment included, as appropriate:

- Baseline nutritional and hydration status indicators that include height, weight, and body mass index (BMI);

- A calculation of calorie, protein, fluid needs based on clinical condition (and calculation of free water for residents being fed by a naso-gastric or gastrostomy tube);

- Adequacy of food and fluid intake, including significant changes in the resident's overall intake in the last 90 days or since the last assessment was completed;

- Weight history, noting substantial changes or insidious weight loss/gain and identifying the etiology of the changes (e.g., fluid or obesity); use of a planned weight change program; impact of obesity/weight loss on overall health;

- New or existing conditions or diagnoses that may affect overall intake, nutrient utilization, and weight stability such as:

  > Malnutrition, dehydration, cachexia, or failure-to-thrive;

  > Decreased kidney function or urine output, renal disease;

  > Decreased thirst perception, increased thirst, change in appetite, anorexia;

  > Cognitive and/or functional impairment, e.g., dysphagia, dependency on the staff for ADLs, inability to communicate needs;

  > Terminal, irreversible or progressive conditions (e.g., incurable cancer, severe organ injury or failure, acquired immunodeficiency syndrome);

  > Constipation, impactions and/or diarrhea;

(Continued)

Figure 18.7 **Stage II—Critical Elements for Nutrition, Hydration, and Tube Feeding Status** *(Continued)*

Assessment (Continued)

> Pressure ulcers and other chronic wounds, fractures;

> COPD, pneumonia, diabetes, cancer, hepatic disease, congestive heart failure, infection, fever, nausea/vomiting, orthostatic hypotension, hypertension;

> Psychiatric disturbances, significant changes in behavior or mood; and

> Lethargy, or confusion.

- A hydration issue/deficit and lab values which may suggest dehydration (such as ratios of blood urea nitrogen to creatinine of 25 or more; or a serum sodium level greater than 148 mmol per L), efforts to address the issue (e.g., IV hydration) and the nature of the deficit:

  > Isotonic dehydration-a balanced loss of water and sodium typically resulting from a decreased intake, refusal to consume food and water, or large volume losses caused by diarrhea or vomiting;

  > Hyponatremic dehydration-a loss of more sodium than water, which has numerous etiologies, but is often due to the use of diuretics; or

  > Hypertonic dehydration-a loss of more water than sodium resulting in elevated serum sodium concentrations is often observed in residents with fever, since insensible water loss exceeds the ability to replace water through oral intake.

- The clinical indication for the use of a naso-gastric or gastrostomy tube, resident's/representative's wishes regarding tube feeding, alternatives tried prior to the insertion of the naso-gastric or gastrostomy tube, plans for removal of a tube, including the functional status of the resident and anticipated level of participation with rehabilitation to improve nutrition, hydration and restore eating skills;

- Factors contributing to or causing the resident to refuse or resist care and alternative efforts to find means to address nutrition and hydration needs;

- Purposeful restriction of fluid intake and/or not consuming all or almost all liquids provided;

- Problems with the teeth, mouth, or gums (for example, oral cavity lesions, mouth pain, decayed teeth, or poorly fitting dentures) that could affect eating; various causes of chewing and swallowing problems;

- A review of medications known to cause a drug/nutrient interaction or having side effects potentially affecting food intake or enjoyment by affecting taste or causing anorexia, increasing weight, causing diuresis, or associated with GI bleeding such as Coumadin or NSAIDs.

Notes:

FORM CMS–20075 (06/07)

DEPARTMENT OF HEALTH AND HUMAN SERVICES
CENTER FOR MEDICARE & MEDICAID SERVICES

(Continued)

Figure 18.7 Stage II—Critical Elements for Nutrition, Hydration, and Tube Feeding Status *(Continued)*

	Notes:
1. Did the facility complete a comprehensive assessment to address nutritional and hydration status and/or use of a naso-gastric or gastrostomy tube? ☐ Yes ☐ No F272 The comprehensive assessment is not required to be completed until 14 days after admission. For newly admitted residents, before the 14–day assessment is complete, the lack of sufficient assessment and care planning to meet the resident's needs should be addressed under F281 (see the Care and Services Meet Professional Standards section). NOTE: The facility may have completed a 5–day assessment for the Medicare beneficiary. Use the 5–day assessment as the comprehensive assessment only if it was completed with the RAPS.	

Care Planning

	Notes:
☐ Determine whether the facility developed a care plan that was consistent with the resident's specific conditions, risks, needs, behaviors, and preferences and current standards of practice and included measurable objectives and timetables with specific interventions/services to: • Prevent the unnecessary use of a naso-gastric or gastrostomy tube; or • Restore eating skills to allow removal of the tube, if possible; and • Prevent or address unplanned weight loss and dehydration with plans to meet the nutritional and fluid needs identified on the assessment. ☐ If the care plan refers to a specific facility treatment protocol that contains details of the treatment regimen, the care plan should refer to that protocol and should clarify any major deviations from or revisions to the protocol for this resident. The treatment protocol must be available to the caregivers and staff should be familiar with the protocol requirements. ☐ Review the care plan to determine whether the plan is based upon the goals, needs, and strengths specific to the resident and reflects the comprehensive assessment. Determine whether the care plan addresses, as appropriate: • Efforts to seek alternatives to address the needs identified in the assessment, if the resident refuses or resists staff interventions to consume foods and/or fluids; • Interventions used to assist with hydration efforts to provide fluid intake between and with meals, including alternative methods of providing fluids (gelatins, soups, broths, frozen drinks, etc.) if concern with fluid intake is identified; NOTE: In general, to determine fluid requirements, multiply the resident's body weight in kg times 30cc (2.2 lbs=1kg). (Assessment and care planning must take into consideration the clinical condition of the resident in order to prevent overhydration which could lead to congestive heart failure or death).	

Figure 18.7 **Stage II—Critical Elements for Nutrition, Hydration, and Tube Feeding Status** *(Continued)*

Care Planning (Continued)

Notes:

- Advance directives and other relevant declarations of wishes regarding aggressive nutritional support which honor the resident's wishes regarding the withholding or withdrawing of undesired interventions such as tube feeding;

- If palliative and/or end of life care is appropriate and goals are consistent with the resident's wishes, interventions to address decreased appetite and dehydration, good mouth care, preservation of resident dignity and promotion of comfort rather than specific food/fluid intake goals;

- Preventive care that promotes a specific amount of fluid intake each day to prevent dehydration rather than treat signs of dehydration when these appear;

- Methods to monitor the intake of foods and fluids daily and when to report deviations;

- The provision of hydration and/or food intake for a resident with cognitive impairment or dysphagia, minimizing aspiration risk, and providing sufficient time and assistance to consume the food and/or fluids, including the degree of staff assistance needed to meet nutritional and hydration needs;

- Interventions that honor individual food preferences and accommodate the resident's fluid restrictions, food allergies and intolerances;

- How often weights are to be monitored if weight falls out of usual body weight parameters;

- Planned weight change program, if appropriate;

- Rehabilitative/restorative interventions and specific measures to promote involvement in improving functional skills;

- Assistive devices needed for eating and drinking skills;

- If the resident is fed by a naso-gastric or gastrostomy tube, the necessary interventions to prevent complications from the tube feeding such as aspiration, dislodgment, infection, pneumonia, fluid overload, fecal impaction, diarrhea, nausea, vomiting; and

- Environmental concerns that may affect accommodating the needs of the resident, such as access to tables and equipment to allow for intake, liberal use of fans or air conditioners in hot weather, appropriate clothing and supplemental efforts to retain body heat in drafts and winter.

☐ If care plan concerns are noted, interview staff responsible for care planning as to the rationale for the current plan of care.

2. **Did the facility develop an interdisciplinary care plan that addresses the provision of care for nutritional, hydration, and/or naso-gastric or gastrostomy tube feeding needs?**

   ☐ Yes ☐ No F279

FORM CMS–20075 (06/07)

DEPARTMENT OF HEALTH AND HUMAN SERVICES
CENTER FOR MEDICARE & MEDICAID SERVICES

(Continued)

Figure 18.7 Stage II—Critical Elements for Nutrition, Hydration, and Tube Feeding Status *(Continued)*

The comprehensive care plan does not need to be completed until 7 days after the comprehensive assessment (the assessment completed with the RAPS). Lack of sufficient care planning to meet the needs of a newly admitted resident should be addressed under F281 (see the Care and Services Meet Professional Standards section). Additionally, lack of physician orders for immediate care (until staff can conduct a comprehensive assessment and develop an interdisciplinary care plan) should be addressed under F271.	**Notes:**

Care and Services Meet Professional Standards

☐ Interview health care practitioners and professionals if the interventions defined or care provided appears not to be consistent with recognized standards of practice, such as: • Observations that indicate that fluids are held to control incontinence episodes, or alternatives are not provided if resident refuses foods and/or fluids served; • Environmental conditions, such as excessive heat, which staff have not evaluated and provided the use of fans or air conditioners in hot weather, or extra fluids; or have not addressed the reduced humidity in cold winter weather; and • Care provided for residents who are at risk of complications from tube feeding, etc. ☐ **Interviews with Health Care Practitioners and Professionals:** If the interventions defined or care provided appear not to be consistent with recognized standards of practice, interview one or more health care practitioners and professionals as necessary (e.g., physician, charge nurse, director of nursing, registered dietitan) who, by virtue of training and knowledge of the resident, should be able to provide information about the causes, treatment and evaluation of the resident's condition or problem. If there is a medical question, contact the physician if he/she is the most appropriate person to interview. If the attending physician is unavailable, interview the medical director, as appropriate. Depending on the issue, ask about: • How it was determined that chosen interventions were appropriate; • Risks identified for which there were no interventions; • Changes in condition that may justify additional or different interventions; • How they validated the effectiveness of current interventions; • How they assure staff demonstrate an understanding of and comply with the facility's system for providing nutrition programs, (for example policies/procedures, staffing requirements, how facility identifies problems and implements action plans, how facility monitors and evaluates the resident's responses, etc.); and	**Notes:**

Figure 18.7 Stage II—Critical Elements for Nutrition, Hydration, and Tube Feeding Status *(Continued)*

Care and Services Meet Professional Standards (Continued)	
• Who monitors for the provision of assistance for encouraging sufficient fluid intake and during meal service, for overall consumption and response to reduced intake, for weight changes, for appropriate treatment regarding tube feedings, and for the frequency of review and evaluation. ☐ In addition, review staffing if observations indicate that meal service is rushed, residents are not properly positioned, offered fluids, or offered timely assistance; there is a lack of programs to offer food and/or fluids between scheduled meal services or residents receiving tube feedings are not provided appropriate care and services. **3. Did the facility implement practices to prevent decline in nutritional parameters, hydration, and/or complications of a naso-gastric or gastrostomy tube feeding that meet professional standards of care?** ☐ Yes ☐ No F281 NOTE: If the care plan addressed the risks and identified needs of the resident, but the care plan was not implemented as written, consider F282 for failure to implement the care plan.	**Notes:**

Care Plan Revision	
Criteria for Compliance: ☐ Determine whether the staff have been monitoring the resident's response to interventions for prevention and/or treatment, have evaluated, and revised the care plan based on the resident's response, outcomes, and needs. ☐ Review the record and interview staff for information and/or evidence that: • Continuing the current approaches meets the resident's needs, if the resident has experienced recurring nutritional or hydration deficits; and • The care plan was revised to modify the prevention strategies and to address the presence and treatment of newly identified nutritional problems. **4. Did the facility revise the care plan as needed?** ☐ Yes ☐ No F280	**Notes:**

Provision of Care and Services	
Criteria for Compliance: ☐ **Compliance with F321, Naso-gastric Tubes**—For a resident who is being fed by a naso-gastric or gastrostomy tube, the facility is in compliance with this requirement, if staff have: • Recognized, assessed, and attempted to correct (to the extent possible) factors placing the resident at risk for tube placement due to not being able to consume food and/or fluids, including specific conditions, causes and/or problems, needs and behaviors;	**Notes:** *(Continued)*

FORM CMS–20075 (06/07)

DEPARTMENT OF HEALTH AND HUMAN SERVICES
CENTER FOR MEDICARE & MEDICAID SERVICES

Figure 18.7 **Stage II—Critical Elements for Nutrition, Hydration, and Tube Feeding Status** *(Continued)*

- Defined and implemented interventions for consuming foods and/or fluids, in accordance with resident needs, goals, and recognized standards of practice;
- Monitored and evaluated the resident's response to the efforts; and
- Revised the approaches as appropriate.

If not, the use of the naso-gastric or gastrostomy tube is avoidable: cite F321.

☐ **Compliance with F322, Naso-gastric Tube**—For a resident who has a naso-gastric or gastrostomy tube, and is at risk of developing complications, and if attempts to restore normal eating skills were provided, the facility is in compliance with this requirement if staff have:

- Recognized and assessed factors placing the resident at risk of developing complications with the use of the tube, including specific conditions, causes and/or problems, needs and behaviors;
- Defined and implemented interventions for services in accordance with resident needs, goals, and recognized standards of practice;
- Addressed the potential for complications;
- Monitored and evaluated the resident's response to efforts and interventions to restore eating skills; and
- Revised the approaches as appropriate.

If not, the resident did not receive treatment and services to prevent complications from tube feeding and restore normal eating skills: cite F322.

☐ **Compliance with F325, Nutrition**—For a resident who has unplanned weight gain or loss, or other nutritional concerns, the facility is in compliance with this requirement, if staff have:

- Recognized and assessed factors placing the resident at risk, including specific conditions, causes and/or problems, needs and behaviors;
- Defined and implemented interventions in accordance with resident needs, goals, and recognized standards of practice;
- Monitored and evaluated the resident's response to the efforts; and
- Revised the approaches as appropriate.

If not, and the resident has unplanned weight loss/gain, and is not maintaining nutritional parameters: cite F325.

☐ **Compliance with F327, Hydration**—For a resident who is not consuming sufficient fluid intake to maintain proper hydration and heath, the facility is in compliance with this requirement, if staff have:

Notes:

FORM CMS–20075 (06/07)

DEPARTMENT OF HEALTH AND HUMAN SERVICES
CENTER FOR MEDICARE & MEDICAID SERVICES

(Continued)

Figure 18.7 **Stage II—Critical Elements for Nutrition, Hydration, and Tube Feeding Status** *(Continued)*

Provision of Care and Services (Continued)

- Recognized and assessed factors placing the resident at risk for dehydration due to not being able to consume fluids, including specific conditions, causes and/or problems, needs and behaviors;
- Defined and implemented interventions for the provision of fluids, in accordance with resident needs, goals, and recognized standards of practice;
- Monitored and evaluated the resident's response to the efforts; and
- Revised the approaches as appropriate.

If not, the lack of sufficient fluids to maintain or improve hydration status is avoidable: cite F327.

☐ **Compliance with F328, Parenteral and Enteral Fluids**—For a resident who is being fed by a naso-gastric or gastrostomy tube, and is receiving enteral fluids, the facility is in compliance with this requirement, if staff have:

- Assessed the type, amount, rate and volume of the formula to be provided;

- Defined and implemented interventions such as:

  > Checking for correct tube placement prior to beginning a feeding, administering medications and after episodes of vomiting or suctioning;

  > Flushing tubing as ordered;

  > Identifying staff responsibilities for the feeding such as who administers, monitors for complications and provides for corrective actions to allay complications;

  > Use equipment and formulas according to manufacturers guidelines and/or infection control policies; and

  > Provides these services in accordance with resident needs, goals, and recognized standards of practice;

- Monitored and evaluated the resident's response to the efforts; and

- Revised the approaches as appropriate.

If not, cite F328.

5. **Did the facility provide care and services to address nutritional and hydration status, prevent complications from the use of naso-gastric or gastrostomy tubes, and restore normal eating skills?**

   ☐ Yes   ☐ No

During the investigation of nutrition, hydration and naso-gastric or gastrostomy tubes, the surveyor may have identified concerns with related outcome, process and/or structure requirements. The surveyor is cautioned to investigate these related requirements before determining whether non-compliance may be present. Some examples of requirements that should be considered include the following (not all inclusive):

Notes:

FORM CMS–20075 (06/07)

DEPARTMENT OF HEALTH AND HUMAN SERVICES
CENTER FOR MEDICARE & MEDICAID SERVICES

(Continued)

Figure 18.7 Stage II—Critical Elements for Nutrition, Hydration, and Tube Feeding Status *(Continued)*

Concerns with Structure, Process, and/or Outcome Requirements Related to Process of Care

☐ **F157, Notification of Changes**—Determine whether staff notified the physician of significant changes in the resident's condition or failure of the treatment plan to prevent or address hydration, weight loss/gain, naso-gastric or gastrostomy tube services/care; or the resident's representative (if known) of significant changes in the resident's condition with these issues.

☐ **F353, Sufficient Staff**—Determine whether the facility had qualified staff in sufficient numbers to assure the resident was provided necessary care and services, based upon the comprehensive assessment and care plan, to provide food/fluids and tube feeding care.

☐ **F385, Physician Supervision**—Determine whether the physician has assessed and developed a treatment regimen relevant to tube feeding, nutritional management, or hydration issues and responded appropriately to the notice of changes in condition.

☐ **F501, Medical Director**—Determine whether the medical director:

- Assisted the facility in the development and implementation of policies and procedures for nutritional management, tube feedings, and fluid requirements, and that these are based on current standards of practice; and

- Interacts with the physician supervising the care of the resident, if requested by the facility, to intervene on behalf of the resident with nutritional and/or fluid issues.

If the surveyor determines that the facility is not in compliance with any of these related requirements, the appropriate F tag should be surveyor initiated.

FORM CMS–20075 (06/07)

DEPARTMENT OF HEALTH AND HUMAN SERVICES
CENTER FOR MEDICARE & MEDICAID SERVICES

In healthcare, there have been many names for quality assurance processes (e.g. CQI, QI, QA, PDCA, LEAN, QAPI). Today, healthcare is realizing that quality is an essential element of organizational strategy, not a single initiative. CMS calls it QAPI (Quality Assessment and Performance Improvement). Your facility probably has some type of quality initiative. Whatever your facility calls your quality initiative, it should have these characteristics:

✓ focus on clients and what they need, rather than on workers or departments and what they do.

✓ be a team approach that is cross departmental

✓ use and evaluate the data

✓ is proactive and continuous. You don't wait for a problem to occur; you continuously look at processes and ways to improve the processes.

✓ contain a performance improvement segment

Quality initiatives use some key terminology. One term is **outcome**. An outcome is the end result of work. In a healthcare environment, a health outcome

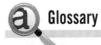 **Glossary**

Outcome
Outcome is the end result of work

Quality Indicators
Quality indicators are measures of outcomes

Figure 18.8 PDSA Worksheet for Testing Change

Aim: (overall goal you wish to achieve)

Every goal will require multiple smaller tests of change

Describe your first (or next) test of change:	Person responsible	When to be done	Where to be done

Plan:

List the tasks needed to set up this test of change	Person responsible	When to be done	Where to be done

Predict what will happen when the test is carried out	Measures to determine if prediction succeeds

Do: Describe what actually happened when you ran the test

Study: Describe the measured results and how they compared to the predictions

Act: Describe what modifications to the plan will be made for the next cycle from what you learned.

Source: Institute for Healthcare Improvement

describes the consequences of clinical interventions. For instance, if members of the healthcare team work together to improve a client's nutritional status, what happens to that client's nutritional status is the outcome of the clinical care plan. **Quality indicators (QIs)** are measures of outcomes. According to CMS, an indicator is "a key clinical value or quality characteristic used to measure, over time, the performance, processes, and outcomes of an organization or some component of healthcare delivery." As you can see by this definition, indicators are designed to facilitate collection and analysis of data. They are objective and measurable.

A general process for implementing QA in healthcare uses two acronyms: FOCUS and PDCA. FOCUS means:

F—Find a process to improve

O—Organize to improve a process

C—Clarify what is known

U—Understand variation

S—Select a process improvement

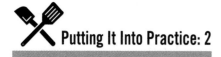

Putting It Into Practice: 2

You have just arrived at your IDT meeting with a flowchart of client weights over the past month. Besides the data, what else would you need to do to demonstrate performance improvement?

(Check your answer at the end of this chapter)

Once you have selected a process to improve, the next acronym relates to the plan itself. PDCA means:

P—Plan: Decide what you will do to improve the process. Decide what information you will collect, and how you will measure outcomes.

D—Do: Make the improvements.

C—Check: Collect and review data, and evaluate how the plan is working.

A—Act: Act on what you have learned. If you have made a successful improvement, make sure it becomes part of your policies and procedures. If not, try an alternate plan.

Quality Assessment and Performance Improvement (QAPI)

Not only are surveyors looking at what you do for quality assurance, they are also looking at how you are using the data for performance improvement. CMS has language in both the hospital and long-term care regulations that facilities must:

✓ develop, implement, and maintain an effective, ongoing, facility-wide, data-driven quality assessment and performance improvement program

✓ involve all departments and services

✓ focus on indicators related to improved health outcomes and the prevention

The Institute for Healthcare Improvement (www.ihi.org) has developed a worksheet that can help you with the Plan, Do, Check/Study, Act for performance improvement. Their tool is shown in Figure 18.8. The Medicare Quality Improvement Community (MedQIC) Website is "a free on-line resource for quality improvement interventions and associated tools, toolkits, presentations, and links to other resources." The Website is funded by CMS to provide a site to share resources based on the CMS scope of work. An example of a tool that is located there to help identify areas for improvement in your facility is shown in Figure 18.9.

A Certified Dietary Manager is involved in many quality management issues. Remember that interdisciplinary effort is a strong focus of quality management and CMS regulations. Thus, neither surveyors nor administrators divide up CMS regulations and hand a section to each manager. The Certified Dietary Manager is often the most accessible person during a survey and you need to understand the regulations, your facility's quality assessment process, and how your data supports your performance improvement.

The long-term care regulation F 325 (September 2008 revisions) requires that a therapeutic diet be provided based upon cleint needs and that client preferences and desires are honored as part of their quality of life. The F 151 requires the facility to give the client a right of refusal of any therapeutic order. The F 242 requires the facility to allow clients to make choices and self-determination. (This applies to hospital client rights as well.) You are expected to ensure that your facility is aware of the client's preferences and desires. How will the client know that he/she has a choice? Review your screening and nutrition assessment information; does it document what the client's preferences and

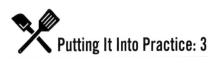

Putting It Into Practice: 3

Your facility has admitted a client on an ordered caloric restriction for diabetic control and thickened liquids for aspiration risk. The client does not want either restriction. If you were in charge, as the day-to-day Certified Dietary Manager in charge of the dining program, what steps would you expect your IDT to take?

(Check your answer at the end of this chapter)

desires are? Interview questions should be specific to inform the client that this is his/her home and the right to make choices will be honored for increased quality of life. As you can see, the Certified Dietary Manager plays a pivotal role in the lives of their clients and in each facility.

Figure 18.9 Worksheet A: Identifying Areas for Improvement

1. **Select one question (from the Facility Assessment Checklist, if applicable) to examine further.**

   Example: Does our facility routinely ask all residents upon admission/readmission if they have pain?

   Question: _____

   _____

2. **Randomly select five (or more) medical records (or other data source, depending on the question) to review. Determine a question that will be asked:**

   Example: Was this resident asked about their pain upon admission/readmission?

   Example: How many call lights were answered within X minutes?

   Question: _____

   _____

3. **Collect data:**

   • Data can help you separate what you think is happening from what is really happening.

   • Data will establish a baseline so you can measure improvement.

   • Data will help you avoid putting solutions in place that will not solve the problem.

   Record findings here:

Case #	Yes	No
1		
2		
3		
4		
5		

4. **If data is not readily available from medical records, what sources did you use to collect your data, and what steps did you take to collect this data?**

   _____

   _____

   _____

   _____

Source: Quality Partners of Rhode Island

END OF CHAPTER

 Putting It Into Practice Questions & Answers

1. What would be the outcome and quality indicator of an improvement plan for a client to gain one pound a week for the next month?

   A. *The outcome would be the client gaining weight. The quality indicator would be one pound a week for the next month.*

2. You have just arrived at your IDT meeting with a flowchart of client weights over the past month. Besides the data, what else would you need to do to demonstrate performance improvement?

   A. *Surveyors not only want to see that you are collecting and tracking data such as client weights but they also want to know how you are using that data. In your IDT, you will want to show that the team is assessing the data and perhaps looking only at those who are nutritionally at risk based on other screening results. Make sure that each team member offers their reasoned opinion based on their role in the facility. The nurse may know about diet intake, the medical director may know about diuretic intake, etc.*

3. Your facility has admitted a client on an ordered caloric restriction for diabetic control and thickened liquids for aspiration risk. The client does not want either restriction. If you were in charge, as the day-to-day Certified Dietary Manager in charge of the dining program, what steps would you expect your IDT to take?

   A. *Work with the medical director, nursing, pharmacist, speech and occupational therapists, and other IDT members to establish specific policies and procedures to honor client right of choice and right to not follow a therapeutic order. Change the wording from 'noncompliant' to client informed choices. Work with the IDT to liberalize and individualize nutrition approaches for your older adult clients, including providing education, informing of risk/benefit, offering alternatives, and monitoring outcome systems. Gather position papers and white papers on client-driven care from The Academy of Nutrition and Dietetics (formerly known as The American Dietetic Association), Medical Director's Association, Association of Nutrition & Foodservice Professionals and the CM/Pioneernetwork symposium on Creating Home II: Food and Dining for guidance. Work to document, for surveyor review, what your efforts have been on behalf of the client.*

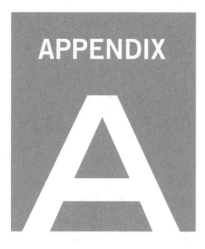

Chapter References and Resources

Chapter 1

- "The International Food Information Council Foundation's 2010 Food & Health Survey," http://www.foodinsight.org/Resources/Detail.aspx?topic=2010_Food_Health_Survey_Consumer_Attitudes_Toward_Food_Safety_Nutrition_Health

- http://fnic.nal.usda.gov/nal_display/index.php?info_center=4&tax_level=1

- http://www.vietnamesecommunity.com/Products/edu_eating.htm/

- "Cultural Diversity—Eating in America Mexican American," http://ohioline.osu.edu/hyg-fact/5000/pdf/5255.pdf

- "Cultural Diversity—Eating in America Middle Eastern," http://ohioline.osu.edu/hyg-fact/5000/pdf/5256.pdf/

- "Cultural Diversity—Eating in America Asian," http://ohioline.osu.edu/hyg-fact/5000/pdf/5253.pdf

- http://www.faqs.org/nutrition/Pre-Sma/Religion-and-Dietary-Practices.html

Chapter 2

- USDA. "Report of the Dietary Guidelines Advisory Committee on the Dietary Guidelines for Americans, 2010." http://www.cnpp.usda.gov/DGAs2010-DGACReport.htm.

- USDA. http://www.myfoodapedia.gov/Default.aspx

- USDA. "What We Eat in America." http://www.ars.usda.gov/Services/docs.htm?docid=13793

- USDA "Food and Nutrition Information Center (Food Sources of Protein)." http://www.ars.usda.gov/SP2UserFiles/Place/12354500/Data/SR22/nutrlist/sr22w203.pdf

Chapter 3

- "Development of the Dietary Guidelines—A Chronology," http://www.cnpp.usda.gov/DGAs2010-DGACReport.htm

- Reinberg, Steven, http://health.msn.com/health-topics/alzheimers-disease/articlepage.aspx?cp-documentid=100261127

- http://apjcn.nhri.org.tw/server/info/books-phds/books/foodfacts/html/data/data2b.html

- USDA Agriculture Research Service. http://www.ars.usda.gov/research/projects/projects.htm?ACCN_NO=415257

Chapter 4

- "Your Digestive System and How It Works," http://digestive.niddk.nih.gov/ddiseases/pubs/yrdd/

Chapter 5

- L.E. Spieth and coauthors, "A Low-glycemic diet in the treatment of pediatric obesity," *Archives of Pediatrics and Adolescent Medicine* 154 (2000): 947-951. http://digestive.niddk.nih.gov/ddiseases/pubs/celiac/#examples
- http://www.kidney.org/atoz/content/dietary_hemodialysis.cfm
- http://www.vcuhealth.org/upload/docs/Transplant/renal_diet.pdf
- http://www.cancer.org/cancer/cancerbasics/cancer-prevalence
- http://www.cancer.gov/cancertopics/pdq/supportivecare/nutrition/Patient
- http://www.mayoclinic.com/health/alzheimers/HQ00217/METHOD=print
- http://www.mayoclinic.com/health/alzheimers-disease/AN02036
- Retelny, Victoria, "G-Free Irony? A Food Fad That Could Be Doing More Harm Than Good," *ADA Times,* Summer 2010, pg. 1. http://www.nhlbi.nih.gov/health/dci/Diseases/Hbp/HBP_WhatIs.html http://diabetes.niddk.nih.gov/dm/pubs/diagnosis/#diagnosis

Chapter 6

- http://nccam.nih.gov/news/camstats/2007/camsurvey_fs1.htm
- http://www.ncahf.org/digest10/10-29.html
- National Health Statistics Reports, Number 12, December 10, 2008. http://www.usp.org/hqi/mmg/index.html?USP_Print
- "Environmental Nutrition," March, 2010, Volume 33, Number 3; http://ods.od.nih.gov/

Chapter 7

- http://www.eatrightnc.org/intranet/downloadManagerControl.php?mode=getFile&elementID=1818&type=5&atomID=704
- http://www.anfponline.org/Events/AMEhandouts/Litchford_NutritionCareProcess.ppt
- "MNT Provider," *American Dietetic Association*, Volume 9, Number 4, August 2010.
- Handy, Linda and Thomsen, Barbara, "Minimum Data Set (MDS) 3.0 as part of new Resident Assessment Instrument (RAI)," ANFP Webinar, August 5, 2010.
- MDS 3.0 RAI Manual and Training Materials. http://www.aahsa.org/MDS3.0_RaiManual
- "MNT Provider," *American Dietetic Association*, Volume 9, Number 3, July 2010.
- http://www.cms.gov/NursingHomeQualityInits/45_NHQIMDS30TrainingMaterials.asp#TopOfPage
- http://www.anfponline.org/CE/nutrition_connection/2008_winter.shtml
- http://www.ucop.edu/ucophome/coordrev/policy/legal-medical-record-policy.pdf

Chapter 8

- http://www.diethistory.com/registration.asp
- http://westone.wa.gov.au/toolbox7/health/shared/resources/cd/communication.htm#cp
- Froschheiser, Lee, "Communication", *Dietary Manager Magazine*, October, 2008, pgs.23-26.
- http://riskfactor.cancer.gov/DHQ/dietcalc/
- http://www.youtube.com/user/CMSHHSgov?feature=mhum#p/u/7/Ereawm4_F7k

Chapter 9

- http://www.dietitians.ca/seniors/pdf/nutrition_screening_eng.pdf
- http://www.epi.umn.edu/let/pubs/img/adol_ch4.pdf
- http://www2.fiu.edu/~nutreldr/SubjectList/N/Nutrition_Screening_Assessment.htm
- http://www.ncbi.nlm.nih.gov/pmc/articles/PMC1694757/pdf/amjph00531-0046.pdf
- https://www.diet.com/store/facts/aging-and-nutrition
- http://pods.dasnr.okstate.edu/docushare/dsweb/Get/Document-2458/T-3120web.pdf
- http://www.ext.colostate.edu/pubs/foodnut/09361.html

Chapter 10

- http://www.fda.gov/Food/LabelingNutrition/ConsumerInformation/ucm078889.htm

Chapter 11

- Department of Health and Human Services, Administration on Aging. "Elder Rights and Resources: Long Term Care Ombudsman Program." Available at www.aoa.gov/eldfam/Elder_Rights/LTC/LTC_pf.asp
- http://www.RD411.com

Chapter 12

- http://www.juiceproducts.org/100juice_in_school.html
- http://www.foodinsight.org/For-Consumers/Healthy-Aging.aspx
- Gregoire, Mary & Spears, Marian, "Foodservice Organizations-A Managerial and Systems Approach," Pearson/Prentice Hall, 2006, pgs. 53-79.

Chapter 13

- http://journal.diabetes.org/diabetesspectrum/00v13n3/pg149f.htm
- http://www.beckydorner.com/uploads/HypertensionCEU-1016.pdf
- Dorner, Becky, et al, "Position of the American Dietetic Association: Individualized Nutrition Approaches for Older Adults in Health Care Communities," *Journal of the American Dietetic Association*, October 2010. pgs. 1549 – 1553.

Chapter 14

- http://people.uncw.edu/gray/curric/sum2000/370L-%20Nursing-Care-Plan.htm
- http://www.dhs.wisconsin.gov/rl_dsl/Publications/care2000.pdf

Chapter 15

- American Dietetic Association, <u>International Dietetics & Nutrition Terminology Reference Manual, Third Edition, 2011</u>, pgs. 279-283.
- Richardson, Brenda E., MA, RD, LD, CD, & American Dietetic Association, "Practitioner Pocket Guide for MDS 3.0 and Nutrition," 2010 DHCC, pgs. 34, 36-50.

Chapter 16

- http://ezinearticles.com/?Culture-Change-and-Dining-Innovations-in-Long-Term-Care&id=1080421
- Handy, Linda, MS,RD, "Culture Change in Dining and Regulator Compliance," *Dietary Manager Magazine*, June 2010, pgs. 14-19.
- http://www.calculturechange.org/services-dining.html

Chapter 17

- "Key Milestones in CMS Programs," http://www.cms.gov/History/Downloads/CMSProgramKeyMilestones.pdf
- Becky Dorner & Associates, Inc. Akron, Ohio, www.beckydorner.com
- "Working with Diverse Cultures" Ohio State University Extension, http://extension.usu.edu/diversity/files/uploads/factsheet704.pdf
- Metcalf, T. (1997) "Listening to your clients," *Life Association News*, 92(7) pgs. 16 - 18. http://www.stfrancis.edu/ba/ghkickul/stu

Chapter 18

- http://cms.gov/manuals/Downloads/som107ap_p_ltcf.pdf
- Handy, Linda, MS, RD, "Surveyor M.O. For Nutritional Status (F 325) Training Manual," www.handydietaryconsulting.com, 2009.
- Handy, Linda, MS, RD, "Deficiency Free in Nutrition Status," *Dietary Manager Magazine*, September, 2008, pgs. 10-15.
- http://cms.gov/manuals/Downloads/som107ap_pp_guidelines_ltcf.pdf
- http://www.mcg.edu/som/fmfacdev/fd_quality.htm
- http://www.aging.state.ks.us/Manuals/QIS/TabIndex.html

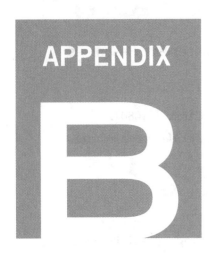

APPENDIX

B Dietary Reference Intakes

Dietary Reference Intakes (DRIs): Recommended Dietary Allowances and Adequate Intakes, Vitamins

Food and Nutrition Board, Institute of Medicine, National Academies

Vitamin A (µg/d)[a]	Vitamin C (mg/d)	Vitamin D (µg/d)[b,c]	Vitamin E (mg/d)[d]	Vitamin K (µg/d)	Thiamin (mg/d)	Riboflavin (mg/d)	Niacin (mg/d)[e]	Vitamin B6 (mg/d)	Folate (µg/d)[f]	Vitamin B12 (µg/d)	Pantothenic Acid (mg/d)	Biotin (µg/d)	Choline (mg/d)[g]
INFANTS													
0 to 6 months													
400*	40*	10	4*	2.0*	0.2*	0.3*	2*	0.1*	65*	0.4*	1.7*	5*	125*
6 to 12 months													
500*	50*	10	5*	2.5*	0.3*	0.4*	4*	0.3*	80*	0.5*	1.8*	6*	150*
CHILDREN													
1 to 3 years													
300	15	15	6	30*	0.5	0.5	6	0.5	150	0.9	2*	8*	200*
4 to 8 years													
400	25	15	7	55*	0.6	0.6	8	0.6	200	1.2	3*	12*	250*
MALES													
9 to 13 years													
600	45	15	11	60*	0.9	0.9	12	1.0	300	1.8	4*	20*	375*
14 to 18 years													
900	75	15	15	75*	1.2	1.3	16	1.3	400	2.4	5*	25*	550*
19 to 30 years													
900	90	15	15	120*	1.2	1.3	16	1.3	400	2.4	5*	30*	550*
31 to 50 years													
900	90	15	15	120*	1.2	1.3	16	1.3	400	2.4	5*	30*	550*
51 to 70 years													
900	90	15	15	120*	1.2	1.3	16	1.7	400	2.4[h]	5*	30*	550*
> 70 years													
900	90	20	15	120*	1.2	1.3	16	1.7	400	2.4[h]	5*	30*	550*
FEMALES													
9 to 13 years													
600	45	15	11	60*	0.9	0.9	12	1.0	300	1.8	4*	20*	375*
14 to 18 years													
700	65	15	15	75*	1.0	1.0	14	1.2	400[i]	2.4	5*	25*	400*
19 to 30 years													
700	75	15	15	90*	1.1	1.1	14	1.3	400[i]	2.4	5*	30*	425*
31 to 50 years													
700	75	15	15	90*	1.1	1.1	14	1.3	400[i]	2.4	5*	30*	425*
51 to 70 years													
700	75	15	15	90*	1.1	1.1	14	1.5	400	2.4[h]	5*	30*	425*
> 70 years													
700	75	20	15	90*	1.1	1.1	14	1.5	400	2.4[h]	5*	30*	425*

(Continued)

Dietary Reference Intakes (DRIs): Recommended Dietary Allowances and Adequate Intakes, Vitamins *(Continued)*

Vitamin A (μg/d)[a]	Vitamin C (mg/d)	Vitamin D (μg/d)[b,c]	Vitamin E (mg/d)[d]	Vitamin K (μg/d)	Thiamin (mg/d)	Riboflavin (mg/d)	Niacin (mg/d)[e]	Vitamin B6 (mg/d)	Folate (μg/d)[f]	Vitamin B12 (μg/d)	Pantothenic Acid (mg/d)	Biotin (μg/d)	Choline (mg/d)[g]
PREGNANCY													
14 to 18 years													
750	**80**	**15**	**15**	75*	**1.4**	**1.4**	**18**	**1.9**	**600**[j]	**2.6**	6*	30*	450*
19 to 30 years													
770	**85**	**15**	**15**	90*	**1.4**	**1.4**	**18**	**1.9**	**600**[j]	**2.6**	6*	30*	450*
31 to 50 years													
770	**85**	**15**	**15**	90*	**1.4**	**1.4**	**18**	**1.9**	**600**[j]	**2.6**	6*	30*	450*
LACTATION													
14 to 18 years													
1,200	**115**	**15**	**19**	75*	**1.4**	**1.6**	**17**	**2.0**	**500**	**2.8**	7*	35*	550*
19 to 30 years													
1,300	**120**	**15**	**19**	90*	**1.4**	**1.6**	**17**	**2.0**	**500**	**2.8**	7*	35*	550*
31 to 50 years													
1,300	**120**	**15**	**19**	90*	**1.4**	**1.6**	**17**	**2.0**	**500**	**2.8**	7*	35*	550*

NOTE: This table (taken from the DRI reports, see www.nap.edu) presents Recommended Dietary Allowances (RDAs) in **bold type** and Adequate Intakes (AIs) in ordinary type followed by an asterisk (*). An RDA is the average daily dietary intake level; sufficient to meet the nutrient requirements of nearly all (97-98 percent) healthy individuals in a group. It is calculated from an Estimated Average Requirement (EAR). If sufficient scientific evidence is not available to establish an EAR, and thus calculate an RDA, an AI is usually developed. For healthy breastfed infants, an AI is the mean intake. The AI for other life stage and gender groups is believed to cover the needs of all healthy individuals in the groups, but lack of data or uncertainty in the data prevent being able to specify with confidence the percentage of individuals covered by this intake.

a   As retinol activity equivalents (RAEs). 1 RAE = 1 μg retinol, 12 μg ß-carotene, 24 μg a-carotene, or 24 μg ß-cryptoxanthin. The RAE for dietary provitamin A carotenoids is two-fold greater than retinol equivalents (RE), whereas the RAE for preformed vitamin A is the same as RE.

b   As cholecalciferol. 1 μg cholecalciferol = 40 IU vitamin D.

c   Under the assumption of minimal sunlight.

d   As a-tocopherol includes RRR a-tocopherol, the only form of a-tocopherol that occurs naturally in foods, and the 2R-stereoisomeric forms of a-tocopherol (RRR-, RSR-, RRS-, and *RSS-a*-tocopherol) that occur in fortified foods and supplements. It does not include the 2S-stereoisomeric forms of a-tocopherol (SRR-, SSR-, SRS-, and SSS a-tocopherol), also found in fortified foods and supplements.

e   As niacin equivalents (NE). 1 mg of niacin = 60 mg of tryptophan; 0–6 months = preformed niacin (not NE).

f   As dietary folate equivalents (DFE). 1 DFE = 1 μg food folate = 0.6 μg of folic acid from fortified food or as a supplement consumed with food = 0.5 μg of a supplement taken on an empty stomach.

g   Although AIs have been set for choline, there are few data to assess whether a dietary supply of choline is needed at all stages of the life cycle, and it may be that the choline requirement can be met by endogenous synthesis at some of these stages.

h   Because 10 to 30 percent of older people may malabsorb food-bound B12, it is advisable for those older than 50 years to meet their RDA mainly by consuming foods fortified with B12 or a supplement containing B12.

i   In view of evidence linking folate intake with neural tube defects in the fetus, it is recommended that all women capable of becoming pregnant consume 400 μg from supplements or fortified foods in addition to intake of food folate from a varied diet.

j   It is assumed that women will continue consuming 400 μg from supplements or fortified food until their pregnancy is confirmed and they enter prenatal care, which ordinarily occurs after the end of the periconceptional period—the critical time for formation of the neural tube.

SOURCES: *Dietary Reference Intakes for Calcium, Phosphorous, Magnesium, Vitamin D, and Fluoride (1997); Dietary Reference Intakes for Thiamin, Riboflavin, Niacin, Vitamin B6, Folate, Vitamin B12, Pantothenic Acid, Biotin, and Choline* (1998); *Dietary Reference Intakes for Vitamin C, Vitamin E, Selenium, and Carotenoids* (2000); *Dietary Reference Intakes for Vitamin A, Vitamin K, Arsenic, Boron, Chromium, Copper, Iodine, Iron, Manganese, Molybdenum, Nickel, Silicon, Vanadium, and Zinc* (2001); *Dietary Reference Intakes for Water, Potassium, Sodium, Chloride, and Sulfate* (2005); and *Dietary Reference Intakes for Calcium and Vitamin D* (2011).These reports may be accessed via www.nap.edu.

Dietary Reference Intakes (DRIs): Tolerable Upper Intake Levels, Vitamins

Food and Nutrition Board, Institute of Medicine, National Academies

Vitamin A (µg/d)[a]	Vitamin C (mg/d)	Vitamin D (µg/d)	Vitamin E (mg/d)[b,c]	Vitamin K	Thiamin	Riboflavin	Niacin (mg/d)[c]	Vitamin B6 (mg/d)	Folate (µg/d)[c]	Vitamin B12	Pantothen- ic Acid	Biotin	Choline (g/d)	Carot- enoids[d]
INFANTS														
0 to 6 months														
600	ND[e]	25	ND	ND	ND	ND	ND	ND	ND	ND	ND	ND	ND	ND
6 to 12 months														
600	ND	38	ND	ND	ND	ND	ND	ND	ND	ND	ND	ND	ND	ND
CHILDREN														
1 to 3 years														
600	400	63	200	ND	ND	ND	10	30	300	ND	ND	ND	1.0	ND
4 to 8 years														
900	650	75	300	ND	ND	ND	15	40	400	ND	ND	ND	1.0	ND
MALES														
9 to 13 years														
1,700	1,200	100	600	ND	ND	ND	20	60	600	ND	ND	ND	2.0	ND
14 to 18 years														
2,800	1,800	100	800	ND	ND	ND	30	80	800	ND	ND	ND	3.0	ND
19 to 30 years														
3,000	2,000	100	1,000	ND	ND	ND	35	100	1,000	ND	ND	ND	3.5	ND
31 to 50 years														
3,000	2,000	100	1,000	ND	ND	ND	35	100	1,000	ND	ND	ND	3.5	ND
51 to 70 years														
3,000	2,000	100	1,000	ND	ND	ND	35	100	1,000	ND	ND	ND	3.5	ND
> 70 years														
3,000	2,000	100	1,000	ND	ND	ND	35	100	1,000	ND	ND	ND	3.5	ND
FEMALES														
9 to 13 years														
1,700	1,200	100	600	ND	ND	ND	20	60	600	ND	ND	ND	2.0	ND
14 to 18 years														
2,800	1,800	100	800	ND	ND	ND	30	80	800	ND	ND	ND	3.0	ND
19 to 30 years														
3,000	2,000	100	1,000	ND	ND	ND	35	100	1,000	ND	ND	ND	3.5	ND
31 to 50 years														
3,000	2,000	100	1,000	ND	ND	ND	35	100	1,000	ND	ND	ND	3.5	ND
51 to 70 years														
3,000	2,000	100	1,000	ND	ND	ND	35	100	1,000	ND	ND	ND	3.5	ND
> 70 years														
3,000	2,000	100	1,000	ND	ND	ND	35	100	1,000	ND	ND	ND	3.5	ND

(Continued)

Dietary Reference Intakes (DRIs): Tolerable Upper Intake Levels, Vitamins *(Continued)*

Vitamin A (µg/d)[a]	Vitamin C (mg/d)	Vitamin D (µg/d)	Vitamin E (mg/d)[b,c]	Vitamin K	Thiamin	Riboflavin	Niacin (mg/d)[c]	Vitamin B6 (mg/d)	Folate (µg/d)[c]	Vitamin B12	Pantothen-ic Acid	Biotin	Choline (g/d)	Carot-enoids[d]
PREGNANCY														
14 to 18 years														
2,800	1,800	100	800	ND	ND	ND	30	80	800	ND	ND	ND	3.0	ND
19 to 30 years														
3,000	2,000	100	1,000	ND	ND	ND	35	100	1,000	ND	ND	ND	3.5	ND
31 to 50 years														
3,000	2,000	100	1,000	ND	ND	ND	35	100	1,000	ND	ND	ND	3.5	ND
LACTATION														
14 to 18 years														
2,800	1,800	100	800	ND	ND	ND	30	80	800	ND	ND	ND	3.0	ND
19 to 30 years														
3,000	2,000	100	1,000	ND	ND	ND	35	100	1,000	ND	ND	ND	3.5	ND
31 to 50 years														
3,000	2,000	100	1,000	ND	ND	ND	35	100	1,000	ND	ND	ND	3.5	ND

NOTE: A Tolerable Upper Intake Level (UL) is the highest level of daily nutrient intake that is likely to pose no risk of adverse health effects to almost all individuals in the general population. Unless otherwise specified, the UL represents total intake from food, water, and supplements. Due to a lack of suitable data, ULs could not be established for vitamin K, thiamin, riboflavin, vitamin B12, pantothenic acid, biotin, and carotenoids. In the absence of a UL, extra caution may be warranted in consuming levels above recommended intakes. Members of the general population should be advised not to routinely exceed the UL. The UL is not meant to apply to individuals who are treated with the nutrient under medical supervision or to individuals with predisposing conditions that modify their sensitivity to the nutrient.

a As preformed vitamin A only.

b As *a*-tocopherol; applies to any form of supplemental *a*-tocopherol.

c The ULs for vitamin E, niacin, and folate apply to synthetic forms obtained from supplements, fortified foods, or a combination of the two.

d ß-Carotene supplements are advised only to serve as a provitamin A source for individuals at risk of vitamin A deficiency.

e ND = Not determinable due to lack of data of adverse effects in this age group and concern with regard to lack of ability to handle excess amounts. Source of intake should be from food only to prevent high levels of intake.

SOURCES: *Dietary Reference Intakes for Calcium, Phosphorous, Magnesium, Vitamin D, and Fluoride* (1997); *Dietary Reference Intakes for Thiamin, Riboflavin, Niacin, Vitamin B6, Folate, Vitamin B12, Pantothenic Acid, Biotin, and Choline* (1998); *Dietary Reference Intakes for Vitamin C, Vitamin E, Selenium, and Carotenoids* (2000); *Dietary Reference Intakes for Vitamin A, Vitamin K, Arsenic, Boron, Chromium, Copper, Iodine, Iron, Manganese, Molybdenum, Nickel, Silicon, Vanadium, and Zinc* (2001); and *Dietary Reference Intakes for Calcium and Vitamin D* (2011). These reports may be accessed via www.nap.edu.

Dietary Reference Intakes (DRIs): Tolerable Upper Intake Levels, Elements

Food and Nutrition Board, Institute of Medicine, National Academies

	Arsenic[a]	Boron (mg/d)	Calcium (mg/d)	Chromium	Copper (µg/d)	Fluoride (mg/d)	Iodine (µg/d)	Iron (mg/d)	Magnesium (mg/d)[b]	Manganese (mg/d)	Molybdenum (µg/d)	Nickel (mg/d)	Phosphorus (g/d)	Selenium (µg/d)	Silicon[c]	Vanadium (mg/d)[d]	Zinc (mg/d)	Sodium (g/d)	Chloride (g/d)
INFANTS																			
0 to 6 months	ND[e]	ND	1,000	ND	ND	0.7	ND	40	ND	ND	ND	ND	ND	45	ND	ND	4	ND	ND
6 to 12 months	ND	ND	1,500	ND	ND	0.9	ND	40	ND	ND	ND	ND	ND	60	ND	ND	5	ND	ND
CHILDREN																			
1 to 3 years	ND	3	2,500	ND	1,000	1.3	200	40	65	2	300	0.2	3	90	ND	ND	7	1.5	2.3
4 to 8 years	ND	6	2,500	ND	3,000	2.2	300	40	110	3	600	0.3	3	150	ND	ND	12	1.9	2.9
MALES																			
9 to 13 years	ND	11	3,000	ND	5,000	10	600	40	350	6	1,100	0.6	4	280	ND	ND	23	2.2	3.4
14 to 18 years	ND	17	3,000	ND	8,000	10	900	45	350	9	1,700	1.0	4	400	ND	ND	34	2.3	3.6
19 to 30 years	ND	20	2,500	ND	10,000	10	1,100	45	350	11	2,000	1.0	4	400	ND	1.8	40	2.3	3.6
31 to 50 years	ND	20	2,500	ND	10,000	10	1,100	45	350	11	2,000	1.0	4	400	ND	1.8	40	2.3	3.6
51 to 70 years	ND	20	2,000	ND	10,000	10	1,100	45	350	11	2,000	1.0	4	400	ND	1.8	40	2.3	3.6
> 70 years	ND	20	2,000	ND	10,000	10	1,100	45	350	11	2,000	1.0	3	400	ND	1.8	40	2.3	3.6
FEMALES																			
9 to 13 years	ND	11	3,000	ND	5,000	10	600	40	350	6	1,100	0.6	4	280	ND	ND	23	2.2	3.4
14 to 18 years	ND	17	3,000	ND	8,000	10	900	45	350	9	1,700	1.0	4	400	ND	ND	34	2.3	3.6
19 to 30 years	ND	20	2,500	ND	10,000	10	1,100	45	350	11	2,000	1.0	4	400	ND	1.8	40	2.3	3.6
31 to 50 years	ND	20	2,500	ND	10,000	10	1,100	45	350	11	2,000	1.0	4	400	ND	1.8	40	2.3	3.6
51 to 70 years	ND	20	2,000	ND	10,000	10	1,100	45	350	11	2,000	1.0	4	400	ND	1.8	40	2.3	3.6
> 70 years	ND	20	2,000	ND	10,000	10	1,100	45	350	11	2,000	1.0	3	400	ND	1.8	40	2.3	3.6

(Continued)

Dietary Reference Intakes (DRIs): Tolerable Upper Intake Levels, Elements *(Continued)*

Arsenic[a]	Boron (mg/d)	Calcium (mg/d)	Chro-mium	Copper (µg/d)	Fluoride (mg/d)	Iodine (µg/d)	Iron (mg/d)	Magne-sium (mg/d)[a]	Manga-nese (mg/d)	Molyb-denum (µg/d)	Nickel (mg/d)	Phos-phorus (g/d)	Sele-nium (µg/d)	Silicon[c]	Vana-dium (mg/d)[d]	Zinc (mg/d)	Sodium (g/d)	Chloride (g/d)
PREGNANCY																		
14 to 18 years																		
ND	17	3,000	ND	8,000	10	900	45	350	9	1,700	1.0	3.5	400	ND	ND	34	2.3	3.6
19 to 30 years																		
ND	20	2,500	ND	10,000	10	1,100	45	350	11	2,000	1.0	3.5	400	ND	ND	40	2.3	3.6
61 to 50 years																		
ND	20	2,500	ND	10,000	10	1,100	45	350	11	2,000	1.0	3.5	400	ND	ND	40	2.3	3.6
LACTATION																		
14 to 18 years																		
ND	17	3,000	ND	8,000	10	900	45	350	9	1,700	1.0	4	400	ND	ND	34	2.3	3.6
19 to 30 years																		
ND	20	2,500	ND	10,000	10	1,100	45	350	11	2,000	1.0	4	400	ND	ND	40	2.3	3.6
31 to 50 years																		
ND	20	2,500	ND	10,000	10	1,100	45	350	11	2,000	1.0	4	400	ND	ND	40	2.3	3.6

NOTE: A Tolerable Upper Intake Level (UL) is the highest level of daily nutrient intake that is likely to pose no risk of adverse health effects to almost all individuals in the general population. Unless otherwise specified, the UL represents total intake from food, water, and supplements. Due to a lack of suitable data, ULs could not be established for vitamin K, thiamin, riboflavin, vitamin B12, pantothenic acid, biotin, and carotenoids. In the absence of a UL, extra caution may be warranted in consuming levels above recommended intakes. Members of the general population should be advised not to routinely exceed the UL. The UL is not meant to apply to individuals who are treated with the nutrient under medical supervision or to individuals with predisposing conditions that modify their sensitivity to the nutrient.

a   Although the UL was not determined for arsenic, there is no justification for adding arsenic to food or supplements.

b   The ULs for magnesium represent intake from a pharmacological agent only and do not include intake from food and water.

c   Although silicon has not been shown to cause adverse effects in humans, there is no justification for adding silicon to supplements.

d   Although vanadium in food has not been shown to cause adverse effects in humans, there is no justification for adding vanadium to food and vanadium supplements should be used with caution. The UL is based on adverse effects in laboratory animals and this data could be used to set a UL for adults but not children and adolescents.

e   ND = Not determinable due to lack of data of adverse effects in this age group and concern with regard to lack of ability to handle excess amounts. Source of intake should be from food only to prevent high levels of intake.

SOURCES: *Dietary Reference Intakes for Calcium, Phosphorous, Magnesium, Vitamin D, and Fluoride* (1997); *Dietary Reference Intakes for Thiamin, Riboflavin, Niacin, Vitamin B6, Folate, Vitamin B12, Pantothenic Acid, Biotin, and Choline* (1998); *Dietary Reference Intakes for Vitamin C, Vitamin E, Selenium, and Carotenoids* (2000); *Dietary Reference Intakes for Vitamin A, Vitamin K, Arsenic, Boron, Chromium, Copper, Iodine, Iron, Manganese, Molybdenum, Nickel, Silicon, Vanadium, and Zinc* (2001); *Dietary Reference Intakes for Water, Potassium, Sodium, Chloride, and Sulfate* (2005); and *Dietary Reference Intakes for Calcium and Vitamin D* (2011). These reports may be accessed via www.nap.edu.

Dietary Reference Intakes (DRIs): Recommended Dietary Allowances and Adequate Intakes, Elements

Food and Nutrition Board, Institute of Medicine, National Academies

Calcium (mg/d)	Chromium (µg/d)	Copper (µg/d)	Fluoride (mg/d)	Iodine (µg/d)	Iron (mg/d)	Magnesium (mg/d)	Manganese (mg/d)	Molybdenum (µg/d)	Phosphorus (mg/d)	Selenium (µg/d)	Zinc (mg/d)	Potassium (g/d)	Sodium (g/d)[g]	Chloride (g/d)
INFANTS														
0 to 6 months														
200*	0.2*	200*	0.01*	110*	0.27*	30*	0.003*	2*	100*	15*	2*	0.4*	0.12*	0.18*
6 to 12 months														
260*	5.5*	220*	0.5*	130*	11*	75*	0.6*	3*	275*	20*	3	0.7*	0.37*	0.57*
CHILDREN														
1 to 3 years														
700	11*	340	0.7*	90	7	80	1.2*	17	460	20	3	3.0*	1.0*	1.5*
4 to 8 years														
1,000	15*	440	1*	90	10	130	1.5*	22	500	30	5	3.8*	1.2*	1.9*
MALES														
9 to 13 years														
1,300	25*	700	2*	120	8	240	1.9*	34	1,250	40	8	4.5*	1.5*	2.3*
14 to 18 years														
1,300	35*	890	3*	150	11	410	2.2*	43	1,250	55	11	4.7*	1.5*	2.3*
19 to 30 years														
1,000	35*	900	4*	150	8	400	2.3*	45	700	55	11	4.7*	1.5*	2.3*
31 to 50 years														
1,000	35*	900	4*	150	8	420	2.3*	45	700	55	11	4.7*	1.5*	2.3*
51 to 70 years														
1,000	30*	900	4*	150	8	420	2.3*	45	700	55	11	4.7*	1.3*	2.0*
> 70 years														
1,200	30*	900	4*	150	8	420	2.3*	45	700	55	11	4.7*	1.2*	1.8*
FEMALES														
9 to 13 years														
1,300	21*	700	2*	120	8	240	1.6*	34	1,250	40	8	4.5*	1.5*	2.3*
14 to 18 years														
1,300	24*	890	3*	150	15	360	1.6*	43	1,250	55	9	4.7*	1.5*	2.3*
19 to 30 years														
1,000	25*	900	3*	150	18	310	1.8*	45	700	55	8	4.7*	1.5*	2.3*
31 to 50 years														
1,000	25*	900	3*	150	18	320	1.8*	45	700	55	8	4.7*	1.5*	2.3*
51 to 70 years														
1,200	20*	900	3*	150	8	320	1.8*	45	700	55	8	4.7*	1.3*	2.0*
> 70 years														
1,200	20*	900	3*	150	8	320	1.8*	45	700	55	8	4.7*	1.2*	1.8*
PREGNANCY														
14 to 18 years														
1,300	29*	1,000	3*	220	27	400	2.0*	50	1,250	60	12	4.7*	1.5*	2.3*
19 to 30 years														
1,000	30*	1,000	3*	220	27	350	2.0*	50	700	60	11	4.7*	1.5*	2.3*
31 to 50 years														
1,000	30*	1,000	3*	220	27	360	2.0*	50	70	60	11	4.7*	1.5*	2.3*

(Continued)

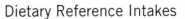
Dietary Reference Intakes (DRIs): Recommended Dietary Allowances and Adequate Intakes, Elements *(continued)*

Calcium (mg/d)	Chromium (µg/d)	Copper (µg/d)	Fluoride (mg/d)	Iodine (µg/d)	Iron (mg/d)	Magnesium (mg/d)	Manganese (mg/d)	Moly-bdenum (µg/d)	Phos-phorus (mg/d)	Selenium (µg/d)	Zinc (mg/d)	Potassium (mg/d)	Sodium (mg/d)ᵍ	Chloride (g/d)
LACTATION														
14 to 18 years														
1,300	44*	**1,300**	3*	**290**	**10**	**360**	2.6*	**50**	**1,250**	**70**	**13**	5.1*	1.5*	2.3*
19-30 years														
1,000	45*	**1,300**	3*	**290**	**9**	**310**	2.6*	**50**	**700**	**70**	**12**	5.1*	1.5*	2.3*
31-50 years														
1,000	45*	**1,300**	3*	**290**	**9**	**320**	2.6*	**50**	**700**	**70**	**12**	5.1*	1.5*	2.3*

NOTE: This table (taken from the DRI reports, see www.nap.edu) presents Recommended Dietary Allowances (RDAs) in **bold type** and Adequate Intakes (AIs) in ordinary type followed by an asterisk (*). An RDA is the average daily dietary intake level; sufficient to meet the nutrient requirements of nearly all (97-98 percent) healthy individuals in a group. It is calculated from an Estimated Average Requirement (EAR). If sufficient scientific evidence is not available to establish an EAR, and thus calculate an RDA, an AI is usually developed. For healthy breastfed infants, an AI is the mean intake. The AI for other life stage and gender groups is believed to cover the needs of all healthy individuals in the groups, but lack of data or uncertainty in the data prevent being able to specify with confidence the percentage of individuals covered by this intake.

SOURCES: *Dietary Reference Intakes for Calcium, Phosphorous, Magnesium, Vitamin D, and Fluoride* (1997); *Dietary Reference Intakes for Thiamin, Riboflavin, Niacin, Vitamin B6, Folate, Vitamin B12, Pantothenic Acid, Biotin, and Choline* (1998); *Dietary Reference Intakes for Vitamin C, Vitamin E, Selenium, and Carotenoids* (2000); *Dietary Reference Intakes for Vitamin A, Vitamin K, Arsenic, Boron, Chromium, Copper, Iodine, Iron, Manganese, Molybdenum, Nickel, Silicon, Vanadium, and Zinc* (2001); *Dietary Reference Intakes for Water, Potassium, Sodium, Chloride, and Sulfate* (2005); and *Dietary Reference Intakes for Calcium and Vitamin D* (2011). These reports may be accessed via www.nap.edu.

Dietary Reference Intakes: Macronutrients

Nutrient	Function	Life Stage Group	RDA/AI* g/d	AMDR[a]	Selected Food Sources	Adverse Effects of Excessive Consumption
Carbohy-drate— Total Digestible	RDA based on its role as the primary energy source for the brain; AMDR based on its role as a source of kilocalories to maintain body weight	**Infants** 0–6 mo 7–12 mo	60* 95*	ND[b] ND	Starch and sugar are the major types of carbohydrates. Grains and vegetables (corn, pasta, rice, pota- toes, breads) are sources of starch. Natural sugars are found in fruits and juices. Sources of added sugars are soft drinks, candy, fruit drinks, and desserts.	While no defined intake level at which potential adverse effects of total digestible carbohydrate was identified, the up- per end of the adequate macronutrient distribu- tion range (AMDR) was based on decreasing risk of chronic disease and providing adequate intake of other nutri- ents. It is suggested that the maximal intake of added sugars be limited to providing no more than 25 percent of energy.
		Children 1–3 y 4–8 y	**130** **130**	45-65 45-65		
		Males 9–13 y 14–18 y 19–30 y 31-50 y 50-70 y > 70 y	**130** **130** **130** **130** **130** **130**	45-65 45-65 45-65 45-65 45-65 45-65		
		Females 9–13 y 14–18 y 19–30 y 31-50 y 50-70 y > 70 y	**130** **130** **130** **130** **130** **130**	45-65 45-65 45-65 45-65 45-65 45-65		
		Pregnancy ≤ 18 y 19-30 y 31-50 y	**175** **175**	45-65 45-65 45-65		
		Lactation ≤ 18 y 19-30 y 31–50 y	**210** **210** **210**	45-65 45-65 45-65		
Total Fiber	Improves laxation, reduces risk of coronary heart disease, assists in maintaining normal blood glucose levels	**Infants** 0–6 mo 7–12 mo	ND ND		Includes dietary fiber naturally pres- ent in grains (such as found in oats, wheat, or unmilled rice) and functional fiber synthesized or isolated from plants or animals and shown to be of benefit to health.	Dietary fiber can have variable compositions and therefore it is dif- ficult to link a specific source of fiber with a particular adverse effect, especially when phytate is also present in the natural fiber source. It is concluded that as part of an overall healthy diet, a high intake of dietary fiber will not produce deleterious effects in healthy individu- als. While occasional adverse gastrointestinal symptoms are observed when consuming some isolated or synthetic fibers, serious chronic adverse effects have not been observed. Due to the bulky nature of fibers, excess consump- tion is likely to be self-limiting. Therefore, a UL was not set for individual functional fibers.
		Children 1–3 y 4–8 y	19* 25*			
		Males 9–13 y 14–18 y 19–30 y 31-50 y 50-70 y > 70 y	31* 38* 38* 38* 30* 30*			
		Females 9–13 y 14–18 y 19–30 y 31-50 y 50-70 y > 70 y	26* 26* 25* 25* 21* 21*			
		Pregnancy ≤ 18 y 19-30 y 31-50 y	28* 28* 28*			
		Lactation ≤ 18 y 19-30 y 31–50 y	29* 29* 29*			

NOTE: The table is adapted from the DRI reports, see www. nap.edu. It represents Recommended Dietary Allowances (RDAs) in **bold type**, Adequate Intakes (AIs) in ordinary type followed by an asterisk (*). RDAs and AIs may both be used as goals for individual intake. RDAs are set to meet the needs of almost all (97 to 98 percent) individuals in a group. For healthy breastfed infants, the AI is the mean intake. The AI for other life stage and gender groups is believed to cover the needs of all individuals in the group, but lack of data prevent being able to specify with confi- dence the percentage of individuals covered by this intake.

a Acceptable Macronutrient Distribution Range (AMDR)[a] is the range of intake for a particular energy source that is associated with reduced risk of chronic disease while providing intakes of essential nutrients. If an individual consumes in excess of the AMDR, there is a potential of increasing the risk of chronic diseases and/or insufficient intakes of essential nutrients.

b ND = Not determinable due to lack of data of adverse effects in.

SOURCE: *Dietary Reference Intakes for Energy, Carbo- hydrate. Fiber, Fat, Fatty Acids, Cholesterol, Protein, and Amino Acids* (2002/2005). This report may be accessed via www.nap.edu

(Continued)

Dietary Reference Intakes: Macronutrients *(Continued)*

Nutrient	Function	Life Stage Group	RDA/AI* g/d	AMDRᵃ	Selected Food Sources	Adverse Effects of Excessive Consumption
Total Fat	Energy source and when found in foods, is a source of *n*-6 and *n*-3 polyunsaturated fatty acids. Its presence in the diet increases absorption of fat soluble vitamins and precursors such as vitamin A and pro-vitamin A carotenoids.	**Infants** 0–6 mo 7–12 mo	31* 30*		Butter, margarine, vegetable oils, whole milk, visible fat on meat and poultry products, invisible fat in fish, shellfish, some plant products such as seeds and nuts, and bakery products.	While no defined intake level at which potential adverse effects of total fat was identified, the upper end of AMDR is based on decreasing risk of chronic disease and providing adequate intake of other nutrients. The lower end of the AMDR is based on concerns related to the increase in plasma triacylglycerol concentrations and decreased HDL cholesterol concentrations seen with very low fat (and thus high carbohydrate) diets.
		Children 1–3 y 4–8 y		30-40 25-35		
		Males 9–13 y 14–18 y 19–30 y 31-50 y 50-70 y > 70 y		25-35 25-35 20-35 20-35 20-35 20-35		
		Females 9–13 y 14–18 y 19–30 y 31-50 y 50-70 y > 70 y		25-35 25-35 20-35 20-35 20-35 20-35		
		Pregnancy ≤ 18 y 19-30 y 31-50 y		20-35 20-35 20-35		
		Lactation ≤ 18 y 19-30 y 31–50 y		20-35 20-35 20-35		
n-6 polyunsaturated fatty acids (linoleic acid)	Essential component of structural membrane lipids, involved with cell signaling, and precursor of eicosanoids. Required for normal skin function.	**Infants** 0–6 mo 7–12 mo	4.4* 4.6*	NDᵇ ND	Nuts, seeds, and vegetable oils such as soybean, safflower, and corn oil.	While no defined intake level at which potential adverse effects of *n*-6 polyunsaturated fatty acids was identified, the upper end of the AMDR is based the lack of evidence that demonstrates long-term safety and human in vitro studies which show increased free-radical formation and lipid peroxidation with higher amounts of *n*-6 fatty acids. Lipid peroxidation is thought to be a component of in the development of atherosclerotic plaques.
		Children 1–3 y 4–8 y	7* 10*	5-10 5-10		
		Males 9–13 y 14–18 y 19–30 y 31-50 y 50-70 y > 70 y	12* 16* 17* 17* 14* 14*	5-10 5-10 5-10 5-10 5-10 5-10		
		Females 9–13 y 14–18 y 19–30 y 31-50 y 50-70 y > 70 y	10* 11* 12* 12* 11* 11*	5-10 5-10 5-10 5-10 5-10 5-10		
		Pregnancy ≤ 18 y 19-30 y 31-50 y	13* 13* 13*	5-10 5-10 5-10		
		Lactation ≤ 18 y 19-30 y 31–50 y	13* 13* 13*	5-10 5-10 5-10		

NOTE: The table is adapted from the DRI reports, see www.nap.edu. It represents Recommended Dietary Allowances (RDAs) in **bold type**, Adequate Intakes (AIs) in ordinary type followed by an asterisk (*). RDAs and AIs may both be used as goals for individual intake. RDAs are set to meet the needs of almost all (97 to 98 percent) individuals in a group. For healthy breastfed infants, the AI is the mean intake. The AI for other life stage and gender groups is believed to cover the needs of all individuals in the group, but lack of data prevent being able to specify with confidence the percentage of individuals covered by this intake.

a   Acceptable Macronutrient Distribution Range (AMDR)ᵃ is the range of intake for a particular energy source that is associated with reduced risk of chronic disease while providing intakes of essential nutrients. If an individuals consumed in excess of the AMDR, there is a potential of increasing the risk of chronic diseases and insufficient intakes of essential nutrients.

b   ND = Not determinable due to lack of data of adverse effects in this age group and concern with regard to lack of ability to handle excess amounts. Source of intake should be from food only to prevent high levels of intake.

SOURCE: *Dietary Reference Intakes for Energy, Carbohydrate, Fiber, Fat, Fatty Acids, Cholesterol, Protein, and Amino Acids* (2002/2005). This report may be accessed via www.nap.edu

Dietary Reference Intakes: Macronutrients *(Continued)*

Nutrient	Function	Life Stage Group	RDA/AI* g/d	AMDR[a]	Selected Food Sources	Adverse Effects of Excessive Consumption
n-3 polyun-saturated fatty acids (*a*-linolenic acid)	Involved with neurological development and growth. Precursor of eicosanoids.	**Infants** 0–6 mo 7–12 mo	0.5* 0.5*	ND[b] ND	Vegetable oils such as soybean, canola, and flax seed oil, fish oils, fatty fish, with smaller amounts in meats and eggs.	While no defined intake level at which potential adverse effects of *n*-3 polyunsaturated fatty acids was identified, the upper end of AMDR is based on maintaining the appropriate balance with n-6 fatty acids and on the lack of evidence that demonstrates long-term safety, along with human in vitro studies which show increased free-radical formation and lipid peroxidation with higher amounts of polyunsaturated fatty acids. Lipid peroxida-tion is thought to be a component of in the development of athero-sclerotic plaques.
		Children 1–3 y 4–8 y	0.7* 0.9*	0.6-1.2 0.6-1.2		
		Males 9–13 y 14–18 y 19–30 y 31-50 y 50-70 y > 70 y	1.2* 1.6* 1.6* 1.6* 1.6* 1.6*	0.6-1.2 0.6-1.2 0.6-1.2 0.6-1.2 0.6-1.2 0.6-1.2		
		Females 9–13 y 14–18 y 19–30 y 31-50 y 50-70 y > 70 y	1.0* 1.1* 1.1* 1.1* 1.1* 1.1*	0.6-1.2 0.6-1.2 0.6-1.2 0.6-1.2 0.6-1.2 0.6-1.2		
		Pregnancy ≤ 18 y 19-30 y 31-50 y	1.4* 1.4* 1.4*	0.6-1.2 0.6-1.2 0.6-1.2		
		Lactation ≤ 18 y 19-30 y 31—50 y	1.3* 1.3* 1.3*	0.6-1.2 0.6-1.2 0.6-1.2		
Saturated and *trans* fatty acids, and choles-terol	No required role for these nutrients other than as energy sources was identified; the body can syn-thesize its needs for saturated fatty acids and cholesterol from other sources.	**Infants** 0–6 mo 7–12 mo	ND ND		Saturated fatty acids are present in animal fats (meat fats and butter fat), and coconut and palm kernel oils. Sources of cholesterol include liver, eggs, and foods that contain eggs such as cheesecake and custard pies. Sources of *trans* fatty acids include stick margarines and foods containing hydroge-nated or partially-hy-drogenated vegetable shortenings.	There is an incremental increase in plasma total and low-density lipoprotein cholesterol concentrations with increased intake of saturated or *trans* fatty acids or with cholesterol at even very low levels in the diet. Therefore, the intakes of each should be minimized while consuming a nutritionally adequate diet.
		Children 1–3 y 4–8 y				
		Males 9–13 y 14–18 y 19–30 y 31-50 y 50-70 y > 70 y				
		Females 9–13 y 14–18 y 19–30 y 31-50 y 50-70 y > 70 y				
		Pregnancy ≤ 18 y 19-30 y 31-50 y				
		Lactation ≤ 18 y 19-30 y 31—50 y				

NOTE: The table is adapted from the DRI reports, see www. nap.edu. It represents Recommended Dietary Allowances (RDAs) in **bold type**, Adequate Intakes (AIs) in ordinary type followed by an asterisk (*). RDAs and AIs may both be used as goals for individual intake. RDAs are set to meet the needs of almost all (97 to 98 percent) individuals in a group. For healthy breastfed infants, the AI is the mean intake. The AI for other life stage and gender groups is believed to cover the needs of all individuals in the group, but lack of data prevent being able to specify with confi-dence the percentage of individuals covered by this intake.

a Acceptable Macronutrient Distribution Range (AMDR)[a] is the range of intake for a particular energy source that is associated with reduced risk of chronic disease while providing intakes of essential nutrients. If an individuals consumed in excess of the AMDR, there is a potential of increasing the risk of chronic diseases and insufficient intakes of essential nutrients.

b ND = Not determinable due to lack of data of adverse effects in.

SOURCE: *Dietary Reference Intakes for Energy, Carbo-hydrate. Fiber, Fat, Fatty Acids, Cholesterol, Protein, and Amino Acids* (2002/2005). This report may be accessed via www.nap.edu

(Continued)

Dietary Reference Intakes: Macronutrients *(Continued)*

Nutrient	Function	Life Stage Group	RDA/AI[a] g/d	AMDR[b]	Selected Food Sources	Adverse Effects of Excessive Consumption
Protein and Amino Acids	Serves as the major structural component of all cells in the body, and functions as enzymes, in membranes, as transport carriers, and as some hormones. During digestion and absorption dietary proteins are broken down to amino acids, which become the building blocks of these structural and functional compounds. Nine of the amino acids must be provided in the diet; these are termed indispensable amino acids. The body can make the other amino acids needed to synthesize specific structures from other amino acids.	**Infants** 0–6 mo 7–12 mo	9.1* **11.0**	ND[c] ND	Proteins from animal sources, such as meat, poultry, fish, eggs, milk, cheese, and yogurt, provide all nine indispensable amino acids in adequate amounts, and for this reason are considered "complete proteins". Proteins from plants, legumes, grains, nuts, seeds, and vegetables tend to be deficient in one or more of the indispensable amino acids and are called 'incomplete proteins'. Vegan diets adequate in total protein content can be "complete" by combining sources of incomplete proteins which lack different indispensable amino acids.	While no defined intake level at which potential adverse effects of protein was identified, the upper end of AMDR based on complementing the AMDR for carbohydrate and fat for the various age groups. The lower end of the AMDR is set at approximately the RDA.
		Children 1–3 y 4–8 y	13 19	5-20 10-30		
		Males 9–13 y 14–18 y 19–30 y 31-50 y 50-70 y > 70 y	34 52 56 56 56 56	10-30 10-35 10-35 10-35 10-35 10-35		
		Females 9–13 y 14–18 y 19–30 y 31-50 y 50-70 y > 70 y	34 46 46 46 46 46	10-30 10-30 10-35 10-35 10-35 10-35		
		Pregnancy ≤ 18 y 19-30 y 31-50 y	71 71 71	10-35 10-35 10-35		
		Lactation ≤ 18 y 19-30 y 31−50 y	71 71 71	10-35 10-35 10-35		

NOTE: The table is adapted from the DRI reports, see www. nap.edu. It represents Recommended Dietary Allowances (RDAs) in **bold type**, Adequate intakes (Als) in ordinary type followed by an asterisk (*). RDAs and Als may both be used as goals for individual intake. RDIs are set to meet the needs of almost all (97 to 98 percent) individuals in a group. For healthy breastfed infants, the AI is the mean intake. The AI for other life stage and gender groups is believed to cover the needs of all individuals in the group, but lack of data prevent being able to specify with confidence the percentage of individuals covered by this intake.

a   Based on 1.5 g/kg/day for infants, 1.1 g/kg/day for 1-3 y, 0.95 g/kg/day for 4-13y, 0.85 g/kg/day for 14-18y, 0.8 g/kg/day for adults, and 1.1 g/kg/day for pregnant (using pre-pregnancy weight) and lactating women.

b   Acceptable Macronutrient Distribution Range (AMDR)* is the range of intake for a particular energy source that is associated with reduced risk of chornic disease while providing intakes of essential nutrients. If an individual consumed in excess of the AMDR, there is a potential of increasing the risk of chronic diseases and insufficient intakes of essential nutrients.

c   ND=Not determinable due to lack of data of adverse effects in this age group and concern with regard to lack of ability to handle excess amounts. Source of intake should be from food only to prevent high levels of intake.

SOURCE: *Dietary Reference Intakes for Energy, Carbohydrate, Fiber, Fat, Fatty Acids, Cholesterol, Protein, and Amino Acids (2002/2005).* This report may be accessed via www.nap.edu

Nutrient	Function	IOM/FNB 2002 Scoring Pattern[a]	Mg/g Protein	Adverse Effects of Excessive Consumption
Indispensable Amino Acids: Histidine Isoleucine Leucine Lysine Methionine & Cysteine Phenylalanine & Tyrosine Threonine Tryptophan Valine	The building blocks of all proteins in the body and some hormones. These nine amino acids must be provided in the diet and thus are termed indispensable amino acids. The body can make the other amino acids needed to synthesize specific structures from other amino acids and carbohydrate precursors.	Histidine	18	Since there is no evidence that amino acids found in usual or even high intakes of protein from food present any risk, attention was focused on intakes of the L-form of these and other amino acid found in dietary protein and amino acid supplements. Even from well-studied amino acids, adequate dose-response data from human or animal studies on which to base a UL were not available. While no defined intake level at which potential adverse effects of protein was identified for any amino acid, this does not mean that there is no potential for adverse effects resulting from high intakes of amino acids from dietary supplements. Since data on the adverse effects of high levels of amino acid intakes from dietary supplements are limited, caution may be warranted.
		Isoleucine	25	
		Leucine	55	
		Lysine	51	
		Methionine & Cysteine	25	
		Phenylalanine & Tyrosine	47	
		Threonine	27	
		Tryptophan	7	
		Valine	32	

NOTE: The table is adapted from the DRI reports, see www. nap.edu

a   Based on the amino acid requirements derived for Preschool Children (1-3 y): (EAR for amino acid ÷ EAR for protein); for 1-3 y group where EAR for protein = 0.88 g/kg/d.

SOURCE: *Dietary Reference Intakes for Energy, Carbohydrate. Fiber, Fat, Fatty Acids, Cholesterol, Protein, and Amino Acids (2002/2005).* This report may be accessed via www.nap.edu

Dietary Reference Intakes: Electrolytes and Water

Nutrient	Function	Life Stage Group	AI	UL[a]	Selected Food Sources	Adverse Effects of Excessive Consumption	Special Considerations
Sodium	Maintains fluid volume outside of cells and thus normal cell function.	**Infants** 0–6 mo 7–12 mo	(g/d) 0.12 0.37	(g/d) ND[b] ND[b]	Processed foods to which sodium chloride (salt)/ benzoate/phosphate have been added; salted meats, nuts, cold cuts; margarine; butter; salt added to foods in cooking or at the table. Salt is ~ 40% sodium by weight.	Hypertension; increased risk of cardiovascular disease and stroke.	The AI is set based on being able to obtain a nutritionally adequate diet for other nutrients and to meet the needs for sweat losses for individuals engaged in recommended levels of physical activity. Individuals engaged in activity at higher levels or in humid climates resulting in excessive sweat may need more than the AI. The UL applies to apparently healthy individuals without hypertension; it thus may be too high for individuals who already have hypertension or who are under the care of a health care professional.
		Children 1–3 y 4–8 y	1.0 1.2	1.5 1.9			
		Males 9–13 y 14–18 y 19–30 y 31–50 y 50-70 y > 70 y	1.5 1.5 1.5 1.5 1.3 1.2	2.2 2.3 2.3 2.3 2.3 2.3			
		Females 9–13 y 14–18 y 19–30 y 31–50 y 50-70 y > 70 y	1.5 1.5 1.5 1.5 1.3 1.2	2.2 2.3 2.3 2.3 2.3 2.3			
		Pregnancy 14-18 y 19-50 y	1.5 1.5	2.3 2.3			
		Lactation 14-18 y 19-50 y	1.5 1.5	2.3 2.3			
Chloride	With sodium, maintains fluid volume outside of cells and thus normal cell function.	**Infants** 0–6 mo 7–12 mo	(g/d) 0.18 0.57	(g/d) ND[b] ND[b]	See above; about 60% by weight of salt.	In concert with sodium, results in hypertension.	Chloride is lost usually with sodium in sweat, as well as in vomiting and diarrhea. The AI and UL are equi-molar in amount to sodium since most of sodium in diet comes as sodium chloride (salt).
		Children 1–3 y 4–8 y	1.5 1.9	2.3 2.9			
		Males 9–13 y 14–18 y 19–30 y 31–50 y 50-70 y > 70 y	2.3 2.3 2.3 2.3 2.0 1.8	3.4 3.6 3.6 3.6 3.6 3.6			
		Females 9–13 y 14–18 y 19–30 y 31–50 y 50-70 y > 70 y	2.3 2.3 2.3 2.3 2.0 1.8	3.4 3.6 3.6 3.6 3.6 3.6			
		Pregnancy 14-18 y 19-50 y	2.3 2.3	3.6 3.6			
		Lactation 14-18 y 19-50 y	2.3 2.3	3.6 3.6			

(Continued)

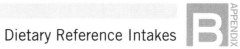

Dietary Reference Intakes: Electrolytes and Water *(Continued)*

Nutrient	Function	Life Stage Group	AI	UL[a]	Selected Food Sources	Adverse Effects of Excessive Consumption	Special Considerations
Potassium	Maintains fluid volume inside/outside of cells and thus normal cell function; acts to blunt the rise of blood pressure in response to excess sodium intake, and decrease markers of bone turnover and recurrence of kidney stones.	**Infants** 0–6 mo 7–12 mo	(g/d) 0.4 0.7	No UL.	Fruits and vegetables; dried peas; dairy products; meats, and nuts.	None documented from food alone; however, potassium from supplements or salt substitutes can result in hyperkalemia and possibly sudden death if excess is consumed by individuals with chronic renal insufficiency (kidney disease) or diabetes.	Individuals taking drugs for cardiovascular disease such as ACE inhibitors, ARBs (Angiontensin Receptor Blockers), or potassium sparing diuretics should be careful to not consume supplements containing potassium and may need to consume less than the AI for potassium.
		Children 1–3 y 4–8 y	 3.0 3.8				
		Males 9–13 y 14–18 y 19–30 y 31-50 y 50-70 y > 70 y	 4.5 4.7 4.7 4.7 4.7 4.7				
		Females 9–13 y 14–18 y 19–30 y 31-50 y 50-70 y > 70 y	 4.5 4.7 4.7 4.7 4.7 4.7				
		Pregnancy 14-18 y 19-50 y	 4.7 4.7				
		Lactation 14-18 y 19-50 y	 5.1 5.1				
Water	Maintains homeostasis in the body and allows for transport of nutrients to cells and removal and excretion of waste products of metabolism.	**Infants** 0–6 mo 7–12 mo	(L/d) 0.7 0.8		All beverages, including water, as well as moisture in foods (high moisture foods include watermelon, meats, soups, etc.).	No UL because normally functioning kidneys can handle more than 0.7 L (24 oz) of fluid per hour; symptoms of water intoxication include hyponatremia which can result in heart failure and rhabdomyolosis (skeletal muscle tissue injury) which can lead to kidney failure.	Recommended intakes for water are based on median intakes of generally healthy individuals who are adequately hydrated; individuals can be adequately hydrated at levels below as well as above the AIs provided. The AIs provided are for total water in temperate climates. All sources can contribute to total water needs: beverages (including tea, coffee, juices, sodas, and drinking water) and moisture found in foods. Moisture in food accounts for about 20% of total water intake. Thirst and consumption of beverages at meals are adequate to maintain hydration.
		Children 1–3 y 4–8 y	 1.3 1.7				
		Males 9–13 y 14–18 y 19–30 y 31-50 y 50-70 y > 70 y	 2.4 3.3 3.7 3.7 3.7 3.7				
		Females 9–13 y 14–18 y 19–30 y 31-50 y 50-70 y > 70 y	 2.1 2.3 2.7 2.7 2.7 2.7				
		Pregnancy 14-18 y 19-50 y	 3.0 3.0				
		Lactation 14-18 y 19-50 y	 3.8 3.8				

Dietary Reference Intakes: Electrolytes and Water *(Continued)*

Nutrient	Function	Life Stage Group	AI	UL[a]	Selected Food Sources	Adverse Effects of Excessive Consumption	Special Considerations
Inorganic Sulfate	Required for biosynthesis of 3'- phosphoadenosine-5'-phosphate (PAPS), which provides sulfate when sulfur-containing compounds are needed such as chondroitin sulfate and cerebroside sulfate.	**Infants** 0–6 mo 7–12 mo **Children** 1–3 y 4–8 y **Males** 9–13 y 14–18 y 19–30 y 31-50 y 50-70 y > 70 y **Females** 9–13 y 14–18 y 19–30 y 31-50 y 50-70 y > 70 y **Pregnancy** 14-18 y 19-50 y **Lactation** 14-18 y 19-50 y	No recommended intake was set as adequate sulfate is available from dietary inorganic sulfate from water and foods, and from sources of organic sulfate such as glutathione and the sulfur amino acids methionine and cysteine. Metabolic breakdown of the recommended intake for protein and sulfur amino acids should provide adequate inorganic sulfate for synthesis of required sulfur-containing compounds.	No UL.	Dried fruit (dates, raisins, dried apples), soy flour, fruit juices, coconut milk, red and white wine, bread, as well as meats that are high in sulfur amino acids.	Osmotic diarrhea was observed in areas where water supply had high levels; odor and off taste usually limit intake, and thus no UL was set.	

NOTE: The table is adapted from the DRI reports. See www.nap.edu. Adequate Intakes (AIs) may be used as a goal for individual intake. For healthy breastfed infants, the AI is the mean intake. The AI for other life stage and gender groups is believed to cover the needs of all individuals in the group, but lack of data prevent being able to specify with confidence the percentage of individuals covered by this intake; therefore, no Recommended Dietary Allowance (RDA) was set.

a   UL = The maximum level of daily nutrient intake that is likely to pose no risk of adverse effects. Unless otherwise specified, the UL represents total intake from food, water, and supplements. Due to lack of suitable data, ULs could not be established for potassium, water, and inorganic sulfate. In the absence of ULs, extra caution may be warranted in consuming levels above recommended intakes.

b   ND = Not determinable due to lack of data of adverse effects in this age group and concern with regard to lack of ability to handle excess amounts. Source of intake should be from food only to prevent high levels of intake.

SOURCE: *Dietary Reference Intakes for Water, Potassium, Sodium, Chloride, and Sulfate.* This report may be accessed via www.nap.edu

Dietary Reference Intakes (DRIs): Recommended Dietary Allowances and Adequate Intakes, Total Water and Macronutrients

Food and Nutrition Board, Institute of Medicine, National Academies

Life Stage Group	*Total* Water[a] (L/d)	Carbohydrate (g/d)	Total Fiber (g/d)	Fat (g/d)	Linoleic Acid (g/d)	*a*-Linolenic Acid (g/d)	Protein[b] (g/d)
INFANTS							
0 to 6 months	0.7*	60*	ND	31*	4.4*	0.5*	9.1*
6 to 12 months	0.8*	95*	ND	30*	4.6*	0.5*	**11.0**
CHILDREN							
1 to 3 yrs.	1.3*	**130**	19*	ND[c]	7*	0.7*	**13**
4 to 8 yrs.	1.7*	**130**	25*	ND	10*	0.9*	**19**
MALES							
9 to 13 years	2.4*	**130**	31*	ND	12*	1.2*	**34**
14 to 18 years	3.3*	**130**	38*	ND	16*	1.6*	**52**
19 to 30 years	3.7*	**130**	38*	ND	17*	1.6*	**56**
31 to 50 years	3.7*	**130**	38*	ND	17*	1.6*	**56**
51 to 70 years	3.7*	**130**	30*	ND	14*	1.6*	**56**
> 70 years	3.7*	**130**	30*	ND	14*	1.6*	**56**
FEMALES							
9 to 13 years	2.1*	**130**	26*	ND	10*	1.0*	**34**
14 to 18 years	2.3*	**130**	26*	ND	11*	1.1*	**46**
19 to 30 years	2.7*	**130**	25*	ND	12*	1.1*	**46**
31 to 50 years	2.7*	**130**	25*	ND	12*	1.1*	**46**
51 to 70 years	2.7*	**130**	21*	ND	11*	1.1*	**46**
> 70 years	2.7*	**130**	21*	ND	11*	1.1*	**46**
PREGNANCY							
14 to 18 yrs.	3.0*	**175**	28*	ND	13*	1.4*	**71**
19 to 30 yrs.	3.0*	**175**	28*	ND	13*	1.4*	**71**
31 to 50 years	3.0*	**175**	28*	ND	13*	1.4*	**71**
LACTATION							
14 to 18 years	3.8*	**210**	29*	ND	13*	1.3*	**71**
19 to 30 years	3.8*	**210**	29*	ND	13*	1.3*	**71**
31 to 50 years	3.8*	**210**	29*	ND	13*	1.3*	**71**

NOTE: This table (take from the DRI reports, see www.nap.edu) presents Recommended Dietary Allowances (RDA) in **bold type** and Adequate Intakes (AI) in ordinary type followed by an asterisk (*). An RDA is the average daily dietary intake level; sufficient to meet the nutrient requirements of nearly all (97-98 percent) healthy individuals in a group. It is calculated from an Estimated Average Requirement (EAR). If sufficient scientific evidence is not available to establish an EAR, and thus calculate an RDA, an AI is usually developed. For healthy breastfed infants, an AI is the mean intake. The AI for other life stage and gender groups is believed to cover the needs of all healthy individuals in the groups, but lack of data or uncertainty in the data prevent being able to specify with confidence the percentage of individuals covered by this intake.

a   *Total* water includes all water contained in food, beverages, and drinking water.

b   Based on g protein per kg of body weight for the reference body weight, e.g., for adults 0.8 g/kg body weight for the reference body weight.

c   Not determined.

SOURCE: *Dietary Reference Intakes for Energy, Carbohydrate, Fiber, Fat, Fatty Acids, Cholesterol, Protein, and Amino Acids* (2002/2005) and *Dietary Reference Intakes for Water, Potassium, Sodium, Chloride, and Sulfate* (2005). The report may be accessed via www.nap.edu.

B Dietary Reference Intakes

Dietary Reference Intakes (DRIs): Acceptable Macronutrient Distribution Ranges

Food and Nutrition Board, Institute of Medicine, National Academies

Macronutrient	Range (Percent of Energy)		
	Children, 1-3 y	Children, 4-18 y	Adults
Fat	30-40	25-35	20-35
n-6 polyunsaturated fatty acid[a] (linoleic acid)	5-10	5-10	5-10
n-3 polyunsaturated fatty acids[a] (a-linolenic acid)	0.6-1.2	0.6-1.2	0.6-1.2
Carbohydrate	45-65	45-65	45-65
Protein	5-20	10-30	10-35

a   Approximately 10 percent of the total can come from longer-chain n-3 or n-6 fatty acids.

SOURCE: *Dietary Reference Intakes for Energy, Carbohydrate, Fiber, Fat, Fatty Acids, Cholesterol, Protein, and Amino Acids* (2002/2005). This report may be accessed via www.nap.edu

Dietary Reference Intakes (DRIs): Acceptable Macronutrient Distribution Ranges

Food and Nutrition Board, Institute of Medicine, National Academies

Macronutrient	Recommendation
Dietary Cholesterol	As low as possible while consuming a nutritionally adequate diet
Trans Fatty Acids	As low as possible while consuming a nutritionally adequate diet
Saturated Fatty Acids	As low as possible while consuming a nutritionally adequate diet
Added Sugars[a]	Limit to no more than 25% of total energy

a   Not a recommended intake. A daily intake of added sugars that individuals should aim for to achieve a healthful diet was not set.

SOURCE: *Dietary Reference Intakes for Energy, Carbohydrate, Fiber, Fat, Fatty Acids, Cholesterol, Protein, and Amino Acids* (2002/2005). This report may be accessed via www.nap.edu

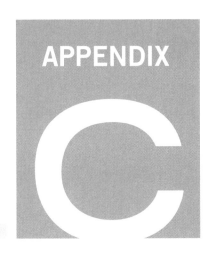

Exchange Lists for Diabetes

The Food Lists

The following chart shows the amount of nutrients in 1 serving from each list.

Food List	Carbohydrate (grams)	Protein (grams)	Fat (grams)	Calories
Carbohydrates				
Starch: breads, cereals and grains; starchy vegetables; crackers, snacks; and beans, peas, and lentils	15	0-3	0-1	80
Fruits	15	—	—	60
Milk • Fat-free, low-fat, 1% • Reduced-fat, 2% • Whole	 12 12 12	 8 8 8	 0-3 5 8	 100 120 160
Sweets, Desserts, and Other Carbohydrates	15	varies	varies	varies
Nonstarchy Vegetables	5	2	—	25
Meat and Meat Substitutes				
Lean	—	7	0-3	45
Medium-fat	—	7	4-7	75
High-fat	—	7	8+	100
Plant-based proteins	varies	7	varies	varies
Fats	—	—	5	45
Alcohol (1 equivalent)	varies	—	—	100

Starch

Cereals, grains, pasta, breads, crackers, snacks, starchy vegetables, and cooked beans, peas, and lentils are starches. In general, 1 starch is:

✓ ½ cup of cooked cereal, grain, or starchy vegetable

✓ ⅓ cup of cooked rice or pasta

✓ 1 oz. of a bread product, such as 1 slice of bread

✓ ¾ oz. to 1 oz. of most snack foods (some snack foods may also have extra fat)

Exchange Lists for Diabetes

Nutrition Tips

✓ A choice on the Starch list has 15 grams of carbohydrate, 0 grams to 3 grams of protein, 0 grams to 1 gram of fat, and 80 calories.

✓ For maximum health benefits, eat three or more servings of whole grains each day. A serving of whole grain is about ½ cup of cooked cereal or grain, 1 slice of whole-grain bread, or 1 cup of whole-grain cold breakfast cereal.

Selection Tips

✓ Choose low-fat starches as often as you can.

✓ Starchy vegetables, baked goods, and grains prepared with fat count as 1 starch and 1 fat.

✓ For many starchy foods (bagels, muffins, dinner rolls, buns), a general rule of thumb is 1 oz. equals 1 serving. Always check the size you eat. Because of their large size, some foods have a lot more carbohydrate and calories than you might think. For example, a large bagel may weigh 4 oz. and equal 4 starch choices.

✓ For specific information, read the Nutrition Facts panel on the food label.

Bread

	Food	Serving Size
	Bagel, large (about 4 oz.)	¼ (1 oz.)
⚠	Biscuit, 2½ inches across	1
☺	Bread • reduced-calorie • white, whole-grain, pumpernickel, rye, unfrosted raisin	2 slices (1½ oz.) 1 slice (1 oz.)
	Chapatti, small, 6 inches across	1
⚠	Cornbread, 1³/₄-inch cube	1 (1½ oz.)
	English muffin	½
	Hot dog bun or hamburger bun	½ (1 oz)
	Naan, 8 inches by 2 inches	¼
	Pancake, 4 inches across, ¼ inch thick	1
	Pita, 6 inches across	½
	Roll, plain, small	1 (1 oz)
⚠	Stuffing, bread	⅓ cup
⚠	Taco shell, 5 inches across	2
	Tortilla, corn, 6 inches across	1
	Tortilla, flour, 6 inches across	1
	Tortilla, flour, 10 inches across	⅓ tortilla
⚠	Waffle, 4-inch square or 4 inches across	1

☺ = More than 3 grams of dietary fiber per serving.

⚠ = Extra fat, or prepared with added fat. (Count as 1 starch + 1 fat.)

[S] = 480 milligrams or more of sodium per serving.

Cereals and Grains

Food	Serving Size
Barley, cooked	⅓ cup
Bran, dry • oat • wheat	¼ cup ½ cup
Bulgur (cooked)	½ cup
Cereals • bran • cooked (oats, oatmeal) • puffed • shredded wheat, plain • sugar-coated • unsweetened, ready-to-eat	½ cup ½ cup 1½ cups ½ cup ½ cup ¾ cup
Couscous	⅓ cup
Granola • low-fat • regular	¼ cup ¼ cup
Grits, cooked	½ cup
Kasha	½ cup
Millet, cooked	⅓ cup
Muesli	¼ cup
Pasta, cooked	⅓ cup
Polenta, cooked	⅓ cup
Quinoa, cooked	⅓ cup
Rice, white or brown, cooked	⅓ cup
Tabbouleh (tabouli), prepared	½ cup
Wheat germ, dry	3 Tbsp.
Wild rice, cooked	½ cup

Tip: An open handful is equal to about 1 cup or 1 oz. to 2 oz. of snack food.

 = More than 3 grams of dietary fiber per serving.

 = Extra fat, or prepared with added fat. (Count as 1 starch + 1 fat.)

 = 480 milligrams or more of sodium per serving.

Starchy Vegetables

	Food	Serving Size
	Cassava	⅓ cup
	Corn	½ cup
	• on cob, large	½ cob (5 oz.)
	Hominy, canned	¾ cup
	Mixed vegetables with corn, peas, or pasta	1 cup
	Parsnips	½ cup
	Peas, green	½ cup
	Plantain, ripe	⅓ cup
	Potato	
	• baked with skin	¼ large (3 oz.)
	• boiled, all kinds	½ cup or ½ medium (3 oz.)
	• mashed, with milk and fat	½ cup
	• French fried (oven-baked)	1 cup (2 oz.)
	Pumpkin, canned, no sugar added	1 cup
	Spaghetti/pasta sauce	½ cup
	Squash, winter (acorn, butternut)	1 cup
	Succotash	½ cup
	Yam, sweet potato, plain	½ cup

✎ **Note:** Restaurant-style French fries are on the Fast Foods list.

 = More than 3 grams of dietary fiber per serving.

 = Extra fat, or prepared with added fat. (Count as 1 starch + 1 fat.)

 = 480 milligrams or more of sodium per serving.

Crackers and Snacks

	Food	Serving Size
	Animal crackers	8
	Crackers	
⚠	• round, butter-type	6
	• saltine-type	6
⚠	• sandwich-style, cheese or peanut butter filling	3
⚠	• whole-wheat regular	2-5 (¾ oz.)
😊	• whole-wheat lower fat or crispbreads	2-5 (¾ oz.)
	Graham cracker, 2½ inch square	3
	Matzoh	¾ oz.
	Melba toast, about 2-inch by 4-inch piece	4 pieces
	Oyster crackers	20
	Popcorn	
⚠ 😊	• with butter	3 cups
😊	• no fat added	3 cups
😊	• lower fat	3 cups
	Pretzels	¾ oz.
	Rice cakes, 4 inches across	2
	Snack chips	
	• fat-free or baked (tortilla, potato), baked pita chips	15-20 (¾ oz.)
⚠	• regular (tortilla, potato)	9-13 (¾ oz.)

Note: For other snacks, see the Sweets, Desserts, and Other Carbohydrates list.

Beans, Peas, and Lentils

The choices on this list count as 1 starch + 1 lean meat.

	Food	Serving Size
😊	Baked beans	⅓ cup
😊	Beans, cooked (black, garbanzo, kidney, lima, navy, pinto, white)	½ cup
😊	Lentils, cooked (brown, green, yellow)	½ cup
😊	Peas, cooked (black-eyed, split)	½ cup
S 😊	Refried beans, canned	½ cup

Note: Beans, peas, and lentils are also found on the Meat and Meat Substitutes list.

😊 = More than 3 grams of dietary fiber per serving.

⚠ = Extra fat, or prepared with added fat. (Count as 1 starch + 1 fat.)

S = 480 milligrams or more of sodium per serving.

Whole Grains

Whole grains and grain products contain the entire grain seed of a plant. They are rich in fiber, vitamins, minerals, and phytochemicals. Here are some tips for including more whole grains in your diet:

✓ Choose whole-grain foods more often. Whole-grain foods include whole-wheat flour, whole oats/oatmeal, whole-grain cornmeal, popcorn, buckwheat, buckwheat flour, whole rye, whole-grain barley, brown rice, wild rice, bulgur, millet, quinoa, and sorghum.

✓ Read food labels carefully. If a product label says "100% whole grain," it must contain at least 16 grams of whole grain per serving. A "whole grain" stamp identifies foods that have at least a ½ serving of whole grains (8 grams of whole grains).

✓ Add several tablespoons of cooked grains to stews, soups, and vegetable salads.

✓ Monitor your blood glucose carefully to find out the effect whole grains have on you.

Fruits

Fresh, frozen, canned, and dried fruits and fruit juices are on this list. In general, 1 fruit choice is:

✓ ½ cup of canned or fresh fruit or unsweetened fruit juice

✓ 1 small fresh fruit (4 oz.)

✓ 2 tablespoons of dried fruit

Nutrition Tips

✓ A choice on the Fruits list has 15 grams of carbohydrate, 0 grams of protein, 0 grams of fat, and 60 calories.

✓ Fresh, frozen, and dried fruits are good sources of fiber. Fruit juices contain very little fiber. Choose fruits instead of juices whenever possible.

✓ Citrus fruits, berries, and melons are good sources of vitamin C.

Selection Tips

✓ Use a food scale to weigh fresh fruits. Practice builds portion skills.

✓ The weight listed includes skin, core, seeds, and rind.

✓ Read the Nutrition Facts on the food label. If 1 serving has more than 15 grams of carbohydrate, you may need to adjust the size of the serving.

✓ Portion sizes for canned fruits are for the fruit and a small amount of juice (1 to 2 tablespoons).

✓ Food labels for fruits may contain the words "no sugar added" or "unsweetened." This means that no table sugar (sucrose) has been added; it *does not* mean the food contains no sugar.

✓ Fruit canned in "extra light syrup" has the same amount of carbohydrate per serving as canned fruit labeled "no sugar added" or "juice pack." All canned fruits on the Fruits list are based on one of these three types of pack. Avoid fruit canned in heavy syrup.

Note: You can count 1/2 cup cranberries or rhubarb sweetened with sugar substitutes as free foods.

Fruit

The weight listed includes skin, core, seeds, and rind.

	Food	Serving Size
	Apple, unpeeled, small	1 (4 oz.)
	Apples, dried	4 rings
	Applesauce, unsweetened	½ cup
	Apricots	
	• canned	½ cup
	• dried	8 halves
	• fresh	4 whole (5½ oz.)
	Banana, extra small	1 (4 oz.)
	Blackberries	¾ cup
	Blueberries	¾ cup
	Cantaloupe, small	⅓ melon or 1 cup cubed (11 oz.)
	Cherries	
	• sweet, canned	½ cup
	• sweet fresh	12 (3 oz.)
	Dates	3
	Dried fruits (blueberries, cherries, cranberries, mixed fruit, raisins)	2 Tbsp.
	Figs	
	• dried	1½
	• fresh	1½ large or 2 medium (3½ oz.)
	Fruit cocktail	½ cup
	Grapefruit	
	• large	½ (11 oz.)
	• sections, canned	¾ cup
	Grapes, small	17 (3 oz.)
	Honeydew melon	1 slice or 1 cup cubed (10 oz.)
	Kiwi	1 (3½ oz.)
	Mandarin oranges, canned	¾ cup
	Mango, small	½ fruit (5½ oz.) or ½ cup
	Nectarine, small	1 (5 oz.)
	Orange, small	1 (6½ oz.)
	Papaya	½ fruit or 1 cup cubed (8 oz.)

(Continued)

 = More than 3 grams of dietary fiber per serving.

 = Extra fat, or prepared with added fat.

 = 480 milligrams or more of sodium per serving.

Fruit *(Continued)*

The weight listed includes skin, core, seeds, and rind.

Food	Serving Size
Peaches	
• canned	½ cup
• fresh, medium	1 (6 oz.)
Pears	
• canned	½ cup
• fresh, large	½ (4 oz.)
Pineapple	
• canned	½ cup
• fresh	¾ cup
Plums	
• canned	½ cup
• dried (prunes)	3
• small	2 (5 oz.)
Raspberries	1 cup
Strawberries	1¼ cup whole berries
Tangerines, small	2 (8 oz.)
Watermelon	1 slice or 1¼ cups cubes (13½ oz.)

Fruit Juice

Food	Serving Size
Apple juice/cider	½ cup
Fruit juice blends, 100% juice	⅓ cup
Grape juice	⅓ cup
Grapefruit juice	½ cup
Orange juice	½ cup
Pineapple juice	½ cup
Prune juice	⅓ cup

 = More than 3 grams of dietary fiber per serving.

 = Extra fat, or prepared with added fat.

 = 480 milligrams or more of sodium per serving.

Get Moving

Increasing physical activity improves blood glucose control, reduces other health risks, and helps with weight management. Here are some tips to help you get started:

✓ Choose an activity you enjoy. Many people enjoy walking because it is easy to start and is free.

✓ Start out with 5 to 10 minutes of physical activity per day, at a pace and distance that feels comfortable. Work up to at least 30 minutes a day of moderate activity five times a week.

✓ Wear comfortable shoes with good traction and shock absorption.

✓ Build exercise into your everyday activities. Take the stairs instead of the elevator. Park your car farther away from the office or store.

✓ Put extra effort into housework and chores, such as washing windows, scrubbing floors, vacuuming, and raking the yard.

✓ Short amounts of activity count. Three 10-minute walks add up to 30 minutes a day.

✓ Have backup plans for bad weather. Walk at the mall or find indoor activities you enjoy, such as walking on a treadmill or following a workout video or fitness TV show.

Milk

Different types of milk and milk products are on this list. However, two types of milk products are found in other lists:

✓ Cheeses are on the Meat and Meat Substitutes list (because they are rich in protein).

✓ Cream and other dairy fats are on the Fats list.

Milks and yogurts are grouped in three categories based on the amount of fat they have: fat-free (skim) low-fat (1%), reduced-fat (2%), or whole. The following chart shows you what 1 milk choice contains:

Food List	Carbohydrate (grams)	Protein (grams)	Fat (grams)	Calories
Fat-free (skim) low-fat (1%)	12	8	0-3	100
Reduced-fat (2%)	12	8	5	120
Whole	12	8	8	160

Nutrition Tips

✓ Milk and yogurt are good sources of calcium and protein.

✓ The higher the fat content of milk and yogurt, the more saturated fat and cholesterol it has.

✓ Children over the age of 2 and adults should choose lower-fat varieties such as skim, 1% or 2% milks or yogurts.

Selection Tips

✓ 1 cup equals 8 fluid oz. or ½ pint.

✓ If you choose 2% or whole-milk foods, be aware of the extra fat.

Milk and Yogurts

Food	Serving Size	Count As
Fat-free (skim) or low-fat (1%)		
Milk, buttermilk, acidophilus milk, Lactaid	1 cup	1 fat-free milk
Evaporated milk	½ cup	1 fat-free milk
Yogurt, plain or flavored with an artificial sweetener	⅔ cup (6 oz.)	1 fat-free milk
Reduced-fat (2%)		
Milk, acidophilus milk, kefir, Lactaid	1 cup	1 reduced-fat milk
Yogurt, plain	⅔ cup (6 oz.)	1 reduced-fat milk
Whole		
Milk, buttermilk, goat's milk	1 cup	1 whole milk
Evaporated milk	½ cup	1 whole milk
Yogurt, plain	1 cup (8 oz.)	1 whole milk

Balanced Energy

A healthy weight is the result of balancing *energy in* and *energy out* of the body. You get energy from the food you eat. Energy is measured in calories. You use energy when you breathe, sit, walk, and move. You stay at the same weight when energy in—the food you eat—is the same as energy out—the energy you use. You gain weight when you take in more energy (calories) than your body uses. This extra energy is stored as unwanted weight. You can lose weight by taking in fewer calories than your body needs or burning off more than you take in. Then your body uses stored energy to meet your needs. Ask your Registered Dietitian to estimate how much energy your body needs. When you balance energy from food and energy used for exercise, you can maintain a healthy weight.

Dairy-Like Foods

Food	Serving Size	Count As
Chocolate milk		
• fat-free	1 cup	1 fat-free milk + 1 carbohydrate
• whole	1 cup	1 whole milk + 1 carbohydrate
Eggnog, whole milk	½ cup	1 carbohydrate + 2 fats
Rice drink		
• flavored, low-fat	1 cup	2 carbohydrates
• plain, fat-free	1 cup	1 carbohydrate
Smoothies, flavored, regular	10 oz.	1 fat-free milk + 2½ carbohydrates
Soy milk		
• light	1 cup	1 carbohydrate + ½ fat
• regular, plain	1 cup	1 carbohydrate + 1 fat
Yogurt		
• and juice blends	1 cup	1 fat-free milk + 1 carbohydrate
• low-carbohydrate (less than 6 grams carbohydrate per serving	⅔ cup (6 oz.)	½ fat-free milk
• with fruit, low-fat	⅔ cup (6 oz.)	1 fat-free milk + 1 carbohydrate

Note: Coconut milk is on the Fats list.

Sweets, Desserts, and Other Carbohydrates

Beverages, Soda, and Energy/Sports Drinks

Food	Serving Size	Count As
Cranberry juice cocktail	½ cup	1 carbohydrate
Energy drink	1 can (8.3 oz.)	2 carbohydrates
Fruit drink or lemonade	1 cup (8 oz.)	2 carbohydrates
Hot chocolate		
• regular	1 envelope added to 8 oz. water	1 carbohydrate + 1 fat
• sugar-free or light	1 envelope added to 8 oz. water	1 carbohydrate
Soft drink (soda), regular	1 can (12 oz.)	2½ carbohydrates
Sports drink	1 cup (8 oz.)	1 carbohydrate

Brownies, Cake, Cookies, Gelatin, Pie, and Pudding

Food	Serving Size	Count As
Brownie, small, unfrosted	1¼-inch square, ⅞-inch high (about 1 oz.)	1 carbohydrate + 1 fat
Cake		
• angel food, unfrosted	½ of cake (about 2 oz.)	2 carbohydrates
• frosted	2-inch square (about 2 oz.)	2 carbohydrates + 1 fat
• unfrosted	2-inch square (about 1 oz.)	1 carbohydrate + fat
Cookies		
• chocolate chip	2 cookies (2¼ inches across)	1 carbohydrate + 2 fats
• gingersnap	3 cookies	1 carbohydrate
• sandwich, with creme filling	2 small (about ⅔ oz.)	1 carbohydrate + 1 fat
• sugar-free	3 small or 1 large (¾-1 oz.)	1 carbohydrate + 1-2 fats
• vanilla wafer	5 cookies	1 carbohydrate + 1 fat
Cupcake, frosted	1 small (about 1¾ oz.)	2 carbohydrates + 1-1½ fats
Fruit cobbler	½ cup (3½ oz.)	3 carbohydrates + 1 fat
Gelatin, regular	½ cup	1 carbohydrate
Pie		
• commercially prepared fruit, 2 crusts	⅙ of 8-inch pie	3 carbohydrates + 2 fats
• pumpkin or custard	⅛ of 3-inch pie	1½ carbohydrates + 1½ fats
Pudding		
• regular (made with reduced-fat milk)	½ cup	2 carbohydrates
• sugar-free or sugar- and fat-free (made with fat-free milk)	½ cup	1 carbohydrate

Candy, Spreads, Sweets, Sweeteners, Syrups, and Toppings

Food	Serving Size	Count As
Candy bar, chocolate/peanut	2 "fun size" bars (1 oz.)	1½ carbohydrate + 1½ fats
Candy, hard	3 pieces	1 carbohydrate
Chocolate "kisses"	5 pieces	1 carbohydrate + 1 fat
Coffee creamer • dry, flavored • liquid, flavored	 4 tsp. 2 Tbsp.	 ½ carbohydrate + ½ fat 1 carbohydrate
Fruit snacks, chewy (pureed fruit concentrate)	1 roll (¾ oz.)	1 carbohydrate
Fruit spreads, 100% fruit	1½ Tbsp.	1 carbohydrate
Honey	1 Tbsp.	1 carbohydrate
Jam or jelly, regular	1 Tbsp.	1 carbohydrate
Sugar	1 Tbsp.	1 carbohydrate
Syrup • chocolate • light (pancake type) • regular (pancake type)	 2 Tbsp. 2 Tbsp. 1 Tbsp.	 2 carbohydrates 1 carbohydrate 1 carbohydrate

Condiments and Sauces

	Food	Serving Size	Count As
	Barbeque sauce	3 Tbsp.	1 carbohydrate
	Cranberry sauce, jellied	¼ cup	1½ carbohydrates
S	Gravy, canned or bottled	½ cup	½ carbohydrate + ½ fat
	Salad dressing, fat-free, low-fat, cream-based	3 Tbsp.	1 carbohydrate
	Sweet and sour sauce	3 Tbsp.	1 carbohydrate

Doughnuts, Muffins, Pastries, and Sweet Breads

Food	Serving Size	Count As
Banana nut bread	1-inch slice (2 oz.)	2 carbohydrates + 1 fat
Doughnut • cake, plain • yeast type, glazed	 1 medium (1½ oz.) 3¾ inches across (2 oz.)	 1½ carbohydrates + 2 fats 2 carbohydrates + 2 fats
Muffin (4 oz.)	¼ muffin (1 oz.)	1 carbohydrate + ½ fat
Sweet roll or Danish	1 (2½ oz.)	2½ carbohydrates + 2 fats

✎ **Note:** You can also check the Fats list and Free Foods list for other condiments.

 = 480 milligrams or more of sodium per serving.

Frozen Bars, Frozen Desserts, Frozen Yogurt, and Ice Cream

Food	Serving Size	Count As
Frozen pops	1	½ carbohydrate
Fruit juice bars, frozen, 100% juice	1 bar (3 oz.)	1 carbohydrate
Ice cream		
• fat-free	½ cup	1½ carbohydrates
• light	½ cup	1 carbohydrate + 1 fat
• no sugar added	½ cup	1 carbohydrate + 1 fat
• regular	½ cup	1 carbohydrate + 2 fats
Sherbet, sorbet	½ cup	2 carbohydrates
Yogurt, frozen		
• fat-free	⅓ cup	1 carbohydrate
• regular	½ cup	1 carbohydrate + 0-1 fat

Granola Bars, Meal Replacement Bars/Shakes, and Trail Mix

Food	Serving Size	Count As
Granola or snack bar, regular or low-fat	1 bar (1 oz.)	1½ carbohydrates
Meal replacement bar	1 bar (1⅓ oz.)	1½ carbohydrates + 0-1 fat
Meal replacement bar	1 bar (2 oz.)	2 carbohydrates + 1 fat
Meal replacement shake, reduced calorie	1 can (10-11 oz.)	1½ carbohydrates + 0-1 fat
Trail mix		
• candy/nut-based	1 oz.	1 carbohydrate + 2 fats
• dried fruit-based	1 oz.	1 carbohydarte + 1 fat

Nonstarchy Vegetables

Vegetable choices include vegetables in this Nonstarchy Vegetables list and the Starchy Vegetables list found within the Starch list. Vegetables with small amounts of carbohydrate and calories are on the Nonstarchy Vegetables list. Vegetables contain important nutrients. Try to eat at least 2 to 3 nonstarchy vegetable choices each day (as well as choices from the Starchy Vegetables list). In general, 1 nonstarchy vegetable choice is:

✓ ½ cup of cooked vegetables or vegetable juice

✓ 1 cup of raw vegetables

If you eat 3 cups or more of raw vegetables or 1½ cups of cooked nonstarchy vegetables in a meal, count them as 1 carbohydrate choice.

Nutrition Tips

✓ A choice on this list (½ cup cooked or 1 cup raw) equals 5 grams of carbohydrate, 2 grams of protein, 0 grams of fat, and 25 calories.

✓ Fresh and frozen vegetables have less added salt than canned vegetables. Drain and rinse canned vegetables to remove some salt.

✓ Choose dark green and dark yellow vegetables each day. Spinach, broccoli, romaine, carrots, chilies, squash, and peppers are great choices.

✓ Brussels sprouts, broccoli, cauliflower, greens, peppers, spinach, and tomatoes are good sources of vitamin C.

✓ Eat vegetables from the cruciferous family several times each week. Cruciferous vegetables include bok choy, broccoli, brussels sprouts, cabbage, cauliflower, collards, kale, kohlrabi, radishes, rutabaga, and turnips.

Nonstarchy Vegetables

Amaranth or Chinese spinach	Jicama
Artichoke	Kohlrabi
Artichoke hearts	Leeks
Asparagus	Mixed vegetables (without corn, peas, or pasta)
Baby corn	Mung bean sprouts
Bamboo shoots	Mushrooms, all kinds, fresh
Bean sprouts	Okra
Beans (green, wax, Italian)	Onions
Beets	😊 Pea pods
Ⓢ Borscht	Peppers (all varieties)
Broccoli	Radishes
😊 Brussels sprouts	Ⓢ Rutabaga
Cabbage (green, bok choy, Chinese)	Sauerkraut
😊 Carrots	Soybean sprouts
Cauliflower	Spinach
Celery	Squash (summer, crookneck, zucchini)
😊 Chayote	😊 Sugar snap peas
Coleslaw, packaged, no dressing	Swiss chard
Cucumber	Tomato
Daikon	Ⓢ Tomatoes, canned
Eggplant	Ⓢ Tomato sauce
Gourds (bitter, bottle, luffa, bitter melon)	Tomato/vegetable juice
Green onions or scallions	Turnips
Greens (collard, kale, mustard, turnip)	Water chestnuts
Hearts of palm	Yard-long beans

Note: Salad greens (like chicory, endive, escarole, lettuce, romaine, arugula, radicchio, watercress) are on the Free Foods list.

 = More than 3 grams of dietary fiber per serving.

 = 480 milligrams or more of sodium per serving.

Meat and Meat Substitutes

Meat and meat substitutes are rich in protein. Foods from this list are divided into four groups based on the amount of fat they contain. These groups are lean meat, medium-fat meat, high-fat meat, and plant-based proteins. The following chart shows you what one choice includes.

	Carbohydrate (grams)	Protein (grams)	Fat (grams)	Calories
Lean meat	—	7	0-3	45
Medium-fat meat	—	7	4-7	75
High-fat meat	—	7	8+	100
Plant-based protein	varies	7	varies	varies

Selection Tips

✓ Read labels to find foods low in fat and cholesterol. Try for 5 grams of fat or less per serving.

✓ Read labels to find "hidden" carbohydrate. For example, hot dogs actually contain a lot of carbohydrate. Most hot dogs are also high in fat, but are often sold in lower-fat versions.

✓ Whenever possible, choose lean meats.

- Select grades of meat are the leanest.
- Choice grades have a moderate amount of fat.
- Prime cuts of meat have the highest amount of fat.

✓ Some types of fish, such as herring, mackerel, salmon, sardines, halibut, trout, and tuna, are rich in omega-3 fats, which may help reduce risk for heart disease. Choose fish (not commercially fried fish fillets) two or more times each week.

✓ Bake, roast, broil, grill, poach, steam, or boil instead of frying.

Lean Meats and Meat Substitutes

	Food	Serving Size
	Beef: Select or Choice grades trimmed of fat: ground round, roast (chuck, rib, rump), round, sirloin, steak (cubed, flank, porterhouse, T-bone), tenderloin	1 oz.
S	Beef jerky	½ oz.
	Cheeses with 3 grams of fat or less per oz.	1 oz.
	Cottage cheese	¼ cup
	Egg substitutes, plain	¼ cup
	Egg whites	2
	Fish, fresh or frozen, plain: catfish, cod, flounder, haddock, halibut, orange roughy, salmon, tilapia, trout, tuna	1 oz.
S	Fish, smoked: herring or salmon (lox)	1 oz.
	Game: buffalo, ostrich, rabbit, venison	1 oz.

(Continued)

S = 480 milligrams or more of sodium per serving (based on the sodium content of a typical 3-oz. serving of meat, unless ½ oz. to 2 oz. is the normal serving size.

Exchange Lists for Diabetes

	Food	Serving Size
S	Hot dog with 3 grams of fat or less per oz. (8 dogs per 14 oz. package) *Note: May be high in carbohydrate.*	1
	Lamb: chop, leg or roast	1 oz.
	Organ meats: heart, kidney, liver *Note: May be high in cholesterol*	1 oz.
	Oysters, fresh or frozen	6 medium
S	Pork, lean • Canadian bacon • rib or loin chop/roast, ham, tenderloin	 1 oz. 1 oz.
	Poultry, without skin: chicken, Cornish hen, domestic duck or goose (well-drained of fat), turkey	1 oz.
	Processed sandwich meats with 3 grams of fat or less per oz.: chipped beef, deli thin-sliced meats, turkey ham, turkey kielbasa, turkey pastrami	1 oz.
	Salmon, canned	1 oz.
	Sardines, canned	2 small
S	Sausage with 3 grams of fat or less per oz.	1 oz.
	Shellfish: clams, crab, imitation shellfish, lobster, scallops, shrimp	1 oz.
	Tuna, canned in water or oil, drained	1 oz.
	Veal: loin chop, roast	1 oz.

Portion Sizes

Portion size is an important part of meal planning. The Meat and Meat Substitutes list is based on cooked weight (4 oz. of raw meat is equal to 3 oz. of cooked meat) after bone and fat have been removed. Try using the following comparisons to help estimate portion sizes:

✓ 1 oz. cooked meat, poultry, or fish is about the size of a matchbox.

✓ 3 oz. cooked meat, poultry, or fish is about the size of a deck of playing cards.

✓ 2 Tbsp. peanut butter is about the size of a golf ball.

✓ The palm of a woman's hand is about the size of 3 oz. to 4 oz. of cooked, boneless meat. The palm of a man's hand is the size of a larger serving.

✓ 1 oz. cheese is about the size of 4 dice.

S = 480 milligrams or more of sodium per serving (based on the sodium content of a typical 3-oz. serving of meat, unless ½ oz. to 2 oz. is the normal serving size.

Medium-Fat Meat and Meat Substitutes

Food	Serving Size
Beef: corned beef, ground beef, meatloaf, Prime grades trimmed of fat (prime rib), short ribs, tongue	1 oz.
Cheeses with 4-7 grams of fat per oz: feta, mozzarella, pasteurized processed cheese spread, reduced-fat cheeses, string	1 oz.
Egg Note: High in cholesterol, so limit to 3 per week.	1
Fish, any fried type	1 oz.
Lamb: ground, rib roast	1 oz.
Pork: cutlet, shoulder roast	1 oz.
Poultry: chicken with skin; dove, pheasant, wild duck, or goose; fried chicken; ground turkey	1 oz.
Ricotta cheese	2 oz. (¼ cup)
⑤ Sausage with 4-7 grams of fat per oz.	1 oz.
Veal, cutlet (no breading)	1 oz.

Smart Supermarket Shopping

✓ Don't shop when you're hungry.

✓ Shop early in the day.

✓ Shop alone.

✓ Use a list.

✓ Cruise the perimeter.

✓ Choose a rainbow of fruits and vegetables.

✓ Go for whole grains.

✓ Be adventurous.

✓ Read food labels.

✓ Skip the "diabetic" food.

High-Fat Meat and Meat Substitutes

These foods are high in saturated fat, cholesterol, and calories and may raise blood cholesterol levels if eaten on a regular basis. Try to eat 3 or fewer servings from this group per week.

Food	Serving Size
Bacon	
⑤ • pork	2 slices (16 slices per lb. or 1 oz. each, before cooking)
⑤ • turkey	3 slices (½ oz. each before cooking)
Cheese, regular: American, bleu, brie, cheddar, hard goat, Monterey jack, queso, and Swiss	1 oz.
⑤ ⚠ Hot dog: beef, pork, or combination (10 per 1 lb.-sized package)	1
⑤ Hot dog: turkey or chicken (10 per 1 lb.-sized package)	1
Pork: ground, sausage, spareribs	1 oz.
Processed sandwich meats with 8 grams of fat or more per oz.: bologna, hard salami, pastrami	1 oz.
⑤ Sausage with 8 grams fat or more per oz.: bratwurst, chorizo, Italian, knockwurst, Polish, smoked, summer	1 oz.

⚠ = Extra fat, or prepared with added fat. (Add an additional fat choice to this food.)

⑤ = 480 milligrams or more of sodium per serving (based on the sodium content of a typical 3-oz. serving of meat, unless ½ oz. to 2 oz. is the normal serving size.

Plant-Based Proteins

	Food	Serving Size	Count As
	"Bacon" strips, soy-based	3 strips	1 medium-fat meat
	Baked beans	⅓ cup	1 starch + 1 lean meat
	Beans, cooked: black, garbanzo, kidney, lima, navy, pinto, white	½ cup	1 starch + 1 lean meat
	"Beef" or "sausage" crumbles, soy-based	2 oz.	½ carbohydrate + lean meat
	"Chicken" nuggets, soy-based	2 nuggets (1½ oz.)	½ carbohydrate + 1 medium-fat meat
	Edamame	½ cup	½ carbohydrate + 1 lean meat
	Falafel (spiced chickpea and wheat patties)	3 patties (about 2 inches across)	1 carbohydrate + 1 high-fat meat
	Hot dog, soy-based	1 (1½ oz.)	½ carbohydrate + 1 lean meat
	Hummus	⅓ cup	1 carbohydrate + 1 high-fat meat
	Lentils, brown, green, or yellow	½ cup	1 carbohydrate + 1 lean meat
	Meatless burger, soy-based	3 oz.	½ carbohydrate + 2 lean meats
	Meatless burger, vegetable- and starch-based	1 patty (about 2½ oz.)	1 carbohydrate + 2 lean meats
	Nut spreads: almond butter, cashew butter, peanut butter, soy nut butter	1 Tbsp.	1 high-fat meat
	Peas, cooked: black-eyed and split peas	½ cup	1 starch + 1 lean meat

 = More than 3 grams of dietary fiber per serving.

Fats

Fats and oils have mixtures of unsaturated (polyunsaturated and monounsaturated) and saturated fats. Foods on the Fats list are grouped together based on the major type of fat they contain. In general, 1 fat choice equals:

✓ 1 teaspoon of regular margarine, vegetable oil, or butter

✓ 1 tablespoon of regular salad dressing

Unsaturated Fats—Monounsaturated Fats

Food	Serving Size
Avocado, medium	2 Tbsp. (1 oz.)
Nut butters (*trans* fat-free): almond butter, cashew butter, peanut butter (smooth or crunchy)	1½ tsp.
Nuts	
• almonds	6 nuts
• Brazil	2 nuts
• cashews	6 nuts
• filberts (hazelnuts)	5 nuts
• macadamia	3 nuts
• mixed (50% peanuts)	6 nuts
• peanuts	10 nuts
• pecans	4 halves
• pistachios	16 nuts

(Continued)

Unsaturated Fats—Monounsaturated Fats *(Continued)*

Food	Serving Size
Oil: canola, olive, peanut	1 tsp.
Olives	
• black (ripe)	8 large
• green, stuffed	10 large

Portion Tip

Your thumb is about the same size and volume as 1 Tbsp. of salad dressing, mayonnaise, margarine, or oil. It is also about the same size as 1 oz. of cheese. A thumb tip is about the size of 1 teaspoon of margarine, mayonnaise, or other fats and oils.

Unsaturated Fats—Polyunsaturated Fats

Food	Serving Size
Margarine: lower-fat spread (30% - 50% vegetable oil, *trans* fat-free)	1 Tbsp.
Margarine: stick, tub (*trans* fat-free), or squeeze (*trans* fat-free)	1 tsp.
Mayonnaise	
• reduced-fat	1 Tbsp.
• regular	1 tsp.
Mayonnaise-style salad dressing	
• reduced-fat	1 Tbsp.
• regular	2 tsp.
Nuts	
• Pignolia (pine nuts)	1 Tbsp.
• walnuts, English	4 halves
Oil: corn, cottonseed, flaxseed, grape seed, safflower, soybean, sunflower	1 tsp.
Oil: made from soybean and canola oil—Enova	1 tsp.
Plant stanol esters	
• light	1 Tbsp.
• regular	2 tsp.
Salad dressing	
🅂 • reduced-fat *Note: May be high in carbohydrate.*	2 Tbsp.
🅂 • regular	1 Tbsp.
Seeds	
• flaxseed, whole	1 Tbsp.
• pumpkin, sunflower	1 Tbsp.
• sesame seeds	1 Tbsp.
Tahini or sesame paste	2 tsp.

🅂 = 480 milligrams or more of sodium per serving.

Exchange Lists for Diabetes

Free Foods

A "free" food is any food or drink choice that has less than 20 calories and 5 grams or less of carbohydrate per serving.

Selection Tips

✓ Most foods on this list should be limited to 3 servings (as listed here) per day. Spread out the servings throughout the day. If you eat all 3 servings at once, it could raise your blood glucose level.

✓ Food and drink choices listed here without a serving size can be eaten whenever you like.

Low-Carbohydrate Foods

Food	Serving Size
Cabbage, raw	½ cup
Candy, hard (regular or sugar-free)	1 piece
Carrots, cauliflower, or green beans, cooked	¼ cup
Cranberries, sweetened with sugar substitute	½ cup
Cucumber, sliced	½ cup
Gelatin: • dessert, sugar-free • unflavored	
Gum	
Jam or jelly, light or no sugar added	2 tsp.
Rhubarb, sweetened with sugar substitute	½ cup
Salad greens	
Sugar substitutes (artificial sweeteners)	
Syrup, sugar-free	2 Tbsp.

Modified-Fat Foods with Carbohydrate

Food	Serving Size
Cream cheese, fat-free	1 Tbsp. (½ oz.)
Creamers • nondairy, liquid • nondairy, powdered	 1 Tbsp. 2 tsp.
Margarine spread • fat-free • reduced-fat	 1 Tbsp. 1 tsp.
Mayonnaise • fat-free • reduced-fat	 1 Tbsp. 1 tsp.
Mayonnaise-style salad dressing • fat-free • reduced-fat	 1 Tbsp. 1 tsp.

(Continued)

Modified-Fat Foods with Carbohydrate *(Continued)*

Food	Serving Size
Salad dressing	
• fat-free or low-fat	1 Tbsp.
• fat-free, Italian	2 Tbsp.
Sour cream, fat-free or reduced-fat	1 Tbsp.
Whipped topping	
• light or fat-free	2 Tbsp.
• regular	1 Tbsp.

Artificial Sweeteners

Sugar substitutes, alternatives, or replacements that are approved by the Food and Drug Administration (FDA) are safe to use. Common brand names include:

✓ Equal and Nutrasweet (aspartame)

✓ Splenda (sucralose)

✓ Sugar Twin, Sweet-10, Sweet'N Low, and Sprinkle Sweet (saccharin)

✓ Sweet One (acesulfame K)

Although each sweetener is tested for safety before it can be marketed and sold, use a variety of sweeteners in moderate amounts.

Condiments

Food	Serving Size
Barbecue sauce	2 tsp.
Catsup (ketchup)	1 Tbsp.
Honey mustard	1 Tbsp.
Horseradish	
Lemon juice	
Miso	1½ tsp.
Mustard	
Parmesan cheese, freshly grated	1 Tbsp.
Pickle relish	1 Tbsp.
Pickles	
Ⓢ • dill	1½ medium
• sweet, bread and butter	2 slices
• sweet, gherkin	¾ oz.
Salsa	¼ cup

(Continued)

Ⓢ = 480 milligrams or more of sodium per serving.

Condiments *(Continued)*

	Food	Serving Size
Ⓢ	Soy sauce, light or regular	1 Tbsp.
	Sweet and sour sauce	2 tsp.
	Sweet chili sauce	2 tsp.
	Taco sauce	1 Tbsp.
	Vinegar	
	Yogurt, any type	2 Tbsp.

Free Snacks

These foods in these serving sizes are perfect free-food snacks.

- ✓ 5 baby carrots and celery sticks
- ✓ ¼ cup blueberries
- ✓ ½ oz. sliced cheese, fat-free
- ✓ 10 goldfish-style crackers
- ✓ 2 saltine-type crackers
- ✓ 1 frozen cream pop, sugar-free
- ✓ ½ oz. lean meat
- ✓ 1 cup light popcorn
- ✓ 1 vanilla wafer

Drinks/Mixes

The foods on this list without a serving size listed can be consumed in any moderate amount.

- ✓ Bouillon, broth, consomme Ⓢ
- ✓ Bouillon or broth, low-sodium
- ✓ Carbonated or mineral water
- ✓ Club soda
- ✓ Cocoa powder, unsweetened (1 Tbsp.)
- ✓ Coffee, unsweetened or with sugar substitute
- ✓ Diet soft drinks, sugar-free
- ✓ Drink mixes, sugar-free
- ✓ Tea, unsweetened or with sugar substitute
- ✓ Tonic water, diet
- ✓ Water
- ✓ Water, flavored, carbohydrate free

Seasonings

Any food on this list can be consumed in any moderate amount.

- ✓ Flavoring extracts (for example, vanilla, almond, peppermint)
- ✓ Garlic
- ✓ Herbs, fresh or dried
- ✓ Nonstick cooking spray
- ✓ Pimento
- ✓ Spices
- ✓ Hot pepper sauce
- ✓ Wine, used in cooking
- ✓ Worcestershire sauce

Note: Be careful with seasonings that contain sodium or are salts, such as garlic salt, celery salt, and lemon pepper.

Ⓢ = 480 milligrams or more of sodium per serving.

Combination Foods

Many of the foods you eat are mixed together in various combinations, such as casseroles. These "combination" foods do not fit into any one choice list. This is a list of choices for some typical combination foods. This list will help you fit these foods into your meal plan. Ask your Registered Dietitian for nutrient information about other combination foods you would like to eat, including your own recipes. A carbohydrate choice has 15 grams of carbohydrate and about 70 calories.

Entrees

Food	Serving Size	Count As
Casserole type (tuna noodle, lasagna, spaghetti with meatballs, chili with beans, macaroni and cheese)	1 cup (8 oz.)	2 carbohydrates + 2 medium-fat meats
Stews (beef/other meats and vegetables)	1 cup (8 oz.)	1 carbohydrate + 1 medium-fat meat + 0-3 fats
Tuna salad or chicken salad	½ cup (3½ oz.)	½ carbohydrate + 2 lean meats + 1 fat

Other Combination Foods

Your home recipes may be different from similar foods listed here. To figure out a recipe's nutrients, follow these steps:

✓ Find the carbohydrate grams, protein grams, fat grams, and calories for each of the recipe ingredients.

✓ Total each of the nutrients.

✓ Divide the totals by the number of servings the recipe yields.

✓ Compare these numbers with the choices in this booklet.

Frozen Meals/Entrees

Food	Serving Size	Count As
Burrito (beef and bean)	1 (5 oz.)	3 carbohydrates + 1 lean meat + 2 fats
Dinner-type meal	generally 14-17 oz.	3 carbohydrates + 3 medium-fat meats + 3 fats
Entree or meal with less than 340 calories	about 8-11 oz.	2-3 carbohydrates + 1-2 lean meats
Pizza • cheese/vegetarian, thin crust • meat topping, thin crust	 ¼ of a 12-inch (4½-5 oz.) ¼ of a 12-inch (5 oz.)	 2 carbohydrates + 2 medium-fat meats 2 carbohydrates + 2 medium-fat meats + 1½ fats
Pocket sandwich	1 (4½ oz.)	3 carbohydrates + 1 lean meat + 1-2 fats
Pot pie	1 (7 oz.)	2½ carbohydrates + 1 medium-fat meat + 3 fats

Salads (Deli-Style)

Food	Serving Size	Count As
Coleslaw	½ cup	1 carbohydrate + 1½ fats
Macaroni/pasta salad	½ cup	2 carbohydrates + 3 fats
Potato salad	½ cup	1½-2 carbohydrates + 1-2 fats

= More than 3 grams of dietary fiber per serving.

 = 600 milligrams or more of sodium per serving (for combination food main dishes/meals).

Soups

	Food	Serving Size	Count As
ⓢ	Bean, lentil, or split pea	1 cup	1 carbohydrate + 1 lean meat
ⓢ	Chowder (made with milk)	1 cup (8 oz.)	1 carbohydrate + 1 lean meat + 1½ fats
ⓢ	Cream (made with water)	1 cup (8 oz.)	1 carbohydrate + 1 fat
ⓢ	• Instant	6 oz. prepared	1 carbohydrate
ⓢ	• with beans or lentils	8 oz. prepared	2½ carbohydrates + 1 lean meat
ⓢ	Miso soup	1 cup	½ carbohydrate + 1 fat
ⓢ	Ramen noodle	1 cup	2 carbohydrates + 2 fats
	Rice (congee)	1 cup	1 carbohydrate
ⓢ	Tomato (made with water)	1 cup (8 oz.)	1 carbohydrate
ⓢ	Vegetable beef, chicken noodle, or other broth-type	1 cup (8 oz.)	1 carbohydrate

Eating Healthy in Restaurants

✓ Plan ahead. Make a list of restaurants near you that offer healthy choices and pick up carryout menus to see what's on the menu.

✓ Ask questions before you place your order: How is the item prepared? Can you substitute items?

✓ Add more vegetables whenever possible.

✓ Avoid items that are "jumbo," "giant," "deluxe," or "super-sized."

✓ Split an entree or dessert with someone.

✓ Put half of your order in a take-home box before you start to eat.

✓ Watch out for hidden extra calories, such as croutons, bacon, or cheese.

✓ Ask for salad dressings, sour cream, and butter on the side.

✓ Don't forget to count calories in beverages.

✓ Walk to and from the restaurant to burn extra calories.

Fast Food

The choices in the Fast Foods list are not specific fast food meals or items, but are estimates based on popular foods. You can get specific nutrition information for almost every fast food or restaurant chain. Ask the restaurant or check its website for nutrition information about your favorite fast foods. A carbohydrate choice has 15 grams of carbohydrate and about 70 calories.

Breakfast Sandwiches

	Food	Serving Size	Count As
ⓢ	Egg, cheese, meat, English muffin	1 sandwich	2 carbohydrates + 2 medium-fat meats
ⓢ	Sausage biscuit sandwich	1 sandwich	2 carbohydrates + 2 high-fat meats + 3½ fats

😊 = More than 3 grams of dietary fiber per serving.

 = 600 milligrams or more of sodium per serving (for fast food main dishes/meals).

Main Dishes/Entrees

Food	Serving Size	Count As
S ☺ Burrito (beef and beans)	1 (about 8 oz.)	3 carbohydrates + 3 medium-fat meats + 3 fats
S Chicken breast, breaded and fried	1 (about 5 oz.)	1 carbohydrate + 4 medium-fat meats
Chicken drumstick, breaded and fried	1 (about 2 oz.)	2 medium-fat meats
S Chicken nuggets	6 (about 3½ oz.)	1 carbohydrate + 2 medium-fat meats + 1 fat
S Chicken thigh, breaded and fried	1 (about 4 oz.)	½ carbohydrate + 3 medium-fat meats + 1½ fats
S Chicken wings, hot	6 (5 oz.)	5 medium-fat meats + 1½ fats

Asian

Food	Serving Size	Count As
S Beef/chicken/shrimp with vegetables in sauce	1 cup (about 5 oz.)	1 carbohydrate + 1 lean meat + 1 fat
S Egg roll, meat	1 (about 3 oz.)	1 carbohydrate + 1 lean meat + 1 fat
Fried rice, meatless	½ cup	1½ carbohydrates + 1½ fats
S Meat and sweet sauce (orange chicken)	1 cup	3 carbohydrates + 3 medium-fat meats + 2 fats
S ☺ Noodles and vegetables in sauce (chow mein, lo mein)	1 cup	2 carbohydrates + 1 fat

Pizza

Food	Serving Size	Count As
S Cheese, pepperoni, regular crust	⅛ of a 14-inch (about 4 oz.)	2½ carbohydrates + 1 medium-fat meat + 1½ fats
S Cheese/vegetarian, thin crust	¼ of a 12-inch (about 6 oz.)	2½ carbohydrates + 2 medium-fat meats + 1½ fats

Sandwiches

Food	Serving Size	Count As
S Chicken sandwich, grilled	1	3 carbohydrates + 4 lean meats
S Chicken sandwich, crispy	1	3½ carbohydrates + 3 medium-fat meats + 1 fat
Fish sandwich with tartar sauce	1	2½ carbohydrates + 2 medium-fat meats + 2 fats
S Hamburger		
• large with cheese	1	2½ carbohydrates + 4 medium-fat meats + 1 fat
• regular	1	2 carbohydrates + 1 medium-fat meat + 1 fat
S Hot dog with bun	1	1 carbohydrate + 1 high-fat meat + 1 fat

(Continued)

 = More than 3 grams of dietary fiber per serving.

S = 600 milligrams or more of sodium per serving (for fast food main dishes/meals).

Sandwiches (Continued)

Food	Serving Size	Count As
Submarine sandwich		
[S] • less than 6 grams fat	6-inch sub	3 carbohydrates + 2 lean meats
[S] • regular	6-inch sub	3½ carbohydrates + 2 medium-fat meats + 1 fat
Taco, hard or soft whell (meat and cheese)	1 small	1 carbohydrate + 1 medium-fat meat + 1½ fats

Salads

Food	Serving Size	Count As
[S] ☺ Salad, main dish (grilled chicken type, no dressing or croutons)	Salad	1 carbohydrate + 4 lean meats
Salad, side (no dressing or cheese)	Small (about 5 oz.)	1 vegetable

Sides/Appetizers

Food	Serving Size	Count As
⚠ French fries, restaurant style	small	3 carbohydrates + 3 fats
	medium	4 carbohydrates + 4 fats
	large	5 carbohydrates + 6 fats
[S] Nachos with cheese	small (about 4½ oz.)	2½ carbohydrates + 4 fats
[S] Onion rings	1 serving (about 3 oz.)	2½ carbohydrates + 3 fats

Desserts

Food	Serving Size	Count As
Milkshake, any flavor	12 oz.	6 carbohydrates + 2 fats
Soft-serve ice cream cone	1 small	2½ carbohydrates + 1 fat

Note: See the Starch list and Sweets, Desserts, and Other Carbohydrates list for foods such as bagels and muffins.

 = More than 3 grams of dietary fiber per serving.

 = Extra fat, or prepared with added fat.

 = 480 milligrams or more of sodium per serving.

Alcohol

✓ In general, 1 alcohol equivalent (½ oz. absolute alcohol) has about 100 calories.

✓ Women who choose to drink alcohol should limit themselves to 1 drink or less per day. The limit is 2 drinks or less per day for men.

✓ To reduce your risk of low blood glucose (hypoglycemia), especially if you take insulin or a diabetes pill that increases insulin, always drink alcohol with food.

✓ While alcohol, by itself, does not directly affect blood glucose, be aware of the carbohydrate (for example, in mixed drinks, beer, and wine) that may raise your blood glucose.

✓ Check with your Registered Dietitian if you would like to fit alcohol into your meal plan.

Alcoholic Beverage	Serving Size	Count As
Beer		
• light (4.2%)	12 fl. oz.	1 alcohol equivalent + ½ carbohydrate
• regular (4.9%)	12 fl. oz	1 alcohol equivalent + 1 carbohydrate
Distilled spirits: vodka, rum, gin, whiskey 80 or 86 proof	1½ fl. oz	1 alcohol equivalent
Liqueur, coffee (53 proof)	1 fl. oz.	½ alcohol equivalent + 1 carbohydrate
Sake	1 fl. oz.	½ alcohol equivalent
Wine		
• dessert (sherry)	3½ fl. oz.	1 alcohol equivalent + 1 carbohydrate
• dry, red or white (10%)	5 fl. oz.	1 alcohol equivalent

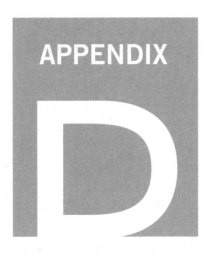

Carbohydrate Counting Choices

When following a carbohydrate counting diet, use the following to help you "count your carbs." Make sure you follow the serving sizes listed.

Food	
Bread, Cereals, Grains	1 Serving = 15 g carbs
Bagel (white or whole wheat)	½ of a small (2 oz.)
Bread (white or whole wheat)	1 slice (1 oz.)
Bun (white or whole wheat)	½ of a small (2 oz.)
Crackers, round butter style	6
Dry cereal, spoon size, bran, frosted	½ cup
Dry cereal, unsweetened	¾ cup
English muffin	½ of a small
Hot cereal (oatmeal, grits, etc.)	½ cup cooked
Macaroni, noodles, pasta or spaghetti	⅓ cup cooked
Pancakes and waffles	1 (4-inch diameter)
Pizza crust, thin	⅛ of a 12-inch pizza
Rice (white or brown)	⅓ cup cooked
Beans and Legumes	1 Serving = 15 g carbs
Baked beans	⅓ cup cooked
Beans (navy, black, pinto, red, etc.)	½ cup cooked
Lentils	½ cup cooked
Starchy Vegetables	1 Serving = 15 g carbs
Baked potato (regular or sweet)	½ medium (4 inches long)
Corn	½ cup cooked
French fries, regular cut	10-15 fries
Peas	½ cup cooked
Winter squash (acorn, butternut, etc.)	1 cup cooked
Vegetable soup	1 cup
Red pasta sauce	½ cup

Food	
Fruits	1 Serving = 15 g carbs
Apple	1 small
Banana	½ medium
Blackberries/Blueberries	¾ cup
Canned fruit (in light syrup or juice)	½ cup
Cantaloupe	1 cup cubed
Cherries	12 to 15
Grapefruit	½ large
Grapes	17 small
Honeydew melon	1 cup
Orange	1 small
Peach	1 small
Pear	1 small
Raspberries	1 cup
Strawberries	1½ cup whole
Watermelon	1¼ cup cubed
100% Fruit Juices	1 Serving = 15 g carbs
Apple juice	½ cup
Cranberry juice	⅓ cup
Grape juice	⅓ cup
Grapefruit juice	½ cup
Orange juice	½ cup
Pineapple juice	½ cup
Dairy Products	1 Serving = 15 g carbs
Milk (skim or 1% fat)	1 cup
Yogurt (plain, light or sugar-free)	1 cup
Sweets and Snacks	1 Serving = 15 g carbs
Cookies	2 small
Animal crackers	8
Mixed nuts	3 oz.
Frozen yogurt, regular	½ cup
Ice cream (light)	½ cup
Popcorn (plain, air-popped or low-fat microwave)	3 cups
Snack chips (fat-free or baked)	15-20 (¾ oz.)
Pretzels	0.75 oz.
Pumpkin seeds (in the shell)	5 oz. (1½ cups)
Pudding (sugar-free)	½ cup

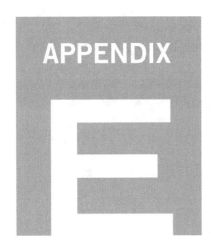

Food Sources of Potassium

Food sources ranked by amounts of potassium and energy per standard food portion and per 100 grams of foods (the Adequate Intake for potassium for adults is 4700 mg)

Food	Standard Portion Size	Calories in Standard Portion[1]	Potassium in Standard Portion (mg)[1]	Calories per 100 grams[1]	Potassium per 100 grams[1] (mg)
Potato, baked, flesh and skin	1 small potato	128	738	93	535
Prune juice, canned	1 cup	182	707	71	276
Carrot juice, canned	1 cup	94	689	40	292
Tomato paste	¼ cup	54	664	82	1014
Beet greens, cooked from fresh	½ cup	19	654	27	909
White beans, canned	½ cup	149	595	114	454
Tomato juice, canned	1 cup	41	556	17	229
Plain yogurt, non-fat	8 oz.	127	579	56	255
Tomato puree	½ cup	48	549	38	439
Sweet potato, baked in skin	1 medium	103	542	90	475
Clams, canned	3 oz.	126	534	148	628
Plain yogurt, low-fat	8 oz.	143	531	63	234
orange juice, fresh	1 cup	112	496	45	200
Halibut, cooked	3 oz.	119	490	140	576
Soybeans, green, cooked	½ up	127	485	141	539
Tuna, yellowfin, cooked	3 OZ.	118	484	139	569
Lima beans, cooked	½ cup	108	478	115	508
Soybeans, mature, cooked	½ cup	149	443	173	515
Rockfish, Pacific, cooked	3 oz.	103	442	121	520
Cod, Pacific, cooked	3 oz.	89	439	105	517

(Continued)

Food	Standard Portion Size	Calories in Standard Portion[1]	Potassium in Standard Portion (mg)[1]	Calories per 100 grams[1]	Potassium per 100 grams[1] (mg)
Evaporated milk, non-fat	½ cup	100	425	78	332
Low-fat chocolate milk, 1%	1 cup	158	425	63	170
Reduced fat chocolate milk, 2%	1 cup	190	422	76	169
Bananas	1 medium	105	422	89	358
Spinach, cooked from fresh or canned	½ cup	21-25	370-419	23	346-466
Tomato sauce	½ cup	29	405	24	331
Peaches, dried, uncooked	¼ cup	96	398	239	996
Prunes, stewed	½ cup	133	398	107	321
Skim milk, non-fat	1 cup	83	382	34	156
Rainbow trout, cooked	3 oz.	128	381	150	448
Apricots, dried, uncooked	¼ cup	78	378	241	1162
Pinto beans, cooked	½ cup	122	373	143	436
Pork loin, center rib, lean, roasted	3 oz.	190	371	223	437
Low-fat buttermilk, 1%	1 cup	98	370	40	151
Low-fat milk, 1%	1 cup	102	366	42	150
Lentils, cooked	½ cup	115	365	116	369
Plantains, cooked	½ cup	89	358	116	465
Kidney beans, cooked	½ cup	112	358	127	405

1. Source: US Department of Agriculture, Agricultural Research Service, Nutrient Data Laboratory. 2009. USDA National Nutrient Database for Standard Reference, Release 22. Available at: http://www.ars.usda.gov/ba/bhnrc/ndl

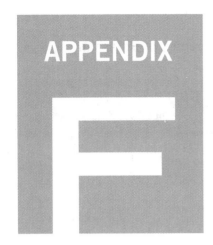

APPENDIX

F

List of Fatty Acids in Fats/Oils

Fats & Oils	Saturated Fatty Acids (grams)	Monounsaturated Fatty Acids (grams)	Polyunsaturated Fatty Acids (grams)
High in Saturated			
Coconut Oil	11.8	0.8	0.2
Palm Kernel Oil	11.1	1.5	0.2
Cocoa Butter	8.1	4.5	0.4
Butter	7.1	3.3	0.4
Palm Oil	6.7	5.0	1.3
Lard	5.0	5.8	1.4
High in Mono-unsaturated			
Olive Oil	1.8	9.9	1.1
Canola Oil	0.9	7.6	4.5
Peanut Oil	2.3	6.2	4.3
High in Polyunsaturated			
Safflower Oil	1.2	1.6	10.1
Corn Oil	1.7	3.3	8.0
Soybean Oil	2.0	3.2	7.9
Cottonseed Oil	3.5	2.4	7.1
Sunflower Oil	1.4	6.2	5.5
Margarine, Liquid	1.8	3.9	5.1
Margarine, Soft Tub	1.8	4.8	3.9

Source: National Institutes of Health

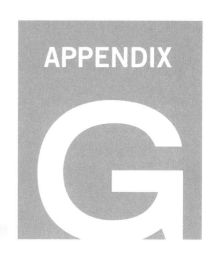

List of Essential and Nonessential Amino Acids

Essential Amino Acids	Nonessential Amino Acids*
Histidine	Alanine
Isoleucine	Arginine
Leucine	Aspartic Acid
Lysine	Cysteine
Methionine	Cystine
Phenylalanine	Glutamic Acid
Threonine	Glutamine
Tryptophan	Glycine
Valine	Proline
	Serine
	Tyrosine

Under some circumstances, one or more of these may become essential.

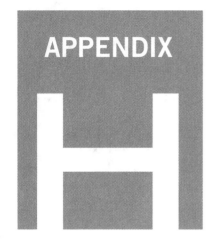

APPENDIX H

Chart to Convert Pounds to Kilograms

lbs	kg	lbs	kg	lbs	kg	lbs	kg	lbs	kg	lbs	kg	lbs	kg	lbs	kg
1	0.45	51	23.13	101	45.81	151	68.49	201	91.17	251	113.85	301	136.53	351	159.21
2	0.91	52	23.59	102	46.27	152	68.95	202	91.63	252	114.31	302	136.99	352	159.66
3	1.36	53	24.04	103	46.72	153	69.40	203	92.08	253	114.76	303	137.44	353	160.12
4	1.81	54	24.49	104	47.17	154	69.85	204	92.53	254	115.21	304	137.89	354	160.57
5	2.27	55	24.95	105	47.63	155	70.31	205	92.99	255	115.67	305	138.35	355	161.03
6	2.72	56	25.40	106	48.08	156	70.76	206	93.44	256	116.12	306	138.80	356	161.48
7	3.18	57	25.85	107	48.53	157	71.21	207	93.89	257	116.57	307	139.25	357	161.93
8	3.63	58	26.31	108	48.99	158	71.67	208	94.35	258	117.03	308	139.71	358	162.39
9	4.08	59	26.76	109	49.44	159	72.12	209	94.80	259	117.48	309	140.16	359	162.84
10	4.54	60	27.22	110	49.90	160	72.57	210	95.25	260	117.93	310	140.61	360	163.29
11	4.99	61	27.67	111	50.35	161	73.03	211	95.71	261	118.39	311	141.07	361	163.75
12	5.44	62	28.12	112	50.80	162	73.48	212	96.16	262	118.84	312	141.52	362	164.20
13	5.90	63	28.58	113	51.26	163	73.94	213	96.62	263	119.29	313	141.97	363	164.65
14	6.35	64	29.03	114	51.71	164	74.39	214	97.07	264	119.75	314	142.43	364	165.11
15	6.80	65	29.48	115	52.16	165	74.84	215	97.52	265	120.20	315	142.88	365	165.56
16	7.26	66	29.94	116	52.62	166	75.30	216	97.98	266	120.66	316	143.34	366	166.02
17	7.71	67	30.39	117	53.07	167	75.75	217	98.43	267	121.11	317	143.79	367	166.47
18	8.16	68	30.84	118	53.52	168	76.20	218	98.88	268	121.56	318	144.24	368	166.92
19	8.62	69	31.30	119	53.98	169	76.66	219	99.34	269	122.02	319	144.70	369	167.38
20	9.07	70	31.75	120	54.43	170	77.11	220	99.79	270	122.47	320	145.15	370	167.83
21	9.53	71	32.21	121	54.88	171	77.56	221	100.24	271	122.92	321	145.60	371	168.28
22	9.98	72	32.66	122	55.34	172	78.02	222	100.70	272	123.38	322	146.06	372	168.74
23	10.43	73	33.11	123	55.79	173	78.47	223	101.15	273	123.83	323	146.51	373	169.19
24	10.89	74	33.57	124	56.25	174	78.93	224	101.60	274	124.28	324	146.96	374	169.64
25	11.34	75	34.02	125	56.70	175	79.38	225	102.06	275	124.74	325	147.42	375	170.10
26	11.79	76	34.47	126	57.15	176	79.83	226	102.51	276	125.19	326	147.87	376	170.55
27	12.25	77	34.93	127	57.61	177	80.29	227	102.97	277	125.65	327	148.32	377	171.00
28	12.70	78	35.38	128	58.06	178	80.74	228	103.42	278	126.10	328	148.78	378	171.46
29	13.15	79	35.83	129	58.51	179	81.19	229	103.87	279	126.55	329	149.23	379	171.91
30	13.61	80	36.29	130	58.97	180	81.65	230	104.33	280	127.01	330	149.69	380	172.37
31	14.06	81	36.74	131	59.42	181	82.10	231	104.78	281	127.46	331	150.14	381	172.82
32	14.51	82	37.19	132	59.87	182	82.55	232	105.23	282	127.91	332	150.59	382	173.27
33	14.97	83	37.65	133	60.33	183	83.01	233	105.69	283	128.37	333	151.05	383	173.73
34	15.42	84	38.10	134	60.78	184	83.46	234	106.14	284	128.82	334	151.50	384	174.18
35	15.88	85	38.56	135	61.24	185	83.91	235	106.59	285	129.27	335	151.95	385	174.63

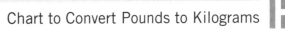

lbs	kg	lbs	kg	lbs	kg	lbs	kg	lbs	kg	lbs	kg	lbs	kg	lbs	kg
36	16.33	86	39.01	136	61.69	186	84.37	236	107.05	286	129.73	336	152.41	386	175.09
37	16.78	87	39.46	137	62.14	187	84.82	237	107.50	287	130.18	337	152.86	387	175.54
38	17.24	88	39.92	138	62.60	188	85.28	238	107.96	288	130.63	338	153.31	388	175.99
39	17.69	89	40.37	139	63.05	189	85.73	239	108.41	289	131.09	339	153.77	389	176.45
40	18.14	90	40.82	140	63.50	190	86.18	240	108.86	290	131.54	340	154.22	390	176.90
41	18.60	91	41.28	141	63.96	191	86.64	241	109.32	291	132.00	341	154.68	391	177.35
42	19.05	92	41.73	142	64.41	192	87.09	242	109.77	292	132.45	342	155.13	392	177.81
43	19.50	93	42.18	143	64.86	193	87.54	243	110.22	293	132.90	343	155.58	393	178.26
44	19.96	94	42.64	144	65.32	194	88.00	244	110.68	294	133.36	344	156.04	394	178.72
45	20.41	95	43.09	145	65.77	195	88.45	245	111.13	295	133.81	345	156.49	395	179.17
46	20.87	96	43.54	146	66.22	196	88.90	246	111.58	296	134.26	346	156.94	396	179.62
47	21.32	97	44.00	147	66.68	197	89.36	247	112.04	297	134.72	347	157.40	397	180.08
48	21.77	98	44.45	148	67.13	198	89.81	248	112.49	298	135.17	348	157.85	398	180.53
49	22.23	99	44.91	149	67.59	199	90.26	249	112.94	299	135.62	349	158.30	399	180.98
50	22.68	100	45.36	150	68.04	200	90.72	250	113.40	300	136.08	350	158.76	400	181.44

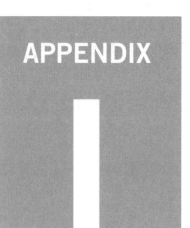

APPENDIX

Complete Glossary

A

10% weight loss in 30 days	Start with the client's weight closest to 180 days ago and multiply it by .90 (or 90%). The resulting figure represents a 10% loss from the weight 180 days ago. If the client's current weight is equal to or less than the resulting figure, the client has lost 10% or more body weight.
5% weight loss in 30 days	Start with the client's weight closest to 30 days ago and multiply it by .95 (or 95%). The resulting figure represents a 5% loss from the weight 30 days ago. If the client's current weight is equal to or less than the resulting figure, the client has lost more than 5% body weight
Absorption	The process by which nutrients pass through the cells of the intestinal tract into the circulatory system
Academy of Nutrition and Dietetics (AND)	Formerly known as The American Dietetic Association (ADA)
Actual Weight	An individual's current weight
Acute Care Facilities	Hospitals or urgent care centers that provide emergency and surgical treatment or care for acute illnesses or injuries
Adequate Intake (AI)	A scientific judgment on the amount of some nutrients for which a specific RDA is not known
Alternative Medicine	Using an unconventional medicinal practice in place of conventional medicine
Alzheimer's Disease	Most common form of dementia marked by loss of cognitive ability
Amino Acids	Building blocks of proteins
Anaphylaxis	A life-threatening allergic reaction that usually shuts down the respiratory system
Anorexia Nervosa	An eating disorder characterized by self-induced starvation and distorted body image
Antibodies	Blood proteins required for an immune response to foreign bodies
Antioxidant	'Anti' means against and 'oxidant' means oxygen so antioxidant prevents oxygen from destroying important substances.
Ascites	Abnormal accumulation of fluid in the abdoomen
Assessment	Analysis based on the subjective and objective data
A-Tags	An identification number of a CMS guideline for general acute care hospitals
Atherosclerosis	When plaque builds up in the arteries

B

Basal Energy Expenditure (BEE)	The energy (calories) needed to maintain basic bodily functions such as breathing, brain function, and keeping the heart beating
Benign	A tumor that is not likely to spread
Body Mass Index (BMI)	A proportion of weight to height
Body Mass Index (BMI)	Number calculated from a person's weight and height. BMI is used as a screening tool to identify possible weight problems for adults. Visit http:// www.cdc.gov/healthyweight/assessing/ bmi/adult_bmi/index.html
BRAT Diet	Used to help the stomach rest after nausea, vomiting, or diarrhea. The diet is comprised of bananas, rice, applesauce, and toast.
Bulimia	An eating disorder involving binging (eating large amounts of food) and then purging (forced vomiting or other methods of getting rid of the food)

C

Care Area Assessment (CAA)	Care Area Assessment is the second component of the RAI and is used to make decisions about areas suggested by the MDS
Caloric Needs Estimate	An estimate of the total amount of calories needed (e.g. for one day) and includes the BEE plus the activity factory and, if needed, an injury factor (Activity Kcal: sedentary, moderate, strenuous)
Calorie	A measurement of heat or energy. Foods that provide energy provide calories.
Calorie Count	Calculation of actual amount consumed from a food record in a 24-hour time period
Cancer	When cells grow at an unrestricted rate or there is excessive multiplication of cells
Cancer Cachexia	Extreme weight loss or body wasting that may not be reversed
Cardiovascular Disease (CVD)	Cardiovascular disease
Care Plan	A written plan for medical care
Care Protocols	Documents that outline a care process related to a specific medical condition
Care Area Triggers (CAT)	Care Area Triggers are related to one or more items in the MDS and are the flags for the interdisciplinary team member
Celiac Disease	Caused by a cell-mediated hypersensitivity to gluten, the protein found in wheat, rye, and barley
Centers for Medicare and Medcaid Services (CMS)	Centers for Medicare and Medicaid Services
Chemical Breakdown	Breakdown of food from digestive juices or enzymes
Chronic Obstructive Pulmonary Disease (COPD)	A group of lung diseases that includes chronic bronchitis, emphysema, and asthmatic bronchitis
Comfort Food	Any food that imparts a unique sense of emotional well-being such as chicken soup
Communication	The exchange of information by writing, speaking, or gestures
Complementary Medicine	Using an unconventional medical practice in addition to conventional medicine
Complementary and Alternative Medicine (CAM)	Complementary and alternative medicines that do not fall within conventional medicine practices

Complementary Protein	Two or more incomplete protein foods, that when eaten within the same day, provide essential amino acids
Complete Protein	Foods that contain all of the essential amino acids
Comprehensive Care Plan (CCP)	Developed by interdisciplinary team that addresses the multifaceted needs of the client
Congestive Heart Failure (CHF)	Inability of the heart to effectively pump blood to the body's organs—can be due to coronary artery disease
Constipation	Passage of small amounts of hard, dry bowel movements usually fewer than three times a week
Conventional Medicine	Medicine practiced by physicians (Medical Doctors—MDs, and Doctors of Osteopathy—DOs) as well as allied health professionals
C-Tags	An identification number of a CMS guideline for small rural or critical access hospitals
Cycle Menu	A menu that repeats itself over a defined period of time

D

Daily Reference Values (DRVs)	Reference intake levels for nutrition labeling for the general public
Diabetes Mellitus	A metabolic disorder marked by high levels of blood glucose resulting from defects in insulin production, insulin action, or both
Diastolic Pressure	The bottom number or the denominator of the blood pressure reading. A tip to remember is that both diastolic and denominator begin with a "d."
Diet	The foods and beverages a person consumes
Diet Manual	Standardized document that specifies therapeutic diets and their application; each facility will specify the diet manual they intend to use
Diet Order	The diet prescribed by the physician for an individual client
Dietary Fiber	A polysaccharide made up of many molecules of sugar; plant materials that are NOT digestible by the body
Dietary Guidelines	Guidelines issued jointly by the U.S. Department of Agriculture (USDA) and the U.S. Department of Health and Human Services (DHHS) to provide advice, promote health, and reduce risk for major chronic diseases
Dietary Reference Intakes (DRIs)	Generic terms that encompass four types of reference values: Estimated Average Requirement, Recommended Dietary Allowance, Adequate Intake, and Tolerable Upper Intake Level.
Dietary Supplement	A product intended to supplement the diet
Digestion	The process of breaking down food into nutrients
Disaccharide	Simple carbohydrate containing two sugar molecules
Diuretics	A class of blood pressure medications that cause increased urine output
Diverticulitis	A disease where the diverticula become inflamed or infected
Diverticulosis	A disease of the intestine where the intestinal walls become weakened and bulge into pockets called diverticula
Drug-Nutrient Interaction	Can lead to nutrient malabsorption or the drug not working effectively
Dysphagia	Difficulty swallowing

E

Edema	Abnormal pooling of fluid in the tissues causing swelling
Electrolyte	Compounds that contain both potassium and chloride. They can separate when in contact with water and are required for fluid balance in the body
Electronic Health Record (EHR)	One of the methods to adopt the full exchange of healthcare information where all records are updated and maintained electronically
Empty Calories	Calories that provide little or no nutrient density
Energy-Yielding Nutrients	Those nutrients that provide energy or calories to the body (carbohydrates, lipids, protein)
Enriched	Adding the B-Vitamins and iron back into refined flour and grain products
Enteral Nutrition	Feeding or formulas, by mouth or by tube, into the gastrointestinal tract
Essential Amino Acids	Cannot be made in the body
Essential Fatty Acid (EFA)	Fatty acids that cannot be made by the body
Essential Nutrient	The six categories of nutrients that we must obtain through food. Not enough of these nutrients can be made in the body

F

Feeding Tube	Presence of any type of tube that can deliver food/nutritional substances/fluids/medications directly into the gastrointestinal system. Examples include, but are not limited to nasogastric tubes, gastrostomy tubes, jejunostomy tubes, percutaneous endoscopic gastrotomy (PEG) tubes
Fixed Menu	A menu that doesn't change from day to day such as what is found in restaurants
Fluoridation	The addition of fluoride to municipal water systems
Food Allergies	An immune response to dietary protein that is either cell mediated or non-cell mediated
Food Frequency Questionnaire	A checklist or questionnaire that tracks how often a client eats each of a variety of foods
Food Intolerance	Does not produce an immune response but may not be tolerated for various reasons, such as lactose intolerance where one cannot digest the milk, sugar, or lactose
Food Record	A diary of food and beverages consumed, usually for a given number of days
Fortified	Foods that have one or more nutrients added
Frame Size	Calculated from the ratio of height to wrist circumference
F-Tags	An identification number of a CMS guideline for long-term care
Functional Foods	Foods that convey health benefits beyond the nutrients.
Gastritis	Inflammation of the stomach lining
Gastroesophageal Reflux Disease (GERD)	Where stomach acid comes up into the esophagus and causes acid indigestion or heartburn
Gastrointestinal Tract (GI Tract)	The tubular organs from the mouth to the anus plus the liver, pancreas, and gallbladder
Glucose	A single sugar used for energy; sometimes call blood sugar or dextrose
Glycogen	A stored form of starch used for quick energy by the body
Gram	A unit of weight. There are 28 grams in one ounce

H

Health Care Communities	The Position Paper of the The Academy of Nutrition and Dietetics (formerly known as The American Dietetic Association): *Individualized Nutrition Approaches for Older Adults in Health Communities* identifies the following as healthcare communities: "assisted living facilities, group homes, short-term rehabilitation facilities, skilled nursing facilities, and hospice facilities."
Health Insurance Portability and Accountability Act (HIPAA)	Standardizes the exchange of healthcare information and assures client/patient privacy and the right to keep information confidential
Hepatic	Relating to the liver
High-Density Lipoproteins (HDL)	The lipoprotein that carries cholesterol away from body organs to the liver—"healthy" cholesterol
Hormones	Chemical messengers such as the thyroid hormone
Hydrogenated	A process of adding hydrogen to oils in order to make them more solid
Hyperglycemia	High blood sugar
Hypertension	Medical condition involving chronic high blood pressure
Hypoglycemia	Low blood sugar

I

I/O (In and Out) Record	A document of all fluids consumed and excreted over a 24-hour time period
Ideal Body Weight (IBW)	An estimate of what would be a healthy weight for an individual according to a standard
Incomplete Protein	Foods that lack either the amount or type of amino acid needed for growth and maintenance of tissues.
Indicators	Pieces of information, such as weight measurement, that might suggest a concern or risk
Inflammatory Bowel Disease (IBD)	A disease that can cause ulceration of the mucosa lining in both the large and small intestine. Two types of IBD are ulcerative colitis and Crohn's disease.
Insoluble Fiber	Outer covering (bran) of plants or fibrous inner parts that are NOT soluble in water (i.e. bran, celery, corn)
Integrative Medicine	Combines conventional practices with CAM practices
Interdisciplinary Team (IDT)	Interdisciplinary team of health professionals that collaborate in the completion of the RAI and other cross-functional responsibilities
Iron-Deficiency Anemia	A condition resulting from insufficient dietary iron intake or blood loss
Irritable Bowel Syndrome (IBS)	Common disorder that affects the large intestine that can cause abdominal pain, bloating, nausea, and diarrhea

J

Jaundice	Yellowing of the skin associated with liver disease

K

Kosher	Fit, proper or in agreement with Religious law. Kosher meat means the animal has been slaughtered in a special way. Usually Kosher foods have been blessed by a Rabbi.

L

Lacto-Vegetarian	A diet excluding all animal foods except dairy.
Lean Body Mass	The weight of all parts of the body not counting the fat (e.g. muscle, bones, and organs)
Learning Objective	A specific, measurable statement of the outcome of a lesson, inservice, or nutrition education session
Lipids	A category that is both fats, such as butter and shortening; and oils, such as olive oil or canola oil
Long Term Care (LTC)	Long-term care
Low-Density Lipoproteins (LDL)	The lipoprotein that carries most of the cholesterol in the blood— "lousy" cholesterol

M

Major Minerals	Calcium, chloride, magnesium, phosphorous, potassium, sodium and sulfur
Malignant	A tumor that is likely to spread
Meal Observation	A tool that helps to identify individuals who are having eating problems such as swallowing, chewing, or self feeding
Mechanical Breakdown	Physical breaking down of food into smaller pieces using teeth, tongue, jaws, and the smooth muscles in the esophagus and stomach
Mechanically Altered Diet	A diet specifically prepared to alter the texture or consistency of food to facilitate oral intake. Examples include soft solids, puréed foods, ground meat, and thickened liquids. A mechanically altered diet should not automatically be considered a therapeutic diet.
Medical Record	Formal, legal account of a client's health and disease
Metabolism	The chemical processes in a cell by which nutrients are used to support life
Metastasis	Transfer of cancer from one part of the body to another organ or part of the body
Minimum Data Set (MDS)	Minimum Data Set is the starting point of the RAI and is a standardized tool for collecting information that is the core of the RAI
Monosaccharide	Simple carbohydrate containing one sugar molecule
Monounsaturated Fatty Acid	A fatty acid that contains one double bond and is found in foods like olive oil, almonds, most hydrogenated margarines
Mucosa	The lining of the mouth, stomach and small intestine that contain tiny glands to produce digestive enzymes
Myocardial Infarction (MI)	Heart attack
MyPyramid	Developed by the USDA and DHHS; provides a personalized plan about how to eat and apply the Dietary Guidelines

N

Natural Foods	Contain no artificial ingredients or added color and are only minimally processed
Nonessential Amino Acid	Is able to be made in the body
Nonverbal Communication	The form of communication without speaking or writing that includes gestures, facial expressions, and body language
Nutrient Density	The amount of nutrients a food contains relative to its calorie (energy) content
Nutrients	Components in food that are essential to good health
Nutrition	The science of how components in food nourish the body
Nutrition Assessment	A comprehensive approach by a Registered Dietitian using multiple data sources to determine nutritional status
Nutrition Care Process (NCP)	New method of a standardized care process to document nutritional data with five steps: ADIME (Assessment, Diagnosis, Intervention, Monitoring, and Evaluation)
Nutrition Screening	A component of Nutrition Assessment meant to identify potential nutrition problems
Nutrition Support	General term describing providing food and liquids to improve nutritional status and supporting good medicine

O

Obesity	Having a body mass index (BMI) of 30 or greater
Objective	Data that is acquired by inspection, examination with only a stethoscope, from a laboratory, and radiologic tests
Organic Foods	Grown without genetic engineering, without use of inorganic hormones, antibiotics, pesticides, herbicides, or fertilizers
Outcome	Outcome is the end result of work
Overweight	Having a body mass index of 25 to 29.9
Ovo-lacto Vegetarian	A diet excluding animal foods except dairy and eggs.

P

Parenteral Nutrition	Administration of simple essential nutrients into a vein
Parenteral/IV Feeding	Introduction of a nutritive substance into the body by means other than the intestinal tract (e.g., subcutaneous, intravenous).
Percent of IBW	A comparison of the actual weight to the ideal body weight
Percent of Weight Change	A proportion of current body weight to usual body weight or weight change over a certain period of time
Physician-Prescribed Weight-loss Regimen	A weight reduction plan ordered by the client's physician with the care plan goal of weight reduction. May employ a calorie-restricted diet or other weight loss diets and exercise. Also includes planned diuresis. It is important that weight loss is intentional.
Phytochemicals	Phyto means plant so these are chemicals in plants thought to provide special health benefits.

Placebo	A substance given in clinical trials that contain no medication or active ingredient
Plan	Recommended actions of the caregiver's to further information, therapy, education or counseling
Polyunsaturated Fatty Acids (PUFA)	A fatty acid that contains more than one double bond and is found in foods like corn oil, soybean oil, soft margarines
Pressure Ulcers, aka Pressure Sores, Decubitus Ulcers	Lesions caused by pressure
Problem Oriented Medical Record (POMR)	A medical record that utilizes a system of collecting, planning data and client care focused on a client's problems
Progress Note	A notation in the medical record by a health professional
Protein-Calorie Nutrition	A name for a group of diseases characterized by both protein and calorie deficiency
Q	
Quackery	A medical treatment that does not perform as claimed and is offered by an untrained or uninformed individual
Quality Indicators (QI)	Quality indicators are measures of outcomes
R	
Resident Assessment Instrument (RAI)	Resident Assessment Instrument consists of three components and is utilized to assess each nursing home or swing bed client's functional capacity and needs
Recommended Dietary Allowance (RDA)	The amount of a nutrient adequate to meet the known nutrient needs of practically all healthy persons.
Renal Failure	When kidneys fail to function normally
RUMBAS Objective	A learning objective that is Relevant, Understandable, Measurable, Behavioral, Attainable, Specific
S	
Saturated Fatty Acid	A fatty acid that is filled with hydrogen making it solid or semisolid at room temperature and is found in foods like butter, cream, coconut oil
Selective Menu	An adaptation of a cycle menu where clients have the opportunity to make choices or selections in advance of meal service
Simple Carbohydrates	Those that are usually found in foods as a sugar and contain one or two molecules of sugar
Single Use Menu	Menus used for special meals that are not repeated
SOAP	A structured type of collecting data that stands for Subjective, Objective, Assessment, and Plan
SoFAS	A new term in the 2010 Dietary Guidelines that refers to solid fats and added sugars
Soluble Fiber	Fiber that forms a gel when combined with water (i.e. fruits, oats, dried beans)
Standard of Practice	Standards for what you normally do that constitute quality in practice
Starch	A polysaccharide made up of many molecules of sugar; plant materials that are digestible

Stroke	When blood vessels bringing oxygen to the brain burst or become clogged
Subjective	Data from the client's point of view or as told by the client or family members
Sundowning Effect	When confusion or disorientation worsens at the end of the day
Systolic Pressure	The top number of the blood pressure reading
T	
Therapeutic Diet	A diet ordered to manage problematic health conditions. Therapeutic refers to the nutritional content of the food. Examples include calorie-specific, low-salt, low-fat, lactose free, no added sugar, and supplements during meals.
The Joint Commission (TJC)	The Joint Commission
Tolerable Upper Intake Level (UL)	The maximum level of a daily nutrient that is considered safe.
Trace Minerals	Minerals needed in less than 100 ml daily
Trans-Fatty Acid	A fatty acid where the hydrogen atoms have been chemically rearranged, found in hydrogen atoms that have been chemically rearranged; and are found in hydrogenated oils, margarines, and shortening
Triglycerides	A common form of fats and foods comprised of three fatty acids and glycerol
Tube Feeding	Enteral feeding given through a tube
Tumors	Growths of cancerous cells
Type 1 Diabetes (T1D)	When the body's immune system destroys pancreatic beta cells and insulin cannot be made
Type 2 Diabetes (T2D)	Begins as insulin resistance where the cells do not use insulin properly. Gradually the pancreas loses the ability to produce any insulin.
U	
U.S. Pharmacopeia (USP)	U.S. Pharmacopeia provides model guidelines for prescription drugs
Unsaturated Fatty Acid	A fatty acid that contains one or more double bonds
V	
Vegan Diet	A diet containing no animal foods.
Verbal Communication	Communicating thoughts, messages, or information by speaking
Written Communication	Communicating thoughts, messages, or information by writing

Index

Page numbers followed by an '*f*' indicate figures

Page numbers followed by an 'f' indicate figures

    Page numbers followed by an '*f*' indicate figures

Page numbers followed by an '*f*' indicate figures

Page numbers followed by an *'f'* indicate figures

NOTES

NOTES

NOTES